MW00345608

Pharmacology and Ototoxicity for Audiologists

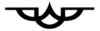

Kathleen C. M. Campbell, PhD

Professor & Director of Audiology Research
Southern Illinois University School of Medicine
Springfield, IL

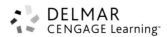

Australia • Brazil • Japan • Korea • Mexico • Singapore • Spain • United Kingdom • United States

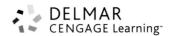

Pharmacology and Ototoxicity for Audiologists
Kathleen C. M. Campbell

Vice President, Health Care Business Unit:
   William Brottmiller

Director of Learning Solutions: Matthew Kane

Acquisitions Editor: Sherry Dickinson

Product Manager: Juliet Steiner

Editorial Assistant: Angela Doolin

Marketing Director: Jennifer McAvey

Marketing Manager: Christopher Manion

Production Director: Carolyn Miller

Production Manager: Barbara A. Bullock

Content Project Manager: Anne Sherman

© 2007 Delmar, Cengage Learning

ALL RIGHTS RESERVED. No part of this work covered by the copyright herein may be reproduced, transmitted, stored or used in any form or by any means graphic, electronic, or mechanical, including but not limited to photocopying, recording, scanning, digitizing, taping, Web distribution, information networks, or information storage and retrieval systems, except as permitted under Section 107 or 108 of the 1976 United States Copyright Act, without the prior written permission of the publisher.

For product information and technology assistance, contact us at
Cengage Learning Customer & Sales Support, 1-800-354-9706

For permission to use material from this text or product,
submit all requests online at **www.cengage.com/permissions**
Further permissions questions can be emailed to
permissionrequest@cengage.com

Library of Congress Control Number: 2006021195

ISBN-13: 978-1-4180-1130-7

ISBN-10: 1-4180-1130-4

Delmar
Executive Woods
5 Maxwell Drive
Clifton Park, NY 12065
USA

Cengage Learning is a leading provider of customized learning solutions with office locations around the globe, including Singapore, the United Kingdom, Australia, Mexico, Brazil, and Japan. Locate your local office at **www.cengage.com/global**

Cengage Learning products are represented in Canada by Nelson Education, Ltd.

To learn more about Delmar, visit **www.cengage.com/delmar**

Purchase any of our products at your local bookstore or at our preferred online store **www.CengageBrain.com**

Notice to the Reader

Publisher does not warrant or guarantee any of the products described herein or perform any independent analysis in connection with any of the product information contained herein. Publisher does not assume, and expressly disclaims, any obligation to obtain and include information other than that provided to it by the manufacturer. The reader is expressly warned to consider and adopt all safety precautions that might be indicated by the activities described herein and to avoid all potential hazards. By following the instructions contained herein, the reader willingly assumes all risks in connection with such instructions. The publisher makes no representations or warranties of any kind, including but not limited to, the warranties of fitness for particular purpose or merchantability, nor are any such representations implied with respect to the material set forth herein, and the publisher takes no responsibility with respect to such material. The publisher shall not be liable for any special, consequential, or exemplary damages resulting, in whole or part, from the readers' use of, or reliance upon, this material.

Printed in the United States of America
3 4 5 6 7 11 10 09

PREFACE

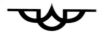

For several years, both clinical audiologists and audiology training programs have been asking for a textbook or a collection of articles on ototoxicity. Many pharmacology books are available; however, none were written to focus on ototoxicity and otoprotective agents, and most assumed a different knowledge base than was provided in audiology training. Further, most of them emphasized clinical applications for nurses, physicians, or pharmacists that were not directly relevant for the field. For clinical audiologists, many of the research articles or medical/basic science texts on ototoxicity and otoprotective agents used terms and concepts they had never been exposed to and had little access to in their clinical practices. Additionally, physicians had largely found that although audiologists' skills in monitoring for ototoxicity had increased, the physicians sometimes had trouble fully communicating with audiologists on patient care issues relating to the various drugs the patients were taking.

WRITTEN BY EXPERTS

The audiologists who wrote for the book were universal in recognizing the need for a book of this kind, particularly in the absence of any similar book on the topic. Perhaps more surprising was the enthusiasm of the leading basic scientists, pharmacologists, PharmDs, and otolaryngologists for a text of this kind specifically written for audiologists. All of the contributors who were contacted, save one who truly couldn't accept at that time, immediately agreed to write the chapter that was requested. Getting his or her first choice of contributors is every author's dream. The contributors were carefully selected in advance. These authors are the individuals lecturing and moving the field forward in their area. Additionally, each author was selected because he or she had a background working with, teaching, and preparing lecture materials for audiologists. Therefore, the authors could target their chapters for the audiology audience for which this book is intended. Making complex material understandable requires both skill and perseverance. Those characteristics are reflected in each chapter.

ORGANIZATION

This book is designed first to take the audiology student, practicing clinical audiologist, or research audiologist through the basic concepts and terminology of pharmacology, including the definition of a drug, the definition of pharmacology, and the various aspects of pharmacology including pharmacokinetics, pharmacodynamics, toxicology, pharmacogenetics, and pharmacogenomics—all concepts that the practicing audiologist should understand in day-to-day practice. The chapters then progress through pharmacotherapeutics and patient care factors and regulatory issues with the Food and Drug Administration (FDA). Because some audiologists will be involved with clinical trials of new drugs that may be either ototoxic or otoprotective, the FDA clinical trials and approval process is also reviewed.

The book then reviews the most common classes of drugs used in otolaryngologic practice and nutraceuticals and herbal supplements and related rules and regulations. A chapter on infection control in the audiology clinic is also included to provide students and practicing clinicians with the information they need to meet current regulatory standards. Although audiologists frequently receive training in auditory anatomy and physiology, most receive little training in the biochemistry of the auditory system and in basic mechanisms of toxicity relevant to the auditory system. That information is essential to understanding the workings of the auditory system in normal and in various pathologic states and to understand the latest research emanating from various labs around the world.

The section on drug-induced and noise-induced ototoxicity provides the audiology student and practicing clinician with a thorough grounding in the most common ototoxins they are likely to encounter in clinical practice and the guidelines for audiologic clinical management for both cochleotoxicity and vestibulotoxicity. The information is detailed enough also to serve as a basis for research audiologists who want to pursue research in the area. The chapters on cancer and the ototoxicity of chemotherapeutics, aminoglycoside antibiotic ototoxicity, loop diuretics, salicylates and other nonsteroidal anti-inflammatory drugs (NSAIDS), quinine, and macrolide antibiotics are written not only to help the audiologist understand the clinical impact of those ototoxins, but also to help him or her understand the basic mechanisms of how those drugs impact the auditory system. Consequently, as new research in these areas evolves, the audiologist will have a basis for putting it in context and understanding it relative to the current knowledge base in each area.

Because many audiologists see patients from industrial settings and because virtually all audiologists see patients with noise-induced hearing loss, the book includes chapters on industrial chemicals and solvents that affect the auditory system and the cellular mechanisms of noise-induced hearing loss. For those doing research in ototoxicity, in many senses, noise is simply another ototoxin with some similar mechanisms of damage. Further, industrial chemicals and solvents can frequently be an overlooked factor in causing or exacerbating hearing loss. Three chapters are directed toward the specific clinical management of cochleotoxicity and vestibolotoxicity, including audiologic monitoring and patient management, mechanisms of vestibular toxicity, and audiologic findings in vestibular toxicity. Those chapters will help the clinician in practice and the audiologist involved in clinical research that includes clinical trials.

The final section of the book reviews some of the most exciting new directions in ototoxicity and pharmacology of the auditory system. This section starts with a chapter on otoprotective and rescue agents, including some of my own research in the area. It is likely that within the next decade, one or more otoprotective agents will be FDA approved for human use. When that happens, the role of the audiologist may change from simply monitoring ototoxin-induced and noise-induced hearing losses as they occur to working with the physician in determining when a protective or rescue agent may prevent permanent hearing loss. There can be no more exciting change in audiologic practice than for audiologists to be able to prevent permanent hearing loss in many thousands of the patients that used to be simply monitored as their hearing and balance deteriorated.

The following chapter presents an equally exciting concept of being able to reverse long-standing hearing loss through hair cell regeneration. Although that treatment is a ways off from FDA approval, the idea that at some point in time, doctors may be able to "cure" most sensorineural hearing loss is incredibly exciting. The audiology students reading this text may see it happen during their careers. Perhaps some of them will become the researchers carrying that work to fruition. The chapter on using drugs to investigate the auditory system is designed to help audiology students, clinicians, and researchers understand how drugs can be used as tools in auditory research.

To understand the research emanating from the auditory research labs around the country, audiologists must first understand the tools employed. A chapter is also included on Web sites regarding drugs, ototoxicity, and hearing loss to assist audiologists in obtaining constantly updated information and to allow them to see the Web sites their patients are probably accessing. Some of the audiologists may decide, after several years of clinical practice, to return for a PhD to move the field forward through "bedside-to-bench-to-bedside research." Translational research needs that combination of skills.

GOING FORWARD

The field needs more audiology researchers with a strong clinical background to become deeply involved in research. The greatest breakthroughs in research frequently emanate from individuals or teams of individuals that combine knowledge in two or more disciplines to generate new ideas. After several years of clinical practice, I obtained my PhD with an emphasis in physiology and electrophysiology in both animals and humans. After my PhD, thanks to a Clinical Investigator Development Award from NIDCD/NIH, I took another five years of chemistry to better understand the mechanisms of ototoxicity I was studying. It is that combination of background and training that has allowed me to develop new protective agents that are now in clinical trials. I have no doubt that the audiology students and clinicians reading this book will have even larger contributions to make to our field. The best advice I can give to anyone embarking on a career is to find a need and fill it. Identify the problem in patient care you would like to change and then embark on a journey to change it. In the clinic, you may be able to improve patient care fairly quickly by using improved monitoring procedures and more informed interactions with patients, pharmacists, and physicians about drugs affecting the patients' hearing and/or balance. In research, the journey may be lengthy, but the results may change long-term outcomes for many thousands of patients. You will likely need friends and collaborators, but you will not find a more fascinating route. To quote Gandhi, "Become the change you wish to see."

ACKNOWLEDGMENTS

I cannot fully express my gratitude to the many contributors of this book. I contacted the leaders in their fields for the various chapter areas and was met with great enthusiasm. They were a huge part of making this product successful.

When I agreed to edit and write this book, I had intended to do all of the organization and clerical support myself. My secretary at the time was overwhelmed with clinical support work, so I didn't even ask. Fortunately, Susie Gentry, a long-time friend and secretary volunteered to help me and at her request had my work added to her job description. I can't imagine how this book would have stayed on schedule without her. She obtained figure permissions, formatted chapters, worked with the authors and the publisher, and basically kept everything moving forward smoothly. She has my heartfelt gratitude.

Lastly I would like to thank my husband Craig. For over thirty years, he has seen me through a masters degree, jobs in two countries, a PhD, five more years of chemistry, the odd hours and travel that accompany a research career—and all with unfailing support. Considering that he proposed to a waitress (a fact he occasionally mentions), his patience is amazing.

ABOUT THE AUTHOR

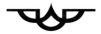

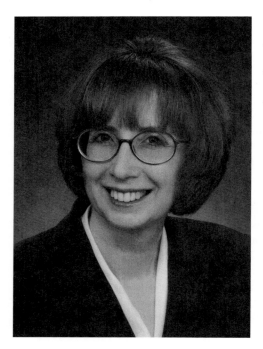

Kathleen C. M. Campbell, PhD, is Professor and Director of Audiology Research at Southern Illinois University (SIU) School of Medicine in Springfield, Illinois. She worked as a full-time clinician for twelve years before and while obtaining her PhD at the University of Iowa. After obtaining her PhD, she studied chemistry for another five years while establishing the first audiology program at SIU School of Medicine, including clinical, teaching, and research programs. Dr. Campbell has directed and provided audiology services for over 30 years in Canada and the United States but now focuses primarily on basic and clinical research. For over 25 years, she has taught audiology not only to audiologists, but also to medical school faculty, residents, and medical students in otolaryngology, pediatrics, neurology, primary care, neonatology, and surgery. She is the author of *Essential Audiology for Physicians* and numerous book chapters and articles.

She previously served on the American Academy of Audiology Board of Directors. She consults in audiology clinical management, in clinical trials of new drugs, and as an expert witness. Dr. Campbell is also a prolific researcher, publishing numerous articles on basic science and clinical topics in various areas of auditory science and auditory disorders. She is a noted lecturer nationally and internationally, focusing on audiologic assessment of auditory disorders and particularly ototoxicity, noise-induced hearing loss, and otoprotective agents.

Dr. Campbell has received an NIH Clinical Investigator Development Award, the James A. Shannon Director's Award from NIH for her research in ototoxicity, and a Special Presidential Citation from the American Academy of Audiology for her work in Professional Practice Standards. She has been named an ASHA Fellow and is in *Who's Who in America*. Dr. Campbell also received the 2004 Copper Black Award for Creative Achievement from American Mensa for her patents in otoprotective agents. She is the first audiologist to receive that award. Dr. Campbell holds a number of patents for otoprotective agents to prevent chemotherapy-induced, aminoglycoside-induced, and noise-induced hearing loss and for agents to reduce other side effects of chemotherapy and radiation. All of her patents are licensed, and clinical trials are in progress.

CONTRIBUTORS

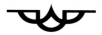

A. U. Bankaitis, PhD, FAAA
Oaktree Products, Inc.
St. Louis, MO

Venkatesh Atul Bhattaram, PhD
Center for Drug Evaluation and Research
U.S. Food and Drug Administration
Rockville, MD

Eric Bielefeld, PhD
Center for Hearing and Deafness
University at Buffalo
Buffalo, NY

F. Owen Black, MD
Legacy Clinical Research and Technology Center
Portland, OR

Richard Bobbin, PhD
Louisiana State University Health Sciences Center
New Orleans, LA

Douglas A. Cotanche, PhD
Harvard Medical School
Children's Hospital Boston
Boston, MA

Hartmut Derendorf, PhD
University of Florida, Gainesville
Gainesville, FL

Robert M. DiSogra, AuD, FAAA
Audiology Associates of Freehold
Freehold, NJ
School of Audiology
Pennsylvania College of Optometry
Elkins Park, PA

Karen Doyle, MD, PhD
University of California, Davis
Davis, CA

Stephen A. Fausti, PhD
VA RR&D National Center for Rehabilitative
Auditory Research
Portland VA Medical Center
Oregon Health and Science University
Portland, OR

Laurence D. Fechter, PhD
Jerry Pettis Memorial Veterans Medical Center
Loma Linda, CA

Jane S. Gordon, MS, CCC-A
VA RR&D National Center for Rehabilitative
Auditory Research
Portland VA Medical Center
Portland, OR

Jaynee A. Handelsman, PhD, CCC-A
University of Michigan Health System
Ann Arbor, MI

Wendy J. Helt, MA, CCC-A
VA RR&D National Center for Rehabilitative
Auditory Research
Portland VA Medical Center
Portland, OR

Donald Henderson, PhD
Center for Hearing and Deafness
University at Buffalo
Buffalo, NY

Bohua Hu, PhD
Center for Hearing and Deafness
University at Buffalo
Buffalo, NY

Xinyan Huang, MD, PhD
Southern Illinois School of Medicine
Springfield, IL

Robert J. Kemp, MBA
Oaktree Products, Inc.
St. Louis, MO

Dawn L. Konrad-Martin, PhD
VA RR&D National Center for Rehabilitative
Auditory Research
Portland VA Medical Center
Oregon Health and Science University
Portland, OR

Sharon G. Kujawa, PhD
Harvard Medical School
Cambridge, MA
Massachusetts Eye and Ear Infirmary
Boston, MA

Brenda L. Lonsbury-Martin, PhD
Loma Linda School of Medicine
Loma Linda, CA

Rajanikanth Madabushi, PhD
University of Florida, Gainesville
Gainesville, FL

Glen K. Martin, PhD
Loma Linda School of Medicine
Jerry Pettis Memorial Veterans Medical Center
Loma Linda, CA

Jonathan I. Matsui, PhD
Harvard University
Cambridge, MA
Children's Hospital Boston
Boston, MA

Sandra L. McFadden, PhD
Western Illinois University
Macomb, IL

Michael M. Meldrum, PhD
University of Florida
Gainesville, FL

Marie Moneysmith, BS
Beverly Hills, CA

Thomas Nicotera, PhD
Center for Hearing and Deafness
University at Buffalo
Buffalo, NY

Tabitha Parent Buck, AuD
A. T. Still University
Mesa, AZ

Susan Pesznecker, RN, BA
Legacy Clinical Research and Technology Center
Portland, OR

David S. Phillips, PhD
VA RR&D National Center for Rehabilitative
Auditory Research
Portland VA Medical Center
Oregon Health and Science University
Portland, OR

Benoit Pouyatos, PhD
Jerry Pettis Memorial Veterans Medical Center
Loma Linda, CA

Jean-Luc Puel, PhD
INM-Hôpital St. Eloi
Montpelier, France

Amir Rafii, MD
University of California, Davis
Davis, CA

Kelly M. Reavis, MS, CCC-A
VA RR&D National Center for Rehabilitative
Auditory Research
Portland VA Medical Center
Portland, OR

Jose A. Rey, PharmD
Nova Southeastern University
Fort Lauderdale, FL

Brenda M. Ryals, PhD
James Madison University
Harrisonburg, VA

Leonard P. Rybak, MD, PhD
Southern Illinois School of Medicine
Springfield, IL

Jochen Schacht, PhD
Kresge Hearing Research Institute
University of Michigan
Ann Arbor, MI

Michael D. Seidman, MD, FACS
Henry Ford Health System
West Bloomfield, MI

William F. Sewell, PhD
Harvard Medical School
Cambridge, MA
Massachusetts Eye and Ear Infirmary
Boston, MA

Henry P. Trahan, AuD
A. T. Still University
Mesa, AZ

Jing Wang, MD, PhD
INM-Hôpital St. Eloi
Montpelier, France

O. T. Wendel, PhD
A. T. Still University
Mesa, AZ

BRIEF CONTENTS

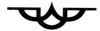

DETAILED CONTENTS

CHAPTER 1

An Introduction to Pharmacology

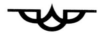

Michael Meldrum, PhD
Associate Professor of Pharmacodynamics
College of Pharmacy, University of Florida
Gainesville, Florida

INTRODUCTION

Since the earliest of times, humans have sought out plant and animal products to aid in their efforts to combat sickness and disease. The earliest of those products was discovered by trial and error, and many of those initial treatments caused more harm than good. Also, many products had religious connotations associated with their use. Since those early times, humans' search for new agents to prevent and treat disease has continued.

The advent of the scientific revolution in the later part of the fourteenth century led the search for a better understanding of normal bodily functions and an effort to understand the physiological basis of disease. Those early scientific endeavors led to an understanding of anatomy and basic concepts of physiology that continue to develop. The evolution of scientific thought and study led to the search for and isolation of plant and animal products that could alter the disease process and maintain life. The isolation by Sertürner (1783–1841) of morphine as the active agent in opium in the early 1800s and the isolation of other plant alkaloids (digitalis, atropine, ephedrine, quinine, and strychnine), which are still used today, increased the interest in and the search for new and more efficient chemicals to alter or prevent the disease process. Suggestions by François Magendie (1783–1855) that the site of a drug's action could be localized to specific organs and studies by Claude Bernard (1813–1878) into the site and action of curare, a muscle poison, were instrumental in the development of basic concepts of drug action. Rudolph Buchheim (1820–1879) continued that development with the establishment of the first Institute of Pharmacology in Estonia in 1847. Buchheim and his student Oswald Schmeideberg (1838–1921) were responsible for the training of John Jacob Abel (1857–1938), the first professor of pharmacology in the United States, and many other original scientists who helped establish pharmacology as a scientific discipline. That new era of scientific discovery led to the evolution of the study of *Matrica Medica* (Latin for "Medical Material")—from the study of medicinal plants and extracts to the development and synthesis of new chemical agents used to treat disease and the birth of modern pharmacology.

"Pharmacology" comes from the combination of the Greek word *pharmakon* meaning "poison" or "drug" and *logos* meaning "the study of or discourse of." Broadly defined, **pharmacology** is the study of the interactions of drugs or chemicals with living systems. This broad definition includes any chemical that interacts with living systems in any manner, thus including a very large number of natural and synthetic chemical compounds. In an effort to make the subject more manageable, efforts have been made to limit the definition. For discussion purposes, *pharmacology* has been defined as "the basic and clinical applied science that concerns itself with the fate and actions of drugs in the body." A **drug,** which will be discussed in more detail later, is defined as "any substance used in the diagnosis, treatment, and prevention of disease."

Pharmacology can be categorized into several separate disciplines, including pharmacokinetics, pharmacodynamics, toxicology, and the disciplines of pharmacogenetics and pharmacogenomics. **Pharmacokinetics** is the study of how drugs are acted upon by physiological functions—essentially what the body does with the drug, including absorption, distribution in the body, biotransformation, and excretion from the body as well as the time course for those actions. **Pharmacodynamics** explores the site of drug action and the mechanism of interaction with physiological systems—essentially the site and effect the drug has on the body and its physiological mechanism of action. **Toxicology** encompasses the toxic or unwanted effects of drugs on physiological systems, including unwanted and nontherapeutic side effects. **Pharmacogenetics,** a more recent branch of pharmacology, analyzes the body's genetic response to specific drugs. Genetic factors can often explain the response when an affected individual shows an abnormal response to a drug. **Pharmacogenomics** is a more recent term to describe the increasing role of genetic information in guiding the choice of drug therapy on an individual basis. In the future, understanding specific gene variations that can be associated with good or poor therapeutic responses to a particular drug therapy will enable individual tailoring of therapeutic choices based on an individual's genetic makeup.

ROLE OF HEALTH PROFESSIONALS

Many health care professionals require a thorough knowledge and understanding of pharmacology. Physicians are particularly trained in the diagnosis of disease and are responsible for determining the particular therapeutic agent to be used in the disease treatment. Therefore, to be effective, physicians need a thorough understanding of pharmacology. Pharmacists also require a very thorough knowledge and understanding of pharmacology and therapeutics because they are legally responsible for the preparation, storage, and dispensing of medications. They serve as a direct resource for physicians regarding the correct choice of appropriate medications and questions about drug interactions. Pharmacists also serve as a direct source of information for patients taking medications. They can explain how the drug is to be used, how it is to be taken, what side effects are possible, and answer other questions about medication use. Pharmacy technicians may complete some of the dispensing functions of pharmacists, but they always work under direct supervision of a pharmacist. The pharmacist checks to make sure the prescription is filled correctly. Nurses and other allied health professionals also need an understanding of pharmacology to participate fully in the health care process. Audiologists can benefit from an understanding of the interactions of drugs with the hearing process, especially those drugs that may adversely affect hearing or balance. While those roles are largely clinical in nature, the role of the pharmacologist is somewhat different. Pharmacologists study drugs to understand the basis for drugs' actions on bodily functions, as well as participate in the discovery and testing of new therapeutic agents.

FEDERAL LEGISLATION AND DRUGS

A **drug** can be defined as "any chemical substance that affects living processes in a positive or negative manner." As that definition encompasses a very wide range of chemical substances, a drug is more traditionally defined as "any substance used in the diagnosis, treatment, or prevention of disease." Legal statutes, which have their basis in federal legislation, also define what a drug is and is not (for an overview, see Milestones in U.S. Food and Drug Law History 1999). In 1906, the **Pure Food and Drug Act** was passed by Congress. For the first time, drug manufacturers were required to list the ingredients of their preparations on labels. The act prevented false and misleading claims about the therapeutic actions of a drug from appearing on the package label. This act also required the registration of preparations containing certain dangerous or addictive drugs (e.g., morphine, heroin, alcohol, cocaine, and opium). The Pure Food and Drug Act, however, covered preparations sold only in interstate commerce and did not regulate therapeutic claims made in advertisements, by salespeople, or by signs in store windows. The 1906 act also established the *United States Pharmacopeia* and the *National Formulary* as official standards for drug preparation and gave the federal government the power to enforce those standards through the Bureau of Chemistry.

In 1927, the Bureau of Chemistry became the Food, Drug, and Insecticide Administration, which became the Food and Drug Administration (FDA) in July 1930. Federal regulation of therapeutic agents continued when, in 1912, Congress passed the **Sherley Amendment,** which prohibited fraudulent therapeutic claims from being made for patent medications.

In 1938, Congress passed the **Federal Food, Drug, and Cosmetic Act.** This act prevented the marketing of new drugs and preparations until they had been properly tested for safety. The act also mandated that labels on medications had to be both accurate and complete.

In 1951, this act was modified by the **Durham-Humphrey Amendment,** which specified how legend (prescription) drugs could be ordered and dispensed. Prescription drugs were required to include the following statement on their label: "Caution: Federal law prohibits dispensing without prescription." That warning is required on all (1) drugs given by injection; (2) drugs that are hypnotic, narcotic, or habit-forming or derivatives of such; (3) drugs deemed, because of toxicity, method of use, or side effects, not safe unless administered by a licensed practitioner; and (4) new drugs limited to investigational use. The amendment also recognized a second group of drugs that is referred to as over-the-counter, or OTC, preparations.

Over-the-counter (OTC) medications are drugs deemed by the FDA to be safely used without direct medical supervision and may, therefore, be sold directly to the public. A drug may exist in both a prescription and OTC formulation. The OTC form is usually available in a lower dose or different formulation than the prescription form.

In 1962, the **Kefauver-Harris Drug Amendment** further regulated medications by requiring drug manufacturers for the first time to prove to the FDA the safety and effectiveness of their products before being allowed to market them. This amendment also required all drugs previously approved between 1938 and 1962 to undergo testing to confirm safety and effectiveness. This testing was initiated in 1968 because of legal challenges and was completed in the mid-1980s. This testing has resulted in those preparations not meeting the safety and effectiveness standards of the FDA being removed from the market.

The **Dietary Supplement Health and Education Act** of 1994 authorized the FDA to regulate the labeling and therapeutic claims of "dietary supplements," but classified them as foods, which means they are not required to undergo testing to prove safety and effectiveness. Herbal medicines are covered under these provisions and are therefore considered "dietary supplements" and are not tested for safety and effectiveness. The act also gave the FDA authority to limit claims of therapeutic effectiveness of dietary supplements.

Source and Uses of Drugs

Drugs come from both natural and synthetic sources. Naturally occurring products provided the early source of drugs and consisted of both plant and animal products. Examples of drugs derived from natural sources are morphine obtained from the opium poppy and insulin isolated from the pancreas of cows and pigs. Penicillin G was isolated and purified from a specific species of mold. The second source of drugs is those that are semisynthetic,

where a natural product is used as the basis for chemical modifications to make a drug safer or more effective. Examples include newer preparations of penicillin that can be taken orally and the modifications made to beef and pork insulin to make them more effective. By far, the greatest number of drugs used today are synthetically made. Chemical synthesis is used to produce the active ingredient; thus, drugs are synthesized from the interaction of chemical components. Examples include antidepressant and antipsychotic medications. Recombinant DNA technologies are also being used to enhance the production of drugs. For example, the gene for the human form of insulin has been isolated and inserted into the genome of *Escherichia coli* bacteria. Those bacteria produce the human form of insulin, which is then isolated and purified and is now used by most patients with type I diabetes.

Drugs are used for three main purposes: (1) to cure disease, (2) for replacement therapy, and (3) to treat disease symptoms. While curing disease is the ultimate goal of medical science and therapeutics, there are relatively few disease conditions where a cure can actually be achieved with drug therapy. Antibiotic therapy, where the offending microorganism can be completely eliminated, is an example of a drug used to cure disease. Another example is elimination of tumors with appropriate drug therapy, which can lead to a cure in some forms of cancer. However, true cures are not common with present drug therapy. Replacement therapy, the second use of drugs, involves the use of hormones administered to replace deficient hormone production in the patient. Often, patients with thyroid hormone deficiencies receive thyroid hormone replacement. Other examples of replacement therapy include the use of growth hormone in children lacking growth hormone; insulin use in diabetics; and L-DOPA, a precursor to dopamine (a central nervous system neurotransmitter that controls movement), which is deficient in Parkinson's disease. The third and major use of drugs is to control or treat symptoms of the disease process. Antihypertensive medications used to treat high blood pressure, cholesterol-lowering drugs used to help prevent heart attacks and strokes, and vasodilators used to help maintain normal blood pressure are examples. Drugs for replacement and treatment of symptoms usually must be used for the duration of the patient's life to prevent the symptoms from returning.

Names of Drugs

During development, drugs are given three distinct drug names. The first is the chemical name, the second is the generic or nonproprietary name, and the third is the trade or proprietary name. The chemical name is a description of the drug's chemical composition and molecular structure. The generic or non-proprietary name is assigned by the manufacturer with approval of the United States Adopted Name Council (USAN) and is the official name listed in the *United States Pharmacopia*. When drugs are marketed to the public, the manufacturer selects and copyrights a trade, brand, or proprietary name for its product. Doing so restricts the use of the trade name to that individual drug company and that individual drug product. For example, the chemical name of Acetaminophen is N-(4-hydroxyphenyl)-acetamide; the generic name is acetaminophen; and it is sold under the trade names of Tylenol, Tempra, Tapanol, and Liquiprin, among others. Since numerous brand or trade names may exist for the same chemical, the use of generic names is recommended when referring to drugs. This use also avoids confusion between some trade names that may be very similar.

GENERAL CONCEPTS CONCERNING DRUG EFFECTS

In a general discussion of how drugs work, it is useful to distinguish between **drug actions** and **drug effects.** The action of a drug is the underlying biochemical or physiological mechanism by which the chemicals produce their responses in living organisms. The effects of a drug are the observed consequences of the drug's actions. An example is penicillin. Penicillin acts to interfere with the synthesis of components of the bacterial cell wall. The effect of penicillin's action on the cell wall results in the death of the bacteria.

This focus on the action of drugs has led pharmacologists to focus on understanding the mechanism of action of drug effects.

One of the most basic principles in the study of pharmacology is that no drug produces a single effect. A drug may produce many effects that result from a single action or many different actions that lead to a single effect. Because drugs can act at multiple sites, all drugs produce multiple effects, some of which are therapeutic and beneficial and some of which are unwanted and not beneficial. Using penicillin again as an example, the desired beneficial therapeutic effect of penicillin is to prevent the growth of bacteria and to limit infection. The undesired effect of treatment with penicillin may be initiation of diarrhea or an allergic response. A drug's primary effect is the **therapeutic effect;** secondary effects are referred to as **side effects.**

There are many examples of drugs that were initially developed for one specific therapeutic action or effect and because another effect became evident during testing, the drug was then marketed for a different use. Minoxidil is an example. It was first developed to relax blood vessels, thus lowering blood pressure. One of the side effects seen with Minoxidil testing was an increase in the growth of hair. Minoxidil is now marketed as Rogaine®, which is available as an OTC topical preparation used for the treatment of male pattern baldness, while Minoxidil as Lonitin® is an orally available prescription medication used as a vasodilator.

A second basic principle of pharmacology is that every drug or chemical produces adverse or unwanted effects. Paracelsus (1493–1541) said, referring to natural therapeutic preparations, that "all substances are poisons, for there is nothing without poisonous qualities, it is only the dose which makes a poison" (Oxford Dictionary of Medical Quotes, 2004). Paracelsus introduced the principle that (1) experimentation was essential in determining the response to chemicals, (2) one should make a distinction between therapeutic and toxic properties of chemicals, (3) dose separated the therapeutic and toxic properties, and (4) there is a degree of specificity of chemicals and their therapeutic and toxic effects. Those ideas served as the foundation for the development of ideas regarding drug mechanisms and effects. Those ideas also served as the basis for the development of the discipline of toxicology.

Mechanisms of Drug Action

The biological effects observed after drug administration are the results of interactions between the chemical and some distinct portion of the organism. This interaction of drugs with specific portions of cells or membranes gives drugs their specificity of action. The term **receptor** has been used to define the constituents of the cell with which the drug interacts to produce its actions. Receptors are usually thought to be proteins that exist on cells or in membranes and act to transfer the binding of a drug to a physiological action that is observed. After attachment of the drug to the receptor, a drug may either initiate a physiological response or prevent the natural response from occurring. An **agonist** is a drug capable of interacting with a receptor to activate a response. An **antagonist** is a drug that can bind to a receptor, but because of its structure, does not activate the receptor completely to produce a response. The binding of the antagonist can, however, prevent an agonist from binding and, therefore, can prevent the normal response to that agonist. (Figure 1-1)

Drug actions are therefore controlled by two aspects of this drug-receptor interaction: **affinity,** which describes how well the drug binds to its receptor, and **efficacy,** which describes how efficient the drug-receptor complex is in producing a response. By definition, an antagonist has a high affinity but an efficacy of zero, while an agonist has both high affinity and high efficacy. Drugs with intermediate levels of efficacy (e.g., when 100 percent of receptors are occupied and the tissue response is submaximal) are referred to as partial agonists. It is this drug receptor interaction that gives drugs their specificity for therapeutic actions, as drugs produce responses only in tissues with the appropriate receptors present. As mentioned previously, all drugs can produce multiple effects. Those multiple effects may be produced by actions at one or more different receptors or multiple receptors in different tissues. The study of those drug-receptor interactions has greatly increased scientists'

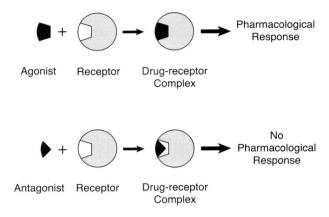

Figure 1-1. Drug Receptor Interactions. Agonists bind to receptors, and the interactions produce a pharmacological response. The binding of an antagonist by itself cannot activate the receptor to produce a response; but it can prevent the agonist from binding, activating the receptor, and producing its effects.

understanding of how drugs work to produce their physiological effects in the body. The efforts of scientists now focus on discovering new receptors and determining the steps that occur between the binding of a drug and the production of the physiological effects. Those efforts will help design more effective and safer medications.

Variability in Response

Even though scientists understand how some drugs interact with receptors, not all individuals respond in the same fashion to the same dose of a drug. Some individuals show a response to very low levels of a drug, while others may require a larger dose to get the same therapeutic action. While scientists understand some of the reasons for that variability, not all variability can be easily explained. Variability between drug responses in patients can be accounted for by the following factors: body weight, size, gender, age, disease states, and genetic factors.

Body weight is an especially significant factor in clinically obese or clinically underweight patients, where the dose of a drug must be altered to account for the difference in body size. That is especially true for drugs that are very lipid- (fat) soluble and accumulate in fat, thus preventing a drug from reaching its normal site of action. For example, during surgery, it is very difficult to maintain the appropriate amount of general anesthetic in the blood of a clinically obese individual. The drugs are very lipid-soluble and have a tendency to accumulate in body fat and then are not available to work in the brain.

Size and *surface area* also play a role in drug response. Chemicals sprayed to help control mosquitoes are an example. Those chemicals can be safely sprayed in the environment because the amounts used are small for the size of a human. However, the amounts are large for the surface area of a mosquito, and the concentration is sufficient to kill the mosquito.

While there are significant differences in how men and women respond physiologically, *gender* has not been widely studied as a factor in drug response variability. It is, however, now receiving increased attention.

Age can also cause variability, especially at the two ends of the scale—the newborn and the elderly. Newborns are particularly sensitive to some drugs and not sensitive to others because the physiological processes the drugs affect are absent or still under development. The elderly are more sensitive to some drugs and less sensitive to others because those same processes affected by the drugs are beginning to slow down. There are significant differences in how drugs are metabolized between infants, where the systems are still developing, and the elderly, where the systems are loosing effectiveness.

The elderly also face another issue, and that is chronic *disease states*. Many diseases change the way normal physiological systems function and therefore will change how the body responds to drugs. That is especially true for those people with chronic disease, especially liver or kidney disease, because those organs are so intimately involved with the metabolism and excretion of drugs.

Perhaps the greatest factor in drug variability is *genetics*. Scientists involved in drug development are constantly trying to predict how well a drug will perform based on an individual's genetic factors. Pharmacogenomics is based on the concept of using genetic information to guide therapeutic decisions.

Genetic factors are by far the major reason for variability in response to drugs.

With over 13,000 prescription drugs available in the United States, it is very important that you understand the rational use of those drugs. It is essential that drugs be used for the purpose prescribed and by the person for whom the prescription was written by a licensed physician. One of the problems with drug use today is that some people are very willing to diagnose the illnesses of a friend or colleague based on their own symptoms. In many circumstances, those same people are willing to give some of their own prescription medication to another person to treat the perceived problem. That practice can lead to life-threatening consequences. All medications have risks associated with them, and the benefit of the medication must outweigh the risks for a particular drug to be useful. The level of risk a person is willing to tolerate should relate to the severity of the disease being treated. For example, cancer drugs can cause significant physiological problems, but the terminal outcome of cancer needs to be weighed against the benefit of being able to cure the cancer. People are willing to accept many more risks with cancer agents than they are for a medication to treat a minor headache.

A second concern of rational drug use is using the medication at the prescribed dose. Most people think that if two aspirin will fix a headache in 30 minutes, three or four will work much faster and be better. Unwanted drug side effects and toxicities increase as the dose of a drug is increased.

Third, many patients expect that every doctor visit should result in a prescription. That is especially true for respiratory infections, where an expectation for an antibiotic prescription exists for all doctors' visits and many patients are disappointed if they do not receive one. Most respiratory infections are viral in nature, and antibiotics have no therapeutic effects on viruses. While the antibiotic may have minimal side effects, the indiscriminant use of antibiotics has led to the problem of antibiotic resistance. The classic example is penicillin. When it was first introduced, penicillin was very effective in killing specific types of bacteria. But with widespread indiscriminant use, many of the bacteria have developed resistance not only to penicillin, but also to many other antibiotics. Rational use of drugs requires them to be used for specific disease processes at the appropriate dose and by the person for whom they were prescribed.

SUMMARY

This chapter considers the historical development of the discipline of pharmacology and the interaction of the subdisciplines of pharmacokinetics, pharmacodynamics, pharmacogenetics, and toxicology. The interactions of drugs with living physiological systems are described. A drug is defined as "a chemical used in the diagnosis, treatment, or prevention of disease." The regulatory environment of drug use and the establishment of regulation by the developing Food and Drug Administration are also discussed. Clinically used drugs come from natural products both plant and animal and from semisynthetic and synthetic sources. Drugs are specifically used to cure disease, as physiological replacements or to treat symptoms of disease. Drugs are discussed using three different names: the chemical name describing the chemical structure, the generic name given to the drug entity by its manufacturer, and the trade or brand name used in promotional advertising. Different drug companies may sell a single generic drug under various trade names.

Drugs may produce multiple actions, and those multiple actions may lead to a variety of effects. Pharmacology is intimately involved with understanding a drug's mechanism of action both for therapeutic and unwanted side effects. All chemical compounds can produce toxic side effects if the concentration of the drug is high enough. The specificity of a drug's actions has a basis in the interaction of drug and receptor molecules found on cells or membranes and the specific interactions of agonists and antagonists. The variability of drug responses in different individuals is based on several factors: body weight; size; gender; age; disease states; and the most important factor, genetics. The rational use of drugs requires them to be used by a specific individual for the specific purpose they were prescribed and at the dose prescribed. Other uses can lead to development of unwanted side effects, which can be lethal.

Notable Figures in Pharmacology

François Magendie (1783–1855) was a French physiologist, a scientist who described the foramen of Magendie, but was best known for his suggestion that physiology should be based on experimental evidence.

Friedrich Wilhelm Adam Sertürner (1783–1841) was a German pharmacist who discovered morphine in 1803. He was the first person to isolate morphine from opium, calling the isolated alkaloid "morphine" after the Greek god of dreams, Morpheus.

Claude Bernard (1813–1878) was a French physiologist and a student of Magendie. Bernard's aim was to continue Magendie's idea of experimentation as the basis of medicine. He dismissed many previous misconceptions, taking nothing for granted. He is also known for his pioneering work on the mechanism of curare and carbon monoxide.

Rudolph Buchheim (1820–1879) established the first Institute of Pharmacology at the University of Dorpot in Estonia, which was later moved to the University of Leipzig.

Oswald Schmeideberg (1838–1921) was a German pharmacologist trained by Buchheim. Schmeideberg established pharmacology as a discipline at the University of Strasburg and was the mentor for a large number of subsequent leaders in pharmacology. He is considered by many to be the father of modern pharmacology.

John J. Abel (1857–1938) trained under Schmeideberg and established the first Department of Pharmacology at the University of Michigan in 1891. In 1893, he moved to Johns Hopkins University as its first Chair of Pharmacology. He is recognized as the American father of pharmacology.

SUGGESTED READINGS

Holmstedt, B., & Liljestrand, G. (Eds.). (1963). *Readings in Pharmacology.* New York: Macmillan.

Leake, C. D. (1975). *An Historical Account of Pharmacology to the Twentieth Century.* Springfield, IL: Charles C. Thomas.

McDonald, P. (2004). *Oxford Dictionary of Medical Quotes.* (p. 76). Oxford, UK: Oxford University Press.

Parascandola, J. (1992). *The Development of American Pharmacology, John J. Abel and the Shaping of a Discipline.* Baltimore: Johns Hopkins University Press.

U.S. Food and Drug Administration, FDA Backgrounder, Milestones in U.S. Food and Drug Law. FDA Backgrounder. (1999). Access: http://www.fda.gov/opacom/backgrounders/miles.html

PHARMACOLOGY TEXTBOOKS

Brunton, L. L., Lazo, J. S., & Parker, K. L. (Eds.). (2006). *Goodman and Gilman's the Pharmacological Basis of Therapeutics* (11th ed.). New York: McGraw-Hill.

Katzung, B. G. (Ed.). (2004). *Basic and Clinical Pharmacology* (9th ed.). New York: McGraw-Hill.

Levine, R. R., Walsh, C. T., & Schwartz, R. D. (2005). *Pharmacology: Drug Actions and Reactions* (7th ed.). London and New York: Taylor & Francis.

Rang, H. P., Dale, M. M., Ritter, J. M., & Gardner, P. (2001). *Pharmacology* (4th ed.). New York: Churchhill Livingstone.

CHAPTER
2

Pharmacodynamics and Pharmacokinetics

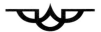

Jose A. Rey, PharmD
Nova Southeastern University—College of Pharmacy

INTRODUCTION

The broad area of pharmacology entails all aspects of all medications and their application for the prevention or treatment of diseases or symptoms of disease. It is not within the scope of this chapter to teach every aspect of pharmacology. Rather, the goal of this chapter is to introduce the basic concepts that the reader needs to continue his or her study of this topic in the focused areas desired and to create a foundation of understanding for the more advanced concepts presented later in this textbook. Many terms may be unfamiliar to the reader. Refer to the Glossary for further explanation or to specialized texts and references in pharmacology as needed. The references for this chapter provide excellent resources and supplemental readings for a continued exploration and understanding of pharmacology.

PHARMACODYNAMICS

Pharmacodynamics is an area of pharmacological study that refers to a drug and its intended target or site of action. It also relates to the drug's mechanism of action, or how it works at the target site. It is the way a medication interacts with the body to elicit a beneficial or, possibly, adverse outcome. So, simply stated, pharmacodynamics is what the drug does to the body. Most but not all drugs interact with molecular targets called receptors. A drug can fit into a receptor, which is usually integrated with a cell's membrane surface, due to its physical, bioelectrical, or chemical qualities. The drug subsequently causes a response that may trigger a multistep process, eventually eliciting the desired positive (or negative) effect. Many receptors (a protein macromolecule) are attached to or integrated into the target cell's membrane surface. However other drugs may target sites or receptors found inside the cell to cause the desired result. There are many different types of receptors. They include transmembrane ion channels (ligand-gated, voltage-gated, and second messenger-regulated); transmembrane receptors linked to intracellular G proteins, which can be both stimulatory or inhibitory, that often use second messengers

such as cyclic adenosine 3′,5′ monophosphate (cAMP); transmembrane receptors linked to cytosolic enzymes (often utilizes phosphorylation such as tyrosine kinase); and intracellular receptors requiring the drug to pass through or be transported into the cell's cytoplasm or nucleus (e.g., steroid hormones affecting DNA-RNA-protein activities). When activated, some receptors initiate a cascade of events and the generation of second messengers to signal or secondarily cause the desired physiologic response. The simplest way to visualize a drug-receptor interaction is to picture how a house key fits into a simple or complex door lock to cause the door to open easily or stay closed (Figure 2-1). The lock will open only in response to one key or a few specific keys. This may be referred to as the lock-and-key model of drug-receptor interactions. It is believed that the body has a natural **ligand** (or key) for every receptor.

Many of these natural ligands are known to science and medicine, while there are still many more to be fully identified. For the purpose of this discussion,

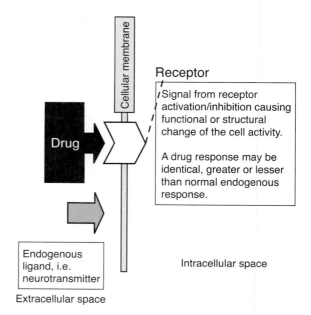

Figure 2-1. A simple representation of a drug-receptor complex on the surface of a cellular membrane and the result of interaction and the way drugs seem to "fit" into a receptor.
A natural, endogenous ligand can also affect receptors. May be referred to as a lock-and-key model.

ligands are agonists that will activate receptors. All neurotransmitters, such as acetylcholine (ACh), dopamine (DA), epinephrine, gamma-amino butyric acid (GABA), glutamate, histamine, norepinephrine (NE), and serotonin (5-HT), are agonists at their respective receptor sites. Although all neurotransmitters are agonists, some activities (or purposes) of these neurotransmitters may be either excitatory (e.g., ACh or glutamate) or inhibitory (e.g., GABA) in their physiologic responses. Some neurotransmitters can be excitatory in some tissues or neurons and inhibitory in others. That may be more a function of the receptor's activity and location than the neurotransmitter itself. Some drugs are receptor agonists that can mimic or enhance the actions of the naturally occurring agonists with similar or identical responses. The over-the-counter decongestant pseudoephedrine is considered a sympathomimetic since it mimics the effect of NE. Therefore, it can be considered an agonist at the NE-responsive alpha-1 receptor.

An antagonist is a drug that can block or reduce the action of the natural agonist or neurotransmitter at the respective receptor site through either direct (competitive) or indirect (e.g., noncompetitive allosteric) methods. Beta-receptor antagonists (also known as beta blockers), for example, are a group of drugs that affect blood pressure and heart rate by blocking the effect of NE (the natural agonist) at its respective binding site on the beta receptor. Other examples of antagonists that an audiologist may encounter in practice are medications used for the treatment of vertigo or Méniere's disease, such as the ACh receptor antagonists scopolamine (Transderm Scop patch) and meclizine (Antivert), the dopamine receptor antagonist prochlorperazine (Compazine), and the histamine

receptor antagonist or "antihistamine" diphenhydramine (Benadryl). Some agents, such as promethazine (Phenergan), can actually block multiple neurotransmitters and have anticholinergic, antidopaminergic, and antihistamine properties all in one product.

Enzymes (also proteins) can be targets of drug action as well. An example is the **non-steroidal anti-inflammatory drug (NSAID)** ibuprofen that inhibits the enzyme cyclooxygenase needed to create inflammatory prostaglandins that can form secondary to muscular injury. Inflammation can signal and promote pain; therefore, ibuprofen is considered an analgesic as well. Another drug that can inhibit prostaglandin formation, which interestingly may also contribute to its ototoxic effects, is acetylsalicylic acid (aspirin). Further discussion regarding aspirin and ibuprofen and their pharmacodynamic, pharmacokinetic, and possible ototoxic effects will be presented in subsequent chapters.

When describing the drug-receptor interaction or the ability of a drug to cause a given response, we often refer to **dose-response curves.** Basically, it is the relationship of the given dose of a drug to its desired therapeutic effect or adverse toxic effect. **Efficacy** can refer to a drug's ability to elicit its maximum response at a given dose, or it can describe a drug's ability to treat a disease state. Efficacy can be used to compare two agents with different pharmacodynamic mechanisms of action. The term **potency** has sometimes been used in place of *efficacy,* although potency should refer to two agents with similar mechanisms of action in the same or very similar class of drugs. Potency refers to the quantity of drug necessary to produce 50 percent of the drug's potential maximal

Note to Audiologists

A medication's ability to be ototoxic may involve both pharmacodynamic and pharmacokinetic properties. For instance, a toxic effect related to a drug's negative action on the auditory hair cells may be increased if the drug is not removed from that particular site (compartment) due to poor elimination or accumulation over time. Whereas drug accumulation (increasing

concentration in the endolymph/perilymph over time) has not been proven to be the reason for the ototoxic effects of the aminoglycosides, perhaps the toxicity observed with aminoglycosides is actually a more pharmacodynamic effect related to direct or indirect damage to the hair cells.

response. A drug X may be considered to be more potent than a comparator drug Y if a lower dose of drug X is required to achieve the same response. This can be restated such that the lower comparative dose generally indicates greater potency. Different potencies between drugs are often corrected by adjusting the doses to achieve similar therapeutic responses. These dose-response curves can be separated by beneficial response and toxic response.

This model can also be used to help describe the therapeutic index of a drug. The **therapeutic index** of a given drug is the ratio of a drug's dangerous, or toxic, dose to its therapeutic, or beneficial, dose (or plasma concentration). A drug with a small ratio generally has a small therapeutic index and usually has what can be referred to as a narrow therapeutic window (Figure 2-2). Thus, that drug is more dangerous to use in the general population. The larger the ratio or index, the safer the medication is considered to be; it is referred to as having a wide therapeutic window (Figure 2-3).

Refer to Figures 2-2, 2-3, and 2-4 for a graphical depiction of the dose-response concept and the therapeutic window concept. Figure 2-4 refers to a different graphical depiction: as a dose of a drug X increases to

Large Therapeutic Index
(Rarely encounter adverse effects at normal treatment doses)

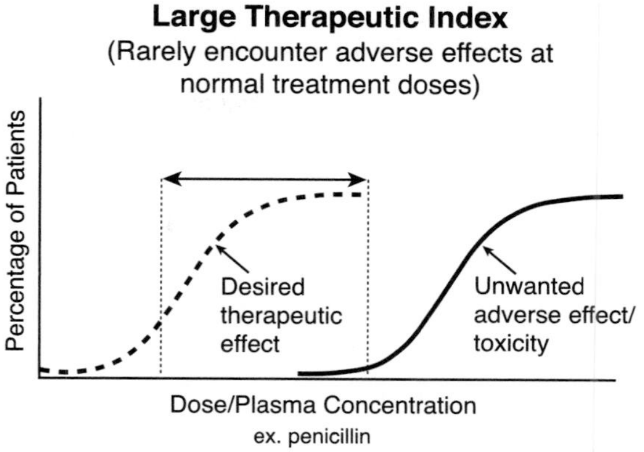

Figure 2-3. The concept of a large therapeutic index, or wide window, between efficacy and toxicity, which some medications have and is generally a good quality to have. This implies that drugs with a large therapeutic index can have efficacy in treating diseases with very minimal risk of toxicity or certain dangerous adverse effects.

achieve a therapeutic response, an incremental increase in the risk for an adverse or toxic effect also occurs. At a certain point or dose, some drugs reach maximal therapeutic benefit; and any further increase in dose may only increase the risk for toxicity. Following the layperson's common line of reasoning, he or she may expect that if one pill of a given medication is good, then two pills are better. Continuing that line of thought, then, three or four pills should continue to treat even more severe symptoms. The reality of the situation is that the person taking more than the recommended amount of medication is risking a possible severe or toxic reaction. That is a common occurrence with individuals who self-medicate with nonprescription and prescription medications based on limited experience or knowledge of drug effects and pharmacology.

There is individual variability in these responses to drugs. Every person is different in both pharmacodynamic and pharmacokinetic characteristics. Even genetic factors and the differences in which a person expresses this genetic variability contribute to the difficulty in predicting a drug response for a specific individual. Most data on a medication is obtained from large numbers of subjects and is expressed as the average response observed in a particular study population.

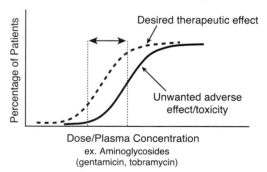

Figure 2-2. The concept of a small therapeutic index, or narrow window between efficacy and toxicity, which some medications have. This implies that for these drugs to have efficacy and positive disease-treating effects, there is a risk, which is sometimes high, of a certain adverse or toxic effect.

Therapeutic Dose-Response versus Dose-Toxicity

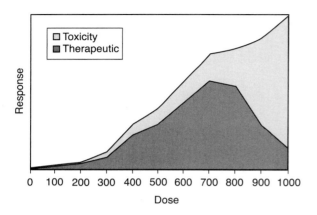

Figure 2-4. Another graphic representation of the concept that although increasing a dose of a medication can increase its efficacy in treating a disease, for some medications, there is a maximal beneficial response; that is, any further increases in dosing may result in toxicity and may actually diminish a medication's effectiveness. This figure refutes the common lay belief that if "taking one pill works well, then taking two pills will work even better." Instead, taking two pills, or doubling the dose, may risk adverse effects.

Some individuals may be very sensitive to a low dose of a medication and have a greater risk for adverse effects. Perhaps those individuals are somehow uniquely sensitive (for audiology, sensitive outer hair cells to low doses of aminoglycosides due to possible genetic factors); or there is a **polymorphism** in the expression of the genetic code, and the receptor in question is not responsive or is dysfunctional. There could be an impairment of the necessary enzyme required to metabolize a specific drug. Impaired renal function can also contribute to a person's response and apparent sensitivity to a normal dose of a drug due to higher-than-expected tissue or plasma concentrations. The potential pharmacokinetic characteristics will be discussed later.

Adverse effects of drugs may not be toxic or even dangerous. Some adverse effects (or side effects) are predictable due to a drug's pharmacological profile. Some drugs bind to more than one type of receptor (as either agonists or antagonists); and although only one specific receptor was the desired target, the other receptors to which a drug binds may be responsible for certain, even predictable adverse effects. An example is the common sedation effect of the antihistamine diphenhydramine (a histamine type-1 receptor antagonist) that is used for the temporary treatment of insomnia. This is also a major cause of the sedation effects from certain antidepressants, such as the tricyclic antidepressants amitriptyline or doxepin, although those drugs' intended effects are to treat depression by affecting a different receptor and transport carrier for NE and serotonin. The antagonism at the histamine receptor is unintended but expected. Other adverse effects of medications, such as the risk for gastrointestinal ulceration and bleeding with NSAIDs, are related to the same mechanism of action (inhibition of prostaglandin synthesis) that the medication uses to cause its intended effects of decreased inflammation and analgesia. This prostaglandin inhibition may also be the cause of NSAID-induced ototoxicity. Inhibition of some types of prostaglandins may result in changes in blood flow to the auditory system. An **iatrogenic adverse effect** is often unpredictable and is usually not dose-related. It may be an allergic reaction that can range in severity from a mild dermatological rash to fatal anaphylactic shock or a hematological reaction affecting red or white blood cell creation. Medication-related hepatic or renal damage may also be iatrogenic and therefore not predictable, but requiring treatment discontinuation.

PHARMACOKINETICS

Pharmacokinetics is an important area of study and research that must be considered when drug therapy is utilized. It involves how a drug moves through the body from the time it is administered (through various routes) and absorbed, where it goes into the body and then to sites of action (distribution), the metabolism of the drug, and finally its excretion or elimination from the body. Each drug has unique characteristics with regard to those parameters. Therefore, each drug may have a different time course in the body that is reflected in different durations of action or exposure to the intended or unintended sites of action.

Absorption

The body has natural defenses to foreign substances, including drugs, and those barriers must be overcome so the medication can be delivered to the body. For delivering a drug, various routes of administration exist:

- Oral

- Sublingual

- **Buccal**

- Rectal

- Topical (dermatologic, nasal, otic, and ophthalmologic)

- Transdermal

- Inhalation

- Intranasal

- Intraocular

- Intratympanic

- Parenteral routes (subcutaneous, intramuscular, and intravenous)

Once a drug is administered, the amount of drug that is absorbed may be determined by factors such as stomach pH, the drug's physical and chemical characteristics (e.g., ionization state, molecular weight, **hydrophilicity,** or **lipophilicity**), other drugs or food that may have been consumed or given at a similar time to drug administration, and possibly even processes related to active drug transport across membranes. A dosage formulation of a drug can be modified to cause a slower-than-normal release of a medication to allow for slower absorption and possible delay in activity. These delayed-release or slow-release formulations are popular in attempting to improve either adverse effects or medication adherence with prescribed regimens. Some medications are not absorbed through the oral route and must be given parenterally, such as the aminoglycosides. By bypassing the gastrointestinal tract, usually 100 percent of the parenterally administered medication is delivered into the blood circulation. **Bioavailability** describes the actual amount of drug that reaches the systemic circulation and is often expressed as a fraction (percentage) of the given dose. Even if a medication is well absorbed through the gastrointestinal tract, it must first travel to the liver via portal circulation and undergo **first-pass metabolism** via the liver before entering into the systemic circulation. That process is an important barrier and defense to toxins that may be accidentally ingested; however, it also can act to diminish the effect of a medication.

Distribution

Once a drug is absorbed and enters into the systemic circulation, it must then be distributed to the target site of action (a specific tissue, organ, or intracellular space). It may still encounter certain barriers to its delivery to the desired target site. Some drugs must cross barriers such as the blood-brain barrier, blood-testes barrier, blood-placental barrier, or blood-labyrinth barrier. Other compartments of interest in audiology are the endolymph and perilymph compartments as sites of drug distribution and possible toxicity if drugs are distributed into these compartments but have delayed or slowed elimination from them. The plasma concentration of a drug is often used to correlate the effect of the drug because accurate determination of tissue or organ drug concentrations is difficult.

A drug's **volume of distribution (Vd)** is a concept that attempts to quantify the relationship (and explain through assumptions and calculations) of the observed concentration of a drug in the body (e.g., plasma or blood) to the amount of drug administered (Vd = X / Cp). Vd attempts to explain the concentration of the drug observed by assuming the uniform amount of fluid it would take to provide the observed concentration (Cp = X/Vd). Of note, the common Vd used to explain and calculate gentamicin dosing regimens is 0.25 L/kg.

As stated earlier, certain parts of the body can be expressed as separate compartments or sites of drug distribution. The systemic circulation is often the principle compartment to be considered; but the brain and even the endolymph/perilymph behave as separate compartments for a drug to be delivered to—either intended, such as antidepressants into the brain, or unintended, such as aminoglycosides in endolymph. Another factor affecting the availability of a drug to a target site is plasma protein binding. Only a free drug (unbound) is capable of diffusing across membranes or interacting with receptors at target sites or organs. Drugs bound to plasma proteins, such as albumin, are generally contained in the vascular compartment. Protein binding is a potential source for drug interactions when two or more drugs with high binding affinity compete for the same protein binding site and can displace one or both medications, essentially allowing for more unbound/free drug (and thus active drug) for target-site activity or toxicity.

Metabolism

As soon as a drug presents itself to the systemic circulation, it begins to be metabolized, usually by the liver, in an attempt to remove the drug from the body. Enzymatic degradation and conversion of the drug molecule take place in an attempt to make the drug more water soluble and available for renal excretion.

The types of metabolism may include Phase I reactions that modify drug structure, usually through hydrolysis, oxidation, or reduction. A popular group of **Phase I hepatic enzymes** includes the microsomal cytochrome P-450 group that mediates a large number of drug metabolic pathways. Another type of hepatic metabolism is Phase II conjugative reactions that act to combine drugs with large, water-soluble polar molecules to enhance a drug's solubility and excretion into the urine. Hepatic metabolism of drugs is a common site for drug-drug interactions. Some drugs may impair or induce the hepatic metabolism of another drug by inhibiting (or inducing) the enzymatic activity of the respective microsomal metabolic processes. Most drug-drug interactions involve phase I metabolic interactions. Hepatic failure can also result in reduced or impaired metabolism and elimination of a drug from the body.

Some medications may be given as an inactivated prodrug and may actually require hepatic metabolism for their conversion to the active moiety of the drug.

Excretion and Elimination

Renal excretion is the major route of final drug elimination from the body with **biliary excretion** being a minor route of elimination. The purpose of hepatic

metabolism is to make the drug molecule more water soluble for easy renal excretion. Renal blood flow, **glomerular filtration rate,** and protein binding all affect renal excretion. Renal function often declines with increasing age, and drug accumulation is possible. Patients with impaired renal function must often have their dosage regimens adjusted to accommodate and account for the decreased ability to eliminate certain drugs, especially certain ototoxic agents such as cisplatin, aspirin, and aminoglycosides.

Other Pharmacokinetic Concepts

The term **clearance (CL)** takes into consideration metabolism and elimination variables such as blood flow and the volume of body fluid cleared per time unit (L/hr, mL/min) and is usually a constant (k) for a given individual and drug. It is due to the contribution of multiple organs (e.g., CL = CL renal + CL hepatic + CL other). The calculation of the CL of a drug takes into account the Vd of a drug and an elimination constant (k) CL = k (Vd). Another term to be addressed and presented is **half-life** ($t_{1/2}$). When discussing the half-life of a medication ($t_{1/2}$ = the time it takes for the drug's concentration in the plasma to decrease by 50 percent), keep in mind that most reported drug half-lives are averaged from population studies. Therefore, the half-life of a drug may be different between two similar individuals. Half-life is determined by parameters such as metabolic rate or clearance rate and Vd, which may be affected by other medications a patient is receiving. The equations for half-life are as follows:

$$t_{1/2} = \frac{0.693 \, (Vd)}{CL}$$

$$t_{1/2} = \frac{\ln 2}{k} = \frac{0.693}{k}$$

The half-life of a drug can be affected by drug-drug interactions; drug-food interactions; metabolic changes; and changes in elimination, such as impaired renal function.

Figure 2-5 demonstrates the combination of some of the discussed pharmacokinetic concepts: absorption of an oral medication, its peak plasma concentration denoting maximum achieved distribution and concentration in plasma, the drug's therapeutic activity above a certain minimal plasma concentration (while staying below a predetermined toxic plasma concentration), the duration of action, and eventually the elimination phase leading to loss of drug activity due to below minimally effective plasma concentrations. Figure 2-6 reflects the concept of steady state and washout period. **Steady state** commonly relates to the point when the amount of drug delivered to the body is the same as the amount of drug being eliminated from the body in one half-life. It generally takes approximately five half-lives at a specific dose of a drug to achieve this steady state. Some drugs do not demonstrate stable plasma levels or clinical efficacy until steady state is achieved. The **washout period** for a drug, assuming the last dose is administered after achieving steady state, is generally equivalent to five half-lives of the drug in question. For example, if a drug with a 24-hour half-life had been administered to a patient for the last month (thirty days) and steady state had been achieved, then once the drug was discontinued, the washout period would be approximately five days before no drug could be

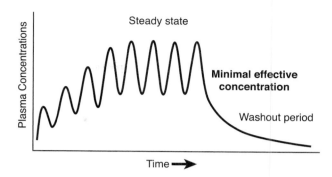

Figure 2-6. Some medications may work relatively fast and after one dose. However, many medications require the achievement of steady state of their plasma concentrations above a certain level to maintain continuous efficacy. Steady state is achieved after approximately five half-lives of a regularly given medication. For example, if a medication had a 24-hour half-life and was given once per day, steady state and consistent efficacy would be achieved after approximately five days of dosing. Also, once a medication is discontinued, it will take approximately five half-lives of the medication to be close to completely eliminated from the body. This has implications in that adverse effects and toxicities may not be resolved immediately upon discontinuation of a medication and for some agents, may actually persist for several days.

detected in plasma. These pharmacokinetic concepts assist the audiologist in predicting whether a potentially dangerous or toxic outcome is likely in a patient predisposed to having drug-related ototoxicity and may provide support for a recommendation to adjust the dosing of a known ototoxic agent. These concepts also allow the clinician to identify factors that can affect drug efficacy and toxicity so as to anticipate potential therapeutic dilemmas in audiological practice.

SUMMARY

The broad science of pharmacology as a whole and the parts related to pharmacodynamics and pharmacokinetics are significant and constantly expanding. The audiologist should consider both the pharmacodynamic and pharmacokinetic properties of all medications. Specific knowledge regarding the historically ototoxic agents and their properties is a recommended and necessary priority of study. Also, familiarity with the pharmacological agents used in sudden hearing loss and balance disorders assists the clinician in both

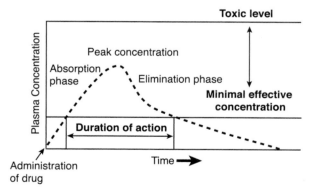

Figure 2-5. In general, an orally given drug must be administered, absorbed into the body's blood supply over a period of time, delivered to a site of action/tissue, then eventually eliminated over a period of time. These are pharmacokinetic aspects of drug handling by the body and the concept that achievement of certain plasma concentrations are needed and can correlate to both efficacy and toxicity. How long a medication will work for a symptom or disease state may be related to the period of time the medication remains above a certain plasma concentration, often referred to as the drug's duration of action.

medication selection and patient counseling. Understanding the characteristics of a medication helps assist in predicting and monitoring clinical outcomes, both positive and negative. These areas of study assist in selecting the correct medication for a given disease state, determining the correct dosage and dosing interval, and determining the possible interactions with other coexisting disease states or other drugs that a patient may be receiving. Understanding the dose-response relationships and the pharmacodynamic effects of varying doses on an individual versus a population norm is important. Knowing the therapeutic indices of medications, whether small or large, will assist in choosing or monitoring medications for both efficacy and toxicity and provide the audiologist with data to support a recommendation for a safer alternative treatment or provide for a margin of safety and monitoring if a medication with a narrow therapeutic window, such as the aminoglycoside gentamicin, is to be used. Medications have a variety of mechanisms of action that may include being agonists or antagonists of a variety of receptors. Other mechanisms of action include enzyme inhibitors that interfere with cell replication and protein synthesis, such as cisplatin, or mechanisms meant for bacterial pathogens that have unfortunate toxicities in humans, such as the aminoglycoside-related effects on hearing and balance. Other considerations, such as the pharmacokinetic aspects of medications, which include the processes and phases of absorption, distribution, metabolism, elimination, and excretion, also assist in determining the specific effects of a medication on a given patient and the necessary changes in dosing and monitoring if one or more of the pharmacokinetic properties change over time. Concepts such as Vd, drug half-life, dose-concentration relationships, and other factors affecting dosing and drug outcomes assist the practicing audiologist in determining a rational and individualized therapeutic regimen for a patient. Currently, most of the pharmacokinetic information available for a specific drug is based on population studies and averages. That information assists in guiding the clinical decision process; but it must be considered along with an individual patient's specific characteristics, such as age, gender, body mass, and coexisting disease states, including hepatic or renal impairment.

Determining an individualized treatment regimen may soon require the incorporation of patient-specific factors such as their genetic expression and polymorphisms. All of the discussed factors are integrated for a given patient to tailor a customized drug treatment and monitoring regimen. An understanding of both pharmacodynamic and pharmacokinetic principles is vital to the safe and efficacious use of medications and for the informed contributions and treatment recommendations of the audiologist as part of the multidisciplinary treatment team.

REFERENCES

Banerjee, A., & Parnes, L. S. (2004). The biology of intratympanic drug administration and pharmacodynamics of round window drug absorption. *Otolaryngologic Clinics of North America, 37*(5), 1035–1051.

Golan D. E., & Tashjian A. H. (Eds.). (2005). *Principles of Pharmacology: The Pathophysiologic Basis of Drug Therapy.* Baltimore: Lippincott Williams & Wilkins.

Hardman, J. G., & Limbird, L. E. (Eds.). (2001). *Goodman and Gilman's The Pharmacological Basis of Therapeutics* (10th ed.). New York: McGraw-Hill.

Harvey R. A., Champe P. C., & Mycek M. J. (Eds.). (2000). *Lippincott's Illustrated Reviews: Pharmacology* (2nd ed.). Baltimore: Lippincott Williams & Wilkins.

Henley, C. M., & Schacht, J. (1988). Pharmacokinetics of aminoglycoside antibiotics in blood, inner-ear fluids and tissues and their relationship to ototoxicity. *Audiology, 27*(3), 137–148.

Julien, R. M. (2001). *A Primer of Drug Action* (9th ed.). New York: Worth Publishers.

Nicolau, D. P., Freeman, C. D., et al. (1995). Experience with a once-daily aminoglycoside program administered to 2,184 adult patients. *Antimicrobial Agents and Chemotherapy, 39*(3), 650–655.

Turnidge, J. (2003). Pharmacodynamics and dosing of aminoglycosides. *Infectious Disease Clinics of North America, 17*(3), 503–528.

Winter, M. E. (Ed.). (1994). *Basic Clinical Pharmacokinetics* (3rd ed.). Vancouver, Washington: Applied Therapeutics, Inc.

CHAPTER
3

Pharmacotherapeutics and Patient Factors

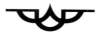

Tabitha Parent Buck, AuD
A.T. Still University—Arizona School of Health Sciences

Henry P. Trahan, AuD
A.T. Still University—Arizona School of Health Sciences

O. T. Wendel, PhD
A.T. Still University—Arizona School of Health Sciences

INTRODUCTION

The term *pharmacotherapeutics* refers to the study of the use of drugs in the treatment of disease. Drug literature contains information that represents average or common responses to pharmacotherapy. Individual variations in patient drug responsiveness are to be expected and must be a consideration in pharmacotherapeutic regimens. For example, two individuals may vary in their responses to the same dose of a given drug, and a single individual's response to a given dose of a drug may vary each time the drug is administered. This represents normal biologic variation. A quantal dose-response curve shown in Figure 3-1 gives a graphic representation of the percentage of a given population that responds to a specific drug dose.

Significant differences in responses to drugs occur frequently and, in many cases, can be predicted. Patients may require alterations in drug dose or exhibit drug effects not commonly associated with a given drug. Those effects are referred to as idiosyncratic drug reactions. The dramatic differences are beyond those that can be accounted for by normal biologic variation. The ability to predict such variations is dependent on understanding a number of factors that may contribute to such significant variations. Variations can result from pharmacokinetic or pharmacodynamic changes in the expected response to a drug because of an individual's age, gender, lifestyle, or genetic background.

The characterization of a drug included as the package insert describes the results of preclinical testing of that agent. As such, that information provides a limited perspective with regard to drug dosage and adverse effects. Most drugs are tested in a young to middle-aged population. Until recent changes occurred in the required testing protocols, the preclinical testing population was predominately young adult males. Preclinical testing affords little opportunity to identify the true extent of biologic variation in other populations that subsequently becomes evident as the drug is marketed. At that point, individual variation may represent an important issue as the agent is used in a large, heterogeneous population. To examine some factors that underlie variations in responses to drugs, this chapter will present information regarding both ends of the life cycle continuum to examine pharmacotherapeutic issues in neonates and infants, as well as in the geriatric population. This chapter also will examine other factors related to variations in responses to drugs, including diet, patient compliance, and genetics.

PATIENT FACTORS RELATED TO LIFE CYCLE

Individuals at each end of the life cycle differ from young and middle-aged adults in some dimensions of both pharmacokinetics and pharmacodynamics. A lack of knowledge about those differences resulted in therapeutic disasters in the past. Simple dosage adjustments, such as taking half a pill, to account for differences in the volume of distribution are not sufficient to accommodate for changes in the way the body handles drugs at the extremes of the age spectrum. Some differences are frequently accounted for

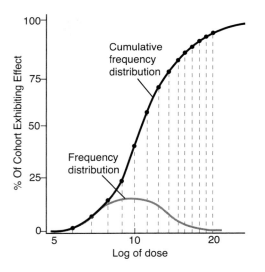

Figure 3-1. Quantal Dose-Response Curve. The quantal dose-response curve graphs the relationship between dose and effect, demonstrating the distribution of minimum doses of a drug required to produce a defined response in a population of subjects. The sigmoidal curve represents the cumulative dose-response relationship when the number of subjects responding is plotted against the log dose.

in the prescribing information and clinicians rely on the drug manufacturers to recommend alterations in drug dosage or utilization. However, understanding some of the basic physiologic and biochemical differences of pediatric and elderly patients will help health care providers make therapeutic decisions and provide informed counseling and referrals when specific information is unavailable.

For purposes of discussion, the age classifications in Table 3-1 will be used. Variables in drug administration (including dose, route of administration, time of administration, and interval between doses) must be considered in relation to patient age. Additionally, there are known differences in absorption, distribution, metabolism, and elimination in the neonatal, infant, and geriatric populations as compared to adolescents and adults. Providing safe and effective drug therapy for patients throughout the life cycle poses a challenge for health professionals. Patients' responses to drugs at normal or even low concentrations may be less predictable and are, in fact, more difficult to study at the extreme ends of the age continuum. As part of the health care team regularly in contact with pediatric and geriatric patients, audiologists should be aware of the potential for variations in drug responsiveness and should refer a patient to the prescribing health care professional if concerns are present.

Neonatal and Infant Populations

Following birth, the pediatric patient goes through changes in physical growth, psychosocial development,

and sensitivity to drugs, with the effects of those changes being most evident in neonates and infants. Due to the complexities of studying drugs in children for safety and efficacy, "it has been estimated that three fourths of the prescription drugs currently marketed in the United States lack full approval by the Food and Drug Administration (FDA) for pediatric use and, therefore, lack specific dosage guidelines for pediatric patients" (Reiss et al., 2002). However, drug therapies are used to treat numerous diseases and conditions in neonates and infants, including treatments for sepsis, respiratory infections, otitis media, and cancers. Therefore, it is important to consider the pharmacokinetic properties of absorption, distribution, metabolism, and elimination that may be influenced by the changing physiological characteristics of the neonatal or infant patient.

Absorption

In pediatric patients, a variety of factors may increase or decrease absorption. Reduced gastric acidity due to immature acid-producing cells in the stomach until the age of three can result in altered absorption or no absorption for drugs given orally. For example, some coated tablets, dependent on a low pH or acidity to be broken down, may pass through the digestive tract unchanged. Absorption of acidic drugs such as phenobarbital and phenytoin would be reduced, while absorption of acid-labile drugs such as penicillin, ampicillin, and erythromycin would be improved by the less acidic pH of the gastrointestinal tract. A constant diet of relatively alkaline foods such as milk may also further reduce stomach acidity. Gastric emptying is slower because peristalsis is irregular. The net result for most orally administered drugs may be a reduced effect as a result of reduced absorption or a delayed onset of the drug effect due to prolonged time before the drug reaches the small intestines, where most drugs are absorbed.

Due to thinner skin and the large disproportionate surface area provided by the skin, topical absorption can be faster in pediatric patients. Although that may seem appealing, systemic toxicity may occur due to enhanced absorption of some applied agents, such as corticosteroids and hexachlorophene. This type of

Table 3-1. Age Classifications of Patients

Age	Classification
Less than 1 month	Neonate
1 month to less than 2 years	Infant
2 years to less than 12 years	Child
12 years to less than 18 years	Adolescent
18 years to less than 65	Adult
65 and older	Geriatric adult

toxicity was evidenced years ago when several infants developed central nervous system toxicity after being bathed in 3% hexachlorophene emulsion to control staphylococcal infections.

Intramuscular (IM) absorption is generally slower and more difficult to predict in pediatric patients since peripheral circulation is easily affected by environmental changes, leading to variations in vasodilation and vasoconstriction. Additionally, there is limited muscle mass, limited blood flow due to low cardiac output or the presence of respiratory distress, and limited mobility in premature neonates that can delay IM drug absorption. Intravenous (IV) drug administration, which is frequently used in hospitalized children, completely bypasses the process of absorption and circumvents the first-pass hepatic effect. Although IV drug administration produces the least variable drug response in pediatric patients of different ages, the limitation of total fluid a neonate can handle by any route must be considered. The proper dilutions and concentrations must be used for the IV drug so that fluid intake of calories still meets the higher metabolic needs of the patient. Rectal administration of drugs may be appropriate for some agents that are available in the proper form. An important variable is the proper introduction of the drug into the inferior and middle rectal veins so the drug reaches systemic circulation and avoids the first-pass effect.

Distribution

Distribution of a drug is dependent on the amount of water or fat in the body and the affinity of the drug for plasma and tissue protein-binding sites. The amount of drug dissolved in body water or fat often determines how much drug will reach the receptor site and how quickly. Variations in drug distribution may be responsible for decreased or adverse drug effects. Three different mechanisms may account for that, as follows:

1. The percentage of total body water decreases with age, and the percentage of total body fat increases with age. The greater proportion of body weight made up of water in pediatric patients can significantly alter the concentration of drugs, such as aminoglycosides, distributed in body water. Ironically, in order to have a drug reach the desired concentration at its site of action, the need may exist for higher doses of water-soluble drugs per unit of weight than would be given to an adult.

2. The distribution of fat-soluble drugs is lower for younger patients due to less body fat, which generally results in increases in plasma concentration.

3. In the pediatric patient, protein binding may be diminished due to a relatively lower protein concentration as a result of liver immaturity and reduced protein production. Diminished protein binding may also be due to decreased affinity of the protein for drug molecules. Those factors can result in a greater proportion of the drug in a pharmacologically active and unbound state, creating a greater-than-expected drug action.

Also, in relation to distribution, the blood-brain barrier of infants is relatively incomplete at birth. Water-soluble compounds that normally do not penetrate this barrier in adults may gain free access to the interstitial fluid of the brain during the initial years of life.

Biotransformation

The body inactivates and promotes elimination of potent drugs through liver enzymes. In pediatric patients under the age of two, the levels of enzymes are decreased because of the immaturity of the liver. The hepatic microsomal drug-metabolizing enzymes are not fully developed and lack the capacity to transform drugs. This difference can result in prolonged half-lives for drugs that undergo inactivation by this system. Age-related changes in metabolism are frequently difficult to predict because of developmental and genetic differences. Intrauterine drug exposure (maternal drug use) and drugs transmitted to infants through breast milk appear to play particularly important roles in determining a neonate's drug metabolizing capabilities, possibly increasing or decreasing the liver production of metabolizing enzymes (Reiss et al., 2002).

Elimination

Renal elimination is the primary pathway of elimination for most drugs. Understanding the structure and function of the kidneys is critical, but is beyond the scope of this chapter. The *Color Atlas of Physiology* by Despopoulos and Silbernagl (2003) provides the foundational information needed in its Chapter 7: Kidneys, Salt, and Water Balance. Renal elimination in neonates and infants is limited due to reduced renal blood flow; immature tubular secretion levels; and reduced glomerular filtration rates, which mature between four and twelve months of age. As a result of reduced renal elimination, there is reduced renal excretion of drugs, as evidenced by prolonged half-lives, lower clearances, longer durations of actions, and potentially more toxicities. In addition, drugs may circulate longer, having more potential to reach toxic levels due to low urine pH and a lower capacity to concentrate urine.

Chloramphenicol Case Example

Chloramphenicol (Chlormycetin) is an effective broad-spectrum antibiotic reserved for use in life-threatening infections because of significant risk of serious adverse effects. The agent provides a classic example of the unique aspects of drug handling in infants where its use may result in the gray baby syndrome. This syndrome initially recognized in the 1950s results from the administration of chloramphenicol to neonates or premature infants and is characterized by vomiting, refusal to nurse, irregular respiration, and cyanosis. These babies rapidly deteriorate, becoming flaccid and turning ashen gray in color. Approximately 40% of these patients die within 48 hours of drug administration.

Two mechanisms are responsible for the gray baby syndrome:

1. The drug is not conjugated with glucuronic acid because glucuronyl transferase is not sufficiently developed in the newborn infant. The development of this important drug-metabolizing enzyme is delayed for three to four weeks following birth.

2. There is inadequate renal excretion of the unconjugated chloramphenicol due to the normal delay in maturation of renal function in the neonate.

Both of those mechanisms cause excessive and toxic plasma concentrations of chloramphenicol, causing blood dyscrasias. The increased plasma concentration of chloramphenicol can also displace bilirubin from plasma protein, resulting in kernicterus. Kernicterus, manifested by a variety of neurologic abnormalities, including hearing deficits, is a condition associated with the accumulation of bilirubin in the central nervous system and occurs in these babies because the blood-brain barrier is incomplete.

Summary of Pediatric Patient Factors

Neonatal and infant patients cannot be treated simply as miniature adults with respect to drug pharmacokinetics due to the various reasons listed above. The dosage cannot simply be cut in half for a patient half the weight of the average adult. These differences make determining appropriate drug doses and routes of administration a complex task, requiring more knowledge, observation of effects, and monitoring for the safe and effective use of medications in the pediatric population.

The Geriatric Population

According to *A Profile of Older Americans: 2003*, published by the Administration on Aging, U.S. Department of Health & Human Services, the growth of the American population in the sixty-five and over age bracket will present increasing challenges related to policymaking, business, and health care provision. The agency's data show that people aged sixty-five and over accounted for just over 12% of the total population in the United States in 2003, with 36 million people in that age bracket. In addition, the population of people aged eighty-five and over grew from 100,000 in 1900 to 4.2 million in 2000. The baby boomers, considered to be those born between 1946 and 1964, will start turning sixty-five years of age in 2011, greatly increasing the number of older adults. The agency's projections indicate that by 2030, people sixty-five and over will account for 20% of the U.S. population, reaching 71.5 million. Decreasing death rates in older populations are likely to make the eighty-five and over population grow dramatically, also.

In the growing geriatric population, the presence of polypharmacy is of major concern. Polypharmacy refers to the use of a number of different drugs concurrently by the same patient. "It is estimated that 70% of the elderly regularly use over-the-counter (OTC) medication as compared to only 10% of the general adult population" (Reiss et al., 2002). A study of long-term care facilities reported by Reiss et al. (2002) found that about 32% of the elderly receive more than eight medications daily and that some receive as many as fifteen medications daily. Polypharmacy increases the risk of drug interactions, with a 50% chance of drug interactions with five or more drugs, rising to a 100% chance of drug interactions with eight or more drugs taken concurrently.

The risk of drug-drug interactions can occur for patients of any age, even if only two medications are taken rather than numerous medications. However, polypharmacy in the elderly increases the risks and complicates the already challenging task of providing safe and effective pharmacologic management for multiple health conditions. Drug-drug interactions account for a small but extremely important proportion of adverse drug reactions because they are predictable and can by avoided or managed. A few factors that increase the frequency of drug-drug interactions are the age of the patient, alterations in physiologic function, the number of drugs prescribed, the number of physicians involved in the patient's care, the number of different pharmacies used, and additional OTC medications being taken. It is not unusual for a physician to be unaware of all the medications a patient is on and the dosages and frequency of administration. That lack of information can be due to compliance issues and inaccuracy in the patient reporting to numerous physicians.

Mechanisms of drug-drug interactions include inhibition or induction of drug metabolism and potentiation or antagonism of the drug action. Only about 10% of potential interactions result in clinically significant consequences. Since those significant consequences can include death or complications that greatly affect the patient's quality of life, it is imperative to consider ways to reduce the instances of drug-drug interactions. Even low-grade morbidity or nonspecific complaints such as confusion, lethargy, depression, weakness, dizziness, and falling should prompt a closer investigation into the patient's use of medications. In the past decade, increased attention to polypharmacy and drug-drug interactions has led to studies of the benefit of therapeutic drug-monitoring databases (Gex-Fabry et al., 1997), computerized prescription entry systems, online prescription screening (Halkin et al., 2001), and the promotion of routine medication reviews between primary care physicians and elderly patients (Fillit et al., 1999).

The technology and increased understanding of drug-drug interactions have the potential to decrease coprescribing of contraindicated drugs and to monitor potential interactions. The challenge now lies in the hands of the administrators, physicians, pharmacists, and patients to adequately and effectively use the technology in hospitals, as well as in community-based practices and pharmacies. Ultimately, the establishment of a universal electronic medical record could offer a viable method for identifying potential drug-drug interactions. All health care providers should have a heightened awareness of the potential for drug interactions and should refer the patient to the prescribing physician when symptoms and concerns show a need.

In addition to the issue of polypharmacy, drug therapy in the geriatric population may also be complicated by changes in pharmacokinetics, sensory impairment (i.e., hearing and vision loss), social isolation, inadequate nutrition, and reduced financial income. To understand basic drug responsiveness in the geriatric population, it is valuable to understand how the changes in the pharmacokinetic properties of absorption, distribution, metabolism, and elimination may be influenced by the changing physiological characteristics.

Absorption

Absorption of drugs via the gastrointestinal tract may be reduced in the geriatric patient due to gradually reduced production of gastric acid. Similar to the changes noted in the pediatric population, this reduction in gastric acid affects how a tablet dissolves in the stomach, allowing some drugs to pass unchanged. Declining motor tone and activity in the gastrointestinal tract results in slower gastric emptying and variable patterns of drug absorption. Furthermore, absorption of drugs via the gastrointestinal tract can be reduced by an abnormally accelerated rate of passage due to the use of stimulant laxatives. Atherosclerotic changes in blood vessels and changes in cardiac output result in reduction of blood perfusion to major organs, including the stomach. Drug absorption from the gastrointestinal tract is dependent on adequate blood supply to the stomach and small intestines. As in the pediatric population, topical absorption is faster because of thinner skin surface and IM absorption is less predictable because peripheral circulation is more affected by environmental factors.

Distribution

The distribution of a drug in an elderly person may differ considerably from that of a younger adult because of a gradual loss of water content in the body. That reduction of water content may diminish the volume of distribution of some water-soluble drugs and increase the blood concentration of a drug beyond target levels. Additionally, the geriatric patient experiences an increase in total body fat due to decreased muscle mass, thus reducing the distribution and activity of fat-soluble medications such as hypnotics and sedatives during the initial time period when the effects would be expected. This difference occurs because the increase in total body fat may provide for a medication to be absorbed into fatty tissue and released more slowly into the bloodstream. As the drugs are released back into the blood stream very slowly over time, extended effects of the medication may be seen. That may explain why the elderly frequently experience cumulative long-term residual effects from the use of drugs, especially those that are central nervous system depressants. The distribution of intramuscularly administered drugs in the elderly is also compromised by the loss of muscle tissue.

A general decrease in the plasma protein-binding capability of drugs may be present in the geriatric patient. It has been speculated that that is the result of reduced serum albumin concentration that accompanies the aging process and may be partially due to reduced protein intake in the diet and/or hepatic or renal disorders. In addition, other substances in the plasma may compete for the protein binding sites. The competing substances may be other drugs or simply chemicals that have accumulated in the plasma due to reduced renal function and thus reduced excretion. Since only the free or unbound drug can diffuse or be transported across membranes to reach receptors, reductions in plasma protein binding can lead to increased therapeutic effects or increased adverse effects.

Biotransformation

Advancing age also produces a decline in the body's ability to transform active drugs into inactive metabolites. Blood flow to the liver, as well as most other major organs, has a tendency to diminish with age. Some studies have reported a 0.5%–1.5% per year reduction in liver blood flow after age twenty-five. That probably has a significant effect on the rate of biotransformation of drugs that are metabolized primarily by the liver. In addition, enzymes produced by the liver are decreased because of the age-related decline in liver function.

Elimination

With aging, there is a gradual reduction in renal function that could significantly affect the safe and effective use of many medications. The reduction in renal function is believed to be secondary to reduced blood flow to the kidneys and/or a loss of intact nephrons. Glomerular filtration rate can be reduced by 40%–50%, while tubular secretion and reabsorption are both decreased due to the reduction in blood flow. That can lead to an accumulation of a drug in the renal system and consequently cause drug toxicity.

Summary of Life Cycle Considerations

The variations in pharmacokinetics discussed above provide general examples of the possible changes that may affect drug responsiveness in the pediatric and geriatric populations. All of those factors may not exist in every patient in those age groups. Conversely, diseases or poor health status of patients throughout the life cycle may result in alterations in drug absorption, distribution, metabolism, and elimination. Conditions that affect body water, adiposity, blood flow, liver function, and kidney function, for example, are not present solely in pediatric and geriatric patients; therefore, disease and general health status must be considered in determining the doses and handling the effects of drugs in patients.

PATIENT FACTORS RELATED TO DIET

Some definitions of the term *drug* are so broad that anything a person puts into the body could be considered a drug, including food such as chocolate. Even without subscribing to such a broad definition of the term, it is important to discuss how diet plays a role in pharmacotherapy. A more accurate definition of drug is a therapeutic substance, other than food, used to aid in the diagnosis, treatment, cure, mitigation, or prevention of disease or other abnormal condition. Drugs and food taken during the same time period can affect one another. The term *food-drug interaction* usually refers to the negative effect of food that is eaten, preventing the desired effect of a medication. Food-drug interactions can occur with OTC drugs as well as prescription medications. Food-drug interactions can cause a variety of side effects. In rare cases, food-drug interactions can be extremely dangerous and even fatal. The magnitude of the effects of food-drug interactions depends on the dosage and form of drug administration (pill versus liquid solution) and the patient's age, sex, body weight, nutrition, general health status, and existing medical conditions. Physicians and pharmacists, as well as package labeling, generally provide warnings regarding food-drug interactions. A physician or pharmacist should be consulted whenever concerns or questions arise about what foods should be avoided, if any, and whether any side effects are likely while taking a drug.

Three major types of food-drug interactions are routinely described: (1) Foods may alter the body's ability to use the drug; (2) Foods may interact with a drug and alter the drug's chemical action in the body; and (3) Food-drug interactions may alter the body's ability to use the particular food and its nutrients. Certain drugs may interfere with the absorption, excretion, or use of one or more nutrients in the body. Drugs can bind with nutrients, resulting in enhanced excretion of the nutrients, interference with nutrient absorption, or decreased conversion of nutrients into usable forms. Over a long period of time, the resulting vitamin and mineral deficiencies can impair health. Poor nutritional status can lead to higher risks for drug toxicity due to reduced ability to excrete some drugs. That creates a vicious cycle of the drug acting on the nutrients, the lack of nutrients affecting the body, and the poor health status leading to adverse reactions to the drug. Some foods, including beverages, may increase or decrease the absorption of a drug into the body. Decreased absorption can reduce the therapeutic effect or delay the effect. Foods may also alter the chemical actions of a drug, causing the drug to lose its therapeutic effect.

Many common warnings regarding food-drug interactions are indicated on drug labels. Common examples include warning against the consumption of alcohol or caffeine while taking a specific drug. For example, alcohol and antihistamines can cause drowsiness and slowed reactions. Caffeine and bronchodilators stimulate the nervous system and should not be taken together. It is often recommended that many drugs be taken with food or milk to avoid stomach irritation. Low-sodium diets are recommended with certain drugs, such as vasodilators and antihypertensive drugs, to improve the effectiveness of the drugs. Anticoagulants should be taken with only moderate consumption of foods high in vitamin K, such as spinach, cauliflower, brussel sprouts, vegetable oil, and egg yolk. The list of recommendations goes on and on.

Ongoing drug development and changes in processed foods and enriched foods can cause new interactions to surface over time. Currently, health care providers should be keenly aware of the potential for food-drug interactions with the use of diuretics, oral antibiotics, anticoagulants, antihypertensives, monoamine oxidase (MAO) inhibitors, and thyroid preparations.

Resources are available for consumers and health care providers through Web sites of the FDA, the Center for Food Safety & Applied Nutrition, and other agencies. Topics relating to food and drugs can be located by using the search function with general keywords such as *food drug interactions* or more specific keywords such as *grapefruit juice* and *drugs* or other combinations of interest. Knowledgeable health care providers, diet-drug histories, appropriate counseling regarding risks, understandable written educational materials for patients, and involvement of dieticians or nutritionists may be the best tools for prevention or reduction in severity of food-drug interactions.

Case Examples

Food-drug interactions are not uncommon and can frequently be understood by recognizing that foodstuff contains many active principles that have the potential to alter the pharmacokinetics and/or the pharmacodynamics of a drug. A relevant food-drug interaction occurs between grapefruit juice and many agents that are clinically important, such as the cholesterol-lowering drugs known as statins, the antihypertensive agents known as calcium channel blockers, the antiarrhythmic agent called amiodarone, and a growing list of other drugs. The intestines contain an enzyme that normally acts to break down drugs as they enter the body. Therapeutic doses of the above-mentioned drugs are calculated to accommodate that breakdown. Grapefruit juice contains a compound that inhibits the enzyme. The concomitant use of grapefruit juice and one of the agents above results in significantly higher drug plasma concentrations because less drug is broken down during absorption from the intestines. Since several of the agents have narrow therapeutic windows, the increase in plasma

concentration may result in significant, potentially life-threatening adverse effects.

Another classic example of a food-drug interaction occurs between dairy products and orally administered tetracycline. Most dairy products contain significant amounts of calcium, and the tetracycline molecule actively binds calcium. When bound with calcium, the tetracycline forms an insoluble crystalline structure that cannot be absorbed. The concomitant administration of tetracycline and dairy products is contraindicated because the tetracycline binds the calcium in the dairy products and forms a nonabsorbable form of tetracycline. That bound form would lead to suboptimal plasma tetracycline levels and reduced ability of the tetracycline to be effective in treating an infection.

PATIENT FACTORS RELATED TO COMPLIANCE

First mentioned by Hippocrates over 2400 years ago, compliance with medical recommendations, especially with pharmacotherapy, represents a complex challenge. The term *compliance* describes the degree to which a patient's behavior matches the medical advice. Noncompliance would, therefore, be defined as any behavior that does not coincide with the therapeutic advice. With reference to pharmacotherapy, compliance is defined as the degree of correlation of the actual dosing history with the prescribed medication therapy, that is, the amount of drug taken versus the amount of drug prescribed. The best medical advice or treatment protocol is only as effective as a patient's motivation and capacity to follow it. Many different factors have been identified as types of noncompliance; and as information from the electronic monitoring of compliance is gathered, several more may be added to the following list.

- Multiple stressors

- Difficulty in the organization of tasks

- Receiving incomplete information from the health care provider

- Not understanding information provided by the health care provider

- Duration of the prescribed therapy

- Financial constraints

- Time constraints

- Diminished mental health status

- Chronic and/or concomitant medical conditions

- Transportation limitations

- Unrealistic expectations of the patient by the caregivers

Studies have shown that noncompliance can range from 20% to an astounding 80%, depending on the kind of treatment (Litt et al., 1980). The rate of compliance is rarely static for any given patient. Compliance will fluctuate over time depending on variables such as the severity of symptoms, external stressors, and family support. On average, patients precisely follow doctors' advice only about half the time. When a treatment regimen is complicated or difficult, such as lifestyle changes to control hypertension or diabetes, compliance is even lower.

Prolonged intervals between dose administrations are the most common deviations from the prescribed drug regimen. Lapses of three days or more are euphemistically referred to as "drug holidays" (Urquhart, 1997). In general, the clinical consequences of a drug holiday depend on the pharmacologic characteristics of a given medication. The extreme deviation of the dosing history from the prescribed drug regimen is cessation of the medication by the patient. This pattern of behavior, called nonpersistence, is not necessarily just another form of noncompliance; it may actually represent a separate problem. Conversely, nonpersistence may also be viewed as the ultimate expression of noncompliance.

Somewhere between noncompliance and nonpersistence is another pattern, which was unknown before the development of electronic medication event monitoring systems; it is referred to as "white coat compliance" (Feinstein, 1990.) The term *white coat compliance* describes poor or partial compliers improving their compliance around the scheduled follow-up visits. In addition to the injurious health care effects of variable compliance, white coat compliance may also introduce diagnostic and therapeutic confusion to the health care provider. White coat compliance must always be considered when a rapidly drug-responsive patient's condition is well-controlled at successive office visits but the desired long-term outcomes of treatment are less than expected or absent. This phenomenon may be thought of as analogous to an audiology patient putting a hearing aid in as he or she walks into an audiology clinic but taking it out when he or she gets back to the car after the appointment. The test results may indicate excellent benefit from the device in the office, but the patient is not receiving the benefit in other settings or adjusting to the hearing aid to receive the desired long-term outcomes.

Compliance involves not only the patient, but also parents and other care providers. According to Buck (1997), the family's beliefs regarding susceptibility to disease, disease severity, and the benefits of treatment will play are role in compliance. Noncompliance can easily become a design for serious consequences, especially in children and adolescents with chronic medical conditions. A child is constantly going through developmental stages that have a profound effect on all behavior, including those related to medication compliance. For example, a child's inability to fully comprehend the benefit to be gained from treatment affects his or her willingness or desire to accept medication. The need for an adolescent to demonstrate independence may affect compliance, as will the denial of illness and the unwillingness to accept cosmetic side effects such as the development of hirsutism (Litt and Cuskey, 1980). The dynamics of a family's interactions also impact compliance. According to Hazzard et al. (1990), parental anxiety and restriction of a child's activity appear to have a greater impact on compliance than more treatment-oriented factors such as frequency of dose administration or tastiness of the medication. Parental anxiety may result in underdosing or overdosing.

The type of illness or disease being treated also affects compliance for pediatric patients. For example, issues must be addressed with families to ensure compliance with short-term therapy as those issues are often quite different from issues for the treatment of chronic disorders. The rate of compliance in the treatment of acute illness in children is believed to be approximately 50% (Buck, 1997). This poor compliance rate has been reported in patients treated for acute otitis media, among other illnesses. Similar rates have been noted for adult patients. Therapy for chronic disorders shows a slight improvement compared to acute illness therapy (Matusi, 1997).

Improving Compliance

Various methods that can be employed to improve compliance include, but are not limited to, patient/family education and the health care provider's choice of regimen. The health care provider must be able to identify the barriers to complying with the prescribed treatment. The patient and the family must be made to comprehend both the necessity for treatment and the method for administering the treatment properly. A thorough discussion of the regimen, tailored to the age and maturity of the patient, and scheduled follow-up visits are the best method to gain patient/family compliance (Buck, 1997). Some health care providers have found that the implementation of a written contract or agreement bolsters compliance (Weinstein, 1995). Older patients also benefit from written instructions. The FDA set a goal that by 2000, 75% of patients should receive written information on how to take their medications and the adverse effects of not following the regimen properly. It is unknown at this time whether that goal has been met.

Educational interventions can now employ a considerable body of research evidence for the development of clear and concise written leaflets for patients. Overall, educational approaches to the problem of noncompliance attempt to improve compliance by promoting knowledge of the condition and treatment plan, as well as providing training in recognition of factors that prevent adherence. It has been suggested that noncompliance problems be discussed at the beginning of therapy and treated as a normal occurrence jointly addressed by the patient, family, and clinical team throughout the treatment plan (Fielding and Duff, 1999). Behavioral interventions have been the most widely used intervention for addressing noncompliance issues. The hypothesis fundamental to behavioral interventions is that some behaviors, such as dietary habits, are difficult to change because they have been established over long periods of time. Lasting change is possible only by breaking down habitual patterns and building new patterns of behavior.

Education appears to be a key to increasing compliance, thus improving therapeutic outcomes and reducing risks. This effort includes educating health care providers to recognize the barriers to compliance and to address them. It also includes the education of patients and caregivers regarding the appropriate drug dose, dosing interval, dietary recommendations/restrictions, possible side effects, benefits of compliance, and risks of noncompliance. The educational efforts aimed at patients should consider some common yet often forgotten factors, such as the patient's sensory perception abilities, memory, proprioception, and dexterity. Vision loss, hearing loss, decreased peripheral sensations, and hand strength can all play a role in how a patient complies with instructions. If a patient cannot clearly hear, read, or remember the instructions or handle the medication bottles or pills, frustration and errors in the therapeutic regimen may occur. One reasonable option to aid in overcoming those problems is to provide the patient with clear, concise written instructions in large print.

PATIENT FACTORS RELATED TO PHARMACOGENOMICS

Pharmacogenetics or pharmacogenomics is the study of how genetic differences affect the encoding of the molecular targets of drugs or the proteins responsible for drug metabolism. These genetic differences can alter expected pharmacotherapeutic effects, causing decreased effectiveness or increased toxicity. Current research estimates that the human genome contains about 3 billion nucleotides, making up 30,000–40,000 genes that may code for approximately 100,000 different proteins (Golan et al., 2005). Many of the proteins are involved in disease processes and also are the targets for drug actions. Although the genomes of any two individuals are about 99.9% identical regardless of race, ethnicity, or geographic origin, that similarity still leaves the possibility of about 3 million differences in individual nucleotides. If one nucleotide in a specific position is exchanged with another nucleotide, the alteration is referred to as a single nucleotide polymorphism, or SNP (pronounced "snip"). The majority of nucleotide variations are SNPs. Other possible variations include insertions, deletions, duplications, and translocations of one or more nucleotides or even entire genes. If the SNPs or other differences affect the amount of a protein or the function of a protein by altering the coding sequences that control gene transcription or messenger ribonucleic acid (mRNA) translation, the nucleotide variation may be pharmacologically important. Research and technology are making it possible to screen patients' genomes for a limited known set of polymorphisms that affect how patients respond to certain medications.

This intersection of traditional pharmaceutical sciences with the scientific study of genes, proteins, and SNPs might hold the key to the creation of personalized drugs with greater efficacy and safety. An anticipated benefit of pharmacogenomics could be drug development accurately targeted to specific diseases based on genetic information, improving therapeutic effects while decreasing damage to healthy cells. The current methods of attempting to match the patient to the right drug and dosage may be improved by prescribing the best available drug therapy based on the individual's genotype. By removing the need to change medications until the patient shows the desired improvement, recovery time could be improved and potential adverse drug reactions could be reduced or eliminated. Advanced screenings for diseases or disease susceptibility may allow for careful monitoring and maximized therapy, as well as lifestyle or environmental changes to lessen the severity or to avoid a genetic disease. Pharmacogenomics also has the potential to allow for more accurate determination of appropriate drug dosages,

better vaccines, improvements in drug discovery and approval processes, and decreases in overall health care costs.

Although there is tremendous potential for pharmacogenomics to improve the way medications are developed and prescribed, barriers still exist. The research is still in its infancy, and it is very complex and time-consuming. Just think of trying to identify and analyze millions of SNPs to determine which one or ones are involved in a given drug response. In addition, knowing that a patient's genetic makeup causes the two available drugs for a condition to be ineffective will not solve the problem if no other drug alternatives are available. Drug companies may not have sufficient incentive to spend hundreds of millions of dollars to bring a drug to market that is needed by only a small portion of the overall population. Some of the tools of pharmacogenomics are in use today, yet much work still must be done and many barriers overcome before the full potential of this intriguing field of study can be reached.

Examples of Pharmacogenomics in Use Today

Researchers doing clinical trials and pharmaceutical companies are using information about the cytochrome P450 (CYP) family of liver enzymes involved in the metabolism of more than thirty different classes of drugs. Genetic variations leading to less active or inactive forms of the CYP enzymes can influence how some drugs are metabolized and can lead to overdoses. Clinical trial researchers screen patients for variations in the cytochrome P450 genes, and pharmaceutical companies screen their chemical compounds to determine how different forms of CYP enzymes function to break down the chemicals ("Pharmacogenomics," 2004).

Currently, physicians can also use a genetic screening to determine if patients have a deficiency in thiopurine methyltransferase (TPMT). If the active form of that protein is not being produced due to genetic variations, the patient cannot break down therapeutic compounds known as thiopurines used to treat common childhood leukemia. Since a small percentage of Caucasians have genetic variants affecting TPMT, the thiopurines can elevate to toxic levels. Therefore, screening for the deficiency and monitoring TPMT activity can assist in determining appropriate thiopurine dosage levels ("Pharmacogenomics," 2004).

SUMMARY

Many patient factors can alter the therapeutic effectiveness of drugs. Factors that can lead to adverse drug reactions include physiologic changes associated with age, drug-drug interactions, food-drug interactions, noncompliance with the prescribed regimen, and genetic factors. Adverse drug reactions may not be immediate or readily detected, especially for patients who are not hospitalized. The entire team of health care providers interacting with patients should be aware of patient factors that can impact drug responsiveness to recognize possible problems and to make appropriate referrals and recommendations.

At the extreme ends of the life cycle continuum, pharmacokinetic changes often reduce the therapeutic effects of a drug or prolong the effects. For example, in both the pediatric and geriatric populations, absorption of orally administered drugs may be lessened, resulting in reduced overall effect of the drug or delayed onset of the desired effect. Reductions in plasma protein binding capabilities can also be seen in both populations, resulting in a greater-than-expected drug action. Additionally, age-related changes in biotransformation of drugs and elimination of drugs may result in prolonged half-lives and potentially more toxicities.

All health care providers should be aware of the growing problems with polypharmacy, especially in the aging population, because the use of multiple drugs concurrently increases the risk of drug-drug interactions. Although drug-drug interactions account for a small proportion of adverse drug reactions, the complications may include confusion, lethargy, depression, weakness, dizziness, and more severe consequences, including death. A patient's diet can also play a role in how the body responds to drugs. The three major types of food-drug interactions are reduction in the body's ability to use the particular food and its nutrients, alteration of the body's ability to use the drug, and alteration of the drug's chemical action in the body. A physician or pharmacist should be consulted whenever concerns or questions arise about drug-drug interactions, foods that should be avoided (if any), and side effects that may be exhibited while taking a drug.

Noncompliance is not a new phenomenon; rather, it is an issue that health care providers have battled for years in all areas of health care. Compliance with the prescribed pharmacotherapeutic regimen can vary dramatically from patient to patient due to numerous factors. Education of health care providers, patients, and caregivers appears to be a key to increasing compliance.

A new direction in pharmacotherapy involves the combination of pharmacology with genetic research. Exploration of pharmacogenomics is currently showing promise as a means for developing drugs accurately targeted to specific diseases, prescribing the best available drug therapy based on an individual's genotype, and establishing advanced screenings for diseases or disease susceptibility. Although research in pharmacogenomics has great potential, many barriers and many factors other than genetics still play a role in the effectiveness of pharmacotherapy. Continued improvements in pharmacotherapy with reductions in morbidity and mortality will continue to rely on research; education of patients and health care providers; teamwork; and the use of technology for postmarketing surveillance of compliance, food-drug or drug-drug interactions, and the sharing of data.

REFERENCES

Administration on Aging, U.S. Department of Health & Human Services. (2003). A profile of older Americans: 2003. Retrieved January 4, 2005, from http://www.aoa.gov/prof/Statistics/profile/2003/profiles2003.asp

Buck, M. L. (1997). Improving compliance with medication regimens. *Pediatric Pharmacotherapy, 3*, 8.

Despopolos, A., & Silbernagl, S. (2003). *Color Atlas of Physiology* (5th ed.). New York: Thieme.

Feinstein, A. (1990). On white-coat effects and the electronic monitoring of compliance. *Arch Intern Med, 150*, 1377–1378.

Fielding, D., & Duff, A. (1999). Compliance with treatment protocols: Interventions for children with chronic illness. *Arch Dis Child, 80,* 196–200.

Fillit, H. M., Futterman, R., Orland, B. I., Chim, T., Susnow, L., Picariello, G. P., Scheye, E. C., Spoeri, R. K., Roglieri, J. L., & Warburton, S. W. (1999). Polypharmacy management in Medicare managed care: Changes in prescribing by primary care physicians resulting from a program promoting medication reviews. *American Journal of Managed Care, 5*(5), 587–594.

Gex-Fabry, M., Balant-Gorgia, A. E., & Balant, L. P. (1997). Therapeutic drug monitoring databases for postmarketing surveillance of drug-drug interactions: Evaluation of a paired approach for psychotropic medication. *Therapeutic Drug Monitoring, 19*(1), 1–10.

Golan, D. E., & Tashjian, A. H. (Eds.). (2005). *Principles of Pharmacology: The Pathophysiologic Basis of Drug Therapy.* Baltimore: Lippincott Williams & Wilkins.

Halkin, H., Katzir, I., Kurman, I., Jan, J., & Malkin, B. B. (2001). Preventing drug interactions by online prescription screening in community pharmacies and medical practices. *Clinical Pharmacology & Therapeutics, 69*(4), 260–265.

Hazzard A., Hutchinson, S. J., & Krawiecki, N. (1990). Factors related to adherence to medication regimens in pediatric seizure patients. *J Ped Psychol, 15,* 543–545.

Litt, I. F., & Cuskey, W. R. (1980). Compliance with medical regimens during adolescence. *Pediatric Clinics of North America, 27,* 3–15.

Matsui, D. M. (1997). Drug compliance in pediatrics: Clinical and research issues. *Pediatric Clinics of North America, 44,* 1–14.

Pharmacogenomics (2004, July 9). Human Genome Project Information. Retrieved December 15, 2004, from http://www.ornl.gov/sci/techresources/Human_Genome/medicine/pharma.shtml

Reiss, B. S., Evans, M. E., & Broyles, B. E. (2002). *Pharmacological Aspects of Nursing Care* (6th ed.). Clifton Park, NY: Thomson Delmar Learning.

Urquhart, J. (1997). The electronic medication event monitor. Lessons for pharmacotherapy. *Clin Pharmacokinet, 32,* 345–356.

U.S. Food and Drug Administration and National Consumers League. *Food & Drug Interactions.* (1998). [Brochure]. Access: http://www.cfsan.fda.gov/~lrd/fdinter.html

Weinstein, A. G. (1995). Clinical management strategies to maintain compliance in asthmatic children. *Ann Allergy Asthma Immunol, 15,* 543–555.

CHAPTER 4

Role of Food and Drug Administration in Drug Development

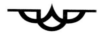

Venkatesh Atul Bhattaram, PhD
Office of Clinical Pharmacology and Biopharmaceutics
Center for Drug Evaluation and Research
U.S. Food and Drug Administration
Rockville, Maryland

Rajanikanth Madabushi, PhD
Department of Pharmaceutics
University of Florida, Gainesville

Hartmut Derendorf, PhD
Department of Pharmaceutics
University of Florida, Gainesville

Disclaimer The views expressed in this review are those of the author (Venkatesh Atul Bhattaram) and do not reflect official policy of the U.S. Food and Drug Administration (FDA). No official support or endorsement by the FDA is intended or should be inferred.

33

INTRODUCTION

Development of new drugs is an extremely challenging process in which both the pharmaceutical industry and the Food and Drug Admnistration (FDA) work closely to ensure the safety and effectiveness of drugs before they are available to the public. The Pharmaceutical Research and Manufacturers of America estimates that, on average, it takes between 10 and 15 years and costs more than $800 million to do the research and testing to bring a new drug to patients. Furthermore, only one in ten of the compounds that enter clinical development is successful (Workman, 2003). The mission of the FDA is to (1) promote and protect public health by helping safe and effective products reach the market in a timely manner, (2) monitor products for continued safety after they are in use, and (3) help the public get the accurate science-based information needed to improve their health (USFDA, 2005b). At the heart of all of the FDA's regulatory activities is a judgment about whether a new product's benefits to users will outweigh its risks. The aim of this chapter is to give an overview of drug law and the role of the FDA in drug development. The chapter will not cover the role of the FDA in the development of biologics and devices.

DRUG LAW

The FDA acts as a public health protector by ensuring that all drugs on the market are safe and effective. Authority to do that comes from the 1938 Federal Food, Drug, and Cosmetic Act, a law that has undergone many changes over the years. Some of the major milestones in the evolution of the U.S. drug law (USFDA, 1999) are discussed in the following sections.

Food and Drugs Act (1906)

This first drug law required only that drugs meet standards of strength and purity. The burden of proof was on the FDA to show that a drug's labeling was false and fraudulent before the drug could be taken off the market.

Federal Food, Drug, and Cosmetic Act (1938)

A bill was introduced in the Senate in 1933 to completely revise the 1906 drug law—widely recognized then as being obsolete. But congressional action was stalled. It took a tragedy in which 107 people died from a poisonous ingredient in Elixir Sulfanilamide to promote passage of revised legislation that, for the first time, required a manufacturer to prove the safety of a drug before it could be marketed (USFDA, 1999).

Durham-Humphrey Amendment (1951)

Until this law was passed, there was no requirement that any drug be labeled for sale by prescription only. The amendment defined prescription drugs as "those unsafe for self-medication and should be used only under a doctor's supervision."

Kefauver-Harris Drug Amendments (1962)

News reports about the role of an FDA medical officer keeping the drug thalidomide off the U.S. market aroused public interest in drug regulation. Thalidomide had been associated with the birth of thousands of malformed babies in western Europe. In October 1962, Congress passed these amendments to tighten control over drugs. Before marketing a drug, firms now had to prove not only safety, but also effectiveness for the product's intended use. In addition, firms were required to send adverse reaction reports to the FDA, and drug advertising in medical journals was required to provide complete information to doctors—the risks as well as the benefits. The amendments also required that informed consent be obtained from the study subjects.

Orphan Drug Act (1983)

Orphans are drugs and other products for treating rare diseases that affects fewer than 200,000 people nationwide (Center for Drug Evaluation and Research, 1998c). These include diseases as familiar as cystic fibrosis, Lou Gehrig's disease, and Tourette's syndrome, and as unfamiliar as Hamburger disease,

Job syndrome, and acromegaly (or gigantism). Some diseases have patient populations of fewer than one hundred. Collectively, however, the diseases affect as many as 25 million Americans, according to the National Institutes of Health (NIH); and that makes the diseases—and finding treatments for them—a serious public health concern (Rados, 2003). Development of new drugs for these diseases may offer little or no profit to the manufacturer, but may benefit people with the diseases. To foster drug development, this law allows drug companies to take tax deductions for about three-quarters of the cost of their clinical studies.

Waxman-Hatch Act, or Drug Price Competition and Patent Term Restoration Act (1984)

This act expedites the availability of less costly generic drugs by permitting the FDA to approve applications to market generic versions of brand-name drugs without repeating the research done to prove them safe and effective. At the same time, the brand-name companies can apply for up to five years' additional patent protection for new medicines they developed to make up for time lost while their products were going through the FDA's approval process.

Generic Drug Enforcement Act (1992)

This law imposes debarment and other remedies for criminal convictions based on activities relating to the approval of Abbreviated New Drug Applications (ANDAs).

PDUFA (1992)

In the Prescription Drug User Fee Act (PDUFA), manufacturers agree to pay user fees for certain new drug applications (NDAs) and supplements, an annual establishment fee, and annual product fees.

FDA Modernization Act (1997)

This act contains some of the most sweeping changes to the Food, Drug, and Cosmetic Act in thirty-five years. Of significant importance to the Center for Drug Evaluation and Research (CDER), an FDA component, was the reauthorization of PDUFA through 2002. The act contains changes in how user fees are assessed and collected. For example, fees are waived for the first application for small businesses, orphan products, and pediatric supplements. The act codifies the FDA's accelerated approval regulations and requires guidance on fast-track policies and procedures.

STAGES OF DRUG DEVELOPMENT AND THE ROLE OF THE FDA

Drug development consists of three distinct stages: (1) discovery/preclinical development, (2) clinical development, and (3) manufacturing/postmarketing development. The various stages of clinical development are traditionally characterized as Phases I, II, and III (Temple, 2000), as shown in Figure 4-1. This terminology is defined in Title 21, Section 312.21 of the Code of Federal Regulations (CFR) (Center for Devices and Radiological Health, 2002a). The CFR is a codification of the general and permanent rules published in the *Federal Register* by the executive departments and agencies of the federal government. Title 21 of the CFR is reserved for rules of the FDA (Center for Devices and Radiological Health, 2002a).

At various stages in the drug development program, meetings are held between sponsors (typically pharmaceutical industry) and the FDA to ensure that enough evidence on drug safety and effectiveness is obtained before making it available to the public. In those meetings, experts from various backgrounds address all potential issues pertaining to drug approval. Briefly, a typical review team, along with project managers, consists of the following:

- Chemists who focus on how the drug is made and whether the manufacturing, controls, and packaging are adequate to ensure the identity, strength, quality, and purity of the product.

- Pharmacologists and toxicologists who evaluate the effects of the drug on laboratory animals in short-term and long-term studies.

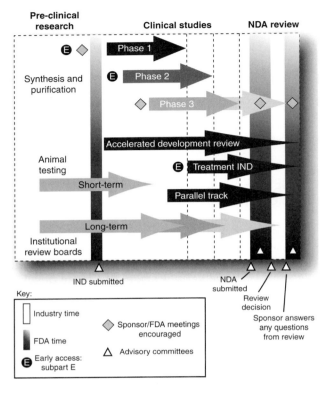

Figure 4-1. An overview of the role of the FDA in the drug development process

- Physicians who evaluate the results of the clinical tests, including what the drug's adverse as well as therapeutic effects are and whether the proposed labeling accurately reflects the effects of the drug.

- Clinical pharmacologists who evaluate the pharmacokinetics (absorption, distribution, metabolism, and elimination) and exposure (drug concentrations and active metabolite) versus response (effectiveness and safety) relationships.

- Statisticians who evaluate the clinical trial designs for each controlled study and conclusions of safety and effectiveness based on the study data.

- Microbiologists who review the microbiological aspects of drug manufacturing to ensure safety of the drug product and public health.

Discovery/Preclinical Research

In the discovery phase, knowledge of biology (receptors or enzymes) and information from drugs in a similar class, if available, are integrated to generate a better compound. The developmental activities at this stage include bioanalytical method development and validation, formulation analyses, toxicity, and pharmacokinetic (PK) and pharmacodynamic (PD) studies in animals. The FDA and International Conference on Harmonisation of Technical Requirements for the Registration of Pharmaceuticals for Human Use (ICH) recommendations provide guidance for pharmacokinetics, toxicokinetics, single and repeat dose toxicity, genotoxicity, carcinogenicity, reproductive toxicity, and impurities (ICH, 1997). The minimum standards for laboratories conducting nonclinical testing is set by the FDA through good laboratory practice (GLP) regulations (Center for Drug Evaluation and Research, 2000).

The sponsors request a meeting(s) with the appropriate clinical division to discuss development plans, data requirements, and any scientific issues that may need to be resolved prior to investigational new drug (IND) submission. At those meetings, the sponsor and FDA discuss and agree on the design of the animal studies needed to initiate human testing.

Clinical Development Phase

During the clinical development phases, the FDA plays at least three major roles:

1. To set general standards for clinical studies to ensure accuracy of the data obtained from the trials. This set of regulations and guidelines are known as good clinical practice (GCP).

2. To protect human subjects participating in the clinical trials. This is achieved by ensuring (1) that

the clinical subjects are not exposed to any unnecessary risks, (2) that the clinical subjects are exposed to the least possible risk given the benefit anticipated from the use of the drug, and (3) that the study participants are aware of the risks through informed consent.

3. To ensure that drugs are safe and effective before approval.

Current federal law requires that a drug be the subject of an approved marketing application before it is transported or distributed across state lines. Because a sponsor will probably want to ship the investigational drug to clinical investigators in many states, it must seek an exemption from that legal requirement. The IND is the means through which the sponsor technically obtains that exemption from the FDA. To conduct the studies in humans, the investigators submit an IND application to the FDA (Center for Devices and Radiological Health, 2004a). The application contains the animal pharmacology/toxicology studies, manufacturing information, clinical protocols, and investigator information. The INDs are of two categories—commercial and noncommercial—and of three types:

* Investigator IND is submitted by a physician who initiates and conducts an investigation and under whose immediate direction the investigational drug is administered or dispensed. A physician might submit a research IND to propose studying an unapproved drug or an approved product for a new indication or in a new patient population.

* Emergency-use IND allows the FDA to authorize use of an experimental drug in an emergency situation that does not allow time for submission of an IND. It is also used for patients who do not meet the criteria of an existing study protocol or if an approved study protocol does not exist.

* Treatment IND is submitted for experimental drugs showing promise in clinical testing for serious or immediately life-threatening conditions while the final clinical work is conducted and the FDA review takes place.

Phase I Study

In the Phase I program, the investigators typically evaluate the tolerance of the drug in healthy subjects at various dose levels. Information on pharmacokinetics and common adverse events is obtained from these studies. The various dose levels for the Phase I studies can be selected based on information such as safety and relationship between drug concentrations and biomarkers from preclinical studies (Aarons et al., 2001; 2005; Derendorf et al., 2000; Mahmood, 2001; Peck et al., 1994; Reigner et al., 1997). However, for drugs that are known to present safety risks to healthy subjects but that may offer substantial benefit to patients (e.g., cancer), these studies are undertaken in patients.

After submission of IND to the FDA, the information is reviewed to determine if there are any safety-related issues that warrant putting the planned clinical trial on hold. A typical process of IND review is shown in Figure 4-2 (Center for Drug Evaluation and Research, 1998a). Following the filing of an IND, unless otherwise stated by the FDA within 30 days, the sponsor can commence the study.

Phase II Study

According to the description in the FDA regulations, a Phase II study is the first controlled clinical study to evaluate the effectiveness of a drug for a specific therapeutic use in patients. The Phase II study enables characterization of relationships between exposure (dose and drug/active metabolite concentrations) and response (Lesko, Rowland, Peck, & Blaschke, 2000; Sheiner, 1997). The information on the dose-response relationship obtained from Phase II trials, in most cases, is used to design Phase III trials. The sponsors request meetings (End of Phase 2 [EOP2] and/or End of Phase 2A [EOP2A]) with the FDA to discuss issues pertaining to evaluating the investigational drug in Phase III trials (Center for Drug Evaluation and Research [CDER], 2001a). At those meetings, issues such as clinical trial design, primary endpoints, dose selection, clinical pharmacology studies, and formulation issues are discussed. The meetings have been found to help sponsors understand the regulatory requirements before a drug is approved.

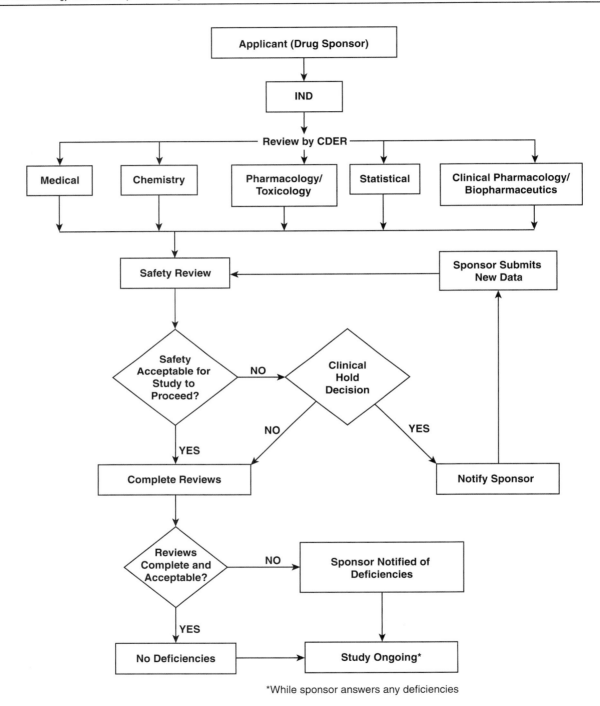

Figure 4-2. A typical review process of an IND

Phase III Study

The FDA regulations describe Phase III trials as the expanded controlled and uncontrolled studies performed after at least some evidence has been found to suggest the evidence of effectiveness. These studies are often conducted in various countries and may involve thousands of patients, depending on the indication being sought. The Phase III trials also may include longer-term safety and effectiveness studies, dose-response analysis, and mortality and morbidity outcomes. Generally, the FDA needs two positive, adequately well-controlled phase III trials that support safety and effectiveness of the drug in the target population prior to approval for marketing in the United States (Center for Drug Evaluation and Research, 1998b; Sahajawalla, 2004). In certain situations, exceptions to this rule have been made for good reasons (Temple, 2002). The results of the Phase III studies are submitted to the appropriate clinical division at the FDA as an NDA. The NDA is reviewed by a team of experts (chemists, clinical pharmacologists, physicians, statisticians, and pharmacologists/toxicologists). A typical NDA review process is shown in Figure 4-3 (Center for Drug Evaluation and Research, 1998a). The team's crucial task is to judge whether the trials have demonstrated that the product's health benefits outweigh its risks. Also, inspections are conducted at the clinical trial and product manufacturing sites aimed at ensuring data integrity and product quality before the drug is made available to the public. These inspections will be conducted by the Division of Scientific Investigation (DSI).

The approval process takes about six months (for priority applications) and ten months (for standard applications). The decision to categorize an application as priority or standard is based on various factors. The application is categorized as priority if the drug product approved would be a significant improvement over marketed products in the treatment, diagnosis, or prevention of a disease. Improvement can be demonstrated, for example, by: (1) evidence of increased effectiveness in the treatment, prevention, or diagnosis of disease; (2) elimination or substantial reduction of a treatment-limiting

drug reaction; (3) documented enhancement of patient compliance; or (4) evidence of safety and effectiveness of a new subpopulation. All nonpriority applications are considered standard applications. Also, issues pertaining to informative labeling are discussed with the sponsors prior to formal approval.

Manufacturing/Postmarketing Development

Once the product license is obtained following an NDA review, postmarketing studies, also known as Phase IV trials, are carried out to resolve any deficiencies or to make promotional claims. Those deficiencies are normally related to dosing recommendations in patients taking concomitant medications, in special populations (e.g., patients with severe renal or hepatic impairment), etc. In certain cases, long-term safety and effectiveness data may be obtained from patients who are followed after completion of the pivotal trial. Through the MedWatch program, the FDA conducts "postmarketing surveillance" of medical products to identify safety concerns and to take necessary action. For example, it was reported in postmarketing studies that patients receiving TOBI (tobramycin solution for inhalation) reported hearing loss, which led to updating the drug label accordingly (WARNING: Ototoxicity) (MedWatch, 2002). In another instance, the FDA notified health care providers about a study showing that children with cochlear implants were at greater risk of developing bacterial meningitis caused by Streptococcus pneumoniae than children in the general population. The FDA issued recommendations to decrease the risk of meningitis in patients with cochlear implant recipients (Center for Devices and Radiological Health, 2002b).

MedWatch reports may prompt the FDA to require manufacturers to conduct postmarketing studies on a product or to make manufacturing facilities available for inspection. MedWatch depends on doctors, dentists, nurses, pharmacists, and other health professionals to pass on to the FDA details of serious adverse reactions and medical product problems. CDER's Division of Pharmacovigilance and Epidemiology (DES) maintains a Spontaneous

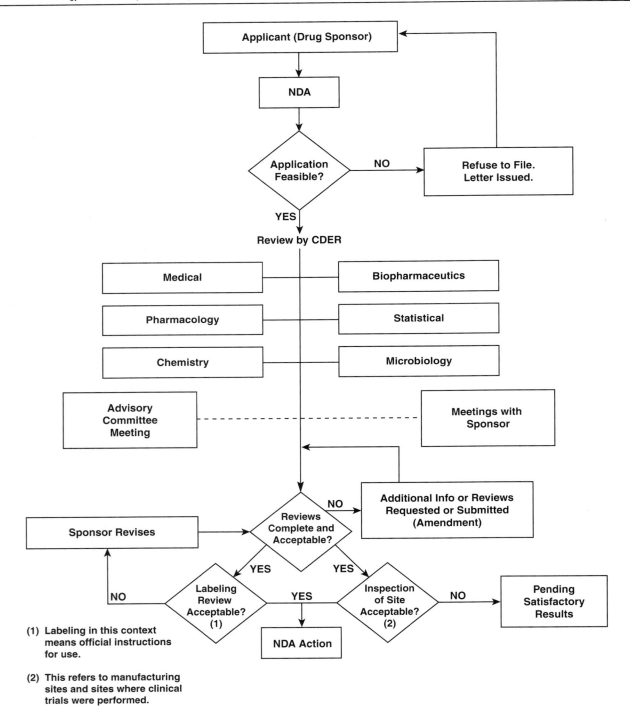

Figure 4-3. A typical review process of an NDA

Reporting System (SRS) that contains the adverse drug reaction reports from hospitals, health care providers, and laypeople. Those reports are sent to the FDA (via MedWatch) directly or to the drug manufacturer before being sent, by regulation, to the FDA by the manufacturer (Center for Drug Evaluation and Research, 1998a).

Some examples of serious adverse reactions are as follows: (Shalala, Henney, & Woodcock, 1995):

- Death—if an adverse reaction to a medical product is a suspected cause of a patient's death

- Life-threatening hazard—if a patient was at risk of dying at the time of the adverse reaction or if it is suspected that continued use of a product would cause death (e.g., pacemaker breakdown or failure of an intravenous pump that could cause excessive drug dosing)

- Hospitalization—if a patient is admitted or has a prolonged hospital stay because of a serious adverse reaction (e.g., a serious allergic reaction to a product such as latex)

- Disability—if the adverse reaction caused a significant or permanent change in a patient's body function, physical activities, or quality of life (e.g., strokes or nervous system disorders brought on by drug therapy)

- Birth defects, miscarriage, stillbirth, or birth with disease—if exposure to a medical product before conception or during pregnancy is suspected of causing an adverse outcome in a child (e.g., malformation in a child caused by the acne drug Accutane or isotretinoin)

- Needs intervention to avoid permanent damage—if use of a medical product required medical or surgical treatment to prevent impairment (e.g., burns from radiation equipment and breakage of a screw supporting a bone fracture). It is not necessary to prove that a medical product caused an adverse reaction; a suspected association is sufficient reason to make a report. For example, the weight-loss drugs Redux (dexfenfluramine) and Pondimin (fenfluramine) were taken off the market after being associated with heart-valve problems.

OTHER TOPICS

Apart from being a regulatory agency, FDA is also actively involved in improving the efficiency of the drug development by improving the existing knowledge in collaboration with experts and by taking lead in various initiatives. Some of the key activities of the FDA are briefly discussed below.

Advisory Committee Meetings

The FDA may especially want a committee's opinion about approval of a new drug; a major new indication for an already approved drug; or a special regulatory requirement being considered, such as a boxed warning in a drug's labeling. The FDA's advisory committees may also consider reports of adverse reactions to an already marketed drug. If severe reactions or deaths are occurring and it's not clear why, the FDA might call a special meeting.

Most members of the FDA's drug advisory committees are physicians whose specialties involve the drugs under the purview of their committee. Other members include registered nurses, statisticians, epidemiologists, and pharmacologists. Consumer-nominated members serve on all committees. As voting members, they must possess scientific expertise to participate fully in deliberations. They must have worked with consumer groups so they can assess the impact of decisions on consumers. Each committee advises a corresponding FDA drug review group. Committees typically meet two to four times a year, but may meet as often as the FDA needs them. The FDA announces upcoming meetings in the *Federal Register*.

Two advisory committee meetings in recent times had a profound impact on public health. One of them, held in September 2004, discussed the risks of suicidality (suicidal thinking and behavior) in children being treated with antidepressants (Center for Drug Evaluation and Research, 2004a). Based on the outcome of the meeting, the FDA asked the manufacturers of all antidepressant drugs to include in their labeling a boxed warning and expanded warning statements that alert health care providers to an increased risk of suicidality in children and adolescents being treated with these agents and additional information about the results of pediatric studies. In

February 2005, another meeting on drugs for arthritis pain (COX-2 inhibitors such as Vioxx, Celebrex, and Valdecoxib) discussed at length the cardiovascular risks associated with those drugs; and recommendations were made to the FDA for further action (Center for Drug Evaluation and Research, 2005a).

Subpart H Regulation

In 1992, Accelerated Approval Subpart H was added to NDA regulations. It is a highly specialized mechanism intended to speed approval of drugs promising significant benefit over existing therapy for serious or life-threatening illnesses. It incorporates elements aimed at making sure that rapid review and approval is balanced by safeguards to protect both the public health and the integrity of the regulatory process. This mechanism may be used when approval can be reliably based on evidence of a drug's effect on a surrogate endpoint or when the FDA determines an effective drug can be used safely only under restricted distribution or use. Usually, a surrogate can be assessed much sooner than an endpoint as survival (e.g., tumor response rates) (Dagher, Johnson, Williams, Keegan, & Pazdur, 2004). In accelerated approval, the FDA approves the drug on the condition that the sponsor studies the actual clinical benefit of the drug. Postmarketing studies would usually be studies already under way. When required to be conducted, such studies must also be adequate and well-controlled (Center for Drug Evaluation and Research, 2004c).

Parallel Track

Parallel track protocols make promising investigational drugs for AIDS and other HIV-related diseases more widely available while the controlled clinical trials essential to establish the safety and effectiveness of new drugs are carried out (USFDA., 2005a). The system established by this policy is designed to make the drugs more widely available to patients with the illnesses who have no therapeutic alternatives and who cannot participate in the controlled clinical trials.

Critical Path Initiative

The FDA has recently issued a document titled "Challenge and Opportunity on the Critical Path to New Medical Products" that describes the venues for improving the current drug development paradigm (USFDA., 2004). The document makes a serious attempt to bring attention and focus to the need for targeted scientific efforts to modernize the techniques and methods used to evaluate the safety, efficacy, and quality of medical products as they move from product selection and design to mass manufacture. This effort is to address the rising public expectations about the prospects of new therapies based on new biomedical discoveries (e.g., sequencing the human genome) and to reduce the number of failures in drug development (Colditz et al., 2004; Griffin & Bollard, 2004; Kelloff & Sigman, 2005; Lesko et al., 2003; Lesko & Woodcock, 2002; Lewin & Weiner, 2004; Petricoin et al., 2002; Salerno & Lesko, 2004; Soares et al., 2004; Weingarten et al., 2005).

SUMMARY

The FDA is responsible for protecting the public health by assuring the safety, efficacy, and security of human and veterinary drugs, biological products, medical devices, the food supply, cosmetics, and products that emit radiation. The FDA is also responsible for advancing the public health by helping to speed innovations that make medicines and foods more effective, safer, and more affordable. The FDA helps the public get accurate science-based information they need to use medicines (drugs) and foods to improve their health. Under current law, all new drugs require proof that they are effective, as well as safe, before they can be approved for marketing. But no drug is absolutely safe. There is always some risk of an adverse reaction. It's when the benefits outweigh the risks that the FDA considers a drug safe enough to approve. Today's policies also allow broader use of some investigational drugs before they are approved for marketing. The FDA participates actively in the drug development process, seeking to provide clear standards and expectations. It also provides advice in the form of guidelines on how to study particular classes of drugs and how to submit and analyze data in a marketing application. The various guidance documents written by experts from the FDA and consultants on clinical, nonclinical, and statistical issues related to drug development are used by the pharmaceutical industry to make decisions. The role of the FDA as described in this chapter is a very simplified version of the complex issues involved in the regulatory process of drug approval. To fully appreciate the role of the FDA in drug development and devices and the latest developments in this field, the readers are urged to visit the FDA Web site (http://www.fda.gov) for more details.

REFERENCES

Aarons, L., Karlsson, M. O., Mentre, F., Rombout, F., Steimer, J. L., & van Peer, A. (2001). Role of modelling and simulation in Phase I drug development. *Eur J Pharm Sci, 13*(2), 115–122.

Center for Devices and Radiological Health, U. (2002a). *Code of Federal Regulations, Title 21, Food and Drugs.* Retrieved March 25, 2005, from http://www.fda.gov/cdrh/aboutcfr.html

Center for Devices and Radiological Health, U. (2002b). *FDA Public Health Web Notification: Risk of Bacterial Meningitis in Children with Cochlear Implants.* Retrieved April 6, 2005, from http://www.fda.gov/cdrh/safety/cochlear.html#1

Center for Devices and Radiological Health, U. (2004a). *21CFR312.23.* Retrieved March 25, 2005, from http://www.accessdata.fda.gov/scripts/cdrh/cfdocs/cfcfr/CFRSearch.cfm

Center for Devices and Radiological Health, U. (2004b). *21CFR312.34.* Retrieved March 25, 2005, from http://www.accessdata.fda.gov/scripts/cdrh/cfdocs/cfcfr/CFRSearch.cfm

Center for Devices and Radiological Health, U. (2004c). *21CFR312.47.* Retrieved March 25, 2005, from http://www.accessdata.fda.gov/scripts/cdrh/cfdocs/cfcfr/CFRSearch.cfm

Center for Devices and Radiological Health, U. (2004d). *21CFR312.82.* Retrieved March 25, 2005, from http://www.accessdata.fda.gov/scripts/cdrh/cfdocs/cfcfr/CFRSearch.cfm

Center for Drug Evaluation and Research, U. (1995). *Guidance for Industry: Content and Format of Investigational New Drug Applications (INDs) for Phase 1 Studies of Drugs, Including Well-Characterized, Therapeutic, Biotechnology-Derived Products.* Retrieved March 23, 2005, from http://www.fda.gov/cder/guidance/phase1.pdf

Center for Drug Evaluation and Research, U. (1998a). *The CDER Handbook.* Retrieved March 23, 2005, from http://www.fda.gov/cder/handbook/

Center for Drug Evaluation and Research, U. (1998b). *Guidance for Industry: Providing Clinical Evidence of Effectiveness for Human Drugs and Biological Products.* Retrieved March 4, 2005, from http://www.fda.gov/cder/guidance/1397fnl.pdf

Center for Drug Evaluation and Research, U. (1998c). *Orphan Drugs.* Retrieved March 25, 2005, from http://www.fda.gov/cder/handbook/orphan.htm

Center for Drug Evaluation and Research, U. (2000). *Guidance for Industry: Good Laboratory Practices.* Retrieved February 23, 2005, from http://www.fda.gov/ora/compliance_ref/bimo/glp/qna.htm

Center for Drug Evaluation and Research, U. (2001a). *Guidance for Industry: IND Meetings for Human Drugs and Biologics Chemistry, Manufacturing, and Controls Information.* Retrieved March 23, 2005, from http://www.fda.gov/cder/guidance/3683fnl.pdf

Center for Drug Evaluation and Research, U. (2001b). *Regulatory Pharmacology and Toxicology Guidance.* Retrieved February 27, 2005, from http://www.fda.gov/cder/PharmTox/guidances.htm

Center for Drug Evaluation and Research, U. (2004a). *Food and Drug Administration: Joint Meeting of the Psychopharmacologic Drugs Advisory Committee and Pediatric Advisory Committee.* Retrieved March 23, 2005, from http://www.fda.gov/ohrms/dockets/ac/04/briefing/2004-4065b1.htm

Center for Drug Evaluation and Research, U. (2004b). *Guidance Documents.* Retrieved March 31, 2005, from http://www.fda.gov/cder/guidance/guidance.htm

Center for Drug Evaluation and Research, U. (2004c). *NDA Supplements Approved under Subpart H.* Retrieved March 23, 2005, from http://www.fda.gov/cder/rdmt/accappr1.htm

Center for Drug Evaluation and Research, U. (2005a). *Food and Drug Administration: Arthritis Advisory Committee and the Drug Safety and Risk Management Advisory Committee.* Retrieved March 23, 2005, from http://www.fda.gov/ohrms/dockets/ac/05/briefing/2005-4090b1.htm

Center for Drug Evaluation and Research, U. (2005b). *MedWatch: The FDA Safety Information and Adverse Event Reporting Program.* Retrieved March 23, 2005, from http://www.fda.gov/medwatch/

Colditz, F., Nyamsuren, O., Niehaus, K., Eubel, H., Braun, H. P., & Krajinski, F. (2004). Proteomic approach: Identification of Medicago truncatula proteins induced in roots after infection with the pathogenic oomycete Aphanomyces euteiches. *Plant Mol Biol, 55*(1), 109–120.

Committee, M. o. t. C. B. M. (2005). Action COST B15: Modeling during drug development: October 1998 to July 2004. *Basic & Clinical Pharmacology & Toxicology, 96,* 149–150.

Dagher, R., Johnson, J., Williams, G., Keegan, P., & Pazdur, R. (2004). Accelerated approval of oncology products: A decade of experience. *J Natl Cancer Inst, 96*(20), 1500–1509.

Derendorf, H., Lesko, L. J., Chaikin, P., Colburn, W. A., Lee, P., Miller, R., et al. (2000). Pharmacokinetic/pharmacodynamic modeling in drug research and development. *J Clin Pharmacol, 40*(12 Pt 2), 1399–1418.

Griffin, J. L., & Bollard, M. E. (2004). Metabonomics: Its potential as a tool in toxicology for safety assessment and data integration. *Curr Drug Metab, 5*(5), 389–398.

ICH. (1997). ICH Consensus guideline on general considerations for clinical trials, *CPMP/ICH/291/95.*

Kelloff, G. J., & Sigman, C. C. (2005). New science-based endpoints to accelerate oncology drug development. *Eur J Cancer, 41*(4), 491–501.

Lesko, L. J., Rowland, M., Peck, C. C., & Blaschke, T. F. (2000). Optimizing the science of drug development: Opportunities for better candidate selection and accelerated evaluation in humans. *Pharm Res, 17*(11), 1335–1344.

Lesko, L. J., Salerno, R. A., Spear, B. B., Anderson, D. C., Anderson, T., Brazell, C., et al. (2003). Pharmacogenetics and pharmacogenomics in drug development and regulatory decision making: Report of the first FDA-PWG-PhRMA-DruSafe Workshop. *J Clin Pharmacol, 43*(4), 342–358.

Lesko, L. J., & Woodcock, J. (2002). Pharmacogenomic-guided drug development: Regulatory perspective. *Pharmacogenomics J, 2*(1), 20–24.

Lewin, D. A., & Weiner, M. P. (2004). Molecular biomarkers in drug development. *Drug Discov Today, 9*(22), 976–983.

Mahmood, I. (2001). Interspecies scaling of maximum tolerated dose of anticancer drugs: Relevance to starting dose for phase I clinical trials. *Am J Ther, 8*(2), 109–116.

MedWatch, U. (2002). *Summary of Safety-Related Drug Labeling Changes Approved by FDA Center for Drug Evaluation and Research (CDER) March 2002.* Retrieved April 6, 2005, from http://www.fda.gov/medwatch/SAFETY/2002/mar02.htm#tobi

Peck, C. C., Barr, W. H., Benet, L. Z., Collins, J., Desjardins, R. E., Furst, D. E., et al. (1994). Opportunities for integration of pharmacokinetics, pharmacodynamics, and toxicokinetics in rational drug development. *J Clin Pharmacol, 34*(2), 111–119.

Petricoin, E. F., 3rd, Hackett, J. L., Lesko, L. J., Puri, R. K., Gutman, S. I., Chumakov, K., et al. (2002). Medical applications of microarray technologies: A regulatory science perspective. *Nat Genet, 32 Suppl,* 474–479.

Rados, C. (2003). Orphan products: Hope for people with rare diseases. *FDA Consumer, 37.*

Reigner, B. G., Williams, P. E., Patel, I. H., Steimer, J. L., Peck, C., & van Brummelen, P. (1997). An evaluation of the integration of pharmacokinetic and pharmacodynamic principles in clinical drug development. Experience within Hoffmann La Roche. *Clin Pharmacokinet, 33*(2), 142–152.

Sahajawalla, G. (2004). *New Drug Development: Regulatory Paradigms for Clinical Pharmacology and Biopharmaceutics* (Vol. 141). New York: Marcel Dekker Inc.

Salerno, R. A., & Lesko, L. J. (2004). Pharmacogenomics in drug development and regulatory decision-making: The genomic data submission (GDS) proposal. *Pharmacogenomics, 5*(1), 25–30.

Shalala, D. E., Henney, J. E., & Woodcock, J. (1995). *From Test Tube to Patient: New Drug Development in the United States.*

Sheiner, L. B. (1997). Learning versus confirming in clinical drug development. *Clin Pharmacol Ther, 61*(3), 275–291.

Soares, H. D., Williams, S. A., Snyder, P. J., Gao, F., Stiger, T., Rohlff, C., et al. (2004). Proteomic approaches in drug discovery and development. *Int Rev Neurobiol, 61*, 97–126.

Temple, R. (2000). Current definitions of phases of investigation and the role of the FDA in the conduct of clinical trials. *Am Heart J, 139*(4), S133–135.

Temple, R. (2002). Policy developments in regulatory approval. *Stat Med, 21*(19), 2939–2948.

FDA. (1999). *Milestones in U.S. Food and Drug Law History.* Retrieved February 23, 2005, from http://www.fda.gov/opacom/backgrounders/miles.html

USFDA. (2004). *Innovation/stagnation: Challenge and Opportunity on the Critical Path to New Medical Products.* Retrieved March 4, 2005, from http://www.fda.gov/oc/initiatives/criticalpath/whitepaper.html#fig2

USFDA. (2005a). *A Drug Review Glossary.* Retrieved March 25, 2005, from http://www.fda.gov/fdac/special/newdrug/bengloss.html

USFDA. (2005b). *FDA's Mission Statement.* Retrieved March 23, 2005, from http://www.fda.gov/opacom/morechoices/mission.html

Weingarten, P., Lutter, P., Wattenberg, A., Blueggel, M., Bailey, S., Klose, J., et al. (2005). Application of proteomics and protein analysis for biomarker and target finding for immunotherapy. *Methods Mol Med, 109*, 155–174.

Workman, P. (2003). How much gets there and what does it do?: The need for better pharmacokinetic and pharmacodynamic endpoints in contemporary drug discovery and development. *Curr Pharm Des, 9*(11), 891–902.

CHAPTER
5

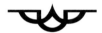

Common Classes of Drugs Used in Otolaryngologic Practice

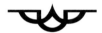

Amir Rafii, MD
Karen Doyle, MD
Department of Otolaryngology—Head and Neck Surgery
University of California, Davis

INTRODUCTION

Otolaryngology is a surgical subspecialty, but there are many otorhinolaryngic diseases for which the initial treatment is medical. This chapter summarizes the drug therapies used in the treatment of the following otorhinolaryngic diseases: allergic rhinitis, head and neck infections (including otitis externa, otitis media, sinusitis, tonsillitis, epiglottitis, and deep neck space infections), inflammatory diseases, Meniere's disease, and gastroesophageal reflux.

ALLERGIC RHINITIS

Allergic rhinitis, inflammation of the nasal mucous membranes, is an extremely common disease, affecting as much as 25% of the U.S. population (Osguthorpe & Derebery, 2003). Because otolaryngologists are trained allergy specialists and because they often treat complications of allergic rhinitis such as otitis media, sinusitis, and nasal polyps, they require particular expertise in the use of the four major classes of medications used in the treatment of allergic rhinitis: topical nasal steroids, **antihistamines,** decongestants, and mast cell stabilizers.

Intranasal Corticosteroids

Topical corticosteroids are considered the first line of therapy and are very effective in the treatment of the symptoms of allergic rhinitis (Hadley, 2003). Many different formulations are available, including triamcinolone, **dexamethasone,** beclomethasone, budesonide, mometasone, and fluticasone (Waddell, Patel, Toma, & Maw, 2003). All of them are significantly better than placebo and equally efficacious as systemic antihistamines in the reduction of the symptoms of allergic rhinitis. Many studies also show that compared to second-generation antihistamines, intranasal corticosteroids are more cost-effective, as well as effective in the treatment of the symptoms of nasal stuffiness, **pruritis** (itching), and sneezing. Intranasal steroids do not produce a significant steroid effect, influence growth and bone metabolism, or compromise ocular function (Benninger & Marple, 2003).

Antihistamines

Histamine is an amine that is stored in high concentrations in mast cells and basophils (Simon, 2004). Histamine is released in response to IgE-mediated (immediate) antigen antibody allergic reactions and causes a variety of effects throughout the body. It plays an important role in allergic rhinitis, **urticaria** (hives), and angioedema (Katzung, 2001). Thus, its effects can range from mild irritation and itching to **anaphylaxis** and death. Histamine also plays a role in the control of acid secretions in the stomach (Katzung, 2001) and has a central nervous system neurotransmitter effect.

Three receptors of histamine have been defined: H1, H2, and H3 (Simon, 2004). H1 receptors mediate the allergic manifestations of the histamine response such as bronchoconstriction and vasodilatation via smooth muscles. The H2 receptor mediates the gastric acid secretion of parietal cells in the stomach. H3 receptors are involved in central nervous system neurotransmission (Katzung, 2001). Thus, blocking the effects of antihistamines could lead to therapeutic effects in a variety of situations.

H1 receptor antagonists are typically divided into two groups: sedating (traditional or first-generation) and nonsedating (second-generation) (Mabry, 1998). They are all competitive antagonists of the H1 receptor (Simon, 2004). **Diphenhydramine** (Benadryl) and **chlorpheniramine** (Chlor-Timetron) are prototypes of the traditional antihistamines (Simon, 2004). Most antihistamines are metabolized in the liver, and their half-lives range from four to twelve hours (Katzung, 2001).

Antihistamines have long been part of the mainstay of the treatment of allergic reactions such as rhinitis and urticaria (Katzung, 2001). Unfortunately, first-generation antihistamines possess a number of undesirable properties, including depression of the central nervous system (Ferguson, 1998). Utilizing this property, some antihistamines (diphenhydramine, pyrilamine, and doxylamine) are marketed as sleep aids or medications for motion sickness (Katzung, 2001). Older antihistamines also interact with sedating drugs such as alcohol and **benzodiazepines.** Antihistamines also have anticholinergic properties (Mabry, 1998). Undesirable effects due to their anticholinergic properties may lead to dry mouth, impotence, blurred vision, double vision, euphoria, hypertension, or constipation. Some antihistamines can promote central nervous system stimulation, resulting in seizures, insomnia, irritability, appetite stimulation, and even hallucinations and psychosis (Ferguson, 1998).

Undesirable effects of the sedating antihistamines led to the development of the second-generation antihistamines that do not readily cross the blood-brain barrier and, therefore, have decreased central nervous system side effects (Ferguson, 1998). Loratadine, **fexofenadine** (Allegra), and **cetirizine** (Zyrtec) are examples of the second-generation antihistamines (Mabry, 1998; Ferguson, 1998). **Azelastine** (Astelin) is the first topically administered antihistamine in the form of a nasal spray (Ferguson, 1998), allowing the drug to provide symptom relief while avoiding systemic action.

Otolaryngologists mainly use antihistamines for the treatment of allergic rhinitis. However, for children, topical nasal steroid sprays control allergic rhinitis symptoms while avoiding the possible loss of alertness and performance associated with antihistamines (Bender & Milgrom, 2004). Antihistamines may be used on an as-needed basis prior to anticipated allergen exposure to treat the symptoms of allergic rhinitis such as itching, sneezing, and **rhinorrhea** (Mabry, 1998). Antihistamines provide very little benefit in the treatment of asthma and anaphylactic emergencies (Simon, 2004). Table 5-1 lists the two classes of antihistamines.

Decongestants

Oral and topically applied decongestants are often used in otolaryngology practice. Decongestants are often used with antihistamines to help relieve nasal obstruction. Topically applied agents consist of phenylephrine and oxymetazoline. Those drugs lead to vasoconstriction of submucosal blood vessels of the nose and work almost immediately (Hadley, 2003). Pseudoephedrine is an example of an oral decongestant (Hadley, 2003). Pseudoephedrine leads to vasoconstriction via release of stored catecholamines, as well as nonselective, direct stimulation of alpha-one adrenergic receptors (Ferguson, 1998). Side effects of

Table 5-1. Classes of Antihistamines

"Sedating" Antihistamines	hydroxyzine (Atarax, Vistaril)
	diphenhydramine (Benadryl)
	dimenhydrinate (Dramamine)
	meclizine (Bonine)
	brompheniramine (Dimetane)
	promethazine (Phenergan)
	chlorpheniramine (Chlor-Trimeton)
	clemastine (Tavist)
	cyproheptadine (Periactin)
	azatadine (Optimine)
	cetirizine (Zyrtec)
"Nonsedating" Antihistamines	fexofenadine (Allegra)
	loratidine (Claritin)
	desloratadine (Clarinex)
[off market]	terfenadine (Seldane)
	astemizole (Hismanal)
Topical	azelastine (Astelin)—nonspecific H1

oral decongestants include, most commonly, insomnia, but also dizziness, headaches, tremor, and nervousness (Ferguson, 1998). Combining oral decongestants with sedating antihistamines may counteract the undesired effects of both products (Hadley, 2003). In fact, oral decongestants are often combined with H1 antagonists, expectorants, and cough suppressants in many over-the-counter products (Hadley, 2003).

Mast Cell Stabilizers

Cromoglycate inhibits the degranulation of mast cells and is available as a nasal spray. It is effective in treating allergic rhinitis, though it requires several days to work. Its major advantage is its lack of adverse effects; its disadvantage is that it requires frequent dosing, up to four to six times per day (Ferguson, 1998).

HEAD AND NECK INFECTIONS

Otolaryngologists treat many bacterial infections such as otitis externa, otitis media, sinusitis, tonsillitis/pharyngitis, epiglottitis, and deep neck space infections.

Choices of antibiotics are complicated not only by the myriad of available agents, but also by the continuing emergence of antibacterial-resistant strains of pathogens. This section briefly presents the pathogens responsible for six common otolaryngologic infections and their symptoms and signs. It also covers the different classes of antibiotics, their mechanisms of action, bacterial targets, and special drugs of choice for important pathogens.

Otitis Externa

Infection of the external auditory canal can occur in the setting of maceration of the skin from water or high humidity, trauma, or contamination. In otitis externa, the canal skin is red and edematous, with purulent drainage and intense pain. If untreated, infection can spread to the skull base (malignant otitis externa) or the pinna (cellulitis or perichondritis). The bacterial species Pseudomonas aeruginosa can usually be cultured from the canal, and other bacteria such as Staphylococcus aureus and other aerobic gram-negative rods may be involved. Topical antibiotic drops are adequate to treat otitis externa in the absence of complications such as cellulitis (Hennley, Denneny, & Holzer, 2000).

Otitis Media

Acute otitis media is a common childhood disease that commonly occurs as a complication of upper respiratory infections, particularly in children. The most common bacteria responsible for acute otitis media are Streptococcus pneumoniae, and the recommended first-line treatment for acute otitis media is oral amoxicillin (Lieberthal et al., 2004). In patients with severe illness, or when Haemophilus influenzae or Moraxella catarrhalis are suspected, amoxicillin/clavulanate should be used (Lieberthal et al., 2004). In healthy children, the vast majority of acute otitis media will resolve without antibiotic treatment, although those children will suffer from more pain and fever than children who receive treatment (Le Saux et al., 2005). Chronic otitis media with effusion in children occurs when pneumatic otoscopy reveals the presence of middle ear fluid without acute symptoms and signs such as pain and fever. Chronic otitis media with effusion usually is a self-limited disease; but when effusion persists for more than three months, surgical treatment with tympanostomy tubes is considered. Pharmacotherapy such as antibiotics, decongestants, and antihistamines are no longer recommended for chronic otitis media with effusion (Rosenfeld et al., 2004). Chronic suppurative otitis media occurs when there is chronic infection of the middle ear and mastoid, with a draining tympanic membrane or tympanostomy tube. Its microbiology differs from acute otitis media in that the most common bacterial species is Pseudomonas aeroginosa, followed by Staphylococcus aureus and anaerobic bacteria (Kenna et al., 1994). In the setting of cholesteatoma, chronic suppurative otitis media is always a surgical disease; but when cholesteatoma is not present, medical therapy with topical or systemic antibiotics directed against Pseudomonas and staphylococcus aureus can be effective.

Sinusitis

Acute and chronic rhinosinusitis are characterized by symptoms of purulent anterior or posterior nasal discharge, nasal congestion, facial pain or pressure, and fever (Lanza & Kennedy, 1997). Disease is detectable by computed tomographic scan. The bacteria Streptococcus pneumoniae, Haemophilus influenzae, and Moraxella catarrhalis are the predominant organisms causing acute sinusitis, while Pseudomonas aeruginosa, Staphylococcus aureus, and anaerobic bacteria can be implicated in chronic sinusitis. For adult sinusitis, antibiotic treatment is recommended for symptoms lasting one week (Mucha & Baroody, 2003). Antibiotic treatment is also recommended for pediatric sinusitis (Wald et al., 2001). Adding intranasal steroids to the treatment results in more rapid resolution (Meltzer et al., 1993).

Tonsillitis

Recurrent pharyngeal and tonsillar infections are usually caused by Group A beta-hemolytic

Streptococcus in adults and children. The infections should be promptly treated with antibiotics that cover this organism (Casey & Pinchichero, 2004).

Epiglottitis

Acute infection of the supraglottis, including the epiglottis, is an airway emergency. Symptoms include fever, drooling, and the so-called "hot potato voice" (Shah, Roberson, & Jones, 2004). In children, emergency intubation secures the airway; and in adults, after fiberoptic laryngoscopy verifies the diagnosis, the airway is secured by intubation or tracheostomy. Haemophilus influenzae type B is the most commonly cultured organism, but there is a trend toward other bacteria being the cause of epiglottitis in adults and children, while epiglottitis has become less common in children (Isaacson & Isaacson, 2003).

Deep Neck Space Infections

Deep neck space abscesses involving the parapharyngeal, retropharyngeal, submandibular, and submental spaces can result from dental, pharyngeal, and other ear/nose/throat infections. These infections are treated with a combination of targeted intravenous antibiotics and surgical drainage, following airway management (Gidley, Ghorayeb, & Stiernberg, 1997). Bacteriology depends on the etiology and can include Streptococcus, Staphylococcus, Bacteroides, gram-negative, and anaerobic species.

BETA LACTAMS: PENICILLINS AND CEPHALOSPORINS

The penicillins and cephalosporins comprise the beta-lactam group of antibiotics, named after the four-membered ring structure that is common to the drugs. This group of medications includes some of the most effective and widely used antibacterials available to the otolaryngologist.

Penicillins bind to penicillin-binding proteins and arrest cell wall synthesis, leading to cell death. Thus, penicillins are bactericidal. They are excreted by the kidneys; thus, kidney function must be considered when dosing. Most penicillins cross the blood-brain barrier when the meninges are inflamed. Allergic reactions to penicillins include urticaria, pruritis, fever, joint swelling, and anaphylaxis. Patients may also develop nausea and diarrhea due to direct irritation or via overgrowth of gram-positive organisms and yeast. Resistance is often mediated by the formation of beta lactamases or penicillinases by microorganisms. Those enzymes hydrolyze the beta-lactam ring, leading to loss of antibacterial activity.

Types of Penicillins

There are four general types of penicillins:

1. Narrow-spectrum penicillinase-susceptible agents (Penicillin G and Penicillin V): **Penicillin G** is the prototype penicillin. It is used mainly against pneumococcal and other streptococcal infections, but it is also active against about half the usual anaerobic organisms of the upper respiratory and gastrointestinal tract. Penicillin G is administered intramuscularly or intravenously, whereas penicillin V is an oral drug. When taken orally, they should not be taken with meals, as gastric acid denatures penicillin V.

2. Very-narrow-spectrum penicillinase-resistant agents (Methicillin, Oxacillin, and **Nafcillin**): These are the drugs of choice for treatment of staphylococcal infections, including Staphylococcus aureus. Otherwise, they do not have an advantage over penicillins against streptococci and pneumococci. Methicillin-resistant staphylococci (MRSA) refer to a growing strain of cells that is resistant to all beta lactams, including this group.

3. Wider-spectrum penicillinase-susceptible agents:

   a. Amino penicillins (**Ampicillin** and Amoxicillin): These have a similar coverage compared to penicillins, but also include gram-negative organisms such as Escherichia coli, Proteus mirabilis, and H. flu (but not Pseudomonas). Ampicillin plays a prominent role in otolaryngologic practice given its coverage of Haemophilus influenzae, which is one of the organisms responsible for sinusitis and ear infections. A higher tendency to develop a rash has been noted with the use of amino penicillins, especially in the setting of mononucleosis.

b. Pipercillin, Ticarcillin: These provide broad coverage, but primarily address gram-negative rods, including Pseudomonas. These drugs are synergistic with aminoglycosides. Given their pseudomonal coverage, they are frequently utilized in the treatment of necrotizing external otitis.

4. Augmented penicillins (Amoxicillin plus Calvulanate (Augmentin), Ampicillin plus Sulbactam (Unasyn), Ticarcillin plus potassium clavulanate (Timentin), Piperacillin plus tazobactam (Zosyn)): As noted, resistance to penicillins is mediated by penicillinases or beta lactamases. Inhibitors of these enzymes (such as clavulanic acid, sulbactam, and tazobactam) may be combined with penicillins to prevent their inactivation. For example, when used in combination, clavulanic acid extends the scope of amoxicillin's activity to Haemophilus influenzae, Moraxella catarrhalis, Staphylococcus aureus, Bacteroides fragilis, and other anaerobes. These combinations are effective in the treatment of sinusitis and ear infections when bacteria are resistant to amoxicillin alone. Timentin and Zosyn add coverage against Pseudomonas aeruginosa.

Cephalosporins

Cephalosporins are also bactericidal, beta-lactam antibiotics that inhibit cell wall synthesis. They are described as first-, second-, third-, or fourth-generation drugs. In general, the higher generations have more gram-negative and less gram-positive coverage. The following are some features of these drugs:

1. First-generation agents **cefazolin** (Ancef) and cephalexin (Keflex): These drugs are active against most gram-positive cocci such as Streptococcus pneumoniae and against Staphylococcus aureus, many strains of Escherichia coli, and Klebsiella

pneumoniae. These agents are frequently used by otolaryngologists against Staphylococcus aureus infections and prophylaxis against surgical infections.

2. Second-generation agents cefuroxime (Ceftin), cefotetan, cefoxitin, cefprozil (Cefzil), and cefaclor (Ceclor). Cefuroxime is the drug of choice for Haemophilus influenzae infections. These agents are valuable in the treatment of Haemophilus influenzae infections encountered in acute ear infections, epiglottitis, and sinusitis.

3. Third-generation agents ceftriaxone (Rocephin), cefotaxime (Claforan), and ceftazadime (Fortaz): This class includes even broader gram-negative coverage, as well as the ability to cross the blood-brain barrier. Oral agents in this group have decreased activity against gram-positive cocci and are not the ideal first-line treatments for untyped otolaryngologic infections. Parenteral agents in this group (ceftriaxone and cefotaxime) retain effective antipneumococcal activity, along with higher activity against Haemophilus influenzae and Neisseria meningitidis. Along with their ability to cross the blood-brain barrier, they are commonly utilized in the setting of meningitis.

4. Fourth-generation agents (Cefepime): These drugs are active against Pseudomonas as well as Staphylococcus aureus. They provide a nonototoxic alternative to aminoglycosides for the treatment of Pseudomonas.

Other Beta-Lactams

Meropenem, Imipenem/Cilastin, Aztreaonam, and Ertapenem are the "other" beta lactams. These drugs are usually used when first-line treatment has been unsuccessful.

AMINOGLYCOSIDES

Aminoglycosides are **bacteriocidal** (causing death to bacteria) inhibitors of protein synthesis. These drugs are important in the treatment of serious infections caused by aerobic gram-negative bacteria, including Escherichia coli, Enterobacter, Klebsiella, Proteus, Pseudomonas, and Serratia species. Aminoglycosides include **gentamicin,** amikacin, tobramycin, streptomycin, kanamycin, neomycin, and spectinomycin. These drugs are well known to the otolaryngologist because they can be ototoxic (and nephrotoxic). They can be used safely by carefully monitoring their dosages, their serum levels, and the patient's renal function.

MACROLIDES

The macrolides, erythromycin, clarithromycin, and azithromycin bind reversibly to the 50S ribosomal subunit in susceptible bacteria, inhibiting RNA-dependent protein synthesis. They are active against most gram-positive and some gram-negative organisms and are most often used as an alternative to penicillins in cases of penicillin allergy. They are frequently used to treat whooping cough, Legionella pneumonia, Corynebacterium (such as diphtheria), and mycoplasma. There is a high incidence of gastrointestinal side effects that include nausea, vomiting, and diarrhea. These antibiotics are known to antagonize the action of clindamycin and should not be used in patients with liver disease.

CLINDAMYCIN

Clindamycin is a unique antibiotic that has specific action against both gram-positive and gram-negative anaerobic bacteria. It inhibits bacterial protein synthesis by binding to the 50S ribosomal subunit. It is frequently used in otolaryngology to treat odontogenic deep neck space infections that include anaerobic organisms.

METRONIDAZOLE

Metronidazole (Flagyl) is another drug specifically used to treat anaerobic (and some fungal) infections.

Its mechanism of action is to inhibit RNA/DNA synthesis. Because it is active only against obligate anaerobes, it is usually used in combination with other antibiotics.

FLUOROQUINOLONES

Quinolones are the only oral drugs with activity against Pseudomonas aeruginosa and, thus, are extremely important for treatment of external ear infections and chronic suppurative otitis media (Gehanno, 1997). They inhibit prokaryotic type II topoisomerases through direct binding to the bacterial chromosome. They have a broad spectrum of activity, including resistant pneumococci, have prolonged half-lives permitting once- or twice-daily dosing, and are well tolerated. Their systemic use in children is limited because they have been shown to cause joint disorders in juvenile animals (Alghasham & Nahata, 2000).

VANCOMYCIN

Vancomycin inhibits bacterial cell wall synthesis by blocking transpeptidation. It has a very specific action only against gram-positive cocci. Its two main uses are to treat methicillin-resistant Staphylococcus aureus infections and to treat clostridial pseudomembranous colitis. It is contraindicated in the presence of renal failure and is rarely ototoxic at high doses (Bailie & Neal, 1988).

SULFONAMIDES

Sulfonamides suppress bacterial growth by inhibiting folic acid synthesis. Combining sulfonamides with trimethoprim, which inhibits dihydrofolate reductase, further suppresses bacterial DNA, RNA, and protein synthesis. These **bacteriostatic** antibiotics have a broad spectrum of action against many gram-positive and gram-negative bacteria, though resistance is common. About 5% of patients have adverse reactions to sulfonamides, ranging from rashes to serious allergic reactions.

INFLAMMATORY DISEASES

Noninfectious inflammatory and autoimmune diseases can affect the head and neck. These conditions, which include Sjogren's disease, sarcoidosis, Wegener's granulomatosis, polyarteritis nodosa, relapsing polychondritis, and autoimmune sensorineural hearing loss are typically treated with oral corticosteroids such as **prednisone** and dexamethasone. Corticosteroids are given acutely for treatment of head and neck diseases such as nasal polyps, chronic sinusitis, sudden sensorineural hearing loss, **Bell's palsy**, and upper airway obstruction and are used perioperatively to prevent swelling and nausea. Dexamethasone (9-fluoro-11b,17,21-trihydroxy-16a-methylpregna-1, 4-diene-3,20-dione) is a synthetic corticosteroid (Hardman & Lindbird, 2001). Synthetic corticosteroids such as dexamethasone and prednisone are primarily used for their anti-inflammatory effects. Corticosteroids cause potent and varied metabolic effects and modify the body's immune responses to diverse stimuli. Dexamethasone is a long-acting glucocorticoid with a half-life of thirty-six to fifty-four hours. Prednisone has a shorter half-life (12 to 36 hours). Corticosteroids are metabolized primarily in the liver and are then excreted by the kidneys (Katzung, 2001).

Dexamethasone is used therapeutically for endocrine disorders, rheumatic disorders, collagen diseases, dermatologic diseases, allergic states, ophthalmic diseases, respiratory diseases, hematologic disorders, neoplastic disease, and edema (Katzung, 2001). In otolaryngology, dexamethasone is given intravenously at the time of surgery to minimize swelling and nausea (Steward et al., 2001). Orally administered prednisone is more commonly used by otolaryngologists to treat inflammatory head and neck diseases such as Bell's palsy (Ramsey et al., 2000; Axelsson et al., 2003), autoimmune or sudden sensorineural hearing loss (Slattery et al., 2005), sarcoidosis (Schwartzbauer & Tami, 2003), and Wegener's granulomatosis (Reinhold et al., 2000).

Adverse reactions to corticosteroids include fluid and electrolyte disturbance, sodium and fluid retention, congestive heart failure in susceptible patients, hypokalemia, hypertension, muscle weakness and loss of muscle mass, osteoporosis, vertebral compression fractures, aseptic necrosis of femoral and humeral heads, and tendon rupture. Gastrointestinal adverse effects may include peptic ulcers with possible perforation and hemorrhage; perforation of the small and large bowel, particularly in patients with inflammatory bowel disease; pancreatitis; abdominal distention; and ulcerative esophagitis. Dermatologic problems may include impaired wound healing; thin, fragile skin; petechiae; ecchymoses; and increased sweating. Neurologic adverse effects include convulsions, increased intracranial pressure with papilledema, headache, and psychic disturbances. Endocrine problems associated with corticosteroids are menstrual irregularities; development of cushingoid state; suppression of growth in children; secondary adrenocortical and pituitary unresponsiveness, particularly in times of stress, as in trauma, surgery, or illness; decreased carbohydrate tolerance; latent diabetes mellitus; increased requirements for insulin or oral hypoglycemic agents in diabetics; and hirsutism. Possible ophthalmic complications are posterior cataracts, increased intraocular pressure, glaucoma, and exophthalmos. Other adverse effects include thromboembolism, weight gain, increased appetite, nausea, and malaise.

MENIERE'S DISEASE

Meniere's disease is characterized by episodic severe vertigo, fluctuating sensorineural hearing loss, tinnitus, and aural fullness. While its cause is unknown, its underlying pathology is characterized by distension of the endolymphatic spaces and cochlea and/or vestibular apparatus. The initial recommended medical treatment of Meniere's disease is adherence to a low-sodium diet and thiazide diuretics (Santos et al., 1993). Klockhoff and Lindblom (1967) found significant improvements in vertigo and hearing loss with hydrochlrothiazide compared to placebo. Likewise, a randomized clinical trial showed that triamterene/hydrochlorothiazide treatment significantly improved vertigo, though hearing and tinnitus were not improved (Van Deelen & Huizing, 1986). Vasodilators such as histamine and betahistine are frequently used in the treatment of Meniere's disease, although their effectiveness is controversial (Schmidt & Huizing, 1992). Both systemic corticosteroids and injections of corticosteroids into the middle ear have been used as treatment for Meniere's disease, but their efficacy has not been demonstrated (Doyle et al., 2004). During acute vertigo episodes, vestibular suppressants such as meclizine and diazepam are essential, along with antiemetics such as scopolamine and prochlorperazine. The vast majority of Meniere's patients function well on their medical regimen, although many will fail medical therapy and will require surgical intervention. Allergy treatment is indicated in patients with less common bilateral disease (Derebery, 1997).

GASTROESOPHAGEAL REFLUX DISEASE

Gastroesophageal reflux disease (GERD) is a very common condition that results from the reflux of stomach acid into the esophagus. Aside from heartburn, GERD may cause multiple symptoms and signs including chest pain, cough, indigestion, laryngitis, rhinitis, and otalgia. Up to 10% of adults experience heartburn daily (Rakel & Bope, 2005). Numerous antacids may be used to decrease or neutralize stomach acid. They include antihistamines that block H2 histamine receptors, such as **cimetidine** (Tagamet), **ranitidine** (Zantac), and **famotidine** (Pepcid). For more mild symptoms, direct antacids such as calcium carbonate (Tums), magnesium hydroxide (milk of magnesia), aluminum hydroxide (Rolaids), and combinations (Maalox and Mylanta) are effective. The introduction of **proton pump inhibitor**s (PPIs) revolutionized the treatment of GERD. **Omeprazole** (Prilosec), **Lansoprazole** (Prevacid), **Pantoprazole** (Protonix), and **Rabeprazol** (Aciphex) are all PPIs. These drugs specifically bind and block ATP-dependent proton pumps (acid-secreting enzymes) of the stomach's parietal cells, significantly reducing acid secretion. PPIs are considered the most appropriate medical treatment for gastroesophageal reflux (Tougas & Armstrong, 1997) given that they help reduce symptoms, heal erosion, and maintain healthy mucosa (Feston, 2004).

SUMMARY

Otolaryngologists employ a variety of therapeutic and symptomatic medications to treat otorhinolaryngic diseases, after careful history, physical examination, and appropriate tests reveal the diagnosis. Even though otolaryngology is a surgical specialty, in many cases, medications may be employed, delaying or negating the need for surgical treatment. Knowledge of appropriate dosages, possible side effects, and drug interactions are required on the part of the prescribing otolaryngologist. Through proper use of the medications summarized in this chapter, otolaryngologists can successfully treat and often cure otorhinolaryngic conditions.

Audiologists need to be familiar with major classifications of medications available to better understand the treatments their patients are receiving. An understanding of those medications also facilitates communication between audiologists and otolaryngologists as they collaborate in assisting patients and possibly in clinical research.

REFERENCES

Alghasham, A. A., & Nahata, M. C. (2000). Clinical use of fluoroquinolones in children. *Annals of Pharmacotherapy, 34*, 347–359.

Axelsson, S., Lindberg, S., & Stjernquist-Desatnik, A. (2003). Outcome of treatment with valacyclovir and prednisone in patients with Bell's palsy. *Ann Otol Rhinol Laryngol, 112*, 197–201.

Bailie, G. R., & Neal, D. (1988). Vancomycin ototoxicity and nephrotoxicity. A review. *Med Toxicol Adverse Drug Exp, 3*, 376–386.

Bender, B., & Milgrom, H. (2004). Comparison of the effects of fluticasone propionate aqueous nasal spray and loratadine on daytime alertness and performance in children with seasonal allergic rhinitis. *Annals of Allergy, Asthma, and Immunology, 92*, 344–349.

Benninger, M. S., Ahmad, N., & Marple, B. F. (2003). The safety of intranasal steroids. *Otolaryngology—Head and Neck Surgery, 129*, 739–750.

Casey, J. R., & Pinchichero, M. E. (2004). Meta-analysis of cephalosporins versus penicillin for treatment of group A streptococcal tonsillopharyngitis in adults. *Clin Infect Dis, 38,* 1526–1534.

Derebery, M. J. (2000). Allergic management of Meniere's disease: An outcome study. *Otolaryngology—Head and Neck Surgery, 122,* 174–182.

Doyle, K., Bauch, C., Battista, R., Beatty, C. Hughes, G. B., Mason, J., Maw, J., & Musiek, F. (2004). Intratympanic steroid treatment: A review. *Otology and Neurotology, 25,* 1034–1039.

Ferguson, B. J. (1998). Cost-effective pharmacotherapy for allergic rhinitis. *Otolaryngologic Clinics of North America, 31,* 91–110.

Feston, J. W. (2004). Therapeutic choices in reflux disease: Defining the criteria for selecting a proton pump inhibitor. *American Journal of Medicine, 117* (5A), 14S–22S.

Gehanno, P. (1997). Multicenter study of the efficacy and safety of oral ciprofloxacin in the treatment of chronic suppurative otitis media in adults. The French Study Group. *Otolaryngology—Head and Neck Surgery, 117,* 83–90.

Gidley, P. W., Ghorayeb, B. Y., & Stiernberg, C. N. (1997). Contemporary management of deep neck space infections. *Otolaryngology—Head and Neck Surgery, 116,* 16–22.

Hadley, J. A. (2003). Cost-effective pharmacotherapy for inhalant allergic rhinitis. *Otolaryngologic Clinics of North America, 36,* 825–836.

Hannley, M. T., Denneny, J. C., & Holzer, S. S. (2000). Use of ototopical antibiotics in treating 3 common ear diseases. *Otolaryngology—Head and Neck Surgery, 122,* 934–940.

Hardman, L. E., & Limbird, J. G. (Eds.). (2001). *Goodman and Gilman's the Pharmacological Basis of Therapeutics* (10th ed.). New York: McGraw-Hill.

Isaacson, G., & Isaacson, D. M. (2003). Pediatric epiglottitis caused by group G beta hemolytic Streptococcus. *Pediatric Infectious Disease Journal, 22,* 846–847.

Katzung, B.G. (2001). *Basic and Clinical Pharmacology.* New York: Lange Medical Books.

Kenna, M. A. (1994). Management of chronic suppurative otitis media. *Otolaryngology Clinics of North America, 27,* 457–472.

Klockhoff, I., & Lindblom, U. (1967). Meniere's disease and hydrochlorothiazide (Dichlotride)—a critical analysis of symptoms and therapeutic effects. *Acta Otolaryngologica, 63,* 347–365.

Lanza, D. C., & Kennedy, D. W. (1997). Adult rhinosinusitis defined. *Otolaryngology—Head and Neck Surgery, 117,* S1–S7.

Le Saux, N., Gaboury, I., Baird, M., Klassen, T. P., Maccormick, J., Blanchard, A., Pitters, C., Sampson, M., & Moher, D. (2005). A randomized, double-blind, placebo-controlled noninferiority trial of amoxicillin for clinically diagnosed acute otitis media in children 6 months to 5 years of age. *CMAJ, 172,* 335–341.

Lieberthal, A. S., Ganiats, T. G., Culpepper, L., Mahoney, M., Miller, F., Runyan, D. K., & Shapiro, N. L. (2004). Diagnosis and management of acute otitis media. Clinical practice guideline. *Pediatrics, 113,* 1451–1465.

Mabry, R. L. (1998). Allergy management for the otolaryngologist. *Otolaryngologic Clinics of North America, 31,* 175–188.

Mucha, S. M., & Baroody, F. M. (2003). Sinusitis update. *Current Opinion in Allergy and Clinical Immunology, 3,* 33–38.

Osguthorpe, J. D., & Derebery, M. J. (1999). Allergy management for the otolaryngologist. *Otolaryngology Clinics of North America, 31,* 1.

Rakel, R. E., & Bope, E. T. (2005). *Conn's Current Therapy.* Philadelphia: Elsevier Saunders.

Ramsey, M. J., DerSimonian, R., Holtel, M. R., & Burgess, L. P. (2000). Corticosteroid treatment for idiopathic facial nerve paralysis: A meta analysis. *Laryngoscope, 110,* 335–341.

Reinhold-Keller, E., Beuge, J., Latza, U., de Groot, K., Rudert, H., Nolli, B., Heller, M., & Gross, W. L. (2000). An interdisciplinary approach to the care of patients with Wegener's granulomatosis: Long-term outcome in 155 patients. *Arthritis Rheum, 43,* 1021–1032.

Rosenfeld, R. M., Culpepper, L., Doyle, K. J., Grundfast, K. M., Hoberman, A., Kenna, M. A., Lieberthal, A. S., Mahoney, M., Wahl, R. A., Woods, C. R., & Yaw, B. (2004). Clinical practice guideline: Otitis media with effusion. *Otolaryngology—Head and Neck Surgery, 130,* S95–S118.

Santos, P. M., Hall, R. A., Snyder, J. M., Hughes, L. F., & Dobie, R. A. (1993). Diuretic and diet effect on Meniere's disease evaluated by the 1985 Committee on Hearing and Equilibrium guidelines. *Otolaryngology—Head and Neck Surgery, 109,* 680–689.

Schmidt, J. T., & Huizing, E. H. (1992). The clinical drug trial in Meniere's disease with emphasis on the effect of betahistine SR. *Acta Otolaryngologica* (Suppl. 497), 1–189.

Schwartzbauer, H. R., & Tami, T. A. (2003). Ear, nose and throat manifestations of sarcoidosis. *Otolaryngology Clinics of North America, 36,* 673–684.

Shah, R. K., Roberson, D. W., & Jones, D. T. (2004). Epiglottitis in the Hemophilus influenzae type B vaccine era: Changing trends. *Laryngoscope, 114,* 557–560.

Simons, F. E. R. (2004). Advances in H1-antihistamines. *New England Journal of Medicine, 21,* 2203–2217.

Slattery, W. H., Fisher, L. M., Iqbal, Z., & Liu, N. (2005). Oral steroid regimens for idiopathic sudden sensorineural hearing loss. *Otolaryngology—Head and Neck Surgery, 132,* 8–10.

Steward, D. L., Welge, J. A., & Myer, C. M. (2001). Do steroids reduce morbidity of tonsillectomy? Meta-analysis of randomized trials. *Laryngoscope, 111,* 1712–1718.

Tougas, G., & Armstrong, D. (1997). Efficacy of H2 receptor antagonists in the treatment of gastroesophageal reflux disease and its symptoms. *Canadian Journal of Gastroenterology, 11* (Suppl. B), 51B–54B.

Van Deelen, G. W., & Huizing, E. H. (1986). Use of a diuretic (Dyazide) in the treatment of Meniere's disease. A double-blind cross-over placebo-controlled study. *ORL Journal Otorhinolaryngology and Related Specialties, 48,* 287–292.

Wald, E. R., Bordley, W. C., Darrow, D. H., Grimm, K. T., Gwaltney, J. M., March, S. M., Senac, M. O., & William P. V. (2001). Clinical practice guideline: Management of sinusitis. *Pediatrics, 108,* 798–808.

CHAPTER

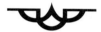

6

Nutraceuticals and Herbal Supplements

*Michael D. Seidman, MD, FACS

Marie Moneysmith
*Henry Ford Health System
Department of Otolaryngology—Head and Neck Surgery
West Bloomfield, MI

INTRODUCTION

East Meets West in Complementary and Integrative Medicine

Complementary and integrative medicine (CIM) can be defined in a variety of ways. The primary definition describes complementary medicine as "any practice that can be used for the prevention and treatment of diseases, but which is not taught widely in medical schools, not generally available in hospitals, and not usually covered by health insurance." Similarly, Andrew Weil, MD, defines integrative medicine as "a healing-oriented medicine that draws upon all therapeutic systems to form a comprehensive approach to the art and science of medicine." CIM is also known as complementary and alternative medicine (CAM).

Some of the more commonly and widely accepted therapies originated in Asia thousands of years ago, while others were developed in Europe and America during the past few decades. There are many examples of CIM therapies, as noted in Figure 6-1.

THE RISE OF COMPLEMENTARY AND ALTERNATIVE THERAPIES

Conventional medicine started approximately 200 years ago, whereas alternative therapies have been present since civilization began. For example, the Bible makes reference to the healing applications of aloe vera. During the mid-

twentieth century, there was a rapid elimination of CIM, as it was often considered to be quackery or charlatanism. As a result, physicians today tend to disregard practices that are not validated by double-blind, randomized, placebo-controlled studies. But clearly it is difficult, if not impossible, to randomize and placebo-control every type of therapeutic intervention.

In spite of the lack of scientific research, there has been an astounding increase in the use of CIM therapies. Americans spent approximately $27 billion in 1998 and $32 billion in 2000 on alternative therapies. Roughly 40%–50% of all Americans have tried some form of alternative therapy, according to a recent report in the *Journal of the American Medical Association*. The concerning aspect of that article is the fact that of the Americans using CIM, 70% do not tell their physicians (Eisenberg et al., 1998). That fact is quite alarming, since many of the herbal supplements, as well as some nutritional supplements, can interfere with common medications, at times with potentially life-threatening effects.

Increasingly, patients are requesting to see a physician who is at least open to considering CIM therapies, particularly where conventional therapies may be less effective. Currently, approximately 75% of medical schools are offering courses on alternative medicine. It is becoming a reality that physicians must learn about CIM. Under the best circumstances, expertise should be utilized from a variety of practitioners and collaborations between physicians and people who practice CIM should become routine. Currently, that is frontier territory, but it might be the best-case scenario for patients.

The Holistic Approach

There continues to be a significant increase in both use and acceptance of CIM by Americans. There are many reasons cited for considering CIM, including dissatisfaction with conventional medicine, which is perceived to be authoritative, expensive, ineffective, and too intent on curing disease rather than focusing on wellness and prevention of disease. Additionally, market-driven forces; the desire of patients to have a more active role in their medical care; and the mere fact that conventional medicine fails to satisfactorily treat chronic ailments such as back pain, fibromyalgia,

- Acupuncture
- Alexander technique
- Biofeedback
- Chiropractic
- Energy healing
- Feldenkrais technique
- Folk remedies
- Homeopathy
- Herbal supplements
- Hypnotherapy
- Imagery
- Magnet therapy

- Massage therapy
- Megavitamin therapy
- Naturopathy
- Neuromuscular therapy
- Prayer
- Reflexology
- Relaxation
- Remote healing
- Rolfing
- Self-help groups
- Spiritual healing by others
- Therapeutic touch

Figure 6-1: Examples of complementary and integrative medicine therapies.

chronic headache, cancer, tinnitus, and vertigo continue to be an impetus for patients to seek out CIM therapies. Thus, many patients who are frustrated with their lack of improvement often consider alternative strategies.

The philosophy for CIM practitioners is not intended to be divisive, but rather collaborative.

CIM practitioners not only rely on the consideration of the body alone, but also embrace the less tangible yet very real effects of the mind and spirit. CIM professionals attempt to mobilize and enhance the healing ability inherent in each person, and they recognize that they are in partnership with their patients and that treatment is directed toward the unique goals and values of each individual.

Prior to the time of René Descartes, the "healing" of patients embraced and acknowledged the inseparability of the body, mind, and spirit. In the 1600s, Descartes initiated the modern-day premise that human health is rooted in tangible science; and he sought to separate the body, mind, and spirit (Figure 6-2). That thinking fostered the current conventional Western medical paradigm that diseases are derived solely from perturbations of cellular and organ dysfunction. CIM, on the other hand, does not necessarily refute this end-stage situation, but, rather, tries to unlock the root cause of those cellular and organ perturbations. Furthermore, the CIM paradigm suggests that the domains of body, mind, and spirit are inseparable and gradually become "out of balance" because of many influences including but not limited to the following: structural and ingrained movement patterns; hormonal, nutritional, and genetic influences; behavioral, stress, and emotional patterns; support and faith; personal past; and environmental factors. Once the threshold of "imbalance" is reached, disease processes are initiated.

Origins in Philosophy

The pre-Descartes era shows the body, mind, and spirit as integral components of health, whereas in the post-Descartes era, those elements were separated.

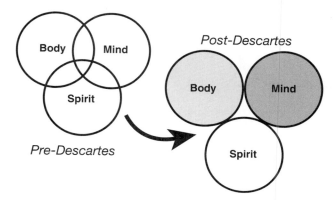

Descartes (in 1600s) initiated thinking of distinct domains of human "construction" and the exactness of science

Figure 6-2: The interrelationship of the body, mind, and spirit in the pre-Descartes era. Descartes suggested that a more scientific and logical approach would be to separate the body, mind, and spirit, which is demonstrated at the right side of the pictorial.

The conventional Western paradigm says that diseases are caused by internal cellular and organ dysfunction (Figure 6-3). As a result, more than 99% of all research funding in the United States is aimed at therapies focused on the body, whereas the mind and spirit are rarely investigated.

Conversely, the holistic or integrative medicine paradigm suggests that the domains of the body, mind, and spirit are inseparable and that disease signals an imbalance (Figure 6-4). Optimal treatment involves addressing all domains together. Clearly, the effects of structural movement patterns and hormonal, nutritional, and genetic forces (as well as personal past, emotion, stress, and behavior patterns) all play a role in the body, mind, and spirit and should not be separated. In the holistic paradigm, it is believed that imbalances of the body, mind, and spirit are the cause of cellular and organ dysfunction. The two-part question then becomes When are cellular and organ changes the result of disease rather than the cause, and are both hypotheses possible?

Conventional western hypothesis: diseases are *caused* by *internal* cellular/organ dysfunction

Post-Descartes

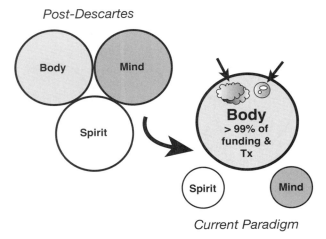

Current Paradigm

Figure 6-3: The separation of body, mind, and spirit (Descartes ideology) and the new complementary integrative paradigm suggesting the importance of the body as a whole, thereby rejoining the consideration of the body, mind, and spirit. The conventional Western paradigm suggests that cellular derangements are responsible for disease processes and does not consider the importance of the mind or spirit. Additionally, the majority of funding is aimed at processes other than the mind and spirit.

Holistic/integrative medicine paradigm-hypotheses: The domains of B-M-S are inseparable and out of balance in disease. Optimal treatment involves addressing all domains *together*.

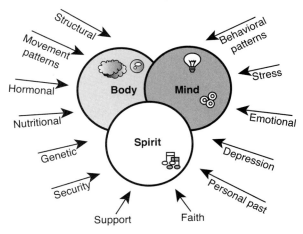

Figure 6-4: The separation of body, mind, and spirit seems illogical and perhaps derangements in body, mind, or spirit cause disease. Other factors that affect the person as a whole need to be considered in the paradigm of complementary and integrative medicine and holistic ideology.

Following the Money: NIH Funding for CIM versus Non-CIM Research

While skepticism is healthy and important, a closed mind prevents the consideration of potentially beneficial therapies. In 1992, because of public pressure, a congressional mandate established the National Center for Complementary and Alternative Medicine (NCCAM) with an initial endowment of approximately $2 million. That figure has grown dramatically; in 2005, the funding pool through NCCAM was approximately $117.7 million.

While $117 million may seem substantial, that figure should be considered in context. The total NIH budget is greater than $16 billion, of which $3 billion is spent on cancer, $1.8 billion is spent on AIDS, and $1.6 billion is spent on allergies and infectious disease. So, clearly, CIM research is not high on the list of priorities.

Consumer spending on CIM therapies, however, grows each year. In 1997, out-of-pocket expenditures for CIM therapies versus conventional services in the United States showed that consumers were spending between $27 and $34 billion per annum; and that amount increases each year. Meanwhile, U.S. physician services were costing $29 billion and an additional $9 billion was spent on hospitalizations in this country. It has also been shown that there were 629 visits to CIM practitioners in 1997—a trend that is growing—whereas visits to primary care physicians during that same year in the United States totaled 386 million, a figure that is declining.

Blending Conventional Medicine with CIM

It is important for medical practitioners to consider integration of conventional medicine and CIM very seriously. There is not only an increase in public interest in alternative therapies, but also a growing awareness of the effectiveness of healing traditions from around the world (such as acupuncture and herbal therapies) on the part of consumers as well as the scientific community.

Generally speaking, chronic health problems respond well to a holistic approach based on state-of-the-art conventional medicine in addition to nutrition, emotional influences, structural abnormalities, energy flow, and belief system. Many disorders simply do not respond well to conventional therapeutic intervention, including tinnitus and vertigo, chronic back pain, arthritis, headache, fibromyalgia, and cancer. It is becoming increasingly clear that the best practices involve providing patients with healing options. Even the most open-minded provider cannot be an expert in all therapies, be aware of all of the options that are available, know what the research supports, and know where to refer people. Providers must be honest with patients, especially when they do not know about a treatment modality. Providers must avoid stating that something is harmful or has no evidence behind it when they have not actually investigated the subject, just as it is essential, above all, that they do no harm.

Alternative Medicine or Mainstream Treatment?

What is considered "alternative medicine" in the United States is very likely mainstream in another country. Hypercholesterolemia is a classic example. Typically, the first line of therapy in the United States is to talk to the patient about dietary modification and then often prescribe a statinlike medication. In Europe, the first line of therapy is also dietary counseling. But that is followed by a recommendation for red yeast rice, an Asian favorite that acts as a statin, and the Ayurvedic remedy gugulipid, derived from the resin of the mukul myrrh tree.

Generally speaking, both of those compounds can successfully lower cholesterol and have a much lower risk/benefit profile than statins. So why is red yeast rice not readily available in the United States? Although it comes from a natural source, the chemical composition of red yeast rice is very similar to statins, a fact that led the pharmaceutical industry to force the Food and Drug Administration (FDA) to order the product be removed from the U.S. market.

SUPPLEMENTS AND THE LAW

To help patients find solutions to health problems, medical professionals need to be aware of the benefits of specific nutraceuticals and herbs, as well as some of the science behind them. In addition, it is important that they understand the Dietary Supplement Health and Education Act of 1994 (DSHEA). The act was designed to allow consumers a certain amount of latitude in the purchase of nutritional supplements and to provide a reasonable degree of safety. The DSHEA law places the responsibility of safety on the manufacturer and specifies the use of literature in connection with sales. It also specifies allowable claims on labels and delineates labeling requirements while establishing regulations for good manufacturing processes.

Many herbs can be used for medicinal purposes. Some of the more common herbs are listed in Table 6-1; it also provides details such as claims information, specific actions when known, contraindications, potential side effects, interactions, and dosages when available.

Drawbacks and Downsides of Herbs

There is always concern about whether a specific supplement contains precisely what the manufacturer claims. Unfortunately, there have been many examples suggesting that that is not always the case. But increasingly, herbal remedies are being sold with standardization information included on the labels. For the time being, the consumer must take the manufacturers at their word because this area is not tightly regulated by the FDA.

Another problem is that most consumers and practitioners have limited or false information about herbs. One of the most reputable references with regard to the medicinal use of herbs is the Complete German Commission E. This commission provides monographs on hundreds of herbs, rating them as either positive or negative. Typically, an herb that is rated positively has reasonable scientific support and data to validate its use. An herb with a negative rating may be ineffective, unsafe, or simply not studied to the extent that sufficient information is available.

Table 6-1. Commonly used supplements

Herbal Supplement	Indications	Actions	Contraindications	Side Effects	Interactions	Dosage
Echinacea	Treatment and prevention of the common cold and flu	Immunostimulant Enhances phagocytosis	Autoimmune or chronic illness Allergy to flowers of the daisy family	Minor gastrointestinal irritation Increased urination Mild allergic reactions	Immune suppressants (i.e, Neoral, Prednisone, Imuran, and Methotreaxate)	Powder extract: 300 mg cap/TID Alcohol tincture (1:5): 3–4 ml TID Juice: 203 ml TID Whole dried root: 102 g TID
Goldenseal	Topical antibiotic for wounds that are not healing well Mouth sores and sore throats	Strong activity against a wide variety of bacteria and fungi	Pregnancy	Gastrointestinal distress Increased nervousness		Cream: cover entire surface of the wound Tincture: swished or gargled Tea: 0.5–1g in a cup of water
Kava Kava	Mild to moderate anxiety Insomnia	Anti-anxiety Mild analgesic Muscle relaxant Anticonvulsant	Pregnancy Nursing mothers Endogenous depression	Mild gastrointestinal irritation Drowsiness Yellowish skin discoloration Balance disturbance Skin rash Enlargement of pupils	Benzodiazepine Buspirone Alcohol Barbiturates Antidepressant Antipsychotic	Standardized extract: 140–240 mg in 2 or 3 divided doses (30%–70% kavalactones)
Ginseng	Tonic Stimulant Diuretic Diabetic impotence	Physiologic effects Lowers blood pressure Depresses CNS activity Stimulates immune system	Coagulopathy Diabetes Insomnia Schizophrenia Cardiac disease	Bleeding Hypotension Hypoglycemia Insomnia	Medications for psychosis and diabetes MAO inhibitors Stimulants Coumadin Caffeine	American: Root: 0.25–0.5 po BID Asian (Panax): 0.6–3 gm 1–3 times daily
Gingko Biloba	Dementia Improved cognitive, sexual, and GI functions Dizziness/Tinnitus	8 CNS blood flow Neuroprotective Free radical 9 capillary fragility	If the patient is on anticoagulants	Anticoagulants Spontaneous bleeding	Cyclosporin SSRIs MAO inhibitors Thiazide diuretics Anticoagulant properties may induce seizures and infertility	120–480 mg/day in 2–33 divided doses
Saw Palmetto	Anti-inflammatory 8 Urinary flow Symptoms of BPH	Inhibits dihydrotestosterone Diuretic Anti-androgenic	Do not take while on prescription BPH treatment	None	Caution with diuretics	160 mg BID

Table 6-1. (continued)

Herbal Supplement	Indications	Actions	Contraindications	Side Effects	Interactions	Dosage
Pygeum Africanum	Symptoms of BPH Anti-inflammatory Diuretic, 9-cholesterol	Antiproliferative effect on fibroblast	None reported	Nausea and abdominal pain	None known	50–200 mg stand ext/day
Guarana	Stimulant, headache, & energy	Sympathomimetic Caffeinelike activities	Cardiac problems Renal disease HTN or hyperthyroidism	8 Heart rate HTN Anxiety Arrythmias	Avoid other stimulants	2x as strong as caffeine
Feverfew	Migraine Rheumatoid arthritis	Inhibits serotonin release	Aster family allergies Avoid during pregnancy	GI upset 6%–15% first week of use	Anticoagulants (inhibit cyclooxygenic)	50 mg–1.2 gm/d equivalent to 0.2–0.6
Hawthorne	Atherosclerosis Arrhythmia	Improves cardiac output and coronary blood flow	Do not use with other inotropes	Mildly sedative	Digitalis Fox Glove	160–900 mg/D
Fox Glove						
Black Cohosh	Menopause Astringent Emmenagogue Diuretic intake Expectorant Vertigo Tinnitus	Estrogen-like action, oxytocic Luteinizing hormone suppression Binds to estrogen receptors	None known	Occasional GI upset Nausea, headache, and dizziness in high doses	None known	Extracts w/alcohol: 40%–60% (v/v) corresponds to 40 mg drug Galenical prep for oral
Garlic	Reduces levels of lipids in blood Prevents age-dependent vascular changes 9 Cholesterol 10%–12%	Antibacterial Antimycotic Lipid-lowering Inhibition of platelet aggregation Prolongation of bleed and clotting time Enhances fibrinolytic activity	None known	GI upset Allergic reactions Odor may pervade breath and skin	Anticoagulants Hypoglycemics	4 g fresh garlic (minced bulb and prep is taken orally)
Pulsatilla	Sedative, headaches Fluid in the ears	Antispasmodic Increases circulation	Avoid during pregnancy			

Table 6-1. (continued)

Herbal Supplement	Indications	Actions	Contraindications	Side Effects	Interactions	Dosage
St. John's Wort	Dizziness/Tinnitus Mild to moderate depression Viral infections Wound healing	Antidepressant Weak MAOI SSRI and DA agonist	Avoid during pregnancy	Photosensitivity	Antidepressants MAOI Antiseizure medications	300 mg TID
Ma Haung	Asthma Bronchial edema (weight loss—not an approved use) Stimulant	Sympathomimetic bronchodilator	Cardiac problems Anxiety Hypertension Angle closure glaucoma Pheochromocytoma Thyrotoxicant	HTN, neurosis, insomnia, palpitations, and hyperglycemia Death	Halothone Cardiac glycosides MAOI Quanethidine Oxytosh	15–30 mg total alkaloid or 300 mg herb/d

Making an Example of Echinacea

The herb Echinacea provides a good example of some of the issues involved in herbal remedies. Echinacea is a very popular herb with a reputation for warding off the common cold and flu type illnesses. What most people do not realize is that there are nine different subtypes of echinacea, including *Echinacea purpurea, Echinacea pallida,* and *Echinacea angustafolia.* Besides each subtype having different health benefits, those benefits vary depending on the part of the plant used. The leaf of *Echinacea purpurea,* for example, has been shown to enhance T- and B-cell functions, whereas the root of that same plant does not. Conversely, the *Echinacea pallida* root has been shown to enhance T- and B-cell function, but the leaf of that same plant does not. Meanwhile, *Echinacea angustafolia* is rated as a negative herb by the German Commission E. Yet on a recent visit to a health food store, there were more than one-hundred bottles of echinacea on the shelves and 95% of them contained *Echinacea angustafolia!*

Why would the market be filled with *Echinacea angustafolia* if it is a negatively rated herb? One explanation is that manufacturers are not doing their homework. Another possibility is that it is a much less expensive or more available herb. Nutritional products that contain *Echinacea purpurea* leaf and *pallida* root are to be considered, both of which have been clearly shown in scientific studies to enhance and activate T- and B-cell functions, to encourage phagocytosis, and to have antibacterial and antiviral properties. Unfortunately, if a study is conducted with a product made from *Echinacea angustafolia,* the results are likely to indicate that it does not work in treating cold or flu symptoms. Studies like that cast doubt on all herbal remedies.

The Limits of Knowledge

Drug/herb interactions are another poorly understood area. Echinacea, for example, may interfere with Neoral, prednisone, Imuran, and methotrexate. Furthermore, consumers and physicians should understand that immunostimulants such as echinacea and the herb goldenseal should not be used for prolonged periods of time. There are also contraindications for patients who have immune disorders or severe infections such as tuberculosis.

When Good Herbs Go Bad

Another area of concern involving herbs is misuse. Ephedra (*Ephedra sinica*), also known by its Chinese name *Ma huang,* is a very popular herb with a long history of use in Asia. Ephedra is an excellent medication for treating asthma and other disorders where bronchodilation is important because it is a known sympathomimetic and bronchodilator. Unfortunately, it also can cause anxiety, hypertension, angle closure glaucoma, insomnia, palpitations, hyperglycemia, and even death. In addition, ephedra has strong interactions with halothane, cardiac glycosides, MAOI, oxytocin, guanethidine, and others.

In recent years, ephedra became a primary ingredient in herbal weight-loss products, as well as energy-boosting supplements and athletic performance enhancers. Product abuse occurred that reportedly contributed to instances of heart attack, stroke, and death. In December 2003, the FDA banned the sale of products containing ephedra. That was the first supplement ban enacted by the DSHEA legislation. Clearly, it is an example of government regulation likely saving lives. But many people are concerned that those regulations can go too far and be applied to less potentially dangerous supplements such vitamins C and E.

Putting Herbs in Perspective

As was mentioned earlier, many times patients do not volunteer information to their physicians regarding their use of CIM therapies. So it is important for health care providers to ask patients specifically about the use of nutraceuticals and herbs. Proven therapeutic options should be discussed. If a viable alternative exists, it should be considered, bearing in mind, of course, that natural does not necessarily mean safe. As always, one needs to be concerned about quality control and standardization and realize that herbal/pharmaceutical interactions do occur with some frequency. It is important to ask what disease or condition is being treated, what the conventional therapeutic option is, what the benefit from the alternatives is, what risks exist, what the cost is, and whether the alternative works? Oftentimes, caution and common sense are enough; but health practitioners who are uninformed about CIM remedies may be their own worst enemy.

Health care professionals should also put nutraceutical safety issues in perspective. According to one study, the average annual mortality rates over the past twelve years show that deaths related to vitamin use occur at approximately one death per year and herbs cause two deaths per year, whereas smoking is responsible for more than 400,000 deaths per year, poor diet is linked to 300,000 deaths each year, and pharmaceutical errors contribute to more than 100,000 deaths each year. Thus, it is not very likely that anyone will be harmed with nutritional or herbal therapies.

As for concerns about the lack of FDA scrutiny of supplements, it is becoming increasingly clear that FDA approval cannot in and of itself guarantee safety, as shown by the recently discovered link between COX-2 inhibitors and an increased risk of heart disease.

THE ABCS OF SUPPLEMENTS

Vitamins and minerals are crucial for many different bodily functions. A number of multivitamins provide the standard vitamins and minerals, but no single pill exists that can provide everything the body needs. Typically, it takes two to four pills a day to obtain the necessary nutrients. Thus, supplements that fit into one pill per day cannot nearly provide the doses necessary to be protective. It is best when the ingredients are natural and minerals are chelated. *Chelating* means that an amino acid is bound to the mineral. Thus, for example, when physicians recommend Tums as a good source of calcium, that is a fallacy. Tums is delivered as a nonchelated calcium—as calcium carbonate, which is the same chemical formula as stone. The absorption of calcium carbonate is approximately 2%–4%. Thus, it is recommended that a chelated calcium such as calcium glycinate, gluconate, or citrate be used. Furthermore, an added benefit is when the supplement is produced in an FDA-inspected laboratory. In addition, antioxidants should have powerful molecular and cellular compounds that are effective and well absorbed. While the standard vitamins C and E are important, it is also necessary to have minerals to support those vitamins. Additionally, certain compounds should be in any antioxidant, including n-acetyl cysteine, resveratrol (grape seed extract), and coenzyme Q10. Obtaining sufficient antioxidant protection may require an additional two to four pills a day.

Many nutrition experts believe that the current vitamin and mineral guidelines are insufficient. The Recommended Dietary Allowances (RDA), or dietary reference intakes (DRIs), were established by the Food and Nutrition Board in 1941. They are considered the best scientific judgment on nutritional allowances and are designed to meet the nutrient needs of most healthy people. While the RDAs are safe and adequate nutrient levels, they are neither minimal requirements nor optimal levels.

To Supplement or Not to Supplement?

Many physicians suggest that people with low stress levels who consume a healthy diet, including five to ten helpings of fruits and vegetables a day, do not need nutritional supplements. It is clear, however, that most of the American population (most of the world population, for that matter) does not follow those guidelines. Even if the guidelines were followed, the levels of supplements required to have a protective or healthful effect could not be easily consumed with a healthy diet.

As Oregon State University's Moret Traber observed, "To obtain enough vitamin E from food to obtain a reduction in the risk of cardiovascular disease and possibly cancer you would need to consume nine tablespoons of olive oil, 75 slices of whole wheat bread, and 40 almonds or 200 peanuts each and every day." Clearly, it is not practical to get sufficient vitamins and minerals from food alone.

Food: Friend and Foe

Furthermore, it is becoming increasingly clear that one must be very careful when it comes to food choices. The dangers of eating farmed salmon, for example, were detailed in a recent report published in *Science* (Hites et al., 2004). Scientists at Indiana University's School of Public and Environmental Affairs analyzed more than two metric tons of farmed and wild salmon from all over the world for organochlorine contaminants. They found that farmed salmon had consistently higher levels of those toxins than wild fish. In addition, the results also showed that European-raised salmon were far more contaminated than those from North or South America. According to the study's risk analysis, eating heavily contaminated salmon could counteract the health benefits of the omega-3 essential fatty acids found in the fish.

HEARING AND CIM

What about hearing and nutrition? Many people are surprised to discover that there is a solid connection, as research has demonstrated. One study supplemented eighteen- to twenty-month-old rats with either oral phosphatidylcholine (lecithin) or a placebo. The subjects were followed for six months and underwent testing that included auditory brainstem responses, flow cytometry to measure reactive oxygen species generation, and mitochondrial DNA deletion studies to assess the effect of supplements on energy production at the molecular level. The studies showed that the lecithin-treated subjects lost approximately 12–15 dB of hearing, while the control group lost approximately 35–40 dB of hearing over the six-month time period. In other words, lecithin had a protective effect on hearing. Production of reactive oxygen species was significantly less in the lecithin group as compared to the placebo-treated group. Additionally, the studies showed that mitochondrial function was significantly enhanced with the lecithin group, which means that the cell produces energy in a safer, more efficient manner (Seidman et al., 2002).

Ongoing studies funded by the NIH are investigating the effects of resveratrol on noise- and age-related hearing loss. The published noise studies have shown that resveratrol is protective from noise-induced hearing loss (Babu et al., 2003). Furthermore, the studies looking at the aging model also are quite encouraging.

Protecting Hearing with Antioxidants

Another study assessed the efficacy of **acetyl-L-carnitine,** an antioxidant that has been shown to restore mitochondrial membrane potential, a measure that significantly declines with age. A laboratory demonstrated that acetyl-L-carnitine reduced age-related hearing loss by enhancing mitochondrial function. Additionally, subjects were treated with **alpha lipoic acid,** a very powerful antioxidant with shown therapeutic benefits for diabetes mellitus and cognitive problems. This specific nutritional supplement has been shown to improve hearing. Together with acetyl-L-carnitine, alpha lipoic acid has been shown to reduce the mitochondrial DNA damage that occurs within the cochlea and the brain (Seidman et al., 2000). Other studies have shown that those compounds will enhance cognitive abilities (Gadaleta et al., 1994) and restore energy levels and mitochondrial function to a more youthful state (Ames et al., 2004).

Calorie Restriction Enhances Effects

In another clinical trial, animals were followed from three months of age to the day they died. One group received a calorie-restricted diet shown to reduce reactive oxygen species generation and to increase life span. For purposes of comparison, a placebo-controlled group was allowed to eat *ad libitum*. Other groups were treated with specific antioxidants, including vitamins E and C and the hormone **melatonin.** This study demonstrated that reactive oxygen species and damage to the mitochondria that occurs with aging leads to presbyacusis. Furthermore, the study demonstrated that caloric restriction and nutrients reduce the progression of age-related hearing loss. It was suspected that a combination therapy would likely provide a synergistic protective effect on presbyacusis and possibly on aging as well (Seidman et al., 2000).

Making Sense of Studies

While important, these single studies do not necessarily change the way doctors practice medicine. Typically, it takes a study, like the one done at the Harvard School of Public Health in 1998, to effect change. That study, involving more than 80,000 women, determined that folic acid and vitamin B6 supplements reduced the risk of heart disease. Conversely, the researchers noted that the opposite scenario—a low intake of folic acid and B6—led to an increased risk of heart disease (Rimm et al., 1998).

While many physicians believe that landmark studies such as that one must be done before existing recommendations can be changed, doing so is not feasible. That type of study costs tens of millions of dollars and takes years to complete. Many other prior studies demonstrated the beneficial effects of increasing folic acid and vitamin B6 intake. Many physicians believed that there was enough evidence to increase the RDA of folic acid from 50 mcg to 400 mcg. But it wasn't until this study came out that the change was actually made. Because of the reluctance to update recommendations, there is a lag of twenty-five to thirty years between research being done in a specific area of nutritional sciences and mainstream guidelines.

Results May Vary

Another complicating factor in establishing uniform guidelines for supplement intake comes from conflicting findings. One example is a two-year study conducted at Wake Forest University that looked at nondisabling stroke in a group of 3,680 adults supplemented with 2.5 mg of folate (a very high dose), 25 mg of B6, and 0.4 mg of B12. That combination lowered homocysteine levels by approximately 2 micromoles per liter, but it had no effect on ischemic stroke, myocardial infarction, or death (Toole et al., 2004).

Conversely, a British study published two years earlier had shown that reducing homocysteine levels by 3 micromoles per liter led to a 24% reduction in the risk of cerebral vascular accidents and a 16% lower risk of myocardial infarction (Wald et al., 2002).

Conflicting research findings are a fact of life in the medical profession. As long as there are scientists and questions to be asked, there will always be a potential disparity in the results. Health care practitioners must review the research and reconcile the discrepancies for their patients. Based on the most recent body of data, all adults should take a good multivitamin, a good antioxidant, and other nutritional supplements. That will protect overall health as well as hearing at a reasonable cost with very little risk and considerable reward.

SUMMARY

Although many CIM remedies have been in existence for thousands of years, there is a lack of randomized, double-blind, placebo-controlled studies supporting their efficacy. As a result, many health care professionals are skeptical and hesitant to recommend CIM modalities. It is clear, however, that there is tremendous public interest in alternative therapies, particularly in those areas that are difficult to treat with conventional medicine. Statistics show that the amount of money the public is spending on CIM is increasing each year. And with increased funding now available from the NIH, preliminary research is showing that certain CIM remedies are appropriate for treating a number of acute and chronic health conditions. Because of that fact, medical professionals need to familiarize themselves with those options. In addition, modalities considered to be "alternative" are actually mainstream and accepted practices elsewhere in the world.

Since the anecdotal evidence outweighs proof from clinical trials in the area of CIM, it is not always easy to determine what works and what does not. That results in herbal products of varying quality and effectiveness. One source of reliable information is Germany's prestigious Commission E, which publishes monographs on hundreds of herbs, reviewing scientific evidence and defining appropriate use.

The United States has nothing similar to Commission E. Consumer protection is provided by the Dietary Supplement Health and Education Act of 1994 (DSHEA), which allows the federal government to remove from the market products that may endanger the public's health.

According to one school of thought, DSHEA could be used to restrict consumers' access to common vitamins and minerals; but thus far that has not occurred.

Then there is the question of whether supplements are necessary. A considerable body of evidence suggests that the answer to that question is yes. While conflicting study results can be confusing to the general public, health care practitioners should be aware of the important role that vitamins, minerals, and other supplements play in overall health. Although the public is encouraged to adopt a healthy lifestyle, engage in stress reduction, eat a nutritious diet, eliminate tobacco use, use alcohol in moderation, and obtain adequate exercise, few people actually follow those guidelines. As a result, vitamin, mineral, and antioxidant supplements not only are necessary, but also are recommended by an increasing number of health authorities. With both public interest and scientific research in CIM on the rise, the profession is certain to experience a great deal of change in the near future. It is essential that health care practitioners remain current in this increasingly evolving field for the sake of the patients and the profession.

REFERENCES

Ames, B. N. (2004). Delaying the mitochondrial decay of aging. *Annals of the New York Academy of Science, 1019*, 406–411.

Eisenberg, D. M., Davis, R. B., Ettner, S. L., Appel, S., Wilkey, S., Van Rompay, M., & Kessler, R. C. (1998). Trends in alternative medicine use in the United States, 1990–1997: Results of a follow-up national survey. *Journal of the American Medical Association, 280*(18), 1569–1575.

Gadaleta, M. N., Petruzalla, V., Daddabbo, L., et al. (1994). Mitochondrial DNA transcription and translation in aged rat: Effect of acetyl-L-carnitine. *Annals of the New York Academy of Science, 717*, 150–160.

Hites, R. A., Foran, J. A., Carpenter, D. O., Hamilton, M. C., Knuth, B. A., & Schwager, S. J. (2004). Global assessment of organic contaminants in farmed salmon. *Science, 303*(5655), 226–229.

Kopke, R. D., Coleman, J. K., Liu, J., Campbell, K. C., & Riffenburgh, R. H. (2002). Candidate's thesis: enhancing intrinsic cochlear stress defenses to reduce noise-induced hearing loss. *Laryngoscope, 112*(9), 1515–1532.

Rimm, E. B., Willett, W. C., Hu, F. B., Sampson, L., Colditz, G. A., Manson, J. E., Hennekens, C., & Stampfer, M. J. (1998). Folate and vitamin B6 from diet and supplements in relation to risk of coronary heart disease among women. *Journal of the American Medical Association, 279*(5), 392–393.

Seidman, M. D. (1997). Nutritional/herbal therapies for the common cold/flu. Retrieved from http://www.bodylangvitamin.com

Seidman, M. D. (2000). Effects of dietary restriction and antioxidants on presbyacusis. *Laryngoscope, 110*(5 Pt 1), 727–738

Seidman, M. D., Babu, S., Tang, W. X., Naem, E., & Quirk, W. S. (2003). Effect of Resveratrol on Acoustic Trauma. *Otolaryngology—Head and Neck Surgery, 129*(5), 463–470.

Seidman, M. D., Khan, M. J., Bai, U., Shirwany, N., & Quirk, W. S. (2000). Biologic activity of mitochondrial metabolites on aging and age-related hearing loss. *American Journal of Otolaryngology, 21*(2), 161–167.

Seidman, M. D., Khan, M. J., Tang, W. X., & Quirk, W. S. (2002). Influence of lecithin on mitochondrial DNA and age-related hearing loss. *Otolaryngology—Head and Neck Surgery, 127*(3), 138–144.

Toole, J. F., Malinow, M. R., Chambless, L. E., Spence, J. D., Pettigrew, L. C., Howard, V. J., Sides, E. G., Wang, C. H., & Stampfer, M. (2004). Lowering homocysteine in patients with ischemic stroke to prevent recurrent stroke, myocardial infarction, and death: the Vitamin Intervention for Stroke Prevention (VISP) randomized controlled trial. *Journal of the American Medical Association, 291*(5), 565–575.

Wald, D. S., Law, M., & Morris, J. K. (2002). Homocysteine and cardiovascular disease: Evidence on causality from a meta-analysis. *British Medical Journal, 325*(7374), 1202.

www.bodylangvitamin.com. See Educational Resources and view the PowerPoint presentation titled "Nutritional/herbal therapies for the common cold/flu".

CHAPTER 7

Mechanisms of Toxicity in the Cochlea (Including Physical, Free Radical: Oxidative and Anti-Oxidative Mechanisms, Protein Interactions, and Defense Mechanisms)

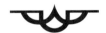

Jing Wang, MD, PhD

Jean-Luc Puel, PhD

Inserm: U 583, INM-Hôpital St Eloi

MONTPELLIER

France

Richard Bobbin, PhD

Kresge Hearing Research Laboratory

Department of Otolaryngology

Louisiana State University Health Sciences Center

533 Bolivar Street, 5th Floor

New Orleans, LA

Acknowledgments: We thank Dr. C. Bonny for the gift of D-JNKI-1. These studies were supported, in part, by the Association pour la Recherche sur le Cancer (ARC), by the Ligue Contre le Cancer (Comité de l'Hérault), and by sanofi-aventis.

INTRODUCTION

Certain cells in the auditory system die during the normal developmental processes. In addition, after maturity, the hair cells and nerve fibers die because of aging processes, intense sound exposure, and the ingestion or exposure to ototoxic drugs and chemicals such as aminoglycosides (e.g., kanamycin, neomycin, and gentamycin), anticancer agents (e.g., cisplatin, cis-diamine-dichloroplatinum II, CDDP), and organic solvents. Most importantly, in mammals, the hair cells and nerve fibers do not regenerate. One of the goals of audiologists is to prevent cell death in the auditory system. That can be accomplished by educating patients and physicians about toxic effects of sound and chemical agents. In addition, hearing can be monitored before and during exposure to document any ill effects. The goal of research in the area is to learn how to prevent cell death by these various toxic agents. That is accomplished first by elucidating the molecular mechanisms whereby the cells die upon exposure to the toxic agent. Once the molecular mechanisms are understood, agents can be administered that prevent the sequence of events that are triggered, leading to eventual cell death. This chapter outlines some of what is known about the mechanisms of cell death and describes treatments that hold promise for preventing cell death in the auditory system.

MECHANISMS OF CELL DEATH

Mechanisms by which cells die have been classified into two general types: necrosis and **programmed cell death (PCD)**. **Necrosis** is considered to be a passive cellular event characterized by the formation of vacuoles in the cytoplasm, swelling of **mitochondria**, dilation of the **endoplasmic reticulum**, cellular debris, and disintegration or a loss of cell membrane integrity and **organelle** membrane integrity (Artal-Sanz & Tavernarakis, 2005). Necrosis is usually due to severe cellular stress or damage induced by mechanical means; lack of blood or a nutritional supply; or exposure to certain toxic organisms, agents, or chemicals.

An example of necrosis is the exposure to extremely high noise intensity (at least 130 dB SPL), which causes direct mechanical destruction of the sensory hair cells and supporting cells in the organ of Corti, most probably by rupture of the cell membrane (Hamernik et al., 1984). PCD, or genetic cell death, is a naturally occurring, active event involving the triggering of a set of molecular events that have been preprogrammed into the **genes** or molecular machinery of the cell (Strasser et al., 2000). An example of PCD is the cell death that occurs normally during embryonic development, where it has been estimated that up to 50% of vertebrate neurons die during this period (Raff et al., 1993). In contrast to necrosis and PCD, after death of an organ or organism, the cells typically undergo autolysis. **Autolysis** is defined as "the breakdown of intracellular structures due to enzymes within the cell that results in the appearance of vacuoles in the cytoplasm with an intact cell membrane."

PROGRAMMED CELL DEATH (PCD) AND CASPASES

Currently, PCD has been classified into three types: apoptotic or nuclear (type 1), autophagic (type 2), and non-lysosomal vesiculate (or cytoplasmic) (type 3) (Clarke, 1990). The most understood pathway is the apoptotic pathway and the one emphasized here (Sperandio et al., 2004). **Apoptosis** is an active cellular process of PCD characterized morphologically by cell shrinkage; membrane blebbing; **chromatin** condensation; intracellular fragmentation associated with membrane-enclosed cellular fragments called apoptotic bodies, causing an increased electron density of the cytoplasm; and fragmentation of the deoxyribonucleic acid (DNA) in the nucleus of the cell (Strasser et al., 2000). Those effects are largely achieved by activation of a **cascade** of events involving the activation of a group of **enzymes** called caspases that cleave proteins (i.e., **proteases**) (Gorman et al., 1998). Caspases represent a family of at least 14 cysteine-dependent and aspartate-specific proteases (Strasser et al., 2000; Stennicke & Salvesen, 2000). Proteases are usually synthesized as **zymogens** that are inactive and must be converted by limited proteolysis into active enzymes. However, the zymogens of some caspases (i.e., initiator caspases) have proteolytic activity that allows them to initiate apoptosis by a mechanism called homo-activation (Stennicke & Salvesen, 2000). That contrasts with hetero-activation, where a protease acts on the caspase zymogen (i.e., pro-caspase) to produce the active caspase molecule. Initiator caspases (e.g., caspase-8, caspase-9, and caspase-10) can start the program sequence, leading to a cascade and amplification of events by activation of a series of effectors or executioner caspases (e.g., caspase-3, caspase-6, and caspase-7) (Strasser et al., 2000). The executioner caspases induce cell death by cleaving proteins necessary for cell survival (e.g., cytoskeletal proteins, DNA-repairing enzymes, cell cycle proteins, and enzymes involved in **signal transduction**) (Artal-Sanz & Tavernarakis, 2005).

APOPTOSIS AND DEATH SIGNALING PATHWAYS

Death Receptor Apoptosis Pathway

The apoptotic program can be initiated by factors acting via an extrinsic (extracellular) or an intrinsic (intracellular) route. The major extrinsic signal pathway that leads to apoptosis of cells involves activation of receptors in the cell membrane that are a subset of the tumor necrosis factor receptor (TNF-R) family (see review by Strasser et al., 2000). The subset members contain intracellular death domains (DD); therefore, they are called death receptors (DRs) (Figure 7-1). Examples of DRs are CD95 (also known as Fas or APO-1), TNF-R1, DR3, DR4, DR5, and NGFRp75. CD95L (Fas L) is a ligand that activates DRs such as CD95. Adapter proteins (e.g., FADD/MORT, TRADD, and RIP) are necessary to link the DRs to the pro-caspase proteins. Once activated, the **death-inducing signaling complex (DISC)** composed of the ligand (e.g., CD95L), receptor (e.g., CD95), and adapter protein (e.g., FADD) recruit and activate pro-caspase molecules (zymogens) and generate the active caspase protein (e.g., caspase 8) (Figure 7-1). Caspase-8 can subsequently activate downstream effector, executioner caspases such as

caspase-3, leading to proteolytic degradation of cellular proteins and to apoptosis (Muzio et al., 1998; Cryns & Yuan, 1998; Strassser et al., 2000). Procaspase-8 activation can be blocked by the endogenous degenerate caspase homologue c-FLIP that acts at the DISC, and the action of activated caspase-8 can be blocked by the caspase inhibitor z-IETD-fmk.

Mitochondrial Apoptosis Pathway

Another cell death pathway that participates in apoptosis is the mitochondrial or intrinsic pathway (Li et al., 1997). The mitochondrial pathway (Figure 7-1) is activated extensively in cells in response to extracellular (e.g., ionizing radiation, chemotherapeutic drugs, and cytotoxic substances) and intracellular triggers (e.g., toxic oxidative stress, DNA damage, and large increases in intracellular and mitochondrial calcium levels). It is characterized by an increase in mitochondrial permeability (i.e., pore formation), a change in the mitochondrial **membrane potential ($\Delta\Psi$m)**, and release of cytochrome c from the mitochondria (Kim et al., 2000). The pathway involves the **Bcl-2 family of proteins**. There are at least 15 members of the Bcl-2 family. They have been divided into three subfamilies: Group I contains Bcl-2 and Bcl-XL that are anti-apoptotic; Group II contains Bax, Bak, and Bok that are pro-apoptotic; and Group III contains Bad, Bid, Bik, and Bim that are pro-apoptotic. Whether a cell undergoes apoptosis is determined by the amount of pro-apoptotic versus anti-apoptotic components in the cell.

Pro-apoptotic Bcl-2 family members such as Bax, Bak, and Bid and anti-apoptotic Bcl-2 family members such as Bcl-2 and Bcl-SL interact at the outer membrane of the mitochondria. If the pro-apoptotic molecules predominate, pores are formed (e.g., Bax in Figure 7-1) in the outer membrane and an array of molecules is released from the intermembrane mitochondrial compartment. Principal among those molecules is the protein cytochrome c, which associates with the apoptotic protease-activating factor (Apaf-1), procaspase-9, and dATP to form the **apoptosome complex.** The binding of cytochrome c to form the apoptosome complex activates procaspase-9, which, in turn, activates downstream effector caspases such

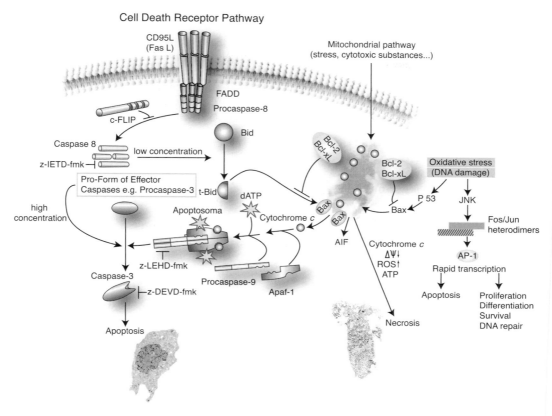

Figure 7-1. A schematic presentation of major apoptotic pathways thought to be active within mammalian hair cells.

The cell death receptor pathway (left side of figure) is triggered through death receptors such as CD95. Binding of CD95 ligand (CD95L) to CD95 induces receptor clustering and, together with adaptor molecules such as FADD, form the death-inducing signaling complex (DISC). The DISC recruits multiple procaspase-8 molecules, resulting in autocatalysis of this procaspase molecule and formation of activated caspase-8. Caspase-8 then activates caspase-3, leading to apoptosis.

The mitochondrial pathway (right side of figure) is activated by extracellular and intracellular triggers. These diverse triggers converge on mitochondria, often through the activation of pro-apoptotic members of the Bcl-2 family (e.g., Bax, Bad, and Bik). Pro-apoptotic proteins interact with anti-apoptotic molecules such as Bcl-2 and Bcl-XL at the outer membrane of the mitochondria. When the pro-apoptotic molecules outnumber the anti-apoptotic molecules, the pro-apoptotic molecules (e.g., Bax) form pores in the outer membrane of the mitochondria. Cytochrome *c* (blue spheres) exits the mitochondria through those pores and enters the cytosol. The cytochrome *c* associates with Apaf-1, procaspase-9, and dATP to form an apoptosome complex. The apoptosome activates procaspase-9, which, in turn, activates downstream effector caspases (e.g., caspase-3). The cell death receptor and mitochondrial cell death pathways converge at the level of pro-caspase-3 activation.

Also shown is a path to necrosis, where cells in which mitochondria have ruptured are at risk for death through a slower nonapoptotic mechanism because of loss of the electrochemical gradient across the inner membrane ($\Delta\Psi$m), production of high levels of reactive oxygen species (ROS), loss of cytochrome *c*, and a rapid decline in ATP production.

Caspase-8 mediates cleavage of Bid to form t-Bid, which translocates to the outer mitochondrial membrane and promotes the formation of pores by Bax.

DNA damage and/or toxic oxidative stress can trigger the activation of the JNK signal transduction pathway (right side of figure). Signal transduction via JNK can induce the phosphorylation of transcription factors such as c-Jun and c-Fos. Activated c-Jun and c-Fos form protein-1 (AP-1), which can trigger rapid transcriptional activity. This transcriptional activity has been implicated in the regulation of many important biological processes including differentiation, proliferation, survival, DNA repair, and apoptosis.

Toxic oxidative stress can also damage DNA and increase levels of P53, a transcription factor. The P53 will activate Bax and induce Bax pore formation in the mitochondrial membrane.

The micrographs at the bottom of the figure show typical necrotic (on the right side) and apoptotic (on the left side) inner hair cells (IHCs).

Adapted from Hengartner, 2000

as caspase-3 and caspase-7, leading to apoptosis (Liu et al., 1996).

The cell death receptor and mitochondrial cell death pathways converge at the level of pro-caspase-3 activation. Activated caspase-9 can be blocked by the caspase-9 inhibitor (z-LEHD-fmk), and activation of caspase-3 can be blocked by the caspase-3 inhibitor (z-DEVD-fmk).

The cell death receptor pathway can recruit the mitochondrial pathway through its product caspase-8. Caspase-8 will proteolytically activate the Bcl-2 family member Bid to form a truncated form of Bid called t-Bid. The t-Bid can be translocated to mitochondria to activate the mitochondrial pathway by allowing the formation of pores in the outer mitochondrial membrane by Bcl-2 family members such as Bax (Kim et al., 2000; Fariss et al., 2005). The actions of t-Bid can be inhibited by Bcl-2 and Bcl-SL.

An additional mechanism for release of caspase-activating proteins such as cytochrome *c* from mitochondria involves **osmotic disequilibrium**, leading to an expansion of the intermembrane space, swelling of the organelle, and subsequent rupturing of the outer membrane (Green & Reed, 1998). Cells in which mitochondria have ruptured are at risk for death through a slower non-apoptotic mechanism resembling necrosis because of loss of membrane potential ($\Delta\Psi$m), production of high levels of reactive oxygen species (ROS) (see later discussion of ROS), and a rapid decline in **adenosine triphosphate (ATP)** production, in addition to the loss of cytochrome *c*.

Role of Death Receptor and Mitochondrial Pathways in the Cochlea

The role of both the death receptor pathway and the mitochondrial pathway in damage to cells in the cochlea and other cells is slowly being elucidated. In other cells (e.g., thymocytes, which are **lymphocytes** derived from the thymus gland), DNA damage and drug-induced damage (e.g., corticosteroids) appear to require the components of the mitochondrial pathway for cell death (Stasser et al., 2000). In contrast, the death receptor pathway relies on activation of the DR by ligands (e.g., CD95L) released from cells such as natural killer and cytotoxic T lymphocytes (Kam et al., 2000).

Aminoglycosides

In the cochlea, the ototoxic aminoglycoside antibiotic neomycin activated caspase-8, caspase-9, and caspase-3 in adult mouse hair cells exposed to the drug (Cunningham et al., 2002). The inhibition of caspase-9, but not inhibition of caspase-8, prevented the activation of caspase-3. Likewise, the ototoxic aminoglycoside antibiotic gentamicin also activated caspase-8, caspase-9, and caspase-3 in the avian basilar papilla (Cheng et al., 2003). In addition, minocycline, a caspase inhibitor, attenuated gentamicin hair cell loss (Corbacella et al., 2004). Further evidence for an involvement of the mitochondrial pathway was obtained in a **transgenic mouse** that overexpresses Bcl-2, an anti-apoptotic protein. In these mice, neomycin did not activate caspase-9 in the hair cells and hair cell survival was significantly increased (Cunningham et al., 2004). These data indicate that the caspase-9 pathway (mitochondrial pathway) for apoptosis is important in aminoglycoside-induced hair cell death. To explain the activation of caspase 8, a component of the death receptor pathway by neomycin, Cunningham et al. (2002) speculate that the neomycin may have acted indirectly on leukocytes present in the hair cell epithelia that, in turn, released death receptor ligands onto the hair cells.

Cisplatin (CDDP) Ototoxicity

Cisplatin (CDDP) is a highly effective and widely used anticancer agent (Trimmer & Essigmann, 1999). The risk of ototoxic and nephrotoxic side effects commonly hinders the use of higher doses that could maximize its antineoplastic effects (Humes, 1999). CDDP has been shown to induce auditory sensory cell apoptosis *in vitro* (Liu et al., 1998; Cheng et al., 1999) and *in vivo* (Teranishi et al., 2001; Alam et al., 2000; Wang et al., 2003a). Both an upstream initiator caspase (i.e., caspase-9) as well as a downstream effector caspase (i.e., caspase-3) were activated in the CDDP-damaged OHCs and some IHCs located in the basal turn of the cochlea (Liu et al., 1998; Devarajan et al., 2002; Watanabe et al., 2003; Zhang et al., 2003; Wang et al., 2003a, 2004). Devarajan et al., (2002) reported CDDP-induced apoptosis in an immortalized cochlear cell line with an increase in caspase-8 and caspase-9 activity, suggesting that both the death receptor and the mitochondrial pathways are involved in CDDP-induced apoptosis of hair cells. In contrast, Wang et al. (2004) did not observe a significant increase in caspase-8 activation in CDDP-treated guinea pig cochleae. Further, local scala tympani perfusion of z-IETD-fmk, a caspase-8 inhibitor, was ineffective in preventing both CDDP-induced hair cell death and hearing loss (Wang et al., 2004). That result suggests that *in vivo* CDDP-induced apoptosis of cochlear cells is caspase-8-independent. Intracochlear perfusion of a caspase-3 inhibitor (z-DEVD-fmk) and a caspase-9 inhibitor (z-LEHD-fmk) dramatically reduced the ototoxic effects of CDDP, as evidenced by a lack of fragmentation of DNA with almost no apoptotic cell death of hair cells or other cell types within the cochlea and almost no loss of hearing (Wang et al., 2004). Altogether, those results suggest that CDDP ototoxicity is mediated through the mitochondrial pathway.

Intense Sound

Morphological features typical of autolysis (i.e., the appearance of vacuoles in the cytoplasm with an intact cell membrane) and of apoptosis (i.e., shrinkage of the cell body, increased electron density of the cytoplasm, and chromatin condensation with an intact cell membrane) are observed in the noise-damaged hair cells (Figure 7-2). Interestingly, individual hair cells sharing both features of autolysis and apoptosis are also seen. Moreover, signs of necrosis (i.e., cellular debris and disintegrated cell membrane) are occasionally seen in the area of the damaged hair cells (Figure 7-2). The presence of those different features indicates that the degeneration of the noise-damaged hair cells involves different mechanisms of cell death, including typical apoptosis, autolysis, and (to a lesser extent) necrosis (Hu et al., 2002; Wang et al., 2002).

Riluzole, a wide-spectrum neuroprotective agent, has been shown to prevent or attenuate apoptotic and necrotic cell death in rat models of spinal cord (Lang-Lazdunski et al., 2000) and retinal (Ettaiche et al., 1999) **ischemia.** In the light of those findings, Wang et al. (2002) examined the potential protective effect of riluzole against noise-induced hearing loss in the cochlea of the adult guinea pig. Intracochlear perfusion of riluzole was found to protect guinea pig cochleas from damage caused by acoustic trauma, as demonstrated by functional tests and by morphometric methods. Riluzole-treated animals showed less compound action potential of the auditory nerve (CAP) threshold elevation and less hair cell loss than noise-exposed controls one month after acoustic trauma (Figure 7-3). The protective effect of riluzole was evident by day 2 and even more pronounced one month after acoustic trauma. **Cytocochleograms** prepared one month after acoustic trauma showed that riluzole treatment (100 μM) protected more than 80% of IHCs and OHCs destined to die.

JNK SIGNALING PATHWAY

Toxic oxidative stress, DNA damage, radiation, and osmotic changes can also trigger the activation of the members of the mitogen-activated protein **kinase** (MAP kinase, MAPK) family such as **c-Jun N-terminal kinases (JNKs)**, also known as stress-activated protein kinase (SAPK) (right side of Figure 7-1) (Davis, 2000; Kyriakis & Avruch, 2001; Zine & VanDeWater, 2004; Dabrowski et al., 2000). Activated JNK molecules **phosphorylate transcription factors** such as c-Jun and c-Fos (Hibi et al., 1993; Xia et al., 1995) and ATF-2. The c-Jun and c-Fos form activation protein-1 (AP-1), which can trigger rapid transcriptional activity and subsequent translation to protein products. AP-1 has been implicated in the regulation of many important biological processes including the **cell cycle** and DNA repair and both signaling for survival and apoptosis (Davis, 2000; Ip & Davis, 1998). Stress induced by UV radiation activates the JNK pathway, which then activates the mitochondrial pathway for apoptosis; however, the mechanisms remain to be elucidated (Davis, 2000). In general, the role of JNK remains unclear since both pro-apoptotic (Bossy-Wetzel et al., 1997; Pirvola et al., 1997) and prosurvival effects of c-Jun activation (Potapova et al., 1997; Doughtery et al., 2002) have been reported.

In the cochlea, the ototoxic aminoglycosides (i.e., neomycin and gentamycin) have been shown to

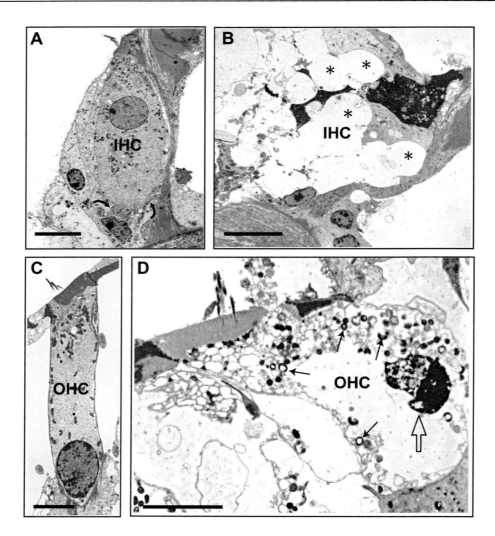

Figure 7-2. Transmission electron micrographs of noise-damaged guinea pig cochlea. **A:** An inner hair cell (IHC) observed in the undamaged region of the organ of Corti 6 hours after acoustic trauma. Both the IHC and its innervations (curve arrows) have a normal appearance. **B:** Typical apoptotic IHC observed 6 hours after trauma. This hair cell shows shrinkage of the cell body and increased electron density of the cytoplasm. The cytoplasmic lateral membrane is preserved. All afferent endings are totally disrupted (asterisks). **C:** Normal appearance of an outer hair cell (OHC) observed 24 hours after acoustic trauma in the undamaged region of the organ of Corti. **D:** In the noise-damaged region of the organ of Corti, a degenerating OHC observed 24 hours after acoustic trauma. Note cellular enlargement, vacuole formation, and organelle disorganization (sign of necrosis), distorted mitochondria (small black arrows), and the electron-dense nucleus due to chromatin compaction (sign of apoptosis) (large white arrow). Scale bars: **A, B** = 10 μm; **C, D** = 5 μm.

Reprinted from *Neuroscience*, 111, Wang et al., Riluzole rescues cochlear sensory cells, 635–648 (2002), with permission from Elsevier.

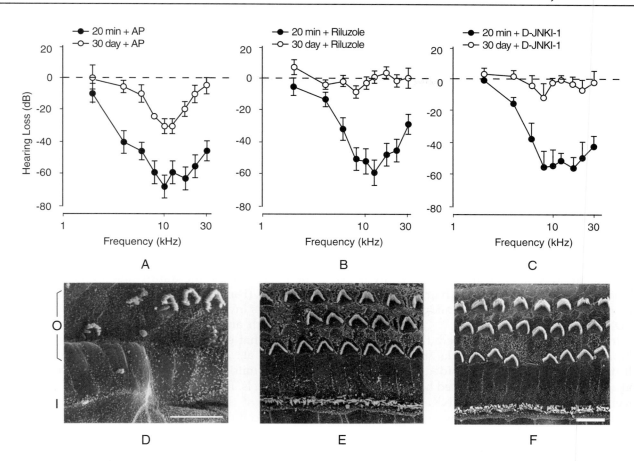

Figure 7-3. Protective effect of riluzole and D-JNKI-1 on noise-induced hearing loss and loss of hair cells in the guinea pig cochlea. **A:** The graphs represent mean audiograms measured 20 minutes (filled circles) and 30 days (empty circles) after acoustic trauma (6 kHz, 120 dB, 30 min) in cochleae perfused with artificial perilymph alone. The average hearing thresholds measured 20 minutes after acoustic trauma were 60–70 dB between 12–16 kHz (Figure 7-2A). There was a partial recovery of CAP thresholds of around 30 dB by the fifth day. This residual impairment at 30 dB represents permanent hearing loss (i.e., permanent threshold shift, PTS). **B:** The immediate elevation of CAP thresholds due to acoustic trauma was not significantly attenuated when the cochlea was perfused with 100 µM riluzole (filled circles). In contrast, a clear improvement in the recovery of CAP thresholds with significantly reduced PTS (empty circle) was observed. **C:** Protection against a permanent hearing loss was clearly observed for the cochlea treated with 10 µM D-JNKI-1, with an initial hearing loss (TTS) that was similar to the contralateral unperfused cochleae at 20 minutes, but with a near complete recovery of hearing function by 30 days postexposure (in **B**). **D:** In the damaged area of the cochleae that received only artificial perilymph, more severe damage was observed in the row of inner hair cells (IHCs) and in the first row of outer hair cells (OHCs) than in the second and the third rows of OHCs. **E:** Direct delivery of 100 µM of riluzole into the scala tympani of the cochlea prevent acoustic trauma-induced hair cell loss. **F:** 10 µM of D-JNKI-1 effectively prevented hair cell loss. Scale bars: **D** and **E** = 25 µm; **F** = 15µM.

Reprinted from *Neuroscience*, 111, Wang et al., Riluzole rescues cochlear sensory cells, 635–648 (2002), with permission from Elsevier; *J. Neuroscience*, 23, 8596–8607 (2003), with permission from the Society for Neuroscience.

activate the JNK pathway; and the inhibitor of the JNK pathway, CEP-1347, attenuated the hair cell damage (Ylikoski et al., 2002). In contrast, a protective role against DNA damage-induced apoptosis is supported by recent studies that have shown that the JNK signal cascade is activated by CDDP and is necessary for the repair of DNA and for cell viability following CDDP treatment (Potapova et al., 1997; Potapova et al., 2001; Hayakawa et al., 1999; Wang et al., 2004). For example, Wang et al. (2004) showed that scala tympani perfusion of D-JNKI-1, a cell-permeable **peptide** that blocks JNK-mediated activation of c-Jun (Bonny et al., 2001), did not prevent the activation and subcellular redistribution of Bax or mitochondrial release of cytochrome *c* and increased the sensitivity of cochlear hair cells to damage by CDDP. That suggests that the JNK pathway is not involved in the CDDP-induced hair cell death, but may have a role in DNA repair and maintenance of CDDP-damaged sensory cells.

Pirvola et al. (2000) reported that the kinase inhibitor CEP-1347, which blocks the MAPK/JNK cell death signal pathway, provided partial protection against sound trauma-induced hearing loss. The novel cell-permeable peptide D-JNKI-1, which blocks the MAPK/JNK signal pathway, was found to be effective in protecting the cochlea against intense sound damage (Wang et al., 2003b). When applied directly into the cochlea, D-JNKI-1 peptide protected the cochlea against permanent hearing loss induced by sound trauma and provided near complete protection of the auditory hair cells (Figure 7-3). Similar results were obtained when D-JNKI-1 was applied onto the round window membrane via an osmotic minipump (Wang et al., 2005). In addition, DJNKI-1 protection was still effective when applied onto the round window 12 hours after acoustic trauma (Wang et al., 2005).

REACTIVE OXYGEN SPECIES (ROS)

Mitochondria serve as the major energy-producing powerhouses of cells by generating ATP. The ATP is generated and oxygen is consumed by a series of chemical reactions utilizing the mitochondrial **electron transport apparatus**. A significant fraction (1%) of molecular oxygen consumed by mitochondria may generate ROS, such as the superoxide anion radical (O_2^-). The mitochondrial O_2^- can then lead to the production of additional ROS, such as hydrogen peroxide (H_2O_2), and the highly reactive hydroxyl radical (OH^-). As protection from the damaging effects of ROS, the mitochondria contain water-soluble and lipid-soluble **antioxidants** (e.g., glutathione, ascorbate, vitamin E, and coenzyme Q) and antioxidant enzymes such as superoxide dismutase, glutathione peroxidase, catalase, thioredoxins, and peroxiredoxin (Heck et al., 2005). **Toxic oxidative stress** results when the concentrations of ROS in the mitochondria increase to levels that are too great to be overcome by the antioxidants and antioxidant enzymes (Fariss et al., 2005). Although the chemical pathways involved in toxic oxidative stress-induced cell death and disease are yet to be defined, it is known that exposure to ROS can induce apoptosis (Zang et al., 2005) and damage lipids, proteins, and DNA in mitochondria and increase intracellular calcium levels. ROS are also capable of damaging components of the electron transport apparatus, thus limiting cellular ATP production and augmenting the production of ROS.

The DNA damage induced by toxic oxidative stress can increase the cytosolic concentration of active p53, a transcription factor also known as a tumor suppressor protein (Figure 7-1) (Schuler & Green, 2005). p53 has been shown to directly activate the pro-apoptotic Bcl-2 protein Bax, leading to Bax pore formation in the outer mitochondrial membrane. Pore formation then leads to an increase in the permeability of the mitochondrial membrane, allowing cytochrome *c* to leave and initiate the mitochondrial apoptotic pathway (Chipuk et al., 2004; Schuler & Green, 2005).

ROS may be important in apoptosis induced by the intrinsic mitochondrial pathway through actions on cardiolipin (see review by Farris et al., 2005). Cardiolipin is a phospholipid that is located in the inner mitochondrial membrane, where it anchors the protein cytochrome *c* so cytochrome *c* can play a role in electron transport. Bound cytochrome c will not be available for release from pores in the outer mitochondrial membrane formed by Bcl-2 family members such as Bax. However, ROS can induce cardiolipin peroxidation and in the process, induce the freeing of cytochrome c from its binding site and allow it to be free to exit the outer mitochondrial membrane through pores and participate in the mitochondrial apoptotic pathway. As mentioned, the Bcl-2 family member t-Bid can be translocated to mitochondria to activate the mitochondrial pathway (Kim et al., 2000; Fariss et al., 2005). Cardiolipin also plays a role in attracting t-Bid to the mitochondria and subsequent Bax pore formation (Fariss et al., 2005). Thus, it appears that ROS can enhance apoptosis by freeing bound cytochrome c and that ROS can be a direct trigger for apoptosis by inducing cardiolipin to attract t-Bid to the mitochondria.

Another important compound is nitric oxide (NO) a **free radical** generated by the mitochondrial enzyme nitric oxide synthase (Ortega et al., 2000). NO can act as an antioxidant and be beneficial to the cell, yet it can also be very disruptive to mitochondria function. That is because of its high reactivity with ROS, such as superoxide, to form a number of reactive nitrogen species (RNS) such as $ONOO^-$, NO_2, and N_2O_3 (Wink et al., 1993; Lipton et al., 1993). RNS are oxidizing agents capable of causing toxic oxidative/nitrosative stress.

In the inner ear, ROS was found to increase substantially after exposure to ototoxins such as aminoglycosides or CDDP (Priuska & Schacht, 1995; Clerici et al., 1996). Previati et al. (2004) report a CDDP-induced expression of genes potentially involved in increasing levels of ROS. After noise exposure in the cochlea, there is an increase in ROS formation (Huang et al., 2000; Ohinata et al., 2000a; Yamane et al., 1995; Ohlemiller et al., 1999; Kaygusuz et al., 2001), an increase in antioxidants such as glutathione (Yamasoba et al., 1998), and oxidative-induced DNA damage (Van Campen et al., 2002).

Genetic deletion of glutathione peroxidase in mice induces a significant increase in sensitivity to noise-induced hearing loss (Ohlemiller et al., 2000), while deletion of superoxide dismutase appears to have a more modest sensitizing effect (McFadden et al., 2001). In addition, exogenous **free radical scavengers** (e.g., glutathione, mannitol, allopurinol, diethyldithiocarbamate, 4-methylthiobenzoic acid, and ebselen) and iron chelators (e.g., deferoxamine) can limit intense sound or cisplatin-induced hearing loss (Ohinata et al., 2000b; Yamasoba et al., 1999, 2005; Pourbakht & Yamasoba, 2003; Dehne et al., 2001; Lynch et al., 2004, 2005; Rybak et al., 2000).

CALCIUM, CALPAINS, AND CATHEPSINS

It has long been known that an increase in the intracellular concentration of calcium is lethal to cells. For example, in the cochlea, the drug thapsigargin, which blocks the transport of calcium into intracellular storage sites and increases levels of free intracellular calcium, results in hair cell loss (Bobbin et al., 2003). The mechanism for the hair cell death appears to be the activation of at least three proteases including caspases, calpains, and cathepsin—all induced by the increased intracellular levels of calcium (e.g., Artal-Sanz & Tavernarakis, 2005; Benjamins et al., 2003; Fernandez-Gomez et al., 2005; Pelletier et al., 2005).

A rise in intracellular calcium will result in calcium uptake by mitochondria. Excessive intracellular calcium can overload mitochondria with calcium and induce an increase in electron transport and an increase in ROS production and induce pore formation accompanied by activation of apoptosis (Fernandez-Gomez et al., 2005).

Increasing intracellular calcium will activate **calpains**, which are calcium-dependent cysteine proteases that are involved in cellular function and that have been implicated in various diseases (Zatz & Starling, 2005; Artal-Sanz & Tavernarakis, 2005). For example, calpain activity will break down cytoskeletal proteins and signal transduction proteins, apoptotic regulatory factors, and caspases, leading to cell death by apoptosis or necrosis (Artal-Sanz & Tavernarakis, 2005; Zatz & Starling, 2005). In addition, calpain activation has been implicated in excitotoxic events triggered by NO (Volbracht et al., 2005). In the cochlea, an increase in calpain activity was reported in hair cells after treatment with the ototoxic aminoglycoside antibiotic gentamicin (Ding et al., 2002).

Activation of calpains will also damage membranes of **lysosomes**, resulting in the release of lysosomal proteolytic enzymes called **cathepsins** (Zatz & Starling, 2005). Cathepsins will induce nonspecific cleavage of various intracellular proteins, and they have been implicated in both apoptosis and necrosis (Artal-Sanz & Tavernarakis, 2005).

Several studies suggest that calpains and cathepsins may have a role in cell death in the cochlea. For instance, leupeptin, an inhibitor of calpains and cathepsins, has been shown to provide some protection of hair cells from acoustic trauma (Wang et al., 1999) and from toxicity due to the aminoglycoside antibiotic gentamicin (Ding et al., 2002), but not from the toxicity due to carboplatin (Wang et al., 1999). Mandic et al., (2003) reported on the possible involvement of calpains in CDDP toxicity in a human melanoma cell line, suggesting a role for calpains in CDDP ototoxicity. However, the lack of a protective effect of calpain inhibitors on CDDP toxicity on auditory hair cells and neurons in culture argues against that hypothesis (Cheng et al., 1999).

In the case of intense sound-induced auditory neuronal cell death, it is not clear if degeneration of the neurons occurs secondarily to the loss of the sensory inner hair cells (IHCs) to which they are connected (loss of supporting cells) or if the neuronal death is due to an excessive release of glutamate (the neurotransmitter of the IHCs) (Stankovic et al., 2004). It is well known that excessive glutamate release in the cochlea can induce excitotoxicity of auditory neurons by overstimulation of AMPA receptors, which leads to calcium overload in the postsynaptic neuron (Ruel et al., 2000). The increase in calcium will lead to the activation of calpains and cathepsins and mitochondrial pore formation with the subsequent activation of caspases. Indeed, intracochlear perfusion of glutamate antagonists during noise exposure prevents 50% of the acute threshold elevation by protecting the auditory neuron nerve endings, but it has no protective effect on the hair cells themselves (Puel et al., 1998).

SUMMARY

Cells have evolved complex biochemical systems that maintain or discard cells in an organ during the life span of the individual. Cell death has been classified into two general types: necrosis and PCD. Necrosis is considered to be a passive cellular event, while PCD is thought to be a naturally occurring, active event involving the triggering of a set of molecular events that have been preprogrammed into the molecular machinery of the cell. An example of PCD is apoptosis. Apoptosis is achieved by activation of a cascade of events involving the activation of a group of enzymes called initiator caspases and executioner caspases. Two pathways utilize caspases to induce apoptosis. They are (1) the death receptor pathway (ligand (CD95L) to DRs (CD95) to adapter proteins (FADD/MORT) to DISC to caspase-8 to caspase-3 to apoptosis) and (2) the mitochondrial pathway (pro-apoptotic molecules predominate to Bax pore formation in the outer membrane to release of cytochrome c to formation of the apoptosome complex (cytochrome c, Apaf-1, procaspase-9, and dATP) to caspase-9 to caspase-3 to apoptosis).

The JNK pathway (activated JNK to phosphorylate transcription factors such as c-Jun and c-Fos to activation protein-1 (AP-1) to rapid transcriptional activity) can lead to either survival signaling or apoptosis through the mitochondrial pathway. ROS and calcium overload can activate the mitochondrial pathway. Calcium overload can also activate calpains and cathepsins, leading to apoptosis and necrosis. Various stresses applied to cells in the cochlea, such as intense sound or toxic drugs, most probably recruit some of these pathways and enzymes. It seems clear that the mitochondrial pathway is important in both aminoglycoside- and CDDP-induced apoptosis of hair cells. On the other hand, ototoxic aminoglycosides and CDDP induce toxic oxidative stress by elevating ROS in the cochlea and activate the JNK cascade. However, there is evidence that the CDDP-induced activation of the JNK pathway is involved in repair and not cell death. Many of the pathways interact with each other, thereby challenging researchers attempting to elucidate pathways involved in response to any given toxic stimulus.

The complexity of the mechanisms involved in cochlear cell death is illustrated by the presence of different morphological phenotypes in noise-damaged hair cells, indicating cell death by apoptosis and necrosis with even autolysis being present. Future research is needed to determine the relative contributions of each of these pathways to drug- and noise-induced hearing loss and discover drugs or other treatments that will prevent cell death in the auditory system.

REFERENCES

Alam, S. A., Ikeda, K., Oshima, T., Suzuki, M., Kawase, T., Kikuchi, T., et al. (2000). Cisplatin-induced apoptotic cell death in Mongolian gerbil cochlea. *Hearing Research, 141,* 28–38.

Artal-Sanz, M., & Tavernarakis, N. (2005). Proteolytic mechanisms in necrotic cell death and neurodegeneration. *FEBS Letters, 579,* 3287–3296.

Benjamins, J. A., Nedelkoska, L., & George, E. B. (2003). Protection of mature oligodendrocytes by inhibitors of caspases and calpains. *Neurochem Res, 28,* 143–152.

Bobbin, R. P., Parker, M., & Wall, L. (2003). Thapsigargin suppresses cochlear potentials and DPOAEs and is toxic to hair cells. *Hearing Research, 184,* 51–60.

Bonny, C., Oberson, A., Negri, S., Sauser, C., & Schorderet, D. F. (2001). Cell-permeable peptide inhibitors of JNK: Novel blockers of beta-cell death. *Diabetes, 50,* 77–82.

Bossy-Wetzel, E., Bakiri, L., & Yaniv, M. (1997). Induction of apoptosis by the transcription factor c-Jun. *EMBO J, 16,* 1695–1709.

Cheng, A. G., Huang, T., Stacher, A., Kim, A., Liu, W., Malgrange, B., et al. (1999). Calpain inhibitors protect auditory sensory cells from hypoxia and neurotrophin-withdrawl induced apoptosis. *Brain Res, 850,* 234–243.

Cheng, A. G., Cunningham, L. L., & Rubel, E. W. (2003). Hair cell death in the avian basilar papilla: Characterization of the in vitro model and caspase activation. *Otolaryngol, 4,* 91–105.

Chipuk, J. E., Kuwana, T., Bouchier-Hayes, L., Droin, N. M., Newmeyer, D. D., Schuler, M., et al. (2004). Direct activation of Bax by p53 mediates mitochondrial membrane permeabilization and apoptosis. *Science, 303,* 1010–1014.

Clarke, P. G. (1990). Developmental cell death: Morphological diversity and multiple mechanism. *Anat Embryol, 181,* 184–213.

Clerici, W. J., Hensley, K., DiMartino, D. L., & Butterfield, D. A. (1996). Direct detection of ototoxicant-induced reactive oxygen species generation in cochlear explants. *Hearing Research, 98,* 116–124.

Corbacella, E., Lanzoni, I., Ding, D., Previati, M., & Salvi, R. (2004). Minocycline attenuates gentamicin induced hair cell loss in neonatal cochlear cultures. *Hearing Research, 197,* 11–18.

Cryns, V., & Yuan, J. (1998). Proteases to die for. *Genes Dev, 12,* 1551–1570.

Cunningham, L. L., Cheng, A. G., & Rubel, E. W. (2002). Caspase activation in hair cells of the mouse utricle exposed to neomycin. *J Neurosci, 22,* 8532–8540.

Cunningham, L. L., Matsui, J. I., Warchol, M., & Rubel, E. W. (2004). Overexpression of Bcl-2 prevents neomycin-induced hair cell death and caspase-9 activation in the adult mouse utricle in vitro. *J Neurobiol, 60,* 89–100.

Dabrowski, A., Boguslowicz, C., Dagrowska, M., Tribillo, I., & Gabryelewicz, A. (2000). Reactive oxygen species activate mitogen-activated protein kinases in pancreatic acinar cells. *Pancreas, 21,* 376–384.

Davis, R. J. (2000). Signal transduction by the JNK group of MAP kinases. *Cell, 103,* 239–252.

Dehne, N., Lautermann, J., Petrat, F., Rauen, U., & de Groot, H. (2001). Cisplatin ototoxicity: Involvement of iron and enhanced formation of superoxide anion radicals. *Toxicol Appl Pharmacol, 174,* 27–34.

Devarajan, P., Savoca, M., Castaneda, M. P., Park, M. S., Esteban-Cruciani, N., Kalinec, G., et al. (2002). Cisplatin-induced apoptosis in auditory cells: Role of death receptor and mitochondrial pathways. *Hearing Research, 174,* 45–54.

Ding, D., Stracher, A., & Salvi, R. J. (2002). Leupeptin protects cochlear and vestibular hair cells from gentamicin ototoxicity. *Hearing Research, 164,* 115–126.

Doughtery, C. J., Kubasiakm, L. A., Prenticem, H., Andreka, P., Bishopric, N. H., & Webster K. A. (2002). Activation of c-Jun N-terminal kinase promotes survival of cardiac myocytes after oxidative stress. *Biochem J, 362*(Pt 3), 561–571.

Ettaiche, M., Fillacier, K., Widmann, C., Heurteaux, C., & Lazdunski, M. (1999). Riluzole improves functional recovery after ischemia in the rat retina. *Invest Ophthalmol Vis Sci, 40,* 729–736.

Fariss, M. W., Chan, C. B., Patel, M., Van Houten, B. V., & Orrenius, S. (2005). Role of mitochondria in toxic oxidative stress. *Molecular Interventions, 5,* 94–111.

Fernandez-Gomez, F. J., Galindo, M. F., Gomez-Lazaro, M., Gonzalez-Garcia, C., Cena, V., Aguirre, N., & Jordan, J. (2005). Involvement of mitochondrial potential and calcium buffering capacity in minocycline cytoprotective actions. *Neuroscience, 133,* 959–967.

Gorman, A. M., Orrenius, S., & Ceccatelli, S. (1998). Apoptosis in neuronal cells: Role of caspases. *Neuroreport, 9,* R49–R55.

Green, D. R., & Reed, J. C. (1998). Mitochondria and apoptosis. *Science, 281,* 1309–1312.

Hamernik, R. P., Turrentine, G., & Wright, C. G. (1984). Surface morphology of the inner sulcus and related epithelial cells of the cochlea following acoustic trauma. *Hearing Research, 16,* 143–160.

Hayakawa, J., Ohmichi, M., Kurachi, H., Ikegami, H., Kimura, A., Matsuoka, T., et al. (1999). Inhibition of extracellular signal-regulated protein kinase or c-Jun N-terminal protein kinase cascade, differentially activated by cisplatin, sensitizes human ovarian cancer cell line. *J Biol Chem, 274,* 31648–31654.

Heck, D. E., Kagan, V. E., Shvedova, A. A., & Laskin, J. D. (2005). An epigrammatic (abridged) recounting of the myriad tales of astonishing deeds and dire consequences pertaining to nitric oxide and reactive oxygen species in mitochondria with an ancillary missive concerning the origins of apoptosis. *Toxicology, 208,* 259–271.

Hengartner, M. O. (2000). The biochemistry of apoptosis. *Nature, 407,* 770–776.

Hibi, M., Lin, A., Smeal, T., Minden, A., & Karin, M. (1993). Identification of an oncoprotein- and UV-responsive protein kinase that binds and potentiates the c-Jun activation domain. *Genes Dev, 7,* 2135–2148.

Hu, B. H., Henderson, D., & Nicotera, T. M. (2002). Involvement of apoptosis in progression of cochlear lesion following exposure to intense noise. *Hearing Research, 166,* 62–71.

Huang, T., Cheng, A. G., Stupak, H., Liu, W., Kim, A., Staecker, H., et al. (2000). Oxidative stress-induced apoptosis of cochlear sensory cells: Otoprotective strategies. *Int J Dev Neurosci, 18,* 259–270.

Humes, H. D. (1999). Insights into ototoxicity. Analogies to nephrotoxicity. *Ann N Y Acad Sci, 884,* 15–18.

Ip, Y. T., & Davis, R. J. (1998). Signal transduction by the c-Jun N-terminal kinase (JNK)—from inflammation to development. *Curr Opin Cell Biol, 10,* 205–219.

Kam, C. M., Hudig, D., & Powers, J. C. (2000). Granzymes (lymphocyte serine proteases): Characterization with natural and synthetic substrates and inhibitors. *Biochemica et Biophysica Acta, 1477,* 307–323.

Kaygusuz, I., Ozturk, A., Ustundag, B., & Yalcin, S. (2001). Role of free oxygen radicals in noise-related hearing impairment. *Hearing Research, 162,* 43–47.

Kim, T. H., Zhao, Y., Barber, M. J., Kuharsky, D. K., & Yin, X. M. (2000). Bid-induced cytochrome *c* release is mediated by a pathway independent of mitochondrial permeability transition pore and Bax. *J Biol Chem, 275,* 39474–39481.

Kyriakis, J. M., & Avruch, J. (2001). Mammalian mitogen-activated protein kinase signal transduction pathways activated by stress and inflammation. *Physiol Rev, 81,* 807–869.

Lang-Lazdunski, L., Heurteaux, C., Mignon, A., Mantz, J., Widmann, C., Desmonts, J., et al. (2000).

Ischemic spinal cord injury induced by aortic cross-clamping: Prevention by riluzole. *Eur J Cardiothorac Surg, 18,* 174–181.

Li, P., Nijhawan, D., Budihardjo, I., Srinivasula, S. M., Ahmad, M., Alnemri, E. S., et al. (1997). Cytochrome *c* and dATP-dependent formation of Apaf-1/Caspase-9 complex initiates an apoptotic protease cascade. *Cell, 91,* 479–489.

Lipton, S. A., Choi, Y. B., Pan, Z. H., Lei, S. Z., Chen, H. S., Sucher, N. J., et al. (1993). A redox-based mechanism for the neuroprotective and neurodestructive effects of nitric oxide and related nitroso-compounds. *Nature, 364,* 626–632.

Liu, W., Staecker, H., Stupak, H., Malgrange, B., Lefebvre, P., & Van de Water, T. R. (1998). Caspase inhibitors prevent cisplatin-induced apoptosis of auditory sensory cells. *Neuroreport, 9,* 2609–2614.

Liu, X., Kim, C. N., Yang, J., Jemmerson, R., & Wang, X. (1996). Induction of apoptotic program in cell-free extracts: Requirement for dATP and cytochrome c. *Cell 86,* 147–157.

Lynch, E. D., Gu, R., Pierce, C., & Kil, J. (2004). Ebselen-mediated protection from single and repeated noise exposure in rat. *Laryngoscope, 114,* 333–337.

Lynch, E. D., Gu, R., Pierce, C., & Kil, J. (2005). Reduction of acute cisplatin ototoxicity and nephrotoxicity in rats by oral administration of allopurinol and ebselen. *Hearing Research, 201,* 81–89.

Mandic, A., Hansson, J., Linder, S., & Shoshan, M. C. (2003). Cisplatin induces endoplasmic reticulum stress and nucleus-independent apoptotic signaling. *J Biol Chem, 278,* 9100–9106.

McFadden, S. L., Ohlemiller, K. K., Ding, D., Shero, M., & Salvi R. J. (2001). The influence of superoxide dismutase and glutathione peroxidase deficiencies on noise-induced hearing loss in mice. *Noise Health, 3,* 49–64.

Muzio, M., Stockwell, B. R., Stennicke, H. R., Salvesen, G. S., & Dixit, V. M. (1998). An induced proximity model for caspase-8 activation. *J Biol Chem, 273,* 2926–2930.

Ohinata, Y., Miller, J. M., Altschuler, R. A., & Schacht, J. (2000a). Intense noise induces formation of vasoactive lipid peroxidation products in the cochlea. *Brain Res, 878,* 163–173.

Ohinata, Y., Yamasoba, T., Schacht, J., & Miller, J. M. (2000b). Glutathione limits noise-induced hearing loss. *Hearing Research, 146,* 28–34.

Ohlemiller, K. K., McFadden, S. L., Ding, D. L., Lear, P. M., & Ho, Y. S. (2000). Targeted mutation of the gene for cellular glutathione peroxidase (Gpx1) increases noise-induced hearing loss in mice. *J Assoc Res Otolaryngol, 1,* 243–254.

Ohlemiller, K. K., Wright, J. S., & Dugan, L. L. (1999). Early elevation of cochlear reactive oxygen species following noise exposure. *Audiol Neurootol, 4,* 229–236.

Ortega, M., & Amaya, A. (2000). Nitric oxide reactivity and mechanisms involved in its biological effects. *Pharmacol, Res, 42,* 421–427.

Pelletier, M., Oliver, L., Meflah, K., & Vallette, F. M. (2005). Caspase-3 can be pseudo-activated by a Ca2+-dependent proteolysis at a non-canonical site. *FEBS Letters, 579,* 2364–2368.

Pirvola, U., Qun, L. X., Virkkala, J., Saarma, M., Murakata, C., Camoratto, A. M., et al. (1997). The Jun kinase/stress-activated protein kinase pathway functions to regulate DNA repair and inhibition of the pathway sensitizes tumor cells to cisplatin. *J Biol Chem, 272,* 14041–14044.

Pirvola, U., Xing-Qun, L., Virkkala, J., Saarma, M., Murakata, C., Camoratto, A. M., et al. (2000). Rescue of hearing, auditory hair cells, and neurons by CEP-1347/KT7515, an inhibitor of c-Jun N-terminal kinase activation. *J Neurosci, 20,* 43–50.

Potapova, O., Basu, S., Mercola, D., & Holbrook, N. J. (2001). Protective role for c-Jun in the cellular response to DNA damage. *J Biol Chem, 276,* 28546–28553.

Potapova, O., Haghighi, A., Bost, F., Liu, C., Birrer, M. J., Gjerset, R., et al. (1997). The Jun kinase/stress-activated protein kinase pathway functions to regulate DNA repair and inhibition of the pathway sensitizes tumor cells to cisplatin. *J Biol Chem, 272,* 14041–14044.

Pourbakht, A., & Yamasoba, T. (2003). Ebselen attenuates cochlear damage caused by acoustic trauma. *Hearing Research, 181,* 100–108.

Previati, M., Lanzoni, I., Corbacella, E., Magosso, S., Giuffre, S., Francioso, F., et al. (2004). RNA expression induced by cisplatin in an organ of Corti-derived immortalized cell line. *Hearing Research, 196,* 8–18.

Priuska, E. M., & Schacht, J. (1995). Formation of free radicals by gentamicin and iron and evidence for an iron/gentamicin complex. *Biochem Pharmacol, 50,* 1749–1752.

Puel, J. L., Ruel, J., Gervais d'Aldin, C., & Pujol, R. (1998). Excitotoxicity and repair of cochlear synapses after noise-trauma induced hearing loss. *Neuroreport, 9,* 2109–2114.

Raff, M. C., Barres, B. A., Burne, J. F., Coles, H. S., Ishizaki, Y., & Jacobson, M. D. (1993). Programmed cell death and the control of cell survival: Lessons from the nervous system. *Science, 262,* 695–700.

Ruel, J., Bobbin, R. P., Vidal, D., Pujol, R., & Puel, J. L. (2000). The selective AMPA receptor antagonist GYKI 53784 blocks action potential generation and excitotoxicity in the guinea pig cochlea. *Neuropharmacology, 39,* 1959–1973.

Rybak, L. P., Husain, K., Morris, C., Whitworth, C., & Somani, S. (2000). Effect of protective agents against cisplatin ototoxicity. *Am J Otol, 21,* 513–520.

Schuler, M., & Green, D. R. (2005). Transcription, apoptosis and p53: Catch-22. *Trends in Genetics, 21,* 182–187.

Sperandio, S., Poksay, K., de Belle, I., Lafuente, M. J., Liu, B., Nasir, J., et al. (2004). Paraptosis: Mediation by MAP kinase and inhibition by AIP-1/Alix. *Cell Death and Differentiation, 11,* 1066–1075.

Stankovic, K., Rio, C., Xia, A., Sugawara, M., Adams, J. C., Liberman, M. C., et al. (2004). Survival of adult spiral ganglion neurons requires erbB receptor signaling in the inner ear. *J Neurosci, 24,* 8651–8661.

Stennicke, H. R., & Salvesen, G. S. (2000). Caspases-controlling intracellular signals by protease zymogen activation. *Biochemica et Biophysica Acta, 1477,* 299–306.

Strasser, A., O'Connor, L., & Dixit, V. M. (2000). Apoptosis signaling. *Annu Rev Biochem, 69,* 217–245.

Teranishi, M., Nakashima, T., & Wakabayashi, T. (2001). Effects of alpha-tocopherol on cisplatin-induced ototoxicity in guinea pigs. *Hearing Research, 151,* 61–70.

Trimmer, E. E., & Essigmann, J. M. (1999). Cisplatin. *Essays Biochem 34,* 191–211.

Van Campen, L. E., Murphy, W. J., Franks, J. R., Mathias, P. I., & Toraason, M. A. (2002). Oxidative DNA damage is associated with intense noise exposure in the rat. *Hearing Research, 164,* 29–38.

Volbracht, C., Chua, B. T., Ng, C. P., Bahr, B. A., Hong, W., & Li, P. (2005). The critical role of calpain versus caspase activation in excitotoxic injury induced by nitric oxide. *J Neurochem, 93,* 1280–1292.

Wang, J., Bonny, C., Ruel, J., Ladrech, S., Meyer, T., & Puel, J. L. (2005). *D-JNKI-1, a potent c-Jun N-terminal kinase (JNK) inhibitor protects against acoustic trauma-induced auditory hair cell death and hearing loss.* Association for Research in Otolaryngology, 28th Mid-Winter Meeting, New Orleans, LA.

Wang, J., Dib, M., Lenoir, M., Vago, P., Eybalin, M., Hameg, A., et al. (2002). Riluzole rescues cochlear sensory cells from acoustic trauma in the guinea pig. *Neuroscience, 111,* 635–648.

Wang, J., Ding, D., Shulman, A., Stracher, A., & Salvi, R. J. (1999). Leupeptin protects sensory hair cells from acoustic trauma. *NeuroReport, 10,* 811–816.

Wang, J., Ladrech, S., Pujol, R., Brabet, P., Van De Water, T. R., & Puel, J. L. (2004). Caspase inhibitors, but not c-Jun NH2-Terminal kinase inhibitor treatment, prevent cisplatin-induced hearing loss. *Cancer Res, 64,* 9217–9224.

Wang, J., Lloyd Faulconbridge, R. V., Fetoni, A., Guitton, M. J., Pujol, R., & Puel, J. L. (2003a). Local application of sodium thiosulfate prevents cisplatin-induced hearing loss in the guinea pig. *Neuropharmacology, 45,* 380–393.

Wang, J., Van De Water, T. R., Bonny, C., de Ribaupierre, F., Puel, J. L., & Zine, A. (2003b). A peptide inhibitor of c-Jun N-Terminal kinase protects against both aminoglycoside and acoustic trauma-induced auditory hair cell death and hearing loss. *J Neurosci, 23,* 8596–8607.

Watanabe, K., Inai, S., Jinnouchi, K., Baba, S., & Yagi, T. (2003). Expression of caspase-activated deoxyribonuclease (CAD) and caspase 3 (CPP32) in the cochlea of cisplatin (CDDP)-treated guinea pigs. *Auris Nasus Larynx, 30*, 219–225.

Wink, D. A., Darbyshire, J. F., Nims, R. W., Saavedra, J. E., & Ford, P. C. (1993). Reactions of the bioregulatory agent nitric oxide in oxygenated aqueous media: Determination of the kinetics for oxidation and nitrosation by intermediates generated in the NO/O_2 reaction. *Chem Res Toxicol, 6*, 23–27.

Xia, Z., Dickens, M., Raingeaud, J., Davis, R. J., & Greenberg, M. E. (1995). Opposing effects of ERK and JNK-p38 MAP kinases on apoptosis. *Science, 270*, 1326–1331.

Yamane, H., Nakai, Y., Takayama, M., Iguchi, H., Nakagawa, T., & Kojima, A. (1995). Appearance of free radicals in the guinea pig inner ear after noise-induced acoustic trauma. *Eur Arch Otorhinolaryngol, 252*, 504–508.

Yamasoba, T., Harris, C., Shoji, F., Lee, R. J., Nuttall, A. L., & Miller, J. M. (1998). Influence of intense sound exposure on glutathione syntesis in the cochlea. *Brain Res, 804*, 72–78.

Yamasoba, T., Pourbakht, A., Sakamoto, T., & Suzuki, M. (2005). Ebselen prevents noise-induced excitoxicity and temporary threshold shift. *Neurosci Lett, 380*, 234–238.

Yamasoba, T., Schacht, J., Shoji, F., & Miller, J. M. (1999). Attenuation of cochlear damage from noise trauma by an iron chelator, a free radical scavenger and glial cell line-derived neurotrophic factor in vivo. *Brain Res, 815*, 317–325.

Ylikoski, J., Xing-Qun, L., Virkkala, J., & Pirvola, U. (2002). Blockage of c-Jun N-terminal kinase pathway attenuates gentamicin-induced cochlear and vestibular hair cell death. *Hearing Research, 166*, 33–43.

Zatz, M., & Starling, A. (2005). Calpains and disease. *N Engl J Med, 352*, 2413–2423.

Zhang, M., Liu, W., Ding, D., & Salvi, R. (2003). Pifithrin-α suppresses p53 and protects cochlear and vestibular hair cells from cisplatin-induced apoptosis. *Neuroscience, 120*, 191–205.

Zhang, Y., Fong, C. C., Wong, M. S., Tzang, C. H., Lai, W. P., Fong, W. F., et al. (2005). Molecular mechanisms of survival and apoptosis in RAW 264.7 macrophages under oxidative stress. *Apoptosis, 10*, 545–556.

Zine, A., & Van De Water, T. R. (2004). The MAPK/JNK signaling pathway offers potential therapeutic targets for the prevention of acquired deafness. *Current Drug Targets - CNS & Neurological Disorders, 3*, 325–332.

CHAPTER

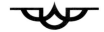

8

Biochemical Bases of Hearing

Sandra L. McFadden, PhD
Assistant Professor
Psychology Department
Western Illinois University

INTRODUCTION

Normal hearing requires the presence of specialized cells that function both independently as they strive to maintain homeostasis in the face of dynamic perturbations in their immediate environment and interactively as they work in concert to achieve integrated tissue-, organ-, and system-specific physiological outcomes. Anatomic and/or physiological abnormalities at any point along the auditory pathway from the periphery to the cortex can impair or prevent normal hearing. As better techniques for studying the fine details of structure and physiology become available and research in the field of auditory science focuses more on the molecular aspects of hearing and hearing loss, it becomes increasingly important to have a basic understanding of biochemical terms and concepts as they relate to the auditory system.

The goal of this chapter is to provide a broad overview of the biochemical bases of hearing to serve as a foundation for appreciating the effects of drugs and other agents on the cochlea and central auditory nervous system (CANS) and, ultimately, on hearing and hearing loss in humans.

Since most drugs that produce temporary or permanent hearing impairment do so by affecting cells and physiological processes in the cochlea, this chapter will focus predominantly on cochlear anatomy and biochemistry. The key cochlear targets of ototoxic drugs are the **outer hair cells** (OHCs)—the "accident prone weaklings of the cochlea" (Hawkins, 1973, 127)—and the cells and processes involved in mechanoelectrical transduction, the process whereby mechanical representations of sound are translated into neural impulses that are conveyed from the cochlea to the CANS via the auditory nerve (AN). Consequently, the primary focus will be on the OHCs, the **inner hair cells** (IHCs), the stria vascularis, the endocochlear potential (EP), and the processes whereby spiral ganglion neurons (SGNs) convert chemical signals into electrical signals that are conveyed to the central nervous system (CNS) by the AN. Damage to the hair cells, stria vascularis, SGNs, and/or AN fibers affects electrophysiological potentials in characteristic ways. Because gross potentials such as the cochlear microphonic (CM),

the summating potential (SP), and the compound action potential (CAP) can be used to detect or monitor the effects of drugs on hearing, the origins of these potentials will be described briefly as well.

Many drugs exert their effects at the neural level. Among the potential targets of drugs in the CANS are cell surface receptors, myelin, neurochemicals or neurotransmitters (NTs), and ion channels involved in electrochemical signaling. Consequently, this chapter will provide a background on those topics as well. To lay the groundwork for sections on mechanoelectrical transduction in the cochlea and electrochemical signaling by SGNs and neurons in the CANS, the chapter will begin with a review of some fundamental features of auditory system anatomy and physiology.

AUDITORY SYSTEM ANATOMY AND PHYSIOLOGY

The outer ear (pinna and external auditory canal), middle ear, cochlea, and SGNs that give rise to the AN comprise the peripheral auditory system; auditory nuclei and fiber tracts in the brainstem (medulla, pons, and midbrain), thalamus, and cortex comprise the CANS. Figure 8–1 shows a simple schematic diagram of the auditory system, summarizing the flow of energy or auditory "information" from the periphery to the CANS and back, via ascending (afferent) and descending (efferent) pathways, respectively.

Afferent Pathways

Sound is collected and shaped in frequency-specific ways by the outer ear, then converted to other forms of energy at subsequent stages of the peripheral auditory system. The tympanic membrane (TM) that separates the outer ear from the middle ear (Figure 8–2) begins the process of transforming acoustic energy into mechanical energy, with sound-induced vibrations that are transmitted directly to the malleus and indirectly to the incus and stapes of the middle ear ossicular chain. Mechanical energy is transmitted from the middle ear to the cochlea, the site of the organ of Corti that contains the IHCs and OHCs, by

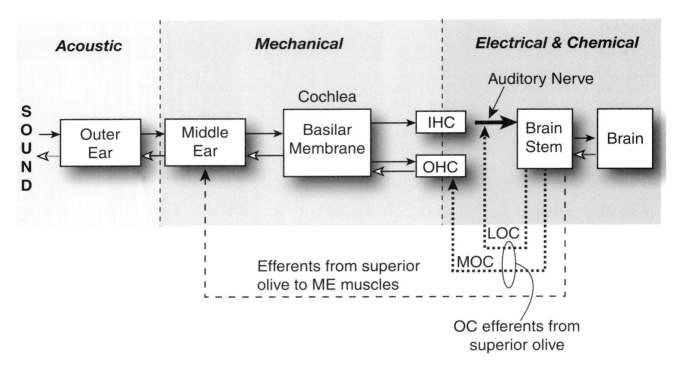

Figure 8-1. The auditory system. The peripheral auditory system consists of the outer ear, middle ear, cochlea, and auditory nerve. The central auditory system consists of auditory regions in the brainstem and brain. Acoustic energy is transformed to mechanical energy by the middle ear and basilar membrane. The hair cells convert mechanical energy into electrical and chemical energy. The auditory nerve is the peripheral nervous system connection between the cochlea and the brain. In addition to feed-forward (afferent) pathways, there are numerous feed-back pathways, represented by arrows pointing to the left. Energy flowing from cochlea to the outer ear is the source of otoacoustic emissions. Three prominent efferent pathways from the superior olive in the brainstem influence peripheral sensitivity and function: a middle ear reflex pathway and two olivocochlear (OC) pathways. The lateral OC (LOC) pathway terminates on afferent fibers beneath IHCs; the medial OC (MOC) pathway innervates outer hair cells (OHCs) directly.

movement of the stapes footplate against the oval window membrane (Figure 8-2). The design of the middle ear allows it to function effectively as an impedance matching transformer so that very little energy is lost in the process of exchanging energy from one medium (air) to another (fluid). In the absence of the middle ear, most of the original sound energy would be lost due to the impedance mismatch between the air in the ear canal and the fluid in the cochlea, and one's hearing sensitivity would be far less acute than it is normally.

Movement of the stapes sets up pressure fluctuations in the cochlear fluids that, in turn, initiate basilar membrane (BM) movement. As illustrated in Figure 8-3, the BM is narrow at the basal end of the cochlea and becomes progressively wider toward the apex, even though the cochlea itself becomes narrower from base to apex. The stiffness and mass gradients of the BM cause it to vibrate in frequency-specific patterns and with place-specific time delays. The stiffer basal end of the BM has a high-frequency resonance and therefore produces the

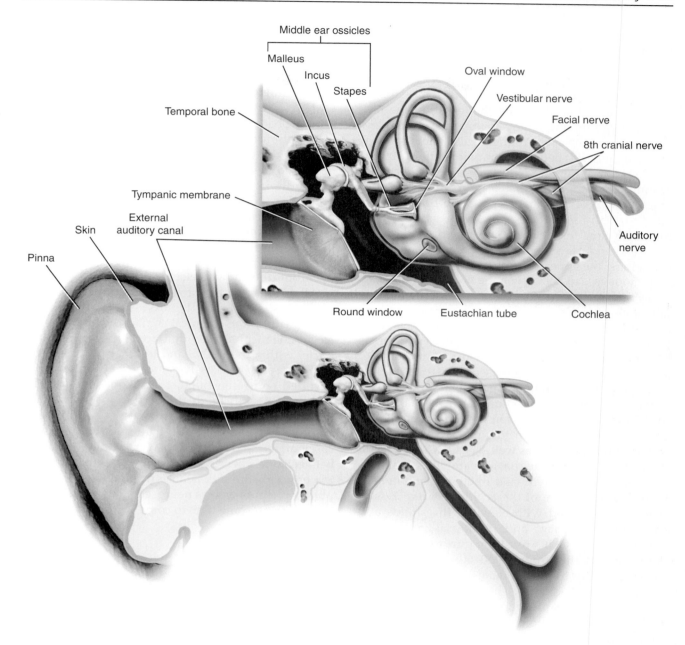

Figure 8-2. The peripheral auditory system. Sound collected by the pinna is funneled down the external auditory canal to the tympanic membrane. Movement of the TM sets the ossicles of the middle ear into motion. Movement of the stapes against the oval window sets up pressure waves in the fluid of the cochlea. The auditory nerve exiting the cochlea joins with the vestibular nerve to form the 8th cranial nerve.

largest amplitude vibrations in response to high-frequency sounds, whereas the more flaccid apical end has a low-frequency resonance and vibrates maximally in response to low-frequency sounds. Consequently, sound frequency is distributed spatially, or tonotopically, along the length of the BM, progressing from high frequencies at the base to low frequencies at the apex. Young, healthy humans hear sound frequencies between approximately 20 Hz and 20,000 Hz. That range of frequency is represented logarithmically along a BM that is approximately 34 mm long (Yost, 1994). Although the entire BM is stimulated virtually simultaneously by pressure waves, there is a time lag between movement of the light basal end and movement of the more massive apical end, giving the appearance of a wave of motion traveling from base to apex when the BM is stimulated.

BM motion indirectly modulates the membrane potentials of IHCs and OHCs in the organ of Corti. Upward movement of the BM leads to hair cell depolarization, or decreased electronegativity, whereas BM movement in the opposite direction leads to hyperpolarization, or increased electronegativity. Changes in membrane potential are associated with important physiological changes in the hair cells: shape and motility changes in the OHCs and modulation of NT release from the basal region of IHCs and presumably OHCs as well. The OHCs are critical elements of a nonlinear cochlear amplifier that contributes to the sensitivity and frequency and temporal resolving powers of the cochlea. Partial loss of OHCs is associated with elevated thresholds and impaired frequency and temporal resolution. Complete loss of OHCs results in pure tone threshold elevations on the order of 50–60 dB, along with impaired ability to discriminate signals in the presence of background noise. The IHCs, in contrast, are the sensory cells responsible for transducing mechanical energy into chemical signals that stimulate the type I SGNs that innervate them. The type I SGNs are **bipolar neurons** of the peripheral nervous system (PNS). Their cell bodies are located in the spiral

ganglion (the term *ganglion* refers to a group of neurons in the PNS, whereas *nucleus* refers to a group of neurons in the CNS); and they give rise to one peripheral process that enters the organ of Corti and one central process, or axon, that projects to the CANS. In response to NT released by the IHC, the type I SGNs generate electrical potentials that convey information from the cochlea to the CANS. When IHCs or the type I SGNs or their nerve fibers are destroyed, fewer channels are available for conveying auditory information from the cochlea to the brain. Loss of all IHCs and/or SGNs results in peripheral deafness (i.e., an inability to hear sounds through normal air conduction pathways). With intact SGNs, IHC loss can be partially overcome with a cochlear implant that stimulates the remaining type I neurons directly with electrical current.

All AN fibers project to the cochlear nucleus (CN) on the ipsilateral side (Figure 8-4). Neurons in the CN transform the chemical signals they receive into electrochemical signals that are conveyed to other nuclei within the CANS and to other regions of the CNS. At each successive nucleus, information is encoded and re-encoded, transformed, processed, and modified through the activity of specialized neurons. How all of those processes culminate in auditory perception is a difficult question that neuroscientists have yet to answer. The relationship between one's perception of sound and the nature of the original stimulus is an intriguing question that philosophers as well as neuroscientists will continue to ponder for some time to come.

Cochlear Ducts

The cochlea consists of a fluid-filled membranous sac (the membranous labyrinth, or cochlear duct) suspended within a fluid-filled bony shell (the osseous labyrinth), coiled into several turns (approximately 2⅝ in humans) from base to apex (Yost, 1994). A cross section through the cochlea reveals three distinct compartments, or ducts (Figure 8-5). The central

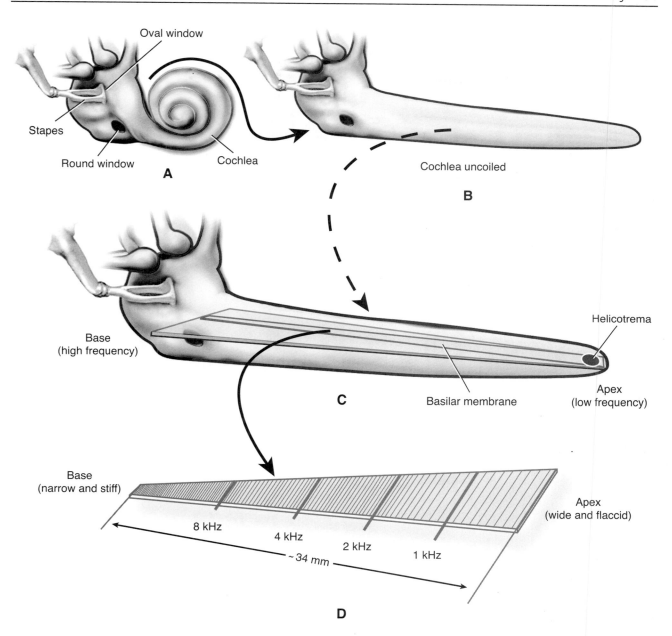

Figure 8-3. The basilar membrane. The cochlea is uncoiled to illustrate several features of the basilar membrane. The BM is narrow and stiff at the base and wide and flaccid at the apex. Frequency is represented logarithmically along a BM that is approximately 34 mm long in humans, with high frequencies represented at the base and low frequencies at the apex.

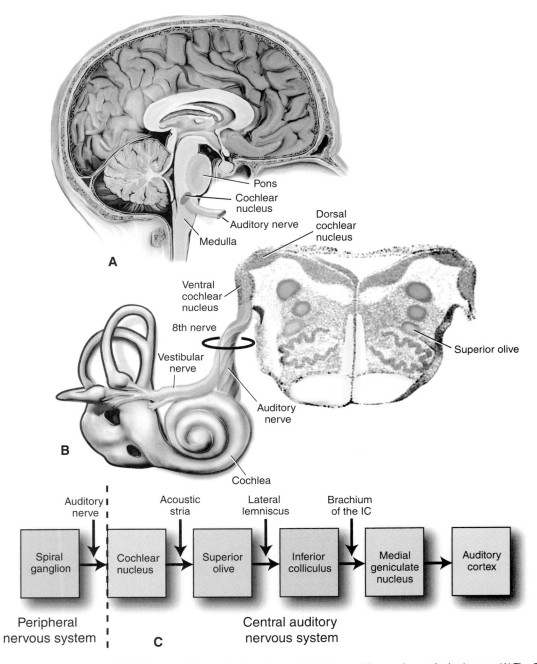

Figure 8-4. The auditory nervous system. The AN conveys information from the cochlea to the cochlear nucleus n the brainstem. (A) The CN is situated on the lateral aspect of the brainstem at the junction between the medulla and the pons. (B) The CN consists of dorsal and ventral divisions, both of which are innervated by AN fibers. The AN travels with the vestibular nerve as the 8th cranial nerve. (C) The AN arises from spiral ganglion neurons located in the spiral ganglion. The AN projects to the first nucleus of the CANS, the CN. The CANS consists of several prominent nuclei and fiber tracts, some of which are illustrated here.

cochlear duct is scala media. Reissner's membrane, a thin and flexible structure consisting of two layers of cells, forms the boundary between scala media and the upper duct, scala vestibuli. The cells comprising the epithelial cell layer facing scala media contain metabolic ion "pumps": **sodium,potassium (Na$^+$, K$^+$)-ATPase** in their basolateral membrane and a **calcium (Ca^{2+})-ATPase** in their apical membrane. It has been proposed that Reissner's membrane plays a role in maintaining the **hydro-ionic homeostasis** of the cochlea through active transport of ions between scala media and scala vestibuli (Petit, Levilliers, & Hardelin, 2001). The BM forms the territorial boundary between scala media and the lower duct, scala tympani. As shown previously in Figure 8-3, scala vestibuli and scala tympani meet at the helicotrema, a small opening at the apex of the cochlea. Inward movement of the stapes footplate at the oval window results in outward movement of the round window membrane into the middle ear cavity.

Most of scala media contains endolymph, a fluid with a chemical composition more similar to intracellular fluid than to other extracellular fluids of the body: a high concentration of K$^+$ ions (157 mM) and a low concentration of Na$^+$ ions (1.3 mM) (Wangemann & Schacht, 1996). The kidney is the only other part of the body with a high K$^+$ fluid in an extracellular space (Durrant & Lovrinic, 1995). Scala vestibuli and scala tympani contain perilymph, a fluid with a composition similar to other extracellular fluids: a high concentration of Na$^+$ (141–148 mM) and a low concentration of K$^+$ (4.2–6.0 mM). Interestingly, scala vestibuli has a slightly higher K$^+$ concentration than scala tympani despite the interconnection of the two fluid compartments at the helicotrema (Wangemann & Schacht, 1996). The human cochlea contains approximately 7.7 μl of endolymph in scala media, 31.5 μl of perilymph in scala vestibuli, and 44.3 μl of perilymph in scala tympani (Igarashi, Ohashi, & Ishii, 1986). Intermixing of endolymph and perilymph is prevented by impermeable barriers formed by tight cell junctions in Reissner's membrane, the reticular lamina, the spiral limbus, and the marginal cell layer of stria vascularis (Slepecky, 1996). The endolymphatic fluid compartment is outlined in Figure 8-5C. The reticular lamina is a plate formed at the top of the organ of Corti by tight junctions between the cuticular plates of hair cells, the heads of inner and outer pillar cells, and the phalangeal processes of Dieter's cells that support the OHCs.

Lateral Wall

Cochlear transduction depends on an electrochemical battery created by the stria vascularis, a highly vascularized region of tissue adjacent to the spiral ligament along the lateral wall of the cochlea (Figure 8-5C). The stria vascularis is responsible for production of endolymph and the EP through integrated activities of three major types of cells: marginal (dark) cells, intermediate cells (melanocytes), and basal cells. A closed intrastrial fluid space exists between the marginal cell layer and the basal cell layer. Tight junctions between marginal cells prevent entry of endolymph from scala media, and the tight junctions between basal cells prevent entry of perilymph from the spiral ligament. **Glucose** and K$^+$ from the perilymph, actively transported into the intrastrial space through gap junctions between fibrocytes in the spiral ligament and basal cells and between basal cells and intermediate cells, are utilized in the production of endolymph and the EP (Slepecky, 1996). Gap junctions are membrane structures that act as conduits for the exchange of small molecules such as nutrients, metabolites, and second messengers between adjacent cells. Mitochondria, intracellular organelles that generate high-energy molecules of ATP, are abundant in the marginal cells of the stria, consistent with the high metabolic demands of ion pumps and cotransporters located in these cells. As in most cells, the most important active transport system in the marginal cells is a Na$^+$,K$^+$-ATPase that uses energy derived from the **hydrolysis** of ATP to exchange three Na$^+$ **ions** for two K$^+$ ions across the cell membrane.

The spiral ligament contains **fibrocytes, epithelial cells,** blood vessels, and **extracellular matrix** material. A highly vascularized region of the spiral ligament, the spiral prominence, bulges into scala media just below the stria vascularis (Figure 8-5C). The spiral ligament is a major source of blood supply to the cochlea, and it plays a critical role in the regulation of fluid and ion composition in the cochlea (Slepecky, 1996).

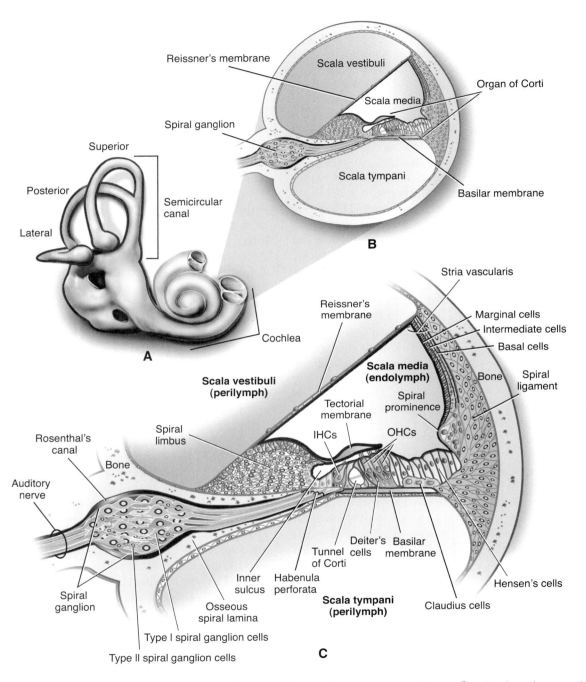

Figure 8-5. A cross section through the cochlea. (A) The cochlea is the auditory portion of the inner ear. (B) A cross section through one portion of the cochlea reveals three fluid-filled compartments. The organ of Corti is located in scala media. (C) An enlarged view shows major elements of the cochlear duct and spiral ganglion. The heavy line in scala media outlines the endolymphatic space. The portion of the organ of Corti below the reticular lamina contains perilymph.

Gap junctions between the supporting cells of the organ of Corti and fibrocytes of the spiral ligament provide a route whereby K$^+$ ions leaving the hair cells can be removed from the perilymph and returned to the stria vascularis. Mutations of several genes coding for gap junction proteins, particularly connexin 26, have been linked to neuroepithelial pathology and nonsyndromic recessive deafness in mice and humans (Petit et al., 2001).

Blood flow is required to supply oxygen and nutrients to cochlear cells and to remove waste products. The major arteries and veins in the human cochlea are illustrated in Figure 8-6. Blood is supplied to the extreme base of the human cochlea by the vestibulo-cochlear artery and to the rest of the cochlea by the spiral modiolar artery, a branch of the anterior inferior cerebellar artery. The veins of scala tympani and scala vestibuli merge into the common modiolar vein for venous drainage. Numerous branches in the form of arterioles and venules supply and drain capillary beds in the cochlea. Since there are no blood vessels in the adult organ of Corti, nutrients and oxygen must be delivered to cells by surrounding fluids.

The stria vascularis is a major target of loop diuretics such as ethacrynic acid (EA). EA induces the formation of edematous spaces in the stria, interferes with strial **adenylate cyclase** and Na$^+$,K$^+$-ATPase activity, and directly inhibits the **Na$^+$,K$^+$,2Cl$^-$ cotransport** system in the basolateral membrane of marginal cells. Inhibition of ion transport mechanisms and Na$^+$,K$^+$-ATPase releases Ca^{2+} via Na$^+$,Ca^{2+} exchange at the cell membrane, and inhibition of oxidative metabolism releases Ca^{2+} sequestered in mitochondria. Those changes are associated with disruption of ion concentrations in marginal cells and the endolymph and with depression of electrophysiologic potentials measured from the cochlea. However, recent evidence suggests that the changes described above are not the primary ototoxic effects of EA. Rather, selective disruption of blood flow in lateral wall vessels may be the initial event that triggers or contributes to subsequent morphologic and enzymatic changes in the stria vascularis (Ding, McFadden, Woo, & Salvi, 2002). Within minutes after IV injection of EA in the chinchilla, blood flow in the

vessels of the spiral ligament and stria vascularis is disrupted, whereas blood flow to other regions of the cochlea and vestibular end organs remains normal. The rapid development of ischemia in the lateral wall is followed by physiological changes: the EP becomes negative within 10 minutes after EA injection; and CAP, SP, and CM decline and become maximally depressed within 30–60 minutes after injection (Ding, Jin, McFadden, & Salvi, 2001). These early physiological changes cannot be attributed to inactivation of stria vascularis enzymes or mitochondrial dysfunction because activity levels of Na$^+$,K$^+$-ATPase, adenylate cyclase, **succinate dehydrogenase,** and **lactate dehydrogenase** remain normal for approximately

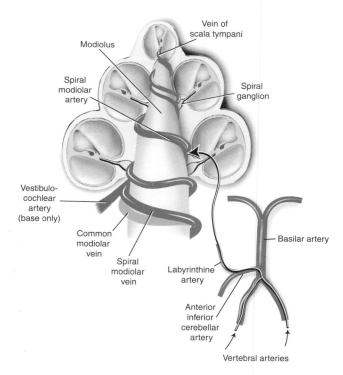

Figure 8-6. Arterial supply and venous drainage of the human cochlea. The human cochlea has two major arteries: the vestibulo-cochlear artery that supplies the basal half of the basal turn and the spiral modiolar artery that supplies the rest of the cochlea. Venous drainage in humans consists of a vein of the scala vestibuli and a vein of the scala tympani, which merge to form the common modiolar vein. (Based on diagram from Axelsson, 1968.)

60 minutes after EA injection (Ding, Jin, McFadden, & Salvi, 2001). Rather, early physiological changes may be a consequence of free radical production during **ischemia** and **reperfusion**. The mechanisms whereby EA selectively targets lateral wall vessels are not known, but the selectivity of the effect implies that there are differences in vessels supplying different regions of the inner ear. Perhaps those regional differences in vessels could be exploited in the design of smart drugs or delivery systems capable of targeting specific tissues of the inner ear for therapeutic purposes.

Organ of Corti

The organ of Corti, situated on top of the BM in scala media, is the site of approximately 12,000 cylinder-shaped OHCs arranged in three parallel rows and approximately 3,500 flask-shaped IHCs arranged in a single row (Yost, 1994). Each hair cell has a bundle of **actin**-filled **microvilli**, the stereocilia, protruding from its apical surface (Figure 8-7). The stereocilia are arranged in rows that are graded by height, with the shortest row located on the modiolar side of the hair cell. A tip link connects each stereocilium to the next taller stereocilium, and lateral links tie adjacent stereocilia together so that the entire bundle moves as a unit (Flock, 1977; Flock, Flock, & Murray, 1977; Pickles, Comis, & Osborne, 1984). The stiff stereocilia pivot at the base, where their tapered rootlets insert into the actin-rich cuticular plate. Mechanically gated ion channels located near the tips of the stereocilia open when the stereocilia bundle is deflected toward the tallest stereocilia and close when the stereocilia bundle is deflected in the opposite direction (Figure 8-8). Mechanical gating of the transduction channels is the basis for rapid changes in hair cell membrane potential and is an important feature underlying the exquisite temporal resolution of the cochlea (Hudspeth, 1997).

The tectorial membrane (TM), an acellular gelatinous structure containing at least three types of **collagen** and various **glycoproteins,** forms a roof over the hair cell region (Figure 8-5C). The stereocilia protruding from the apical surface of the OHCs are embedded in the underside of the TM, and that physical coupling influences stereocilia movement in response to acoustic stimulation. The TM is necessary for a "second resonance" of the BM, as shown by mice lacking ∝-tectorin, one of the major noncollagenous proteins of the TM (Anagnostopoulos, 2002). In *Tecta*-null mice, the TM is detached from the spiral limbus. BM responses are tuned but less sensitive than normal and the CM shows abnormal phase and symmetry, indicating a role of ∝-tectorin in normal gain and timing of cochlear feedback. Whereas the TM is involved in OHC stereocilia deflection, fluid motion in the endolymph in the subtectorial space appears to be the sole impetus for deflection of IHC stereocilia.

Studies of mice with genetically induced hearing loss have led to the identification of several "unconventional" (nonmuscle-like) myosin proteins in stereocilia and other regions of the hair cells (McFadden, 2001; Petit et al., 2001). **Myosins** are molecular motors that, upon interaction with actin filaments, utilize energy from the hydrolysis of ATP to generate mechanical force that moves them in one direction along actin filaments (see reviews by Rodriguez & Cheney, 2000; Sellers, 2000; Titus, 2000; Wu, Jung, & Hammer, 2000). Myosins consist of three regions: a conserved **N-terminal** head (or motor) domain that contains both ATP-binding and **actin-binding sequences:** a **light chain**-binding neck region containing the binding site for **calmodulin** or other calcium-binding proteins and a **C (carboxyl) terminus,** or tail domain, that is different for each myosin class. The tail domain serves in **dimerization**, membrane binding, protein binding, and/or enzymatic activities. Mutations affecting myosin genes underscore the importance and complexity of myosin and actin organization in the normal cochlea, as each of the mutations produces a different nonsyndromic hearing impairment. For example, Shaker-1 mice with a mutation of the *myo7a* gene (*sh-1*) that encodes **myosin VIIA protein** have disorganized stereocilia bundles (Gibson et al., 1995). Myosin VIIA may be involved in membrane trafficking in the IHCs as well as in maintaining stereocilia integrity. Interestingly, Richardson et al. (1997) found that cochlear explants from Shaker-1 mice do not take up aminoglycosides, implicating myosin VIIA in some aspect of uptake across the apical surface of the hair cell. A mutation of *myo6* leads to fusion of stereocilia in the Snell's

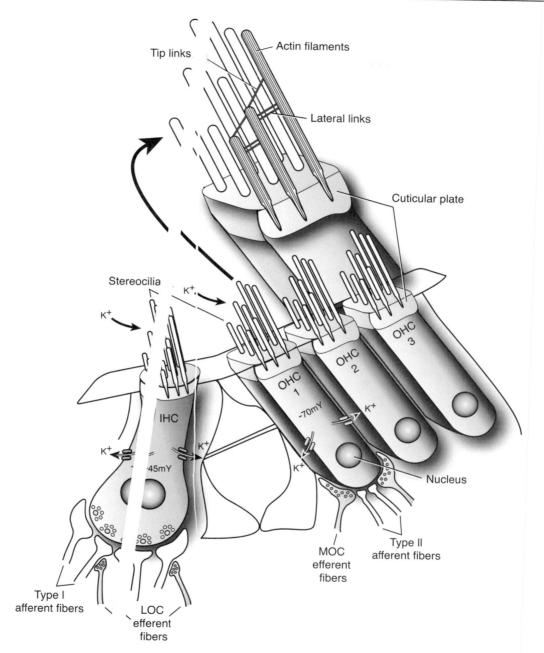

Figure 8-7. Hair cells of the cochlea. Stiff actin-filled stereocilia protrude from the apical surface of the hair cells and form bundles that are tied together by lateral links and tip links. Stereocilia rows are graded in height, with the shortest stereocilia facing the modiolus. Deflection of stereocilia toward the lateral wall opens channels for potassium (K^+) current. The IHCs and OHCs have different innervation patterns. IHCs are heavily innervated by type I afferent fibers, and the afferents are contacted by LOC efferent fibers. The OHCs are sparsely innervated by type II afferent fibers and heavily innervated by large terminals of MOC efferent fibers. Channels in the basolateral membrane of the hair cells permit efflux of K^+ into the perilymph down a concentration gradient.

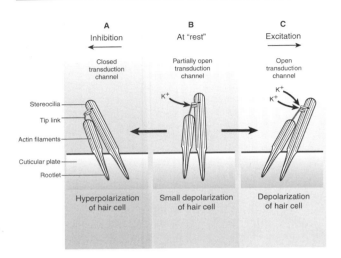

Figure 8-8. Stereocilia deflection causing changes in the membrane potentials of hair cells. Transduction channels located near the tips of stereocilia are mechanically gated. Deflection toward the shortest stereocilia is inhibitory because it closes the channels tightly and the membrane becomes hyperpolarized as K^+ leaves the cell through channels in the basolateral membrane (Figure 8-7). Deflection toward the tallest stereocilia is excitatory because it pulls the channels open and the influx of K^+ depolarizes the membrane. At rest, approximately 5%–15% of the channels are open, resulting in a standing current through the hair cell and a slight depolarization.

waltzer mouse (Avraham, 1997). Myosin VI is a particularly interesting myosin because it moves backward relative to all other known myosins (i.e., toward the cell body rather than away from it). Shaker-2 mice with a *myo15* mutation have OHC and IHC stereocilia that are only about one-tenth their normal length, and the actin filaments extend far beneath the apical surface of the hair cell (Liang et al., 1999; Probst et al., 1998). Several other unconventional myosins have been identified recently. For current information on these and other proteins and gene mutations associated with hearing impairment, the interested reader is referred to the Web site maintained by The Jackson Laboratory: http://www.informatics.jax.org.

Spiral Ganglion Neurons (SGNs) and Afferent Innervation

OHCs are innervated by a small number of peripheral processes from **type II SGNs** located in the spiral ganglion in Rosenthal's canal and by a large number of medial olivocochlear (MOC) efferent fibers (more about them later). IHCs are innervated by peripheral projections from approximately 30,000 type I SGNs. Each type I nerve fiber innervates only one IHC (or two in the human cochlea), and each IHC is innervated by up to twenty type I nerve fibers (Webster, 1992). Thus, there is a remarkable divergence of information from the IHCs to the spiral ganglion and the CANS.

There are many important differences between type I and type II SGNs. As noted above, the peripheral processes of type II SGNs are highly branched so that each type II SGN innervates a large number of OHCs. In contrast, the peripheral processes of type I SGNs typically innervate only one IHC. Differences in the innervation patterns of type I and type II SGNs are illustrated in Figure 8-9. Type I SGNs are far more numerous, comprising 90%–95% of the SGN population and their cell bodies and processes are larger than those of type II SGNs. Fiber size is one factor influencing neural transmission, with large diameter processes conducting electrical potentials more rapidly and over longer distances than small diameter processes. The central processes and portions of the peripheral processes of type I SGNs (up to the spiral lamina, where they pass through openings in the bony ledge to enter the organ of Corti) are usually myelinated, whereas type II SGNs and their processes are unmyelinated. As you will see later, myelination is a second factor influencing neural signaling, with myelinated fibers conveying action potentials (APs), rapid and transient reversals of membrane potential, more rapidly than unmyelinated fibers. In animals, the cell bodies of type I SGNs tend to be myelinated as well, which has implications for spatial and temporal summation of electrical potentials and for rapid transmission of potentials to the central AN processes.

The peripheral processes of SGNs enter the cochlea through tiny holes, the **habenula perforatae**, in the osseous spiral lamina located beneath the medial portion of the BM (Figure 8-9). The osseous spiral lamina is a bony ledge projecting from the modiolus, a bony central canal that houses nerve fibers and blood vessels. It is also the site of **Rosenthal's canal,** where the spiral ganglion cell bodies are located. The central processes of the SGNs

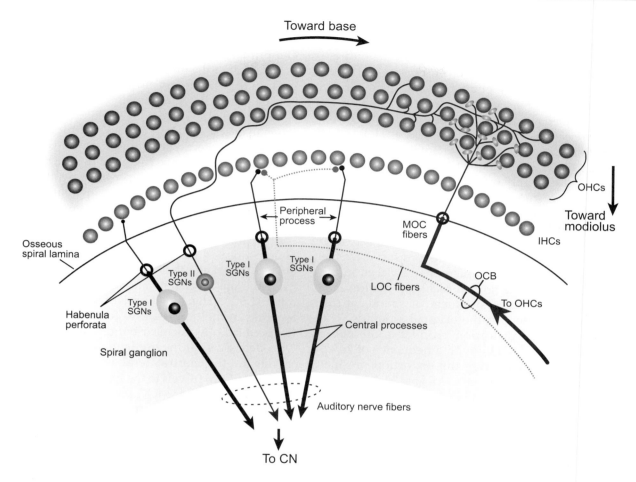

Figure 8-9. Innervation patterns in the organ of Corti. Three rows of OHCs and one row of IHCs are innervated by efferent and/or afferent fibers. IHCs are innervated directly by type I afferents; OHCs are innervated directly by type II afferents and MOC efferent fibers. Each large type I SGN innervates only one or two IHCs, whereas a single small type II SGN innervates multiple OHCs. The central processes of SGNs form the auditory nerve that projects to the cochlear nucleus. The peripheral processes of SGNs enter the organ of Corti through habenula perforata, holes in the osseous spiral lamina beneath the medial portion of the basilar membrane. The type I SGNs tend to be fully myelinated up to the habenula perforata, whereas type II SGNs are unmyelinated. Axons of the olivocochlear bundle (OCB) also enter the organ of Corti through the habenula perforata. Large fibers of the medial efferent system synapse with OHCs, mainly on the modiolar side. The MOC fibers are myelinated up to the habenula perforata. Small unmyelinated fibers of the lateral efferent system synapse on the afferent fibers beneath the IHCs.

gather together in the modiolus to form the AN, which travels with the vestibular nerve as the 8th cranial nerve to the brainstem. The auditory portion of the 8th nerve enters the CN at the junction between the medulla and the pons (Figure 8-4).

The Efferent Pathways

It is common to think of the auditory system as a unidirectional feed-forward system in which information ascends from the auditory periphery to the cortex. However, there are also many feedback pathways and instances of reverse energy transmission in the auditory periphery, represented by the bidirectional arrows in Figure 8-1. The reverse pathway from the cochlea to the middle ear and the outer ear is the source of otoacoustic emissions (OAEs), originally described as "cochlear echoes" by Kemp (1980). OAEs arise from the activity of OHCs (Hofstetter, Ding, Powers, & Salvi, 1997; Hofstetter, Ding, & Salvi, 1997; Tratwein, Hofstetter, Wang, Salvi, & Nostrant, 1996) and reflect the normal nonlinear functioning of the cochlear amplifier. A common method for testing OAEs is to present pairs of pure tones, f_1 and f_2, at a fixed frequency ratio (typically, $f_2/f_1 = 1.2$) and level ratio (typically, $L_1 = L_2 + 10$ dB), then record the resulting sounds produced by the cochlea, using a sensitive microphone placed in the ear canal. Because the normal cochlea is nonlinear, it will generate distortion products, or sounds at frequencies not present in the original stimulus. The largest amplitude distortion product is the **cubic distortion product (CDP)** with a frequency of $2f_1$-f_2; consequently, that is often the distortion product measured clinically. Normal OAEs are indicative of healthy OHCs, whereas reduced or absent OAEs are associated with OHC loss or dysfunction. The frequency-specific nature of CDP OAEs makes them particularly well suited for detecting early basal (high-frequency) OHC damage from ototoxic drugs.

Three Efferent Pathways from the Brainstem

Descending pathways originating in the CANS include the three illustrated in Figure 8-1: an efferent pathway to the middle ear and two efferent pathways to the cochlea. Those efferent pathways allow the CANS to influence peripheral sensitivity and function.

Efferent projections from neurons in the superior olivary region of the brainstem to the middle ear muscles comprise the motor arm of a middle ear acoustic reflex (AR) that is activated in response to high-level sound and prior to self-vocalization. Reflex contraction of the stapedius muscle increases the stiffness of the ossicular chain and attenuates transmission of low-frequency sounds (below about

1.2 kHz in humans) from the middle ear to the cochlea by about 5–30 dB (Durrant & Lovrinic, 1995). The primary function of the middle ear AR appears to be to reduce the masking effects of one's own voice because the middle ear muscles contract *prior* to self-vocalizations in humans and animals (Borg & Counter, 1989). Protection from some types of acoustic overstimulation can be an added benefit of the AR, but protection is limited because of the time it takes for the reflex to be triggered by external sound.

Two anatomically and physiologically distinct efferent pathways originate from neurons in the superior olivary region of the brainstem and project to the cochlea (Guinan Jr., 1996; Warr, 1992; Warr, Guinan Jr., & White, 1986). MOC fibers arise from neurons located in the region of the medial superior olive (MSO). Lateral olivocochlear (LOC) fibers arise from neurons located in and near the lateral superior olive (LSO). The MOC and LOC efferents gather together in the brainstem to form large bundles of fibers called olivocochlear bundles (OCB). A crossed OCB decussates at the midline of the brainstem and travels to the contralateral cochlea, whereas an uncrossed OCB travels to the ipsilateral cochlea. LOC efferents outnumber MOC efferents in most species, but the actual numbers and proportion of LOC to MOC fibers vary greatly. LOC fibers comprise 52%–54% of the entire OCB in guinea pigs and rats; 75%–80% in gerbils, chinchillas, squirrel monkeys, and mustached bats; and 100% in horseshoe bats (Azeredo et al., 1999; Iurato et al., 1978; Warr, 1992; Warr et al., 1986). The OC fibers travel within the inferior vestibular nerve into the internal auditory canal, where they branch off to enter the modiolus at the cochlear base. Efferent fibers enter the cochlea through the habenula perforatae and travel to their sites of termination. As illustrated schematically in Figures 8-8 and 8-10, LOC efferents terminate on the type I afferent nerve fibers beneath the IHCs, whereas MOC efferents synapse directly with OHCs. MOC neurons supply the OHCs with large, **vesiculated** terminals at specialized regions of the OHC base, mainly on the modiolar side (Robertson, Harvey, & Cole, 1989; Spoendlin, 1985; Warr & Guinan, 1979).

Differences between LOC and MOC efferents provide some clues regarding their function. MOC fibers projecting to the cochlea are large and myelinated, whereas LOC fibers are small and unmyelinated. LOC fibers are more complex neurochemically. The differences in myelination and neurochemical complexity suggest that the MOC system is involved in rapid, dynamic feedback to the OHCs, whereas the LOC system provides slow-acting and more general modulation of afferent fiber activity and cochlear output.

Both olivocochlear reflex loops are primarily "intracochlear" loops because LOC and MOC neurons tend to project back to the same cochlea that provided their excitatory input (Warr, 1992; Warr & Beck, 1996). The input and output pathways for the two reflex loops are illustrated schematically in Figure 8-10. Arrow size is roughly proportional to the size or prominence of the fiber tract. As illustrated in the top panel, LOC neurons receive their input from the ipsilateral cochlea via the ipsilateral ventral CN, and nearly all LOC neurons project back to the ipsilateral cochlea. In some species, a small number of LOC neurons (about 15% in cats) project to the contralateral cochlea. However, most animals, including rats, bats, guinea pigs, chinchillas, and gerbils, have very small or no contralateral LOC projections (Warr, 1992). Whereas the LOC system is almost exclusively intracochlear, the MOC system in most animals consists of a large intracochlear component and a smaller intercochlear component. This is illustrated in the bottom panel of Figure 8-10. Most MOC neurons receive their input from the contralateral cochlea via the contralateral ventral CN, and most MOC neurons project back to the same cochlea that activated them. Thus, the largest component of the MOC pathway is a crossed (or "double-crossed" if one considers the input arm of the loop) intracochlear pathway. A smaller number of MOC neurons project to the cochlea on the ipsilateral side via an uncrossed MOC pathway (Warr, 1992; Guinan, 1996). Intercochlear MOC and LOC loops provide the only neural routes by which the activity of one cochlea can influence the activity of the opposite cochlea (Liberman, 1989; Warren & Liberman, 1989). It is the smaller uncrossed MOC intercochlear loop that is activated

in contralateral efferent suppression studies (Mott, Norton, Neely, & Warr, 1989). In those studies, OAE, CM, or CAP amplitudes in one ear can be decreased by sound delivered to the opposite ear, indicating a functional *uncrossed* MOC pathway.

Although the OC efferents have been studied since Rasmussen first described them in 1942 and it is obvious that they provide pathways whereby the CANS can influence cochlear activity, their functional significance is still a mystery. It is most likely that the efferents are involved in attentional processes and in enhancing signal-to-noise ratios in difficult listening situations. A secondary effect of OC efferents is protection from damage caused by acoustic overstimulation. That role has been most clearly demonstrated by studies in which efferent feedback to one ear is entirely eliminated by transection of the OCB as it enters the internal auditory canal (Zheng, Henderson, Hu, Ding, & McFadden, 1997; Zheng, Henderson, McFadden, & Hu, 1997).

Do Medial Olivocochlear (MOC) Efferents Influence Uptake of Aminoglycosides?

There is some evidence that MOC fibers play a role in the chain of events leading to OHC loss from ototoxic drugs such as aminoglycoside antibiotics. Kohonen (1965) first noted that the distribution of MOC fibers in the guinea pig cochlea was correlated with OHC susceptibility to neomycin, kanamycin, and framycetin. Basal OHCs were more vulnerable than apical OHCs, corresponding to the declining base-to-apex gradient in MOC innervation; and Row 1 OHCs were more vulnerable than Row 2 or 3 OHCs, again corresponding to the density of MOC efferent terminals. Direct evidence of a link between MOC innervation and OHC susceptibility to aminoglycosides comes from MOC stimulation and lesions experiments (Brown, 1972; Brown & Daigneault, 1973; Capps & Duvall, 1976; Daigneault, Pruett, & Brown, 1970). Capps and Duvall (1977) observed far less kanamycin-induced OHC loss in cochleas of chinchillas with lesions of the crossed MOC fibers than in unlesioned controls. The greatest saving afforded by elimination of MOC fibers was seen in Row 1 OHCs,

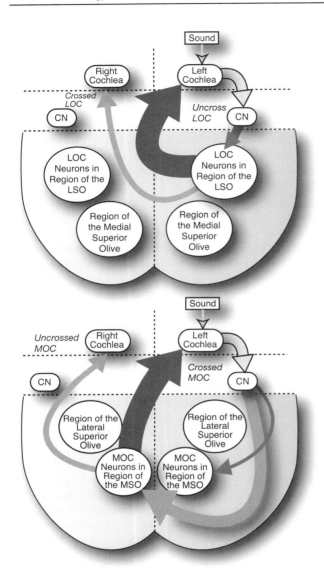

Figure 8-10. Two olivocochlear reflex arcs. The top panel illustrates the LOC pathway that influences afferent nerve fiber activity; the bottom panel illustrates the MOC pathway that influences OHC activity. Arrow size is roughly proportional to the size or prominence of the fiber tract. Light arrows show input pathways to the brainstem; dark arrows show pathways from the brainstem to the cochlea. The largest proportion of LOC and MOC fibers are intracochlear because they project back to the cochlea that provided their initial input. The LOC system is almost exclusively intracochlear. In contrast, about one-third of the MOC system is intercochlear, with an uncrossed pathway projecting from the medial region of the superior olive to the ipsilateral cochlea.

where losses averaged 14% in deefferented ears versus 66% in normal ears! Differences between normal and deefferented ears were also significant, although less pronounced, in OHC Rows 2 and 3.

The mechanisms to account for decreased kanamycin-induced OHC loss after deefferentation are not known. One possibility is that efferent fiber activity normally affects either the local chemical milieu or properties of the hair cell membrane in a way that promotes uptake of aminoglycosides. That idea is interesting in light of experimental data showing that aminoglycoside uptake by bacterial cells decreases as membrane potentials are reduced and that reduction of the EP protects guinea pigs from gentamicin ototoxicity (Takada, Bledsoe, & Schacht, 1985). There is evidence that MOC fibers exert a **tonic influence** on OHC membrane potentials (Zheng, Henderson, McFadden, Ding, & Salvi, 1999; Zheng, McFadden, Henderson, Ding, & Burkard, 2000). It is conceivable that reduced OHC membrane potential in MOC-lesioned ears accounts for decreased uptake of aminoglycosides and relative protection.

COCHLEAR TRANSDUCTION

The role of the cochlea is to convert mechanical energy into electrical energy, a process known as mechanoelectrical transduction. The major players in that process are the BM, the hair cells, the stria vascularis, and type I SGNs (Figure 8-5C). The process depends on the driving forces of a K^+ concentration gradient and the EP, both created by the stria vascularis. Because an understanding of the transduction process requires a basic knowledge of bioelectrical potentials, this section will begin with an overview of resting potentials (RPs) in the cochlea, or voltages that exist in the absence of acoustic stimulation. Although the EP is considered here because it is independent of acoustic stimulation, it is important to note that the mechanisms responsible for the EP are different from those giving rise to the RPs of the hair cells (and as will be shown in a later section, the RPs of neurons). Specifically, the EP is created by metabolic processes in the stria vascularis, and it is maintained at a relatively constant value whether or not acoustic stimulation occurs. Hair cell potentials, in contrast, arise through ion separations maintained by barriers to ion flow. Barrier permeability and ion flow change rapidly in hair cells in response to acoustic stimulation, giving rise to stimulus evoked potentials (EVPs).

Resting Potentials (RPs) of the Cochlea

Electrical potentials, also called potential differences, voltages, or electrical gradients, are created by the separation of charges. The potential energy created by charge separation is proportional to the magnitude of the charges and inversely proportional to the distance between them. When a pathway is provided for charges to move down an electrical gradient, their movement is current. This basic idea is represented by Ohm's law, $I = V/R$, which simply states that the amount of current (I) at a given point in time depends on the voltage (V) applied and the nature of the current path, or resistance (R), across which the potential difference exists. A current path with low resistance (or conversely, a high conductance) allows a large current to flow, whereas a current path with high resistance limits current flow. In an electrical circuit with infinite resistance (in the form of an open switch or an impermeable membrane barrier, for example), no current flows regardless of the voltage. Ohm's law is useful for describing events in linear electrical systems, where the value of R is independent of V. In bioelectrical systems such as nerve cells, however, R can vary as a function of V and voltages change rapidly in response to ion movement. Those issues will be expanded on later in relation to ion channels in the membranes of hair cells and neurons.

To understand the RPs of the cochlea, it may be helpful to envision a hypothetical experiment in which a high-impedance glass micropipette recording electrode is slowly advanced through the cochlea. The experiment is shown schematically in Figure 8-11. A second electrode placed in the vascular system outside the cochlea serves as the reference electrode (arbitrarily defined as 0 mV). Potential differences between the reference electrode and the recording electrode are displayed on an oscilloscope, which

shows voltage (in mV) on the y-axis as a function of time on the x-axis. The RPs of the cochlea are positive or negative DC potentials (i.e., unidirectional shifts in voltage from the baseline).

When the electrode passes through the osseous labyrinth and enters the perilymph in scala tympani, a DC shift of +7 mV or less occurs (Johnstone & Sellick, 1972). The electrical potential changes very little as the electrode passes through the BM into the fluid surrounding the organ of Corti (still perilymph), but when the electrode enters a hair cell, the potential abruptly becomes negative (approximately -70 mV if the electrode has entered an OHC or approximately -45 mV if the electrode has entered an IHC) (Cody & Russell, 1987; Dallos, Santos-Sacchi, & Flock, 1982). When the electrode passes through the reticular lamina at the top of the organ of Corti and enters the endolymph in scala media, the potential abruptly reverses to a high positive value (around +80 mV) (Bosher, 1979; Peake, Sohmer, & Weiss, 1969). Finally, when the recording electrode crosses Reissner's membrane and enters the perilymph of scala vestibuli, the potential abruptly decreases again, to approximately +2 to +5 mV (Johnstone & Sellick, 1972). If the electrode path led to the stria vascularis, a highly unusual positive intracellular potential would be recorded from the marginal cells, even in the absence of endolymph.

The RPs that are recorded from different regions of the cochlea arise through mechanisms involving fluids with very specific ionic compositions and barriers that prevent the free flow of ions. Movement of a charged particle across time and space is electrical current. Whereas negatively charged electrons are the carriers of current in electrical systems, both positively and negatively charged ions (cations and anions, respectively) perform that role in biological systems. Like other charged particles, ions are repelled by like charges and attracted by unlike charges. Thus, a positively charged ion (such as K^+) is attracted to a negatively charged region and repelled by a positively charged region (such as the endolymphatic space with an EP of +80 mV). Unless its movement is impeded or prevented (by closed ion channels, for instance), the ion will move down the electrical gradient until the electrical gradient is abolished.

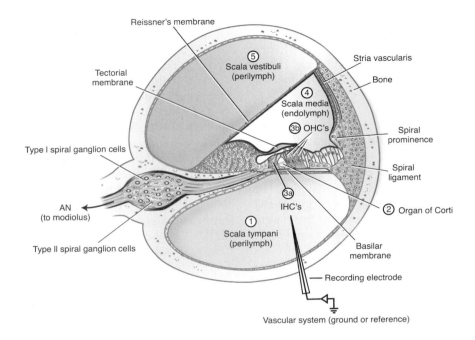

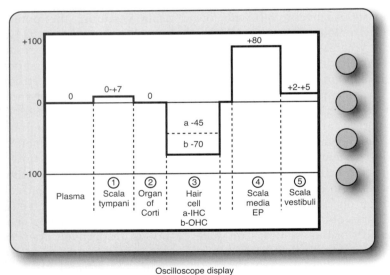

Oscilloscope display

Figure 8-11. Resting potentials of the cochlea. Potential differences are recorded between a reference electrode in the vascular system outside the cochlea and a recording electrode as it moves through the cochlea (top panel). DC potentials are displayed on an oscilloscope (bottom panel). Voltages are positive in the fluid spaces of the cochlea and negative inside the hair cells. The resting potential of an IHC is on the order of -45 mV, compared to about -70 mV for OHCs. The large +80 mV potential measured from scala media is the EP, created and maintained by the stria vascularis. The difference between the positive value of the EP and the negative value of the hair cell potential constitutes the battery for driving the transduction process in the electrical model of Davis (1965). However, the hair cell potential is less important than the concentration gradients for potassium (see text).

In biological systems, current flow is under the influence of concentration, or diffusion, forces as well as electrical forces. Unless movement is impeded or prevented, ions will diffuse from a region of high concentration to a region of low concentration. Thus, K^+ will be inclined to move from a region of high concentration in the endolymph to a region of low concentration in the intracellular fluid of the hair cell. Ionic current will flow until the concentration gradient is either abolished or counterbalanced by an equal but opposite electrical gradient. The electrical potential required to balance a given concentration gradient and prevent current flow in a system that permits free movement of the ion in question is called the equilibrium potential.

Equilibrium is reached in a biological system when electrical forces and concentration gradients are balanced. At equilibrium, there is no net movement of ions even when there is no barrier to their movement because the concentration forces and electrical forces just oppose each other. That is what happens at the peak of an AP when the equilibrium potential for Na^+ is reached and current flow across the membrane momentarily stops before reversing direction. The RPs in the cochlea are not equilibrium potentials, but rather potentials that exist because barriers prevent ion movement and maintain charge separation. Charges will move if or when the barriers become permeable. As will be shown later, that is what happens during mechanoelectrical transduction in hair cells and when APs are generated by neurons.

The Endocochlear Potential (EP)

Although the EP is a DC potential that exists in the absence of acoustic stimulation, it is different from the RPs of the hair cells because it is created by active processes in the stria vascularis and maintained at a fairly constant value (+80 mV) irrespective of acoustic stimulation. When the EP was discovered, it was thought to arise from the concentration gradient between the endolymph and the perilymph. However, early experiments refuted that. Tasaki et al. (1959) showed that positive electrical potentials could be recorded from the marginal cells of the stria vascularis even after Reissner's membrane was destroyed and the K^+ concentration gradient was abolished. Konishi et al. (1968) showed that decreasing the K^+ concentration gradient by injecting potassium chloride into the perilymph had little effect on the EP amplitude. The EP decreased significantly following surgical or drug-induced damage to the stria vascularis (Davis et al., 1958; Sewell, 1984) or anoxia (Bosher, 1979; Johnstone & Sellick, 1972; T. Konishi, 1979). Those results indicated that the EP is a metabolic potential generated by energy-consuming activities of cells in the stria vascularis. Although all details of the process are still not understood, it appears that electrogenic pumps located in the marginal cells of the stria vascularis actively secrete K^+ and extract Na^+ in order to maintain the ionic composition of the endolymph (Kuijpers & Bonting, 1970).

Hair Cell Mechanoelectrical Transduction

Figure 8-12 summarizes the key elements and events of mechanoelectrical transduction. Mechanically gated ion channels at the tips of the stereocilia are opened and closed by back-and-forth movement of the stereocilia (Figure 8-8). When the BM moves toward scala vestibuli, nonselective cation channels at the stereocilia tips are pulled open, allowing positively charged ions to enter. Because K^+ is the most abundant cation in the endolymph, most current into the hair cell is carried by that ion.

Influx of K^+ ions from the endolymph depolarizes the hair cell, whereas efflux of K^+ through the basolateral membrane into the perilymph when the stereocilia ion channels are closed leads to hyperpolarization. The IHC potential is a graded response, as shown in Figure 8-13. BM movement (hence, stereocilia deflection and K^+ current) is graded according to stimulus intensity, with low-level acoustic stimulation producing small BM vibrations (hence, limited stereocilia deflections and small currents) and high-level stimulation producing large BM excursions (hence, large stereocilia displacements and large currents). Small K^+ current changes produce correspondingly small shifts in the IHC membrane potential, whereas large K^+ currents produce larger shifts in membrane potential. Cycles of back-and-forth

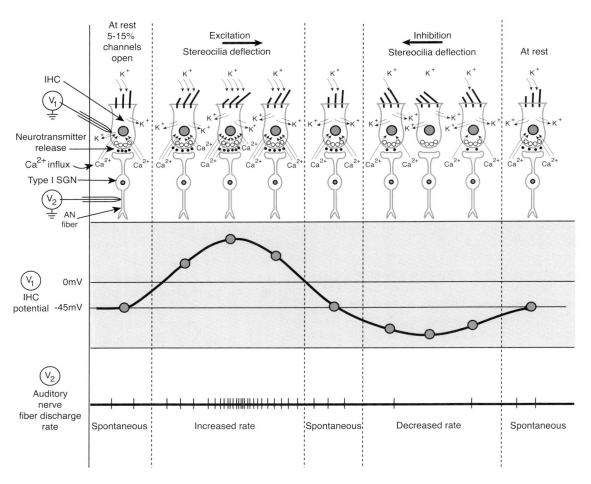

Figure 8-12. Mechanoelectrical transduction. The top panel shows an inner hair cell innervated by a type I spiral ganglion neuron. Stereocilia are deflected back and forth as the basilar membrane moves up and down in response to acoustic stimulation, which opens nonselective cation channels. Cations (primarily K[+]) move into the hair cell down electrical and concentration gradients. Selective ion channels in the basolateral membrane of the hair cell permit efflux of K[+] into the perilymph down a concentration gradient. Calcium channels in the basolateral membrane of the hair cell permit entry of Ca2[+], a necessary precursor for the fusion of synaptic vesicles to the hair cell membrane and exocytosis of neurotransmitter into the synaptic cleft. As stereocilia are deflected toward the tallest row, apical channels open and K[+] current into the hair cell increases; as the stereocilia move in the opposite direction, channels close and apical K[+] current decreases. The membrane potential recorded from the hair cell is shown in the middle panel. The bottom panel shows the discharge rate of the auditory nerve fiber. Membrane potential varies as a function of stereocilia deflection. The discharge rate of the AN fiber increases above a "spontaneous" level when more NT is released by the depolarized IHC and decreases below the spontaneous level when less NT is released by the hyperpolarized IHC.

stereocilia deflection result in cyclic changes in membrane potential.

Davis (1965) modeled the hair cell transduction process as an electrical circuit powered by two batteries, one associated with the +80 mV EP in scala media

that "pushes" K[+] into the hair cell and the other associated with the negative intracellular potential that "pulls" K[+] into the hair cell. As batteries connected in series, the EP and the intracellular potential of the hair cell would result in a large electrical gradient acting to drive K⁺ through transduction channels (approximately 125 mV for IHCs and 150 mV for OHCs). The main limitation of the Davis model is that it ignores the concentration gradients acting on K⁺. When K⁺ concentration gradients are considered in conjunction with electrical gradients, it becomes apparent that the electronegativity of the hair cell interior makes little difference to the influx of K⁺ from the endolymph (Salt & Konishi, 1986). Rather, the electrical potential of the EP and the K⁺ concentration gradient between the endolymph and the hair cell cytoplasm comprise an electrochemical battery that drives K⁺ current into the hair cell. Concentration gradients must also be considered to account for the outward K⁺ current through selective voltage-gated K⁺ channels in the basolateral membrane of the hair cell (Figure 8-7). Whereas the electrical gradient between

the hair cell and the perilymph would favor influx of K⁺, the concentration gradient promotes K⁺ efflux from the hair cell.

For OHCs, changes in membrane potential in response to depolarizing or hyperpolarizing current produce changes in cell length (Brownell, Bader, Bertrand, & de Ribaupierre, 1985). Cyclic contraction and elongation of the OHCs pumps energy back into the BM system. Whether that has a dampening or an amplifying effect on BM motion may depend on the phase of OHC motility relative to BM vibration. The amount of OHC length change is proportional to the gain of the cochlear amplifier. The MOC efferent system can modulate the activity of OHCs and the motion of the BM and, hence, the output of the AN fibers (Zheng et al., 1999). Prestin, a motor protein expressed only in the lateral membrane of OHCs, is

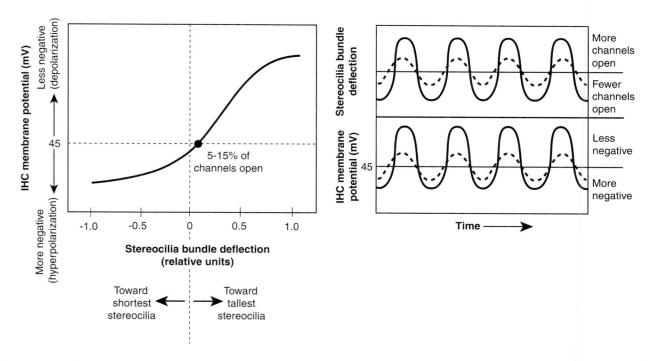

Figure 8-13. Relationship between stereocilia deflection and hair cell membrane potential. The panel on the left shows IHC membrane potential (mV) as a function of stereocilia bundle deflection (in relative units where zero represents an "upright" position). The panel on the right shows stereocilia bundle deflection and IHC membrane potential as a function of time as the ear is stimulated with a low-level tone (dashed line) or a high-level tone (solid line).

the putative OHC motor (Zheng, Madison, Oliver, Fakler, & Dallos, 2002).

Hair Cell Electrochemical Transduction and Spiral Ganglion Neuron (SGN) Activity

Depolarization of the hair cell membrane triggers the opening of **V-gated** Ca^{2+} **channels** and entry of Ca^{2+} into the basolateral region of the hair cell. In the presence of Ca^{2+}, synaptic vesicles containing an excitatory NT (probably glutamate or a similar amino acid) fuse to the plasma membrane of the hair cell and release their contents through **exocytosis**. Otoferlin, a calcium-binding protein expressed only in the IHCs of the mature cochlea, appears to be involved in the fusion of synaptic vesicles to the IHC membrane (Yasunaga et al., 1999). Binding of the excitatory IHC NT to receptors on the afferent nerve fiber membrane opens ligand (chemical)-gated channels through which positively charged ions enter and depolarize the afferent fiber membrane. That depolarization is passively conveyed to a membrane site where an AP, or "spike," is generated.

The number of APs generated by a neuron in a given period of time is referred to as its spike rate or discharge rate. "Driven" discharge refers to APs generated in response to acoustic stimulation, and "spontaneous" discharge refers to APs generated in the absence of suprathreshold acoustic stimulation. Increased NT release from the depolarized IHC increases the discharge rate of the type I SGNs, as illustrated in the bottom panel of Figure 8-11. In the absence of acoustic stimulation, approximately 5%–15% of the stereocilia ion channels are open at any given time, resulting in a "standing current" of K^+ through the hair cell (Crawford & Fettiplace, 1981; Hudspeth & Corey, 1977; Russell, Cody, & Richardson, 1986). This depolarizing bias probably accounts for the "spontaneous" activity of AN fibers. Spontaneous activity is significantly decreased in chronically deefferented ears (Zheng et al., 1999), suggesting a role of LOC fibers in modulating AN fiber reactivity to the IHC NT.

When IHCs are hyperpolarized, they release less NT and the SGNs generate APs at a rate below their spontaneous level. Thus, cycles of alternating depolarization and hyperpolarization of IHCs produce patterned bursts of NT release and SGN discharge. The rate of discharge and pattern of activity across the population of AN fibers carry information about the frequency, intensity, and temporal aspects of the acoustic stimulus to the CANS.

Stimulus Evoked Potentials (EVPs)

Stimulus EVPs are typically recorded using low-impedance electrodes that pick up electrical activity from large groups of cells. The electrodes for recording EVPs may be inserted directly into the site of interest (AN or a specific CANS nucleus, for instance), in which case they are called local field potentials; or they may be placed at sites distant from the source, in which case they may be referred to as gross potentials. Examples of gross potentials include the CM, SP, and CAP recorded from transtympanic or ear canal electrodes and auditory brainstem responses (ABRs) recorded from surface electrodes (typically used with humans) or subdermal needle electrodes (commonly used with experimental animals). EVPs are typically quantified in terms of response amplitude (e.g., peak-to-peak voltage or peak voltage relative to a baseline level) and latency (time lag from stimulus onset to a defined portion of the response). The EVPs are graded responses, meaning that their amplitudes vary in proportion to stimulus level over a range of sound pressure levels (SPLs), from threshold to a level that produces saturation or rollover of the response (Figure 8-14). It is customary in electrophysiology to obtain input-output functions that show response parameters (amplitude and latency) as a function of stimulus input level for each of the evoked responses. In normal ears, amplitudes generally increase and latencies decrease with increases in stimulus SPL. Computerized time averaging of responses is usually required to separate electrical activity that is entrained to an acoustic stimulus from "random" background activity. Figure 8-15 shows an electrophysiology recording that includes the CM, SP, and CAP. Specialized recording or data analysis techniques can be used to look separately at each component of the response.

The CM is an AC (time-varying) potential that follows the moment-by-moment movement of the BM and therefore the frequency and amplitude of the acoustic stimulus (Figure 8-15). As described previously, BM motion is associated with the opening and closing of ion channels in the stereocilia of the hair cells. The resulting changes in current flow through the hair cells produce voltage fluctuations that are recorded as the CM. CM amplitude is influenced by OHC loss but not IHC loss (Trautwein et al., 1996) and is therefore a useful measure for evaluating OHC function.

The SP is a DC potential that lasts as long as the stimulus (Figure 8-15) and mimics the temporal envelope of BM displacement (Zheng et al., 1998). Whether the SP is positive or negative depends on stimulus parameters, recording site, and recording techniques (Dallos, Schoeny, & Cheatham, 1970). The source of the SP has been debated for decades, but

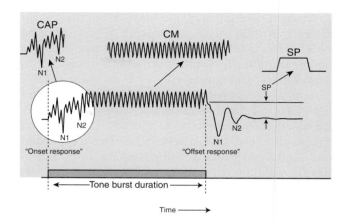

Figure 8-15. Example of a gross potential response to a tone burst. The evoked response consists of three components: the compound action potential generated by the type I spiral ganglion cells, the cochlear microphonic generated by the OHCs, and the summating potential predominated by IHC activity. The CAP consists of two prominent negative peaks, N1 and N2, that are generated at both the onset and the offset of the tone.

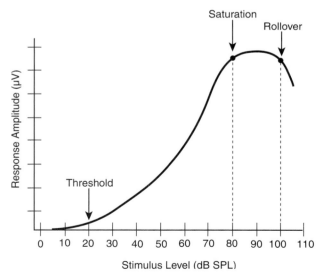

Figure 8-14. Input-output function for a stimulus evoked potential. The amplitude of the response typically increases as a function of stimulus level. Threshold is defined as "the stimulus level that produces a criterion response." At high stimulus levels, the function becomes nonlinear as the response saturates and, in some cases, "rolls over."

two recent studies with chinchillas provide compelling evidence that the IHCs are the major contributors to SPs recorded from the round window. Zheng, Ding, McFadden, and Henderson (1997) recorded SP, CAP, CDP OAEs, and CM from chinchillas with two types of cochlear lesions. One group of chinchillas had basal IHC and SGN loss secondary to surgical transection of the AN. The second group had temporary damage to the afferent nerve terminals beneath the IHCs, caused by application of **kainic acid** to the round window membrane. In both groups, the CM, CDP OAEs, and OHC numbers were all normal, whereas CAP was abolished at the frequencies tested. The amplitude of the SP was reduced by 60%–80% at stimulus levels below 80 dB SPL in animals with 40%–50% loss of IHCs and SGNs. In animals with intact IHCs but damaged afferent synapses, the SP was normal at low to moderate stimulus levels and enhanced at high stimulus levels. The fact that the SP is reduced by IHC loss but not by afferent synapse disruption suggests that the SP could be a valuable clinical tool for differential diagnosis of cochlear pathology.

Durrant, Wang, Ding, and Salvi (1998) used a different chinchilla model to examine the contribution of IHCs to the SP. They recorded SP from chinchillas before and after IP administration of carboplatin. In chinchillas—and apparently *only* in chinchillas—carboplatin preferentially kills IHCs and SGNs rather than OHCs (Ding, McFadden, & Salvi, 2002; Takeno, Harrison, Mount, Wake, & Harada, 1994; Wake, Takeno, Ibrahim, & Harrison, 1994). This unique animal model has provided unprecedented opportunities for studying the effects of IHC loss in animals with normal OHCs. The results of the experiment by Durrant et al. (1998) showed that IHCs are the major contributors to the SP at low to moderate stimulus levels, with a smaller contribution by OHCs.

The CAP consists of two prominent negative peaks, referred to as N1 and N2 (Figure 8-15), produced by the synchronous depolarization of SGN fibers in response to acoustic stimulation. The exact location of the N1 and N2 generators is still a matter of debate. However, it is likely that in humans, N1 arises from the peripheral processes of SGNs, whereas N2 arises from the midportion of the intracranial segment of the AN, accounting for the latency difference (approximately 1 ms) between them. When pure tones are used to elicit the CAP, response threshold, amplitude, and latency can be determined over a range of frequencies to evaluate the functional integrity of the auditory system up to and including the AN. Alternatively, clicks can be used to elicit the CAP for more rapid assessment of cochlear function that is less frequency-specific. Once threshold is reached, CAP amplitude grows linearly over a range of about 40–50 dB; then it saturates and rolls over at very high levels. The amplitude of the N1 and N2 peaks is proportional to the number of AN fibers contributing to the response, and the width of the response is inversely proportional to the synchrony of neural activity. The latency of the response decreases with stimulus level, from approximately 2 ms at low SPLs to approximately 1 ms at high SPLs for N1. Responses to high-frequency stimuli are more synchronized and have shorter latencies than responses to low-frequency stimuli. Common findings in patients with ototoxicity are elevated thresholds and decreased amplitude of the CAP for clicks and high-frequency stimuli due to loss of OHCs in the basal region of the cochlea.

Effects of Inner Hair Cell/Spiral Ganglion Neuron (IHC/SGN) Loss

OHCs are typically the most vulnerable elements of the cochlea, being the first cells to succumb to ototoxicity, acoustic overexposure, and aging. Consequently, the effects of selective OHC loss on auditory function have been known for many years. In contrast, the effects of selective IHC loss are only now being determined. Studies using carboplatin-treated chinchillas have led to the surprising discovery that threshold measures are remarkably insensitive to IHC and SGN loss (Burkard, Trautwein, & Salvi, 1997; Hamernik, Ahroon, Jock, & Bennett, 1998; Jock, Hamernik, Aldrich, Ahroon, Petriello, & Johnson, 1999; McFadden, Kasper, Ostrowski, Ding, & Salvi, 1998). Even substantial losses (>50%) of SGNs and IHCs have little effect on behavioral thresholds or on thresholds of the CAP, inferior colliculus (IC) EVPs, or ABR. Thus, it is important to realize that normal auditory thresholds do not imply a normal cochlea or normal hearing! On the other hand, elevated thresholds are consistently associated with OHC abnormalities.

Whereas thresholds are minimally affected by IHC and SGN loss, the amplitude of the CAP decreases in proportion to IHC/SGN loss. Responses from CANS regions are generally decreased by IHC/SGN loss as well, but that is less predictable. In some cases, EVPs from the IC and the auditory cortex are actually enhanced in amplitude after carboplatin treatment (McFadden et al., 1998; Qiu, Salvi, Ding, & Burkard, 2000). Estimates of temporal processing in the IC, using the amplitude modulation following response, show little to no change with IHC/SGN loss (Arnold & Burkard, 2002). Susceptibility to masking at the level of the IC is increased slightly; but the time course of recovery from masking, which is prolonged in proportion to OHC loss, is not altered by IHC/SGN loss (McFadden et al., 1998).

The CM, SP, and CAP provide different but interrelated perspectives on peripheral auditory system functioning. For example, if the SP and CAP amplitudes are decreased but CAP thresholds and CM are normal, IHC loss should be suspected. On the other hand, if CAP thresholds are elevated and CAP and CM amplitudes are depressed, OHC loss is the most likely cause. A normal SP accompanied by normal CM but reduced CAP amplitude points to abnormalities localized to the SGNs or their processes. Stimulus EVPs from CANS nuclei and recordings from single AN fibers and single neurons in various CANS nuclei provide a different perspective on auditory system functioning. All of those potentials reflect the electrochemical properties of living cells.

NEURAL ELECTROCHEMICAL SIGNALING

The neuron is the essential "signaling device" of the nervous system, conducting electrical impulses and releasing chemicals that affect the electrical, chemical, and gene transcription behaviors of other cells. The SGNs are PNS neurons that convey information to CNS neurons, specifically to neurons located in the dorsal and ventral divisions of the CN. Whereas all type I SGNs have very similar physical properties and discharge patterns, neurons in different regions of the CANS are both physically and functionally diverse. Despite the diversity, all neurons share some common features that will be emphasized here.

Figure 8-16 illustrates the principal regions of a "typical" neuron: dendrites, cell body (also called the soma or perikaryon), and the axon. The dendrites and the cell body generally receive input from other neurons at axondendritic and axosomatic synapses, respectively; and they generate graded potentials (potentials that vary in initial size according to the intensity of the input signal) in response. Graded potentials can summate spatially and temporally, they can add or subtract algebraically, and they decay exponentially as they are conducted over time and space to adjacent regions of the membrane (Figure 8-17). Graded potentials that depolarize the cell membrane are called excitatory postsynaptic potentials (EPSPs); those that hyperpolarize the membrane are called inhibitory postsynaptic potentials (IPSPs).

The membrane is the key to understanding neuron function. The typical neural membrane is a lipid bilayer, about 5 nm thick, with embedded structural proteins and other proteins that serve as pumps, channels, cell surface receptors, and enzymes. The channel proteins are relatively selective for particular ions, and they can be gated closed and/or open by either voltage changes (V-gated channels) or chemicals (ligand-gated channels). Ligand-gated ion channels are generally associated with either ionotropic (ion-channel-linked) or **metabotropic (G-protein-linked)** cell surface receptors. The binding of a ligand to an ionotropic receptor causes a change in protein conformation that directly opens an ion channel in the membrane. The short time course of channel opening makes this receptor mechanism most suitable for rapid intercellular signaling. G-protein-linked receptors act indirectly via "second messengers" such as **cyclic nucleotides** or **phosphoinositides**. Although metabotropic receptors are slow compared to ionotropic receptors, they are very important for signal amplification. Examples have already been shown of V-gated channels and ionotropic ligand-gated receptors in the peripheral auditory system: V-gated Ca^{2+} channels on the hair cell membrane and **neurotransmitter-gated receptors** on the afferent fibers beneath the IHCs.

The types and densities of channel and receptor proteins vary from cell to cell and from one region of a cell to another. For instance, the dendrites and cell bodies of neurons typically have ligand-gated receptors, whereas the axon has a high density of V-gated ion channels. The **axon hillock,** located at the junction between the cell body and the axon (Figure 8-16), has an exceptionally high density of V-gated Na^+ channels, giving it the lowest threshold for generating APs (Figures 8-17 and 8-18). Because APs are most easily generated at the axon hillock, this region is referred to as the trigger zone or spike initiation zone of the neuron. Membranes of myelinated axons have a high density of V-gated channels at the **nodes of Ranvier,** regions where the thick myelin sheath is interrupted (Figures 8-17 and 8-18), and a low density of channels at internodal regions beneath the myelin sheath. Channel and receptor densities are

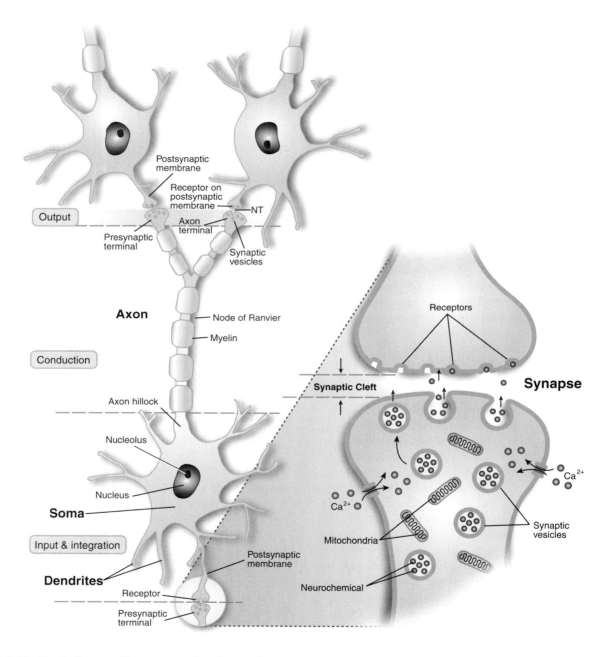

Figure 8-16. A "typical" neuron. The neuron consists of a soma from which dendrites and an axon extend. The dendrites and soma constitute an "input and integration" region, whereas the axon is considered a "conduction" region that conveys action potentials to the terminal where neurotransmitter is stored in synaptic vesicles. Many, but not all, are myelinated, which increases conduction velocity. The synaptic region is enlarged to show synaptic vesicles and mitochondria in one terminal. When the terminal membrane depolarizes, voltage-gated calcium channels open. The influx of Ca^{2+} leads to fusion of the vesicles to the terminal membrane, followed by exocytosis of a "packet" of NT into the synaptic cleft. The NT diffuses across the cleft to bind to receptors on the postsynaptic membrane.

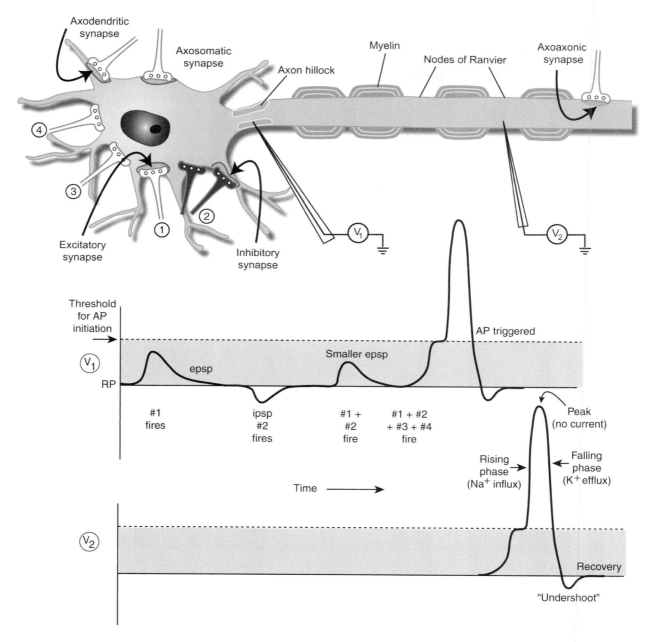

Figure 8-17. Graded potentials and action potentials. A neuron receives numerous inputs from other neurons. Synapses are defined according to regions involved (axodendritic, axosomatic, and axoaxonic) and according to their effects (excitatory or inhibitory). Excitatory synapses produce depolarizing changes called EPSPs; inhibitory synapses produce hyperpolarizing IPSPs. EPSPs and IPSPs are graded potentials that can summate over space and time, dissipate with time and distance, and add together algebraically. If depolarization exceeds a threshold level, an AP can be triggered. Unlike graded potentials that decrease over time and distance, the AP is a propagated reversal of membrane potential of constant magnitude. The AP consists of a rising phase due to Na+ influx, a peak reached at the equilibrium potential for Na+, a falling phase due to K+ efflux, and a recovery period (see text).

not fixed, but can change (up- or down-regulate) in response to local changes in myelin and the surrounding neurochemical environment. Thus, damage to a segment of myelin may be followed by an increase in the density of ion channels in the damaged region of the axon, with compensatory or ameliorative functional consequences for neural conduction. If remyelination occurs, channel density in the repaired region will decrease.

Neurons have a negative RP close to the equilibrium potential for K^+. The RP of the neuron arises because the membrane is selectively permeable to various ions, and those ions are in different concentrations inside and outside the cell. Intracellular fluid has a high concentration of K^+, a low concentration of Na^+, a high concentration of chloride (Cl-), and a large number of protein anions. In contrast, the extracellular fluid, like the perilymph surrounding SGNs, contains a low concentration of K^+, a high concentration of Na^+, and a high concentration of chloride (Cl-). In the resting neuron, the membrane is about 25 times more permeable to K^+ than to Na^+. Since K^+ is the only ion that is relatively free to move across the membrane at low values of membrane potential, the RP is dictated primarily by K+ movement.

EPSPs depolarize the membrane, and this activates (opens) Na^+ channels, resulting in immediate influx of Na^+ into the cell. The influx of Na^+ depolarizes the membrane further and opens yet more Na^+ channels. If the resulting Na^+ current depolarizes the membrane beyond a threshold level, an AP will be triggered (Figure 8-17). The AP entails dramatic changes in Na^+ and K^+ channel permeabilities and currents due to immediate activation and slow inactivation (time- and V-dependent closing) of Na^+ channels and delayed opening of K^+ channels. As illustrated in Figure 8-17, the AP consists of a rising phase of depolarization induced by Na^+ influx, a peak when the equilibrium potential for Na^+ is reached and inward Na^+ current ceases, followed by a falling phase of repolarization induced by K^+ efflux and recovery of the RP. At the peak of the AP, Na^+ permeability has increased by a factor of about 500 and the membrane is about 20 times more permeable to Na^+ than to K^+; Na^+ channel inactivation has

begun, and K^+ channels are opening. During membrane repolarization, a brief "undershoot" period occurs because K^+ conductance is still high and Na^+ channels are still inactivated. While Na^+ channels are inactivated, it is not possible to trigger another AP; this is called the relative refractory period. Once Na^+ channels become deactivated (normally closed) and K^+ channel permeability returns to normal, the membrane is capable of generating another AP. Although the theoretical upper limit on AP generation is close to 1,000 spikes/sec, the practical upper limit is around 200 spikes/sec in mammals.

Once the threshold for triggering an AP has been reached, a regenerative wave of opening and closing of V-gated ion channels moves along the excitable axon membrane. Axons that are wrapped with myelin conduct APs more rapidly than unmyelinated axons because APs are generated only at nodes of Ranvier, regions in which the myelin sheath is thin and the density of V-gated Na^+ channels is high, rather than continuously down the axon (Figure 8-18).

Myelin

Most nerve fibers, including the axons of type I SGNs and MOC neurons, are wrapped in layers of myelin formed by specialized glial cells: Schwann cells in the PNS and oligodendrocytes in the CNS. Myelin is formed by differentiation of the glial cell plasma membrane in response to specific, but largely unidentified, signals from larger-caliber axons and axon/glial cell interactions (Garbay, Heape, Sargueil, & Cassagne, 2000; Jessen & Mirsky, 1999). In the PNS, all Schwann cells have the potential to form a myelin sheath, but only those that come in contact with axons having a diameter of more than 0.7 μm will actually myelinate the axon. Once a one-to-one relationship has been established between a single Schwann cell and an axon, the unit is surrounded by a **basal lamina** secreted by the Schwann cell, and the plasma membrane spirally envelopes the axon. As the internal mesaxon rotates around the axon, the cytoplasm of the Schwann cell condenses and forms both compact and noncompact regions (Bunge, Bunge, & Bates, 1989). Compaction is a critical feature of normal

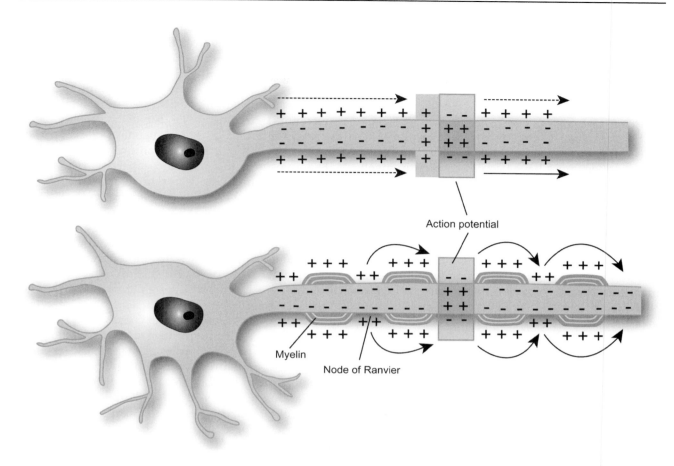

Action potential

Myelin

Node of Ranvier

Figure 8-18. Propagated APs in unmyelinated and myelinated axons. In the unmyelinated axon, the AP is propagated continuously to the terminal region. In the myelinated axon, the AP is generated only at the nodes of Ranvier, resulting in "saltatory" conduction. The density of ion channels is much higher in nodal versus internodal regions.

myelin function and has been shown to be mediated in the PNS by proteins **P0** and **peripheral myelin protein 22** (PMP22) (D'Urso, Ehrhardt, & Muller, 1999; Menichella et al., 2001).

The myelin sheath provides a high-resistance/ low-capacitance insulation that increases the conduction velocity of neural impulses while conserving both space and energy (Morell, Quarles, & Norton, 1989). The electrical properties of myelin derive from its unusually high lipid-to-protein ratio: approximately 70–80% lipids and 20–30% proteins. Although

PNS and CNS myelin contain similar lipids, the myelin in those two systems can be differentiated based on myelin-specific protein composition. While PNS myelin contains nearly 60% glycoproteins (e.g., P0, myelin-associated glycoprotein (MAG), and PMP22) and 20%–30% myelin basic proteins (MBPs), CNS myelin is composed of 60–80% MBPs and proteolipid proteins (PLPs) and only a small proportion of glycoproteins. The functional roles of the region-specific proteins have not been completely elucidated. However, studies of PNS myelin in mouse and rat knockout models have shown that some proteins, such as P0, are necessary for both the formation and maintenance of myelin, while others, such as MAG and PMP22, are important primarily for myelin maintenance (Carenini, Montag, Cremer, Schachner, & Martini, 1997; D'Urso et al., 1999; Schachner & Bartsch, 2000).

It is important to understand that myelin is not simply an inert insulation material for axons. A large number of enzymes have been discovered in myelin that point to an active role in intracellular metabolism and transport, including neutral protease, **cAMP-stimulated kinase**, **Ca^{2+}/calmodulin-dependent kinase**, **phosphoprotein phosphatases**, **acyl-CoA synthetase**, enzymes involved in the metabolism of structural lipids and **glycerol phospholipid** synthesis, and enzymes implicated in membrane transport (including Na$^+$,K$^+$-ATPase) (Banik, Hogan, & Hsu, 1985; Morell et al., 1989). Similarly, glial cells themselves are beginning to be appreciated as active elements in cellular homeostasis. In the cochlea, **glutamine synthetase** is expressed by Schwann cells in the osseous spiral lamina and satellite glial cells in the spiral ganglion (and in those cells only), suggesting a role in protecting the cochlea from excitotoxicity by limiting perilymphatic glutamate concentrations (Eybalin, Norenberg, & Renard, 1996).

Toxic disorders of myelin can be produced by agents such as diptheria toxin, **organotoxins** such as hexachlorophene and triethyltin, copper deficiency, and lead poisoning (Garbay et al., 2000; Quarles, Morell, & McFarlin, 1989; Roncagliolo, Benitez, & Eguibar, 2000). Disruption or destruction of myelin impairs the speed of conduction and neural synchrony that can then lead to a number of motor deficits and sensory impairment, including hearing impairment.

Neurochemicals and Neurotransmitters (NTs)

When the AP reaches the terminal region of the axon, depolarization triggers a series of events culminating in the release of NTs from membrane-bound vesicles into the synaptic space separating the presynaptic cell from the postsynaptic cell (Figure 8-16). The NT can bind to **autoreceptors** on the cell that released it (the presynaptic cell) and/or diffuse across the synapse to bind to specialized receptors on the postsynaptic cell membrane. Receptor binding initiates specific membrane or cellular events. As discussed in the previous section, NT binding can lead to the opening of membrane ion channels either directly (ionotropic receptors) or indirectly (metabotropic receptors). Excitatory NTs typically open channels that permit influx of cations (usually Na$^+$ or Ca^{2+}) or, less frequently, efflux of anions (usually Cl-). Examples are glutamate and aspartate, two similar excitatory amino acids found in the cochlea and CANS. Glutamate or a similar amino acid is likely to be the NT released by IHCs and by AN fibers at their synapses with CN neurons. Inhibitory NTs typically open channels that permit efflux of K$^+$, but they can also increase influx of Cl-. Examples are glycine and gamma-amino butyric acid (GABA), the "universal inhibitory NT" formed from glutamic acid in a reaction catalyzed by glutamic acid decarboxylase (GAD). GABA is found in the cochlea and throughout the CANS. In the primary auditory cortex (AI), GABA plays important roles in shaping the response properties of neurons via ionotropic GABA$_A$ and metabotropic GABA$_B$ receptor subtypes (Wang, McFadden, Caspary, & Salvi, 2002). The effects of endogenous GABA were deduced by comparing response properties of AI neurons before and after iontophoretic application of selective receptor antagonists: bicuculline to block GABA$_A$ receptors and/or CGP35348 to block GABA$_B$ receptors. After application of bicuculline, many AI neurons had significantly increased spontaneous and driven discharge rates, dramatically decreased thresholds, and expanded excitatory response areas on both high- and low-frequency sides. CGP35348 enhanced the effects of bicuculline but had no clear effect alone, suggesting a modulatory role of local GABA$_B$ receptors. The results suggest that GABA-mediated inhibition contributes significantly to intensity and frequency coding in AI.

Neurochemistry of Lateral Olivocochlear (LOC) and Medial Olivocochlear (MOC) Efferents

Acetylcholine (ACh), the first NT to be identified (in the early 1920s) is the primary neurotransmitter of the OCB (Fex & Altschuler, 1986; Schwarz, Schwarz, & Hu, 1989; Wiet, Godfrey, Ross, & Dunn, 1986); thus, the OCB is a "cholinergic" system. Activities of enzymes associated with ACh synthesis and degradation (i.e., choline acetyltransferase (ChAT) and acetylcholinesterase (AChE), respectively) show clear gradients in their distributions along the cochlea (Godfrey et al., 1986). ChAT and AChE activities are consistently greater in the IHC region than in the OHC region, corresponding to the greater number of LOC efferent fibers in the OCB. In both IHC and OHC regions, AChE activities along the cochlea decline from base to apex; ChAT activities peak in the middle turn and decline more in the apex than in the base. The fact that OCB transection leads to a total loss of ChAT activity in the organ of Corti indicates that the OCB is the sole source of ACh activity in the cochlea (Godfrey & Ross, 1985).

Although both LOC and MOC neurons react positively for AChE and to antisera against ChAT, it appears that different cholinergic receptor subtypes mediate ACh effects at MOC and LOC efferent synapses. It appears that only the **muscarinic** subtype of ACh receptors exist at LOC/afferent fiber synapses. In contrast, the cholinergic receptor subtype at the MOC/OHC synapse appears to be an α-9/α-10-containing nicotinic ACh (nACh) receptor with unusual pharmacological properties (Lioudyno et al., 2002; Oliver et al., 2001; Rothlin et al., 2003; Weisstaub, Vetter, Elgoyhen, & Katz, 2002). Activation of this receptor causes the opening of nonselective ionotropic cation channels, resulting in Ca^{2+} influx and subsequent activation of calcium-dependent K^+ channels in the OHC cell membrane. The result is hyperpolarization of the OHC and an increase in auditory thresholds. The α-9/α-10 nACh receptor and the α-9 subunit can be blocked by numerous agents, including both muscarinic and nicotinic receptor antagonists and aminoglycosides (Katz et al., 2000; Lioudyno, Verbitsky, Holt, Elgoyhen, & Guth, 2000; Oliver et al., 2001; Rothlin et al., 2000; Rothlin et al., 2003; Verbitsky, Rothlin, Katz, & Elgoyhen, 2000; Weisstaub et al., 2002).

Only the LOC system contains **enkephalins, dynorphin,** and **dopamine** (Altschuler, Reeks, Fex, & Hoffman, 1988; Mulders & Robertson, 2004;

Altschuler & Fex, 1986). It has been proposed that neurochemicals such as dopamine play a role in protection and repair of afferent dendrites after injury (d'Aldin et al., 1995).

SUMMARY

The chapter provides a broad overview of biochemical concepts as they relate to cells of the cochlea and neurons of the PNS and CNS to familiarize the reader with major structures and biochemical processes underlying normal hearing. The aim is to provide the background necessary for understanding the effects of drugs and other agents on the cochlea and CANS. There are numerous targets for ototoxic agents in the auditory system. Among the most vulnerable elements in the peripheral auditory system are the cochlear hair cells (particularly the OHCs), the stria vascularis, and the type I spiral ganglion cells. The glial cells that ensheath the SGNs in myelin can also be damaged by ototoxic agents, resulting in reduced conduction velocity and dysynchronous firing of AN fibers as myelin unravels or disintegrates. Clinical measures that are sensitive to drug-induced cochlear dysfunction include OAEs, CMs, SPs, CAPs, the ABR, and EVPs recorded from CANS nuclei. OHC dysfunction can be detected by measuring CDP OAEs, CM potentials, or thresholds of most EVPs. IHC dysfunction rarely occurs without OHC loss, and mild to moderate losses of IHCs (or SGNs) have little or no effect on auditory thresholds. Loss of IHCs and/or SGNs reduces the number of channels supplying input to the CANS, so their loss results in diminished amplitude of the CAP. In addition, IHC loss reduces the SP. Drugs that affect the stria vascularis or the metabolic activities of strial cells disrupt cochlear function by reducing or abolishing the EP, the electrochemical battery that drives the cochlear transduction process.

Cochlear transduction involves the conversion of BM movement into electrical potentials in the hair cells. Hair cell depolarization occurs when mechanically gated channels are pulled open by deflection of the stereocilia toward the lateral wall; and hyperpolarization occurs when the stereocilia are deflected in the opposite direction, toward the modiolus. Current through the hair cells is carried primarily by potassium ions, which are abundant in the endolymph of scala media above the hair cells and in low concentration in the perilymph that bathes the hair cell bodies beneath the reticular lamina. OHCs are motile elements of a cochlear amplifier. Changes in membrane voltage cause OHCs to contract or elongate, and their movement pumps energy back into the BM system that, depending on phase, can either enhance or dampen BM movement. Graded changes in IHC membrane potential produce corresponding graded changes in neurochemical release. The excitatory NT of the IHC (glutamate or a similar amino acid) binds to ionotropic receptors on the membrane of the type I AN fiber beneath it, leading to depolarization that can trigger APs. LOC efferent activity modulates the excitability of the type I fibers. APs generated by the type I SGNs are conveyed to the CN of the CANS via the AN portion of the 8th cranial nerve.

There are many CNS targets of ototoxic agents as well, including cell surface receptors, myelin, neurochemicals, and ion channels (i.e., structures and processes involved in electrochemical signaling). Drugs or ototoxic agents can affect auditory function by impairing the ability of neurons to generate or conduct APs or by interfering with their ability to signal other cells at chemical synapses. Synaptic transmission is triggered by depolarization of the terminal membrane, which opens voltage-gated calcium channels. In the presence of calcium, synaptic vesicles containing NTs fuse to the membrane and release their contents into the synaptic cleft. Binding of the NT to ionotropic receptors on the postsynaptic membrane opens ion channels, resulting in transmembrane currents that produce excitatory or inhibitory postsynaptic potentials; binding to metabotropic receptors initiates intracellular events in the postsynaptic cell. A variety of NTs serve the auditory system, including amino acid NTs at the hair cell/afferent fiber synapse and ACh at the terminals of both lateral and medial olivocochlear efferent fibers in the cochlea. Both excitatory and inhibitory NTs are utilized by neurons in the CANS, giving rise to complex neural response properties.

Obviously, there are many important aspects of cellular and cochlear biochemistry that could not be mentioned in this chapter and others that deserve far more detail than could be given here. Readers are encouraged to pursue their interests in this area by availing themselves of the many excellent reviews on individual topics that have been written in recent years.

REFERENCES

Altschuler, R. A., Reeks, K. A., Fex, J., & Hoffman, D. W. (1988). Lateral olivocochlear neurons contain both enkephalin and dynorphin immunoreactivities: Immunocytochemical co-localization studies. *J Histochem Cytochem, 36*(7), 797–801.

Anagnostopoulos, A. V. (2002). A compendium of mouse knockouts with inner ear defects. *Trends Genet, 18*(10), 499.

Arnold, S., & Burkard, R. (2002). Inner hair cell loss and steady-state potentials from the inferior colliculus and auditory cortex of the chinchilla. *J Acoust Soc Am, 112*(2), 590–599.

Avraham, K. B. (1997). Motors, channels and the sounds of silence. *Nat Med, 3*(6), 608–609.

Azeredo, W. J., Kliment, M. L., Morley, B. J., Relkin, E., Slepecky, N. B., Sterns, A., et al. (1999). Olivocochlear neurons in the chinchilla: A retrograde fluorescent labelling study. *Hearing Research, 134*(1–2), 57–70.

Banik, N. L., Hogan, E. L., & Hsu, C. Y. (1985). Molecular and anatomical correlates of spinal cord injury. *Cent Nerv Syst Trauma, 2*(2), 99–107.

Borg, E., & Counter, S. A. (1989). The middle-ear muscles. *Sci Am, 261*(2), 74–80.

Bosher, S. K. (1979). The nature of the negative endocochlear potentials produced by anoxia and ethacynic acid in the rat and guinea-pig. *Journal of Physiology (London), 293,* 329–345.

Brown, R. D. (1972). Influence of chronic treatment with neomycin and kanamycin on N 1 suppression produced by contralateral olivo-cochlear bundle stimulation in cats. *Acta Otolaryngol, 73*(4), 335–340.

Brown, R. D., & Daigneault, E. A. (1973). Neomycin: Ototoxicity and the cochlear efferents. *Acta Otolaryngol, 76*(2), 128–135.

Brownell, W. E., Bader, C. R., Bertrand, D., & de Ribaupierre, Y. (1985). Evoked mechanical responses of isolated cochlear outer hair cells. *Science, 227,* 194–196.

Bunge, R. P., Bunge, M. B., & Bates, M. (1989). Movements of the Schwann cell nucleus implicate progression of the inner (axon-related) Schwann cell process during myelination. *J Cell Biol, 109*(1), 273–284.

Burkard, R. F., Trautwein, P. A., & Salvi, R. (1997). The effects of click level, click rate, and level of background masking noise on the inferior colliculus potential (ICP) in the normal and carboplatin-treated chinchilla. *J Acoust Soc Am, 102*(6), 3620–3627.

Capps, M. J., & Duvall, A. J., 3rd. (1976). Ototoxicity and the olivocochlear bundle. *Trans Sect Otolaryngol Am Acad Opthamol Otolaryngol, 82*(3 Pt 1), 283–284.

Carenini, S., Montag, D., Cremer, H., Schachner, M., & Martini, R. (1997). Absence of the myelin-associated glycoprotein (MAG) and the neural cell adhesion molecule (N-CAM) interferes with the maintenance, but not with the formation of peripheral myelin. *Cell Tissue Res, 287*(1), 3–9.

Cody, A. R., & Russell, I. J. (1987). The response of hair cells in the basal turn of the guinea-pig cochlea to tones. *Journal of Physiology, 383,* 551–569.

Crawford, A., & Fettiplace, R. (1981). An electrical tuning mechanism in turtle cochlear hair cells. *Journal of Physiology (London), 315,* 377–422.

Daigneault, E. A., Pruett, J. R., & Brown, R. D. (1970). Influence of ototoxic drugs on acetylcholine-induced depression of the cochlear N1 potential. *Toxicol Appl Pharmacol, 17*(1), 223–230.

d'Aldin, C., Eybalin, M., Puel, J. L., Charachon, G., Ladrech, S., Renard, N., et al. (1995). Synaptic connections and putative functions of the dopaminergic innervation of the guinea pig cochlea. *Eur Arch Otorhinolaryngol, 252*(5), 270–274.

Dallos, P., Santos-Sacchi, J., & Flock, A. (1982). Intracellular recordings from cochlear outer hair cells. *Science, 218*(4572), 582–584.

Dallos, P., Schoeny, Z. G., & Cheatham, M. A. (1970). Cochlear summating potentials: composition. *Science, 170*(958), 641–644.

Davis, H. (1965). A model for transducer action in the cochlea. *Cold Spring Harbor Symposia on Quantitative Biology, 30,* 181–189.

Davis, H., Deatherage, B. H., Rosenblut, B., Fernandez, C., Kimura, R., & Smith, C. A. (1958). Modification of cochlear potentials by streptomycin poisoning and by extensive venous obstruction. *Laryngoscope, 68,* 596–627.

Ding, D., Jin, X., McFadden, S. L., & Salvi, R. J. (2001). Changes in cochlear potentials and enzyme activities after ethacrynic acid injection are secondary to stria vascularis ischemia. Abstract obtained from *Assoc Res Otolaryngol,* Abstract No. 20635.

Ding, D., McFadden, S. L., Woo, J. M., & Salvi, R. J. (2002). Ethacrynic acid rapidly and selectively abolishes blood flow in vessels supplying the lateral wall of the cochlea. *Hearing Research, 173*(1–2), 1–9.

Ding, L., McFadden, S. L., & Salvi, R. J. (2002). Calpain immunoreactivity and morphological damage in chinchilla inner ears after carboplatin. *J Assoc Res Otolaryngol, 3*(1), 68–79.

Durrant, J. D., & Lovrinic, J. H. (1995). *Bases of Hearing Science* (3rd ed.). Baltimore: Williams & Wilkins.

Durrant, J. D., Wang, J., Ding, D. L., & Salvi, R. J. (1998). Are inner or outer hair cells the source of summating potentials recorded from the round window? *J Acoust Soc Am, 104*(1), 370–377.

D'Urso, D., Ehrhardt, P., & Muller, H. W. (1999). Peripheral myelin protein 22 and protein zero: A novel association in peripheral nervous system myelin. *J Neurosci, 19*(9), 3396–3403.

Eybalin, M., Norenberg, M. D., & Renard, N. (1996). Glutamine synthetase and glutamate metabolism in the guinea pig cochlea. *Hearing Research, 101*(1–2), 93–101.

Fex, J., & Altschuler, R. A. (1986). Neurotransmitter-related immunocytochemistry of the organ of Corti. *Hearing Research, 22,* 249–263.

Flock, A. (1977). Physiological properties of sensory hairs in the ear. In E. Evans & J. Wilson (Eds.),

Psychophysical and Physiology of Hearing. London and New York: Academic Press.

Flock, A., Flock, B., & Murray, E. (1977). Studies on the sensory hairs of receptor cells in the inner ear. *Acta Otolaryngol, 83*(1–2), 85–91.

Garbay, B., Heape, A. M., Sargueil, F., & Cassagne, C. (2000). Myelin synthesis in the peripheral nervous system. *Prog Neurobiol, 61*(3), 267–304.

Gibson, F., Walsh, J., Mburu, P., Varela, A., Brown, K. A., Antonio, M., et al. (1995). A type VII myosin encoded by the mouse deafness gene shaker-1. *Nature, 374*(6517), 62–64.

Godfrey, D. A., & Ross, C. D. (1985). Enzymes of acetylcholine metabolism in the rat cochlea. *Ann Otol Rhinol Laryngol, 94*(4 Pt 1), 409–414.

Guinan Jr., J. J. (1996). Physiology of olivocochlear efferents. In P. Dallos, A. N. Popper, & R. R. Fay (Eds.), *The Cochlea* (pp. 435–502). New York: Springer-Verlag New York, Inc.

Hamernik, R. P., Ahroon, W. A., Jock, B. M., & Bennett, J. A. (1998). Noise-induced threshold shift dynamics measured with distortion-product otoacoustic emissions and auditory evoked potentials in chinchillas with inner hair cell deficient cochleas. *Hearing Research 188*(1–2), 73–82.

Hawkins, J. E., Jr. (1973). Comparative otopathology: Aging, noise, and ototoxic drugs. *Adv Otorhinolaryngol, 20,* 125–141.

Hofstetter, P., Ding, D., Powers, N., & Salvi, R. J. (1997). Quantitative relationship between carboplatin dose, inner and outer hair cell loss and reduction in distortion product otoacoustic emission amplitude chinchillas. *Hearing Research, 112,* 199–215.

Hofstetter, P., Ding, D. L., & Salvi, R. J. (1997). Magnitude and pattern of inner and outer hair cell loss in chinchilla as a function of carboplatin dose. *Audiology, 36,* 301–311.

Hudspeth, A. J. (1997). How hearing happens. *Neuron, 19*(5), 947–950.

Hudspeth, A. J., & Corey, D. P. (1977). Sensitivity, polarity, and conductance change in the response of vertebrate hair cells to controlled mechanical stimuli. *Proceedings of the National Academy of Sciences of the United States of America, 74*(6), 2407–2411.

Igarashi, M., Ohashi, K., & Ishii, M. (1986). Morphometric comparison of endolymphatic and perilymphatic spaces in human temporal bones. *Acta Otolaryngol, 101*(3–4), 161–164.

Iurato, S., Smith, C. A., Eldredge, D. H., Henderson, D., Carr, C., Ueno, Y., et al. (1978). Distribution of the crossed olivocochlear bundle in the chinchilla cochlea. *Journal of Comparative Neurology, 182,* 57–76.

Jessen, K. R., & Mirsky, R. (1999). Schwann cells and their precursors emerge as major regulators of nerve development. *Trends Neurosci, 22*(9), 402–410.

Jock, B. M., Hamernik, R. P., Aldrich, L. G., Ahroon, W. A., Petriello, K. L., & Johnson, A. R. Evoked-potential thresholds and cubic distortion product otoacoustic emissions in the chinchilla following carboplatin treatment and noise exposure. *Hearing Research 96*(1–2), 179–190.

Johnstone, B. M., & Sellick, P. M. (1972). Dynamic changes in cochlear potentials and endolymph concentrations. *Journal of the Oto-Laryngological Society of Australia, 3*(3), 317–319.

Katz, E., Verbitsky, M., Rothlin, C. V., Vetter, D. E., Heinemann, S. F., & Elgoyhen, A. B. (2000). High calcium permeability and calcium block of the alpha9 nicotinic acetylcholine receptor. *Hearing Research, 141*(1–2), 117–128.

Kemp, D. T. (1980). Towards a model for the origin of cochlear echoes. *Hearing Research, 2*(3–4), 533–548.

Kohonen, A. (1965). Effect of some ototoxic drugs upon the pattern and innervation of cochlear sensory cells in the guinea pig. *Acta Otolaryngol* (Suppl. 208), 201–270.

Konishi, T. (1979). Some observations on negative endocochlear potential during anoxia. *Acta Otolaryngol, 87,* 506–516.

Konishi, T., & Kelsey, E. (1968). Effect of sodium deficiency on cochlear potentials. *Journal of the Acoustical Society of America, 43,* 462–470.

Kuijpers, W., & Bonting, S. L. (1970). The cochlear potentials. II. The nature of the cochlear endolymphatic resting potential. *Pflügers Arch, 320,* 359–372.

Liang, Y., Wang, A., Belyantseva, I. A., Anderson, D. W., Probst, F. J., Barber, T. D., et al. (1999). Characterization of the human and mouse unconventional myosin XV genes responsible for hereditary deafness DFNB3 and shaker 2. *Genomics, 61*(3), 243–258.

Liberman, M. C. (1989). Rapid assessment of sound-evoked olivocochlear feedback: Suppression of compound action potentials by contralateral sound. *Hearing Research, 38*(1–2), 47–56.

Lioudyno, M. I., Verbitsky, M., Glowatzki, E., Holt, J. C., Boulter, J., Zadina, J. E., et al. (2002). The alpha9/alpha10-containing nicotinic ACh receptor is directly modulated by opioid peptides, endomorphin-1, and dynorphin B, proposed efferent cotransmitters in the inner ear. *Mol Cell Neurosci, 20*(4), 695–711.

Lioudyno, M. I., Verbitsky, M., Holt, J. C., Elgoyhen, A. B., & Guth, P. S. (2000). Morphine inhibits an alpha9-acetylcholine nicotinic receptor-mediated response by a mechanism which does not involve opioid receptors. *Hearing Research, 149*(1–2), 167–177.

McFadden, S. L. (2001). Genetics and age-related hearing loss. In P. R. Hoff & C. V. Mobbs (Eds.), *Functional Neurobiology of Aging* (pp. 597–603). San Diego: Academic Press.

McFadden, S. L., Kasper, C., Ostrowski, J., Ding, D., & Salvi, R. J. (1998). Effects of inner hair cell loss on inferior colliculus evoked potential thresholds, amplitudes and forward masking functions in chinchillas. *Hearing Research, 120*(1–2), 121–132.

Menichella, D. M., Arroyo, E. J., Awatramani, R., Xu, T., Baron, P., Vallat, J. M., et al. (2001). Protein zero is necessary for E-cadherin-mediated adherens junction formation in Schwann cells. *Mol Cell Neurosci, 18*(6), 606–618.

Morell, P., Quarles, R. H., & Norton, W. T. (1989). Formation, structure, and biochemistry of myelin. In G. Siegel, B. Agranoff, R. W. Albers, & P. Molinoff (Eds.), *Basic Neurochemistry* (4th ed., pp. 109–136). New York: Raven Press.

Mott, J. B., Norton, S. J., Neely, S. T., & Warr, W. B. (1989). Changes in spontaneous otoacoustic emissions produced by acoustic stimulation of the contralateral ear. *Hearing Research, 38*(3), 229–242.

Mulders, W. H., & Robertson, D. (2004). Dopaminergic olivocochlear neurons originate in the high frequency region of the lateral superior olive of guinea pigs. *Hearing Research, 187*(1–2), 122–130.

Oliver, D., Ludwig, J., Reisinger, E., Zoellner, W., Ruppersberg, J. P., & Fakler, B. (2001). Memantine inhibits efferent cholinergic transmission in the cochlea by blocking nicotinic acetylcholine receptors of outer hair cells. *Mol Pharmacol, 60*(1), 183–189.

Peake, W., Sohmer, J., & Weiss, T. (1969). Microelectrode recordings of intracochlear potentials. *M.I.T. Research Laboratory of Electronics: Quarterly Progress Report, 94*, 293–304.

Petit, C., Levilliers, J., & Hardelin, J. P. (2001). Molecular genetics of hearing loss. *Annu Rev Genet, 35*, 589–646.

Pickles, J. O., Comis, S. D., & Osborne, M. P. (1984). Cross-links between stereocilia in the guinea pig organ of Corti, and their possible relation to sensory transduction. *Hearing Research, 15*(2), 103–112.

Probst, F. J., Fridell, R. A., Raphael, Y., Saunders, T. L., Wang, A., Liang, Y., et al. (1998). Correction of deafness in shaker-2 mice by an unconventional myosin in a BAC transgene. *Science, 280*(5368), 1444–1447.

Qiu, C., Salvi, R., Ding, D., & Burkard, R. (2000). Inner hair cell loss leads to enhanced response amplitudes in auditory cortex of unanesthetized chinchillas: Evidence for increased system gain. *Hearing Research, 139*(1–2), 153–171.

Quarles, R. H., Morell, P., & McFarlin, D. E. (1989). Diseases involving myelin. In G. Siegel, B. Agranoff, R. W. Albers, & P. Molinoff (Eds.), *Basic Neurochemistry* (4th ed., pp. 697–714). New York: Raven Press.

Richardson, G. P., Forge, A., Kros, C. J., Fleming, J., Brown, S. D., & Steel, K. P. (1997). Myosin VIIA is required for aminoglycoside accumulation in cochlear hair cells. *J Neurosci, 17*(24), 9506–9519.

Robertson, D., Harvey, A. R., & Cole, K. S. (1989). Postnatal development of the efferent innervation of the rat cochlea. *Developmental Brain Research, 47*, 197–207.

Rodriguez, O. C., & Cheney, R. E. (2000). A new direction for myosin. *Trends in Cell Biology, 10*, 307–311.

Roncagliolo, M., Benitez, J., & Eguibar, J. R. (2000). Progressive deterioration of central components of auditory brainstem responses during postnatal development of the myelin mutant taiep rat. *Audiol Neurootol, 5*(5), 267–275.

Rothlin, C. V., Katz, E., Verbitsky, M., Vetter, D. E., Heinemann, S. F., & Elgoyhen, A. B. (2000). Block of the alpha9 nicotinic receptor by ototoxic aminoglycosides. *Neuropharmacology, 39*(13), 2525–2532.

Rothlin, C. V., Lioudyno, M. I., Silbering, A. F., Plazas, P. V., Casati, M. E., Katz, E., et al. (2003). Direct interaction of serotonin type 3 receptor ligands with recombinant and native alpha 9 alpha 10-containing nicotinic cholinergic receptors. *Mol Pharmacol, 63*(5), 1067–1074.

Russell, I. J., Cody, A. R., & Richardson, G. P. (1986). The responses of inner and outer hair cells in the basal turn of the guinea-pig cochlea and in the mouse cochlea grown in vitro. *Hearing Research, 22,* 199–216.

Salt, A. N., & Konishi, T. (1986). The cochlear fluids: Perilymph and endolymph. In R. A. Altschuler, R. P. Bobbin, & D. W. Hoffman (Eds.), *Neurobiology of Hearing: The Cochlea* (pp. 109–122). New York: Raven Press.

Schachner, M., & Bartsch, U. (2000). Multiple functions of the myelin-associated glycoprotein MAG (siglec-4a) in formation and maintenance of myelin. *Glia, 29*(2), 154–165.

Schwarz, D. W., Schwarz, I. E., & Hu, K. (1989). Transmitter neurochemistry of the efferent neuron system innervating the labyrinth. *J Otolaryngol, 18*(1), 28–31.

Sellers, J. R. (2000). Myosins: A diverse superfamily. *Biochim Biophys Acta, 1496*(1), 3–22.

Sewell, W. F. (1984). The effects of furosemide on the endocochlear potential and auditory nerve fiber tuning curves in cats. *Hearing Research, 14,* 305–314.

Slepecky, N. B. (1996). Structure of the Mammalian Cochlea. In P. Dallos, A. N. Popper, & R. R. Fay (Eds.), *The Cochlea* (pp. 44–129). New York: Springer-Verlag New York, Inc.

Spoendlin, H. (1985). Anatomy of cochlear innervation. *American Journal of Otolaryngology, 6,* 453–467.

Takada, A., Bledsoe, S., Jr., & Schacht, J. (1985). An energy-dependent step in aminoglycoside ototoxicity: Prevention of gentamicin ototoxicity during reduced endolymphatic potential. *Hearing Research, 19*(3), 245–251.

Takeno, S., Harrison, R. V., Mount, R. J., Wake, M., & Harada, Y. (1994). Induction of selective inner hair cell damage by carboplatin. *Scanning Electron Microscopy, 8,* 97–106.

Tasaki, I., & Spyropoulos, C. S. (1959). Stria vascularis as source of endocochlear potential. *Journal of Neurophysiology, 22,* 149–155.

Titus, M. A. (2000). Getting to the point with myosin VI. *Curr Biol, 10*(8), R294–R297.

Tratwein, P., Hofstetter, P., Wang, J., Salvi, R., & Nostrant, A. (1996). Selective inner hair cell loss does not alter distortion product otoacoustic emissions. *Hearing Research, 96,* 71–82.

Verbitsky, M., Rothlin, C. V., Katz, E., & Elgoyhen, A. B. (2000). Mixed nicotinic-muscarinic properties of the alpha9 nicotinic cholinergic receptor. *Neuropharmacology, 39*(13), 2515–2524.

Wake, M., Takeno, S., Ibrahim, D., & Harrison, R. (1994). Selective inner hair cell ototoxicity induced by carboplatin. *Laryngoscope, 104,* 488–493.

Wang, J., McFadden, S. L., Caspary, D., & Salvi, R. (2002). Gamma-aminobutyric acid circuits shape response properties of auditory cortex neurons. *Brain Res, 944*(1–2), 219–231.

Wangemann, P., & Schacht, J. (1996). Homeostatic mechanisms in the cochlea. In P. Dallos, A. N. Popper, & R. R. Fay (Eds.), *The Cochlea* (pp. 130–185). New York: Springer-Verlag New York, Inc.

Warr, W. B. (1992). Organization of olivocochlear efferent systems in mammals. In D. B. Webster, A. N. Popper, & R. R. Fay (Eds.), *The Mammalian Auditory Pathway: Neuroanatomy* (Vol. 1, pp. 410–448). New York: Springer-Verlag.

Warr, W. B., & Beck, J. E. (1996). Multiple projections from the ventral nucleus of the trapezoid body in the rat. *Hearing Research, 93*(1–2), 83–101.

Warr, W. B., & Guinan, J. J. (1979). Efferent innervation of the organ of Corti: Two separate systems. *Brain Research, 173,* 152–155.

Warr, W. B., Guinan Jr., J. J., & White, J. S. (1986). Organization of the olivocochlear system. In R. A. Altschuler, R. P. Bobbin & D. W. Hoffman (Eds.), *Neurobiology of Hearing: The Cochlea* (pp. 333–348). New York: Raven Press.

Warren, E. H., 3rd, & Liberman, M. C. (1989). Effects of contralateral sound on auditory-nerve responses. I. Contributions of cochlear efferents. *Hearing Research, 37*(2), 89–104.

Webster, D. B. (1992). An Overview of Mammalian Auditory Pathways with an Emphasis on Humans. In D. B. Webster, A. N. Popper, & R. R. Fay (Eds.), *The Mammalian Auditory Pathway: Neuroanatomy* (Vol. 1, pp. 1–22). New York: Springer-Verlag.

Weisstaub, N., Vetter, D. E., Elgoyhen, A. B., & Katz, E. (2002). The alpha9alpha10 nicotinic acetylcholine receptor is permeable to and is modulated by divalent cations. *Hearing Research, 167*(1–2), 122–135.

Wiet, G. J., Godfrey, D. A., Ross, C. D., & Dunn, J. D. (1986). Quantitative distributions of aspartate aminotransferase and glutaminase activities in the rat cochlea. *Hearing Research, 24*(2), 137–150.

Wu, X., Jung, G., & Hammer, J. A., III. (2000). Functions of unconventional myosins. *Curr Opin Cell Biol, 12*(1), 42–51.

Yasunaga, S., Grati, M., Cohen-Salmon, M., El-Amraoui, A., Mustapha, M., Salem, N., et al. (1999). A mutation in OTOF, encoding otoferlin, a FER-1-like protein, causes DFNB9, a nonsyndromic form of deafness. *Nat Genet, 21*(4), 363–369.

Yost, W. (1994). *Fundamentals of Hearing: An Introduction* (3rd ed.). San Diego: Academic Press, Inc.

Zheng, J., Madison, L. D., Oliver, D., Fakler, B., & Dallos, P. (2002). Prestin, the motor protein of outer hair cells. *Audiol Neurootol, 7*(1), 9–12.

Zheng, X. Y., Ding, D. L., McFadden, S., & Henderson, D. (1997). Evidence that inner hair cells are the major source of cochlear summating potentials. *Hearing Research, 113,* 76–88.

Zheng, X. Y., Henderson, D., Hu, B. H., Ding, D. L., & McFadden, S. (1997). The influence of the cochlear efferent system on chronic acoustic trauma. *Hearing Research, 107*(1–2), 147–159.

Zheng, X. Y., Henderson, D., McFadden, S. L., Ding, D. L., & Salvi, R. J. (1999). Auditory nerve fiber responses following chronic cochlear de-efferentation. *J Comp Neurol, 406*(1), 72–86.

Zheng, X. Y., Henderson, D., McFadden, S. L., & Hu, B. H. (1997). The role of the cochlear efferent system in acquired resistance to noise-induced hearing loss. *Hearing Research, 104*(1–2), 191–203.

Zheng, X. Y., McFadden, S. L., Henderson, D., Ding, D. L., & Burkard, R. (2000). Cochlear microphonics and otoacoustic emissions in chronically de-efferented chinchilla. *Hearing Research, 143*(1–2), 14–22.

CHAPTER
9

Infection Control in the Audiology Clinic

A. U. Bankaitis, PhD, FAAA,
Oaktree Products, Inc.

Robert J. Kemp, MBA,
Oaktree Products, Inc.

INTRODUCTION

Audiological practice exposes both clinicians and patients to potentially infectious microorganisms that can, under the right conditions, cause disease. Although the need for infection control may have been unrecognized twenty years ago, the standards of practice for audiologists have changed; and effective infection control procedures are recognized as part of routine audiological practice (Roeser, 2003). It is beyond the scope of this chapter to provide an in-depth review of infection control plan requirements and subsequent protocols and procedures specific to audiology. The purpose of this chapter is to provide an overview of microbiology and disease transmission concepts for purposes of presenting a rationale for infection control in the audiology clinic. Fundamental concepts pertinent to an effective infection control strategy will also be presented. For information beyond the scope of this chapter, the reader is referred to available references addressing infection control in the audiology clinic in more detail (Bankaitis & Kemp, 2003, 2004, 2005).

MICROBIOLOGY

Microbiology is the study of living organisms that cannot be readily seen with the naked eye. While these microorganisms may not be visually detectable, they are found in relative abundance throughout the environment. A wide variety of microorganisms currently exist; however, most organisms may be classified into one of four categories. In order of increasing complexity, microorganism categories include viruses, bacteria, fungi, and parasites (Murray, Kobayashi, Pfaller, & Rosenthal, 1994a). A fifth, relatively new microorganism category (prions) has also emerged.

Viruses

Viruses represent the smallest known organisms consisting of genetic material in the form of either deoxyribonucleic acid (DNA) or ribonucleic acid (RNA), but not both. The genetic material is encased in a protective protein coat referred to as a capsid (Bankaitis & Schountz, 1998). Unlike other microorganisms, viruses

are not able to reproduce or metabolize independently; rather, these microorganisms are designed to take over the genetic machinery of other cells for purposes of reproduction. When a virus takes over a cell's genetic machinery, the once healthy cell is reprogrammed to produce new viral particles called virions that break off from the now-infected cell to bond and eventually infect other cells (Bankaitis & Kemp, 2003; Bankaitis & Kemp, 2004). Vaccines represent solutions containing certain elements or properties of a virus that are meant to trick the immune system into thinking the body is infected with a virus. Exposure to a vaccine triggers the immune system to produce antibodies that will most likely protect the body in the event a future encounter with the actual virus occurs. Figure 9-1 shows an image of a hepatitis B virus (HBV).

Bacteria

Bacteria (singular: bacterium) are life forms consisting of a single DNA molecule suspended in cytoplasm encased within a thin cell wall. Depending on the structural and chemical properties of the cell wall,

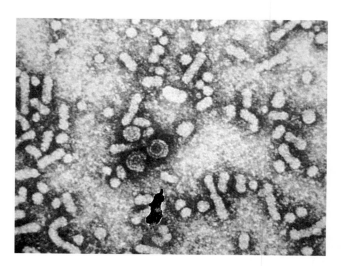

Figure 9-1.   Electron micrograph of HBV. Courtesy of the Centers for Disease Control and Prevention.

bacteria may be either gram-positive or gram-negative. There is a tendency of gram-positive cell bacteria to be more complex, and to have a greater potential for causing disease (Murray, Kobayashi, Pfaller, Rosenthal, Lepine, & Progulske-Fox, 1994). In contrast to viruses, bacteria are generally much larger microorganisms (Murray, Kobayashi, Pfaller, & Rosenthal, 1994a) and are capable of independently executing all of the functions and processes necessary for survival. Furthermore, natural or synthetic substances known as antibiotics are relatively effective in combating infections caused by bacteria; however, they are not effective in treating a viral infection or disease states associated with a viral source (Bankaitis & Kemp, 2003; Bankaitis & Kemp, 2004). Figure 9-2 shows an image of the bacterium *Staphylococcus aureus.*

Fungi

Fungi (singular: fungus) represent a diverse group of organisms divided into two general forms: yeast and mold (Murray, Kobayashi, Pfaller, & Rosenthal, 1994b). Fungi will thrive or grow only in wet or damp areas since a moist environment is needed by the organism to secrete enzymes that allow the fungus to break down organic (e.g., wood or paper) or nonorganic (e.g., metal or glass) materials. Although there are over one hundred thousand identified species, only *Candida albicans* (*C. albicans*) is considered part of the normal human flora, with approximately one hundred species associated with disease (Peters & Filles, 1995). Fungal infections may be superficial and localized to the skin, hair, or nails; or they can cause systemic disease such as disseminated candidiasis, a condition spread through the bloodstream and affecting many organs (Murray, Kobayashi, Pfaller, & Rosenthal, 1994c). Figures 9-3 and 9-4 illustrate two different yet common fungi.

Parasites

Parasites are organisms that exist and function at the expense of a host organism without contributing to the survival of the host. These organisms are capable of causing serious disease in humans and animals. By definition, the category of microorganisms referred to as viruses are considered a form of parasite since viruses also take over and use the host cell's machinery for survival and reproduction (Murray, Kobayashi, Pfaller, & Rosenthal, 1994d). Given the complexity of viruses, they are differentiated by general parasites and considered a separate entity.

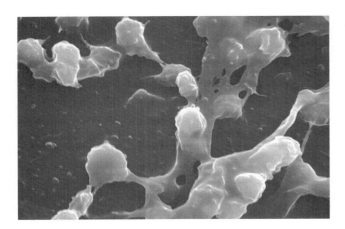

Figure 9-2. Electron micrograph of *Staphylococcus aureus* bacteria. Courtesy of Rodney M. Donlan, PhD, and Janice Carr and the Centers for Disease Control and Prevention.

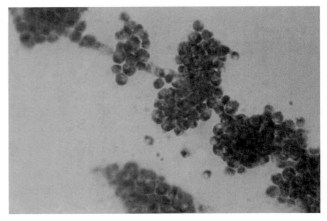

Figure 9-3. Photomicrograph of the fungus *Candida albicans.* Courtesy of Dr. Gordon Roberstad and the Centers for Disease Control and Prevention.

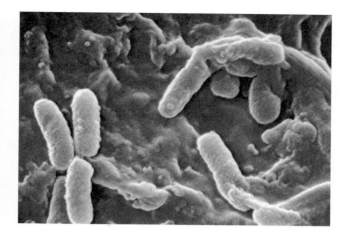

Figure 9-4. Scanning electron micrograph of the fungus *Pseudomonas aeruginosa.* Courtesy of the Centers for Disease Control and Prevention.

Prions

Prions refer to a newer and more mysterious class of infectious agents linked to the neurodegenerative disease referred to as variant Creutzfeldt-Jakob disease (vCJD); bovine spongiform encephalopathy (BSE, or mad cow disease); and chronic wasting disease (CWD) observed in elk, mule, and deer (National Center for Infectious Diseases, 2002). It is currently believed that prions consist of an abnormal protein particle with none of the associated cellular components seen in bacteria and viruses. At this time, the mechanism in which prions cause associated disease is not clear. Humans are thought to be exposed to prions by ingesting diseased meat and/or handling contaminated objects following medical procedures such as surgery. Much more needs to be learned in this emerging area in microbiology.

REQUISITES FOR POTENTIAL DISEASE TRANSMISSION

The process of infection is a very complex development that varies according to the specific type of microorganism that infects the body. From an audiological perspective, the actual process of disease manifestation is not as important as identifying those factors that will facilitate or promote disease transmission. Regardless of whether a microorganism will ultimately manifest in the form of a disease, in order for disease transmission to occur, microorganisms must gain access to a susceptible host (i.e., human body). That is accomplished via a two-tiered process involving a mode of transmission followed by a subsequent route of transmission.

Mode of Transmission

Mode of transmission refers to the means by which a potentially infectious microorganism is transferred from its temporary resting place to the vicinity of the human body. As outlined in Figure 9-5, the main modes of microbial transmission include contact, vehicles, airborne, and vectorborne transmission.

Contact Transmission

Contact transmission represents the most frequent means of disease transmission in the audiology clinic. This type of transmission results in the transfer of a microorganism by way of touching or coming in contact with contaminated objects. Contact transmission may occur in three different ways, including direct, indirect, and droplet contact. **Direct contact transmission** involves physical transfer of a microorganism to a susceptible host in the absence of intervening objects, barriers, or conditions. For example, direct contact transmission may occur when an audiologist touches a patient's ear with an unwashed hand. In that instance, the variety of microbes residing on the surface of the audiologist's unwashed hand is directly transferred to the surface of the patient's ear. In contrast, **indirect contact transmission** occurs when a microorganism is transferred from its temporary resting place to a susceptible host via a secondary surface. This type of transmission usually occurs when an individual is exposed to a contaminated instrument or object. For instance, an audiologist who reuses an immittance probe tip used on a previous patient without properly cleaning and then

1. Contact Transmission: a manner of spreading disease through microbial exposure by way of touching or coming in contact with potentially infectious objects.

    a. Direct Contact Transmission: a type of contact transmission where microbial exposure occurs by coming in direct contact with potentially infectious microbes without intervening persons, barriers, or conditions.
    b. Indirect Contact Transmission: a type of contact transmission where microbial exposure occurs by coming in secondary contact with contaminated objects.
    c. Droplet Contact Transmission: a type of contact transmission where exposure to microbial droplets expelled briefly in the air come in direct or indirect contact with mucous membranes lining the eyelids, nose, mouth.

2. Vehicle Transmission: a manner of potentially spreading disease through ingestion of or exposure to contaminated substances including food, water, blood, or body substances.

3. Airborne Transmission: a manner of spreading diseases through microbial exposure suspended in the air as droplet residue or dust particles.

4. Vectorborne Transmission: a manner of spreading disease whereby insects or animals carrying a pathogenic agent transfer disease by interacting with a susceptible host.

Figure 9-5. Four main modes of microbial transmission and associated subcategories. Reprinted with permission from Bankaitis, A. U. and Kemp, R. J. (2004). *Infection control in the audiology clinic.* Boulder, CO: Auban, Inc.

sterilizing the tip indirectly transfers the microorganisms residing on the tip into the ear canal of the current patient. Lastly, **droplet contact transmission** occurs when a microorganism expelled from an individual comes in contact with the mucosal lining of the eyelids, nose, or mouth of a susceptible individual. This typically occurs when an individual coughs, sneezes, or breathes on another individual.

Vehicle, Airborne, and Vectorborne Transmission

Vehicle transmission involves the transfer of a microorganism to a susceptible host via contaminated food or water. Ingesting food contaminated with *Salmonella* or drinking water contaminated with

legionellosis can result in varying degrees of food poisoning. In contrast, **airborne transmission** occurs when a microorganism is disseminated throughout the air in the form of either droplet nuclei (residue of evaporated droplets suspended in the air) or dust particles. This form of transmission differs from droplet transmission in that airborne transmission involves a larger area. Whereas droplet contact occurs within the proximity of approximately 3 feet, airborne transmission encompasses 3 feet of air space. Lastly, **vectorborne transmission** entails the transfer of a microorganism via an animal or insect. The most recognized examples of vectorborne transmission include ticks transmitting Lyme disease and mosquitoes transmitting malaria.

Route of Transmission

Once a microorganism is transferred to the vicinity of the human body, it must gain entry into the human body for purposes of growth and reproduction. **Route of transmission** refers to the specific portal of entry whereby a microorganism gains access into the human body. Traditional routes of transmission include orifices of the body—the nose, eyes, ears, and mouth (Bankaitis & Kemp, 2003; Bankaitis & Kemp, 2004). Although the epithelial layer of the skin and other linings typically serve as natural barriers to microorganisms, skin that is dry, chapped, or cracked or that contains cuts, scrapes, and nicks also serves as portals of entry for microorganisms. Upon entry into the human body, whether the microorganism manifests in the form of a localized infection or systemic disease depends on a number of factors. A variety of microbes have the potential to cause disease in individuals with varying degrees of immunocompromise. A fairly comprehensive list of microbes and corresponding diseases relative to the audiology clinic is listed in Table 9-1.

Once a microorganism has gained entry into the body, the audiologist is no longer in a position to influence the disease process. The audiologist's influence on the potential disease process occurs proactively, at the level of the clinical environment, by eliminating common modes and potential routes of transmission within the confines of audiological practice. That is accomplished by creating an effective infection control strategy designed to minimize the risk of disease transmission.

INFECTION CONTROL

Infection control refers to the conscious management of the environment for the purposes of minimizing or eliminating the potential spread of disease (Bankaitis & Kemp, 2003). It is based on two fundamental principles: (1) Infection control is geared toward eliminating or minimizing risk of infection from any potentially infectious agent; and (2) Infection control incorporates a mind-set that assumes every patient, bodily fluid, substance, or agent is potentially infectious (Bankaitis & Kemp, 2004, 2005). With regard to the first principle, it is critical for the audiologist to understand that the concept of infection control is not limited to only those pathogens that may be perceived as more aggressive isolated to preventing exposure to a specific disease (i.e., HIV/AIDS, hepatitis B, etc). Rather, infection control assumes that every microbe is potentially infectious.

With regard to the second principle, the concept of infection control is based on the premise that every patient is a potential carrier of an infectious disease, every bodily fluid is potentially infectious, and any microorganism is potentially infectious. Infection control is not a process that is subjectively implemented based on arbitrary factors Regardless of how remote a possibility may seem, infection control involves the application of task-specific procedures that are consistently executed with each patient every time, regardless of the circumstance. Every aspect of audiological practice must be assessed and scrutinized from the perspective of identifying potential modes of microbial transmission and then implementing appropriate and effective infection control procedures designed to eliminate or reduce the potential for cross contamination. That process is particularly critical for those audiologic procedures that involve insertion of objects and/or instrumentation into the ear canal since the ear represents a common route for microorganisms to gain access to the body. Prior to reviewing basic infection control guidelines, a better appreciation for the relevance of infection control to audiology is warranted.

Relevance of Infection Control to Audiology

There are many reasons why an audiologist must implement profession-specific infection control protocols in the clinical environment. The most definitive justification stems from the fact that infection control represents a federally mandated requirement overseen and enforced by the Occupational Safety & Health Administration (OSHA). Failure of compliance results in citations and significant fines. Beyond

Table 9-1. Overview of diseases or microorganisms, corresponding microbial category of the causative agent, and associated complications relative to the audiology clinic.

Disease	Microbial Category	Complications
AIDS	virus (HIV)	wide range of opportunistic infections causing malaise, hearing disorders, systemic infection, death
Aspergillus	fungus	cutaneous infection
Candida	fungus	candidiasis; cutaneous disease of the skin and nails; mucosal infection of the oral, esophageal, bronchial, and/or vaginal surfaces; systemic infection; meningitis; endocarditis; pulmonary infection
Chicken pox	virus	conjunctivitis, shingles, encephalitis
Coag neg staphylococcus	bacterium	folliculitis, furuncles, boils, carbuncles, bacteremia, endocarditis, pneumonia, osteomyelitis
Common cold	virus	cough, occasional low-grade fever, malaise
Cytomegalovirus	virus	mild flu-like symptoms, moderate to severe generalized infection, liver or spleen damage, sensorineural hearing loss, visual impairment, cognitive dysfunction
Hepatitis B (HBV)	virus	flu-like symptoms, jaundice, fever, liver damage, death
Herpes simplex	virus	herpectic conjunctivitis, pain, discomfort, suppurative inflammation of digits
Herpes zoster	virus	painful vesicular eruptions, discomfort
Influenza	virus	respiratory infection, fever, chills, headache, myalgia, cough, sore throat
Otitis externa	bacterium, fungus	itchy, dry ear canal skin; redness; edema; pain
Pseudomonas aeruginosa	bacterium	bacteremia, endocarditis, chronic otitis externa, alignant otitis, externa, pulmonary infections, eye infections
SARS	prion	fever, headache, body aches, discomfort, dry cough, respiratory distress, death
Staphylococcus aureus	bacterium	folliculitis, furuncles, boils, carbuncles, bacteremia, endocarditis, pneumonia, osteomyelitis
Streptococcal infection	bacterium	pneumonia, suppurative inflammation, endocarditis, kidney problems
Tuberculosis	bacterium	persistent, dry cough; chronic lung infection; malaise; weakness; loss of appetite; weight loss; fever; chills; night sweats

Source: Bankaitis, A.U. and Kemp, R.J. (2004). Infection Control in the Audiology Clinic (page 24). Boulder, CO: Auban. Reprinted with permission from Auban, Inc.

the legal obligations, the nature of the profession is inherently associated with a high degree of disease exposure. The services provided by an audiologist and the corresponding infection control principles that he or she chooses to apply or ignore can influence not only his or her own health, but also the overall health and well-being of patients and coworkers. The following sections serve as a brief overview of factors supporting the need for infection control in the audiology clinic.

Nature and Scope of Audiology

The profession of audiology involves a significant degree of direct and indirect contact with multiple patients and multiple objects. Many diagnostic assessments and rehabilitative procedures require the handling of instruments, objects, or devices that have been inserted into and removed from the external auditory canal or worn over the ears of different patients. The audiologist often provides diagnostic and rehabilitative services to pediatric and geriatric patient populations that, by virtue of their age, are immunocompromised and, therefore, susceptible to potentially infectious agents. Other factors such as socioeconomic status, nutritional status, history of pharmacological intervention, exposure to chemotherapy, or presence of underlying disease such as diabetes or HIV/AIDS also influence the integrity of an individual's immune system. Based on the populations served and the types of services provided by the audiologist, the nature of the profession inherently creates an environment where microorganisms may be readily transferred to a susceptible host.

Furthermore, the scope of practice in audiology has significantly changed in the last several decades, and many audiologists are involved in procedures associated with increased risk of exposure to blood or other bodily fluids. The audiologist is commonly involved in intraoperative monitoring procedures that require interaction in an operating room (OR) environment. Many clinicians perform vestibular assessments that, on occasion, can cause patients to become nauseous and physically sick. Given the importance of an unoccluded external auditory canal, the scope of practice in audiology has expanded to include cerumen management. Cerumen is not necessarily an infectious agent unless it is contaminated with blood, dried blood, or mucous (Kemp, Roeser, Pearson, & Ballanchanda, 1996). Given the color and viscosity of cerumen, it is difficult to determine whether it is contaminated with blood or mucous by-products through visual inspection. Since the audiologist is not in a position to determine with predictable accuracy its contents, cerumen should be treated as an infectious substance (Kemp, Roeser, Pearson, & Ballanchanda, 1996). As more of these procedures are performed by audiologists, the incidence of exposure to blood and other bodily fluids and the subsequent risk of exposure to bloodborne pathogens substantially increase (Kemp & Bankaitis, 2000).

Microbial Contamination of Medical Instruments and Hearing Aids

While intraoperative monitoring or vestibular testing procedures may be perceived as having a higher likelihood for exposure to a potentially infectious microorganism, every aspect of audiological practice is associated with potential disease transmission. That has been clearly indicated in several studies that have consistently recovered a broad range of potentially infectious bacterial and fungal microorganisms from ordinary objects that come in contact with patients. Breathnach, Jenkins, and Pedler (1992) found that the majority of physicians' stethoscopes were significantly contaminated with *Staphylococcus aureus*, a bacterium that can cause serious infections in immunocompromised individuals. Within the context of audiology, initial evidence has similarly found that ordinary objects handled in the clinical environment are significantly contaminated with potentially infectious microorganisms. Bankaitis (2002) detected light to heavy amounts of bacterial and/or fungal growth on custom hearing aid surfaces removed from the ears of adult patients. While the predominant recovered organism was *Staphylococcus*, each of the ten hearing aids was contaminated by a unique combination of bacterial and/or fungal microbial growth including *Acinetobacter lwoffi, Lactobacillus, Pseudomonas aeruginosa, Enterobacter, Aspergillus flavus,* and *Candida parapsilosis*. In other words, no two hearing aids exhibited the same bacterial and fungal compositions. That finding is of significance in that audiologists handling more than one hearing aid over the course of a day who do not apply appropriate infection control procedures can inadvertently introduce a foreign microorganism into the ear canal of a patient via a contaminated hearing aid. The potential consequences may not seem evident until the concept of an opportunistic infection is appreciated.

It is important to clarify some potential misconceptions about the physiological role of cerumen in terms of how its presumed function may influence infection control practices. Cerumen has been characterized to possess antimicrobial properties (Meyerhoff & Caruso, 1991; Roland & Marple, 1997), and the concern is that clinicians may assume that cerumen will be effective in neutralizing any potentially infectious bacteria and/or fungi regardless of what contaminated objects may be inserted in the ear. On the contrary, the relative effectiveness of cerumen in inhibiting microbial growth from bacteria, fungi, and other microorganisms has not been supported by histopathological, histochemical, or morphological studies (Roeser & Roland, 1992). From a more conservative standpoint, assuming that cerumen *does* provide some degree of antimicrobial protection, its efficacy will most likely be uniquely challenged by those patients wearing hearing aids, ear protection, or cell phone earpieces a significant portion of the day since occlusion of the ear canal creates a darker and moister internal environment (Bankaitis & Kemp, 2003, 2004). As the ear canal retains moisture, the ear canal's pH level changes to more neutral or more alkaline levels, which are more conducive to bacterial and/or fungal growth (Jahn & Hawke, 1992). Furthermore, the external auditory canal remains more prone to infection than any other skin surface (Jahn & Hawke, 1992). Based on those circumstances, it is important to place the potential antimicrobial role of cerumen in the proper perspective.

Concern for Opportunistic Infections

Virtually all cells in the body are vulnerable to infection from microbes that can, given the right opportunity, cause significant disease. For the individual with an intact immune system, common microorganisms found in abundance throughout the environment are typically held in check and do not cause disease. On the contrary, the very same microorganisms can cause serious and sometimes life-threatening complications in individuals with varying degrees of immunosuppression. By definition, **opportunistic infections** originate from commonplace organisms that do not produce infection in individuals with intact immune systems, but, instead, take the opportunity to infect a body with a disabled immune system (Bankaitis, 1996). For instance, *Staphylococcus* is a bacterium that resides on the surface of the skin and is found in abundance throughout the environment. Because of its ubiquitous nature, this bacterium may be falsely considered harmless since a logical deduction may lead to the conclusion that if a bacterium was truly potentially harmful, a greater incidence of associated infection and disease would be reported.

Unfortunately, that logic creates a false sense of security since it ignores the foundational principles of opportunistic infections. For example, despite its universal nature and regardless of the fact that *Staphylococcus* does not readily cause disease in most individuals, the bacterium accounts for a high percentage of hospital-acquired infections (Murray, Kobayashi, Pfaller, & Rosenthal, 1994e). According to the Centers for Disease Control and Prevention (CDC), it has been estimated that approximately 2 million patients will contract a hospital-acquired, or nosocomial, infection each year; of those patients, 20,000 will die as a direct result of the infection, while the infection will indirectly contribute to the deaths of another 80,000 individuals (Maki, 1995; Pitter, Mourouga, and Perneger, 1999).

It may seem paradoxical for a common, seemingly innocuous microorganism such as *Staphylococcus* to be associated with a high percentage of hospital-acquired infections. To fully appreciate this relationship, the typical profile of a hospital patient needs to be considered. The hospital setting is comprised of a particularly vulnerable cohort of individuals with some degree of immunocompromise; in other words, hospitals typically admit patients who are sick due to a number of reasons. Whether due to age, medical complications, pharmacological interventions, or socioeconomic factors, sick patients exhibit some degree of immunocompromise; and the hallmark of immunosupression is susceptibility to otherwise innocuous microorganisms. While the emergence of hospital-acquired infections has been attributed to various factors, one of the more commonly cited reasons includes the failure of health care personnel to follow basic infection control procedures, such as hand washing between patient contacts (Weinstein, 1998). Those same principles apply to the audiology clinic. An audiologist who does not wash his or her hands at appropriate times or neglects to clean and disinfect hearing aid surfaces properly can inadvertently cross-contaminate objects that ultimately come in contact with patients. A proactive strategy, including adherence to established hand-washing protocols (Figure 9-6), must be implemented and followed to minimize or reduce the possibility of the inadvertent spread of disease.

Ear is a Natural Orifice

Taking all of the reviewed factors into consideration, an equally critical point to keep in mind is that the ear is a natural orifice of the body, serving as a portal of entry for microorganisms to gain access into the human body. The audiologist's inserting reusable items that have not been properly cleaned and disinfected or sterilized or contaminated hearing aids into a susceptible patient's ear provides an easy route for microorganisms to gain access to the body. Under the right conditions, the lack of infection control protocols in the audiology clinic can result in a patient developing an opportunistic infection that manifests at the level of the external auditory canal or even systemically resulting in a more global disease. The onset of the infection or disease may not necessarily manifest immediately following microbial exposure. Unfortunately, the lack of precision regarding exposure to a microorganism and subsequent disease manifestation can create a misleading assumption that audiologists' practices in the clinic have no effect on the overall health of a patient. Nevertheless, clinical circumstances clearly implicate the potential for disease transmission to occur at the level of the audiology clinic. It is, therefore, imperative for the audiologist to proactively minimize inadvertent transmission of potentially infectious microbes from patient to patient, clinician to patient, and patient to clinician.

> - Remove all jewelry including rings, bracelets, and watches
> - Start water and place an appropriate amount of hospital-grade, liquid antibacterial soap in the palm of the hand
> - Lather the soap, scrubbing the palms, backs of hands, and wrists for a minimum of 10 seconds
> - Thoroughly rinse hands with running water
> - With the water running, retrieve an accessible clean disposable paper towel and dry hands with the paper towel
> - Turn the water off with the used paper towel and without making direct contact with the faucet with clean, bare hands
> - Dispose of the paper towel in the appropriate waste container

Figure 9-6. Sample hand-washing protocol for the audiology clinic. Reprinted with permission from Bankaitis, A. U. and Kemp, R. J. (2004). *Infection control in the audiology clinic.* Boulder, CO: Auban, Inc.

Infection Control Principles

In response to the AIDS epidemic, during the mid to late 1980s, the CDC issued a number of recommendations and guidelines for minimizing cross infection of bloodborne diseases to health care workers. The guidelines were based on the principle that every patient is assumed to be a potential carrier of and/or susceptible host for an infectious disease. Eventually, the pronouncements were officially formalized into the Universal Blood and Bloodborne Pathogen Precautions (CDC, 1987). More commonly referred to as universal precautions, the general pronouncements included the following:

- Appropriate personal barriers (gloves, masks, eye protection, gowns) must be worn when performing procedures that may expose personnel to infectious agents.

- Hands must be washed before and after every patient contact and after glove removal.

- "Touch" and "splash" surfaces must be precleaned and disinfected.

- Critical instruments must be sterilized.

- Infectious waste must be disposed of appropriately.

(CDC, 1987)

Originally, the universal precautions were intended to protect health care workers from blood. However, the precautions have since been interpreted to safeguard workers against all potentially infectious body substances. While the universal precautions specifically mention exposure to blood, semen, vaginal secretions, and other bodily fluids containing visible blood, audiologists handling equipment, devices, or instruments contaminated with cerumen should treat the substance as infectious (CDC, 1989; Kemp & Bankaitis, (2000). Furthermore, all patients should be considered potential carriers of or susceptible hosts to infectious disease. As such, the infection control is regarded as standard patient care for every patient and such procedures should be followed universally.

The universal precautions developed and made available by the CDC are straightforward; however, each pronouncement is briefly reviewed in the following section. For more detailed information and samples of corresponding audiology infection control protocols, see Bankaitis & Kemp, 2004, 2005.

Appropriate Personal Barriers

Appropriately fitting gloves, either latex or nonlatex, must be incorporated in an infection control program. The importance of knowing when to wear gloves and understanding their intended use is critical. In the audiology clinic, gloves should be worn when the risk of encountering infectious substances is high. Gloves come in a variety of sizes. The fit of the glove should be tight, adhering very closely to the skin. When the correct sized glove is worn, the audiologist is able to easily manipulate objects, items, and instruments throughout the appointment. Gloves that are too large are ineffective, as the looseness of the material interferes with audiology procedures. Gloves are considered one-time-use items. They should not be reused, nor should the same pair of gloves be used with two different patients. Using gloves inappropriately in this manner will lead to cross contamination.

Safety glasses and disposable masks are necessary when there is risk of splash or splatter of potentially infectious material or when the clinician/patient is at risk of airborne contamination. Masks, as well as appropriate attire and head covers, must be worn in the OR environment. When bedside testing is performed on hospital patients with tuberculosis (TB), special TB masks are necessary, as indicated by OSHA, when the diagnosed patient has not been on an antibiotic regimen for 10 days. After 10 days on antibiotics, the patient is no longer contagious. Gowns should be worn during vestibular testing to protect clothing in the event a patient becomes sick.

Hand Hygiene

Hand hygiene represents the single most important procedure for effectively limiting the spread of infectious disease. Initially, washing hands with soap and water was the only recognized hand-washing technique. Recently, the CDC has endorsed the use of no-rinse degermers as an alternative method of washing hands when access to a sink with running water may not be readily available or convenient (CDC, 2002). These products should be used only in situations where access to a sink is not available and only when the hands are not visibly soiled. In general, hand hygiene should commence at the beginning of the patient appointment; immediately after removing gloves; prior to and after eating, drinking, smoking, or applying lotion or makeup; and after using bathroom facilities. Within the context of the audiology clinic, certain procedures require the clinician to wash his or her hands more often.

Touch and Splash Surfaces Must Be Precleaned and Disinfected

A **touch surface** refers to an area that may come in direct or indirect contact with hands, and typically includes horizontal surfaces such as countertops, workbenches, services areas, tables, and the armrests of chairs. A **splash surface** refers to an area that may be hit with blood, bodily fluids, or other secretions from a potentially contaminated source. A work surface on which a patient may sneeze or a surface that may come in contact with contaminated instruments used during cerumen-management procedures are examples of splash surfaces.

Both types of surfaces must be properly cleaned and disinfected after use and prior to reuse with a different patient. **Cleaning** involves removing gross contamination without killing germs. For example, horizontal surfaces must be wiped with a clean paper towel or a disinfectant towelette to ensure that all gross contamination is removed prior to initiating disinfecting procedures. In contrast, **disinfecting** is a process in which varying degrees of germs are killed. There are different levels of disinfection that vary according to how many and what specific germs are killed. Household disinfectants kill a limited number of germs commonly found in the household. In contrast, hospital-grade disinfectants are much stronger and kill a larger number and variety of germs. Depending on the specific disinfectant brand and the specific testing conducted by various product manufacturers, different hospital-grade disinfectants kill different combinations of microorganisms. Given the number of available products, an exhaustive or even partial list of which chemicals or brands have been found to kill specific microorganisms isn't practical. The critical issue for audiologists is to ensure that hospital-grade disinfectants rather than household disinfectants are incorporated in infection control protocols implemented in patient care settings, including clinics, hospitals, and private practice facilities where audiology services are provided (Rutala, 1990).

Critical Instruments Must Be Sterilized

Critical instruments refer to those instruments that are invasive and directly introduced into the blood stream (i.e., needles); noninvasive instruments that come in contact with mucous membranes and/or bodily substances (i.e., curette used for cerumen removal); or noninvasive instruments that penetrate skin surfaces from use or misuse (i.e., curette used for cerumen removal). Those instruments must be cleaned and sterilized prior to reuse. The process of **sterilization** involves killing 100% of vegetative microorganisms, including associated endospores. When microbes are challenged, they revert to the more resistant life-form called a spore (Kemp & Bankaitis, 2000). Sterilants, by definition, must neutralize and destroy spores because if a spore is not killed, it may become vegetative again and cause disease. Whereas disinfection may kill some germs, sterilization, by definition, kills all germs and associated endospores every time.

Infectious Waste Must Be Disposed of Appropriately

There is no epidemiologic evidence to suggest that hospital-grade waste is any more infective than residential waste or that hospital waste disposal practices have caused disease in the community (CDC, 2002). Therefore, identifying wastes for which special precautions are indicated remains a matter of judgment. The most practical approach to infectious waste is to identify those materials that represent sufficient potential risk of causing infection during handling and/or disposal for which some special precautions may be sensible (CDC, 2002). Special precautions apply to microbiology laboratory waste; pathology waste; blood specimens; blood products; and sharp instruments such as needles, scalpel blades, and razor blades. According to the CDC, while any item that has made contact with blood or bodily secretions may be potentially infectious, it is not normally considered practical or necessary to treat all such waste as infectious (Garner & Simmons, 1983).

For the audiology environment, most waste contaminated with ear discharge or cerumen can be placed in regular waste receptacles and discarded through regular disposal procedures. In the event that certain waste may be contaminated with excessive cerumen or mucous, the material should be placed in a separate impermeable bag before being discarded in the regular trash. That practice will separate the contaminated waste from the rest of the trash and minimize the chance of maintenance or cleaning personnel coming in casual contact with it. It is not likely that materials containing significant amounts of blood or bodily fluids would be encountered in the audiology clinic. In such circumstances, however, materials containing significant amounts of blood should be disposed of in impermeable bags labeled with the symbol for biohazard waste and disposed of by a waste hauler licensed for medical waste disposal.

SUMMARY

A variety of microorganisms can cause infection or varying degrees of disease in susceptible individuals. Viruses, bacteria, fungi, parasites, and the newly identified prions continually seek a resource for growth and reproduction. The human body represents an ideal host for those microorganisms, and it is the job of the immune system to neutralize such pathogens. Unfortunately, immune systems are not always working at an efficient capacity; different factors (including an individual's age, health, diet, and environment) influence the system's integrity. For many individuals, the immune system is effective in preventing disease or infection. However, many individuals possess some degree of immunocompromise and, therefore, are more susceptible to ubiquitous organisms.

There are many steps to the disease process. However, for a disease to arise, microorganisms require both a mode and a route of transmission in order to gain access to a susceptible host (i.e., human body). There are several different modes of microbial transmission, including ingesting contaminated food or being bitten by an infected insect such as a tick or mosquito. Within the context of the audiology clinic, the most common mode of microbial transmission involves making direct contact with another individual or making direct or indirect contact with a contaminated object. Once a microorganism is transferred to the vicinity of the human body, it seeks a portal of entry into the body. Common routes of microbial transmission involve natural orifices of the body, including the ear. Given the nature and scope of audiological practice, the clinical environment is associated with a high degree of disease transmission. As such, infection control is a relevant aspect of clinical practice.

Understanding the justification for an infection control strategy within the context of the audiology clinic is important to motivate implementation of such procedures. First and foremost, infection control is a federally mandated program required of all health care providers, including audiologists. Second, the nature of audiology involves a notable degree of contact with multiple patients and multiple objects. Given the scope of audiological practice, exposure to potentially infectious microorganisms and bodily substances has substantially increased, making infection control a more important issue. Third, objects ordinarily encountered in the audiology clinic, including hearing aids, have been shown to be contaminated with significant amounts of bacterial and/or fungal microorganisms that are not inherent to the population as a whole. Considering the populations served by audiologists, exposing patients to microorganisms that can readily cause opportunistic infections is a significant concern since inappropriate infection control procedures may put a patient's health at risk.

While it may appear straightforward, infection control is a process whereby the clinical environment is intentionally manipulated and managed for purposes of eliminating or significantly reducing the potential spread of disease. The process begins with the mind-set that all patients are potential carriers of an infectious disease and that any and all microorganisms and bodily fluids (including cerumen) are potentially infectious. By applying established infection control guidelines specifically to audiological practice, audiologists are executing a proactive approach to minimizing the potential for disease transmission. For more information on infection control requirements and audiology-specific protocols and procedures, refer to available texts written by the authors.

REFERENCES

Bankaitis, A. E. (1996). Audiological changes attributable to HIV. *Audiology Today, 8*(6), 7–9.

Bankaitis, A. E., & Schountz, T. (1998). HIV-related ototoxicity. *Seminars in Hearing, 19*(2), 155–63.

Bankaitis, A. U. (2002). What's growing on your patients' hearing aids? *The Hearing Journal, 55*(6), 48–56.

Bankaitis, A. U., & Kemp, R. J. (2003). *Infection Control in the Hearing Aid Clinic.* Boulder, CO: Auban.

Bankaitis, A. U., & Kemp, R. J. (2004). *Infection Control in the Audiology Clinic.* Boulder, CO: Auban.

Bankaitis, A. U., & Kemp, R. J. (2005). *Infection Control in the Audiology Clinic* (2nd ed.). St. Louis: Auban.

Breathnach, A. S., Jenkins, D. R., & Pedler, S. J. (1992). Stethoscopes as possible vectors of infection by staphylococci. *British Medical Journal, 305,* 1573.

CDC. (1987). Recommendations for prevention of HIV transmission in healthcare settings. *Morbidity and Mortality Weekly Report, 36*(2S).

CDC. (1989). Guidelines for prevention of transmission of human immunodeficiency virus and Hepatitis B to health-care and public-safety workers. *Morbidity and Mortality Weekly Report, 38.*

CDC. (2002). Guideline for hand hygiene. *Morbidity and Mortality Weekly Report, 51*(RR16), 1–44.

Garner, J. S., & Simmons, B. P. (1983). Guideline for isolation precautions in hospitals. *Infection Control, 4,* 245–325.

Jahn, A. F., & Hawke, M. (1992). Infections of the external ear. In C. Cummings, J. F. Fredrickson, L. Harker, C. Krause, & C. Schuller (Eds.), *Otolaryngology - Head and Neck Surgery* (2nd ed., pp. 2787–2794). St. Louis: Mosby-Year Book.

Kemp, R. J., & Bankaitis, A. U. (2000). Infection control. In H. Hosford-Dunn, R. J. Roeser, & M. Valente (Eds.), *Audiology: Practice Management* (pp. 257–272). New York: Thieme Medical Publishers.

Kemp, R. J., Roeser, R. J., Pearson, D. W., & Ballachanda, B. P. (1996). *Infection Control for the Professions of Audiology and Speech Language Pathology.* Olathe, KS: Iles Publications.

Maki, D. G. (1995). Nosocomial infection in the intensive care unit. In J. E. Parrillo & R. C. Bone (Eds.), *Critical Care Medicine: Principles of Diagnosis and Management* (pp. 893–954). St. Louis: Mosby.

Meyerhoff, W. I., & Caruso, V. G. (1991). Trauma and infections of the external ear. In M. Paparella, D. Shumrick, J. Gluckman, & W. L. Meyerhoff (Eds.), *Otolaryngology* (3rd ed., pp. 1227–1236). Philadelphia: WB Saunders.

Murray, P. R., Kobayashi, G. S., Pfaller, M. A., & Rosenthal, K. S. (1994a). Introduction to microbiology. In P. R. Murray, G. S. Kobayashi, M. A. Pfaller, & K. S. Rosenthal (Eds.), *Medical Microbiology,* (2nd ed., pp. 1–5). St. Louis: Mosby-Year Book.

Murray, P. R., Kobayashi, G. S., Pfaller, M. A., & Rosenthal, K. S. (1994b). Fungal biology and classification. In P. R. Murray, G. S. Kobayashi, M. A. Pfaller, & K. S. Rosenthal (Eds.), *Medical Microbiology,* (2nd ed., pp. 46–50). St. Louis: Mosby-Year Book.

Murray, P. R., Kobayashi, G. S., Pfaller, M. A., & Rosenthal, K. S. (1994c). Opportunistic mycoses. In P. R. Murray, G. S. Kobayashi, M. A. Pfaller, & K. S. Rosenthal (Eds.), *Medical Microbiology,* (2nd ed., pp. 431–437). St. Louis: Mosby-Year Book.

Murray, P. R., Kobayashi, G. S., Pfaller, M. A., & Rosenthal, K. S. (1994d). Parasitic classification. In P. R. Murray, G. S. Kobayashi, M. A. Pfaller, & K. S. Rosenthal (Eds.), *Medical Microbiology,* (2nd ed., pp. 51–57). St. Louis: Mosby-Year Book.

Murray, P. R., Kobayashi, G. S., Pfaller, M. A., & Rosenthal, K. S. (1994e). Stapylococcus. In P. R. Murray, G. S. Kobayashi, M. A. Pfaller, & K. S. Rosenthal (Eds.), *Medical Microbiology,* (2nd ed., pp. 166–179). St. Louis: Mosby-Year Book.

Murray, P. R., Kobayashi, G. S., Pfaller, M. A., Rosenthal, K. S., Lepine, G., & Progulske-Fox, A. (1994). Bacterial structure. In P. R. Murray, G. S. Kobayashi, M. A. Pfaller, & K. S. Rosenthal (Eds.), *Medical Microbiology,* (2nd ed., pp. 6–16). St. Louis: Mosby-Year Book.

National Center for Infectious Diseases (2002). Update 2002: Bovine spongiform encephalopathy and variant Creutzfeldt-Jakob disease. Retrieved July, 2005 from http://www.cdc.gov/ncidod/diseases/cjd/bse_cjd.htm

Peters, W., & Gilles, H. M. (1995). *Colour Atlas of Tropical Medicine and Parasitology.* London: Mosby-Wolfe, Inc.

Pitter, D., Mourouga, P., Perneger, T. V., & Members of the Infection Control Program. (1999). Compliance with handwashing in a teaching hospital. *Annals of Internal Medicine, 130,* 126–130.

Roeser, R. (2003). Foreword. In A. U. Bankaitis & R. J. Kemp (Authors). *Infection Control in the Hearing Aid Clinic,* (pp. vii–ix). Boulder, CO: Auban.

Roeser, R. J., & Roland, P. S. (1992). What audiologists must know about cerumen and cerumen management. *American Journal of Audiology,* (November) 27–34.

Roland, P. S., & Marple, B. F. (1997). Disorders of the external auditory canal. *Journal of the American Academy of Audiology, 8,* 367–378.

Rutala, W. A. (1990). APIC guideline for selection and use of disinfectants. *American Journal of Infection Control, 17*(52), 99–117.

Weinstein, R. A. (1998). Nosocomial infection update. *Emerging Infectious Diseases, 4*(3), 416–420.

CHAPTER 10

Cancer and Ototoxicity of Chemotherapeutics

Leonard P. Rybak, MD, PhD
Southern Illinois University School of Medicine
Department of Surgery, Division of Otolaryngology
Springfield, Illinois

Xinyan Huang, MD
Southern Illinois University School of Medicine
Springfield, Illinois

Kathleen C. M. Campbell, PhD
Southern Illinois University School of Medicine
Springfield, Illinois

INTRODUCTION

This chapter discusses cancer and its treatment with chemotherapy. It is important for the audiologist to be aware that certain anticancer drugs cause hearing loss, while others do not. This chapter provides a brief overview of how cancer cells form tumors. It outlines general mechanisms by which antitumor drugs kill tumor cells. Detailed information about the chemical structure, pharmacology, and mechanisms of action against cancer cells and major toxicity are provided. The effects of the platinum-containing anticancer drugs cisplatin and carboplatin on hearing and on the structures of the inner ear are delineated. Additional information about the vinca alkaloids and difluoromethylornithine (DFMO) and their effects on hearing is explained. This material should be of great benefit in counseling cancer patients about drugs they are given and ways the drugs might cause hearing loss. Knowledge about the effects of these drugs on the inner ear will help the audiologist to determine appropriate rehabilitation strategies.

UNDERSTANDING CANCER

Cell growth and maturation are normal events in organ development during embryogenesis, growth, and tissue repair and remodeling after injury. Dysregulation of those processes can result in loss of control over cell growth, differentiation, and spatial confinement. Cancer represents a spectrum of diseases characterized by abnormal growth and invasion of cells. The process of tumor growth and development is a result of stepwise alterations in cellular function. Those phenotypic changes confer proliferative, invasive, and metastatic potential that are the hallmarks of cancer. The loss of cellular growth control is the result of a series of genetic changes in the cells of cancer. The changes include overriding the normal program for cell differentiation and death and favoring an increase in cell proliferation and life span. Cancer progression involves additional changes that result in establishment of a blood supply, migration, invasion, and metastasis within the

patient host (Hahn & Weinberg, 2002; Hill, 2001; Fidler, 2004).

Under experimental conditions, molecular alteration in expression or function of at least three genes is required to alter important cellular functions and cause transformation and tumor development from normal human cells (Weinberg, 1994). One important requirement for neoplastic transformation and tumor formation is increased cell proliferation. A second requirement is increased cell life span, or immortalization. Cells normally stop proliferating and reach the end of their life in a finite number of cell divisions. The life-span limit of normal cells has been shown to be associated with a gradual shortening of the ends of chromosomes (i.e., **telomeres,** which consist of multiple repeats of specific deoxyribonucleic acid (DNA) sequences and protein). In contrast, cancer cells do not exhibit shortening of the telomeres, which is attributable to increased expression of an enzyme called **telomerase.** Third, cancer cells exhibit a decreased rate of apoptosis, which is programmed cell death. Genes in which alterations result in a gain of function are referred to as **oncogenes,** whereas genes in which deletions or mutations result in loss of control function are defined as **tumor suppressor genes**. Altered expression of different combinations of oncogenes and tumor suppressor genes may result in increased proliferation and life span and decreased cell death, leading to tumor formation.

Cancer and the Cell Cycle

The growth and division of cells, normal and tumor, pass through four different phases of *cell cycle* (Figure 10-1). **Mitosis** occupies a discrete phase (M) of the cell cycle. It is defined as the usual process of somatic reproduction of cells consisting of a sequence of modifications of the nucleus that result in the formation of two daughter cells with exactly the same chromosome and nuclear DNA content as that of the original cell. Following the division, the cell enters the G1 phase (G = gap), which is then followed by DNA synthesis, the S phase. After completion of the DNA synthesis, the cell then enters the G2 phase (premitotic interval) before the initiation of the next mitosis. In most dividing cells, the periods for S, G2, and M phases are of relatively constant duration. Variation of the length of the cell cycle generally occurs in the G1 phase. When the proliferating cells stop dividing, they do so in the G1 phase. A prolonged G1 phase, or resting phase, is commonly termed G0.

The molecular mechanisms controlling cell cycle are being rapidly elucidated. The cell cycle is regulated by a series of protein known as **cyclins, cyclin-dependent kinases,** and **cyclin-dependent kinases inhibitors** (CKIs) that participate in activating and inactivating phosphorylation events on selected proteins. Those events regulate biochemical pathway or **checkpoints** that control mitogenic and growth inhibitory signals and that coordinate the orderly sequence of cell cycle transition. There are two important checkpoints in the cell cycle: at G1/S, when cells must commit to and then complete DNA synthesis, and at G2/M, when cells must commit to and then complete mitosis. The cyclins act as positive regulators of the activity of the cyclin-dependent kinases, whereas the CKIs act as negative regulators.

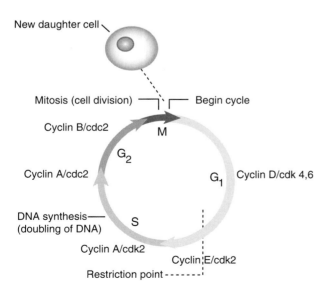

Figure 10-1. A diagram of the cell cycle

These checkpoints are controlled by various genes, which are frequently disrupted in cancer cells (Pietenpol & Kastan, 2004).

Tumor Growth

Tumor growth depends on three factors: (1) the growth fraction, which is defined as a proportion of tumor cells in the mitotic phase at a given time; (2) the cell cycle time, which is quite variable but usually in the range of 2–3 days for human tumors, which is not faster than normal cells; and (3) the rate of cell loss. Usually, renewal of normal cells is accompanied by cell loss, an active process known as programmed cell death, or apoptosis. When cell loss is reduced, tumor formation can occur. This reduction in cell loss seems to be the major factor in the production of most tumors.

Types of Chemotherapeutic Agents

The purpose of cancer chemotherapy is to prevent cancer cells from proliferating, invading, metastasizing, and ultimately killing the host. Most chemotherapeutic agents currently in use exert their effect primarily on cell multiplication and tumor growth. In addition to differences in the biochemical mechanism of action, antineoplastic agents differ in the point in the cell cycle at which they act. The agents can be grouped on the basis of their effects on phases of the cell cycle (Skeel, 1999). This classification is not absolute; it is likely that more than one mechanism is involved and that multiple intracellular sites might be implicated.

1. Phase-specific drugs. The agents that are most active against cells in a specific phase of the cell cycle. Drugs that inhibit DNA synthesis, such as methotrexate, are called S phase-specific, whereas plant alkaloids, such as vincristine, arrest mitosis during metaphase.

2. Cell cycle-specific (or phase-nonspecific) drugs. The agents that are effective in cells that are actively in cycle but that are not dependent on the cell being in a particular phase. Most of the alkylating agents and the antitumor antibiotics exert a direct effect on

DNA; thus, their activities are not dependent on the phase of the cell cycle.

3. Cell cycle-nonspecific drugs. A third group of drugs that appears to be effective whether cancer cells are in cycle or are resting.

CISPLATIN

Cisplatin is a commonly used chemotherapeutic agent that has unique chemical and pharmacological properties. It also exhibits toxic effects on the inner ear and kidney. Its features are discussed in detail below.

Structure and Pharmacokinetics

Cisplatin is the standard of the platinum compound. It has a square planar inorganic platinum (Pt) molecule consisting of a divalent Pt(II) central atom and four ligands of *cis* positioned pairs of chlorine atoms or amine groups (Figure 10-2). The chloride ligands of cisplatin with the +2 oxidation state can be exchanged for nucleophilic atoms in the biologic milieu, including the nitrogens of the DNA bases.

Cisplatin's *cis* geometry is crucial for cytotoxic activity with the ability to form certain stereospecific cross-links. Cisplatin reacts with nitrogen atoms of DNA and preferentially forms covalent bonds with N7 of the purine guanine by hydrolytic displacement of chlorine atoms, as shown in Figure 10-3.

The extremely reactive intrastrand and interstrand crosslinked Pt-DNA adducts formed by the covalent bonds inhibit DNA replication, with subsequent induction of apoptosis via activation or modulation of signaling pathway (Kartalou & Essigmann, 2001; Boulikas & Vougiouka, 2003; Reedijk, 2003).

Following an intravenous bolus administration of 100 mg/m^2 of cisplatin, initial peak plasma concentrations of 3 to >5 μg/ml are archived, with this value declining to 0.2 μg/ml at 2 hours (Patton et al., 1983). The clearance of cisplatin follows a triphasic pattern, with an initial plasma half-life ($t_{1/2}$) of 20–30 minutes, a second phase $t_{1/2}$ of 60 minutes, and a terminal $t_{1/2}$ of more than 24 hours (Himmelstein et al., 1981). More than 90% of cisplatin is bound to serum protein, and this cisplatin-protein complex is biologically inactive (Gormley et al., 1971). About 25% of a dose of cisplatin is eliminated from the body during the first 24 hours, with renal clearance for more than 90%. Cisplatin preferentially concentrates in the liver, kidneys, and large and small intestines, with low penetration of the central nervous system (Vermorken et al., 1984).

Clinical Considerations

Since introduced in 1970s, cisplatin has been widely used clinically against a variety of cancer and remains unrivaled in efficacy against germ cell, ovarian, endometrial, cervical, urothelial, head and neck, lung, and brain cancers (Sturgeon, 2004; Boulikas & Vougiouka, 2004). However, cisplatin is systemically toxic and predictably ototoxic (Hartmann & Lipp, 2003). Cisplatin has the highest ototoxic potential among all platinum compounds, and cisplatin is the most ototoxic compound in clinical use (Anniko & Sobin, 1986; Hartmann & Lipp, 2003).

The incidence for irreversible ototoxicity varies depending on the dose regimen and the method used to define ototoxicity (Moroso & Blair, 1983). Patients with cisplatin-induced ototoxicity generally present with tinnitus and high-frequency hearing loss. Tinnitus has been reported in 2%–36% of patients receiving cisplatin treatment. Often, the tinnitus is transient, lasting from a few hours up to a week after cisplatin therapy (Moroso & Blair, 1983). The incidence of hearing loss among patients treated with cisplatin has been reported to be as low as 11% and as high as 91%, with

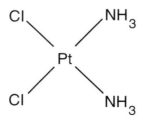

Figure 10-2. Structural formula for cisplatin

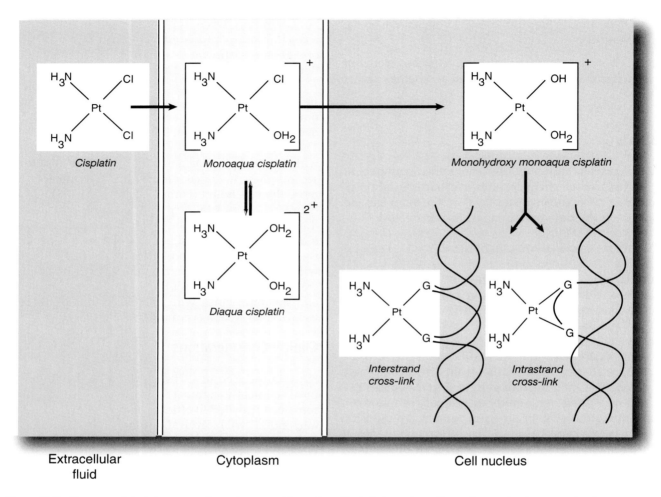

Figure 10-3. Transport of cisplatin across cell membranes and formation of hydrolysis products. The cisplatin molecule crosses the plasma membrane and is transformed within cystoplasm into positively charged monoaqua and monohydroxy-monoaqua species, which are reactive and interact with nuclear DNA, resulting in the formation of interstrand and intrastrand cross-link (Kartalou & Essigmann, 2001). Reprinted from the *Hearing Research*, 203, van Ruijven, de Groot, Hendrikson, Smoorenburg, Immunohistochemical detection of platinated DNA, 113–121 (2005), with permission from Elsevier.

the overall incidence of hearing loss of 69%, usually in the 4000–8000 Hz range (Moroso & Blair, 1983). The more recent studies reported a 40%–60% incidence of ototoxicity (Bokemeyer et al., 1998; de Jongh et al., 2003; Li et al., 2004). In patients with head and neck cancer treated with cisplatin, about half develop hearing loss (Blakley et al., 1994).

Risk Factors for Ototoxicity

There is substantial variability in susceptibility to cisplatin-induced ototoxicity. Risk factors affecting the severity of cisplatin ototoxicity are intravenous bolus administration or high cumulative dosage of cisplatin (Vermorken et al., 1983; Kopelman et al., 1988;

Waters et al., 1991; Bokemeyer et al., 1998), young age (Li et al., 2004) or advanced age (Helson et al., 1978; Laurell & Jungnelius, 1990), renal insufficiency (Schaefer et al., 1985; Hallmark et al., 1992; Bokemeyer et al., 1998), preexisting hearing loss (Melamed et al., 1985; Bokemeyer et al., 1998), anemia (Blakley et al., 1994; de Jongh et al., 2003), and coadministration of high-dose vincristin (Bokemeyer et al., 1998). Ototoxicity of cisplatin also appears to be enhanced by prior cranial irradiation (Granowetter et al., 1983; Schell et al., 1989; Blakley et al., 1994).

Cisplatin ototoxicity is dose-related. A standard cisplatin dose was 50 mg/m^2 early after its introduction. Subsequent cisplatin treatment regimens have been developed using higher doses (100–120 mg/m^2 = high dose and 150–225 mg/m^2 = very high-dose regimens). The increased-dosage regimens have resulted in a higher incidence of hearing loss than that observed with the lower dosage of 50 mg/m^2, as well as some different perspectives on cisplatin-induced hearing loss. In a study of 54 patients with metastatic cancer receiving high-dose cisplatin, Laurell and Jungnelius (1990) found that 81% of the patients had significant elevations of air-conduction hearing threshold (15 dB or more at one frequency and 10 dB or more in three frequencies). After therapy, which ranged from one to seven courses, 41% of the patients had significant deterioration of hearing in the speech frequency range of 500–2000 Hz. Twenty-five percent of patients lost 25% or more of their remaining high-frequency hearing (3000–8000 Hz) after each course treatment. Preexisting hearing loss did not seem to predispose to ototoxicity, but advanced age was slightly associated with risk of hearing loss. The audiogram after the first course did not predict future deterioration of hearing during treatment with high-dose protocols. In the study, the ototoxic risk was determined more by the amount of the single dose than by the cumulate dose levels. No ototoxicity effects were seen at a peak plasma concentration of less than 1 µg/L.

In a recent large retrospective study, de Jongh et al. (2003) found that 42% of 400 patients receiving 70–85 mg/m^2 cisplatin, with median cumulative dose of 420 mg, incurred symptomatic ototoxicity. In contrast, cisplatin ototoxicity was developed in only 20% of patients receiving a low-dose cisplatin

therapy (Vermorken et al., 1983; Waters et al., 1991), but 75%–100% of patients receiving a very high-dose regimen (Vermorken et al., 1983; Pollera et al., 1988; Kopelman et al., 1988; Waters et al., 1991; Ekborn et al., 2004). Furthermore, it has been shown that the best predictor of cisplatin ototoxicity is cumulative dose in both clinical and animal studies (Bokemeyer et al., 1998; Klis et al., 2002; Li et al., 2004). The critical cumulative dose of cisplatin has been reported as 3–4 mg/kg body weight (Moroso & Blair, 1983). Bokemeyer et al. (1998) as well as others (Park, 1996; Waters et al., 1991; Li et al., 2004) have found that the incidence of ototoxicity increased dramatically when the total cumulative dose exceeds 400 mg/m^2. In addition, patients with renal insufficiency, a poor renal creatinine clearance, have increased risk of cisplatin ototoxicity because the serum active cisplatin levels increase (Bokemeyer et al., 1998).

Cisplatin-induced ototoxicity is age-dependent. It has been shown that a greater sensitivity to cisplatin ototoxicity exists for both older and pediatric patients once a critical cumulative dose of cisplatin has been reached. Li et al. (2004) demonstrated that children younger than five years of age are most susceptible to cisplatin ototoxicity. A logistic regression model predicts that about 40% of the children younger than five years would develop moderate to severe hearing loss when they receive a cumulative dose of 400 mg/m^2, compared with the 5% risk among children between fifteen and twenty years of age. Helson et al. (1978) reported that patients aged eight to twenty years or older than forty-six years of age who received a high cumulative dose of cisplatin (> 400 mg/m^2) developed a more severe hearing loss than that incurred by patients twenty-one to forty-five years old. Ototoxic reactions appear to be more likely in patients with low serum albumin and in those with anemia (Blakley et al., 1994; de Jongh et al., 2003).

Cisplatin-induced hearing loss is usually bilateral and appears first at high frequencies. Progression to lower frequencies (it can progress all the way to 250 Hz) may occur with continued therapy. The hearing loss is usually symmetric, but may be asymmetric and may not appear until several days after treatment. Patients may experience some degree of reversibility; but, in general, hearing loss is permanent. Particularly when the hearing loss is profound, it appears to be permanent (Vermorken et al., 1983; Kopelman et al., 1988). Kopelman et al. (1988) reported that all of nine patients complained of decreased hearing (10 dB or more at one or more frequencies) following very high-dose cisplatin administration (150–225 mg/m²). After one dose of cisplatin, 67% (6/9 patients) failed to respond in the range of 9000–20000 Hz, 89% experienced a threshold shift at 8000 Hz, and 78% demonstrated a threshold shift at 6000 Hz. Following the second dose, no measurable hearing in the range of 9000–20000 Hz was obtained in any of the eight patients remaining in the study and 88%, 75%, and 50% exhibited a threshold shift at 4000 Hz, 3000 Hz, and 2000 Hz, respectively.

Characteristics of Cisplatin Ototoxicity

The hearing loss may be gradual, progressive, and cumulative or may present suddenly. Word recognition scores may be markedly reduced when cisplatin ototoxicity occurs. In a study of thirty-nine patients with head and neck cancer receiving intravenous bolus infusion of cisplatin therapy (100 mg/m² for six courses), Blakley and Myers (1993) described several patterns of hearing loss. Following cisplatin treatment, twenty-one patients (54%) had no hearing loss or mild hearing loss (40 dB or less in one frequency or 30 dB or less in three or more frequencies between 250 and 4000 Hz), fourteen (36%) had rapid early hearing loss (after the first dose of cisplatin), and four (10%) had slow and progressive hearing loss. Ninety percent of significant hearing loss occurred in the early treatment. When early hearing loss occurred and treatment was continued, the speech frequencies were eventually affected in 71% of patients.

Because the hearing loss tends to occur at higher frequencies, it may escape detection with conventional audiometry. Cochlear toxicity may be detected earlier with high-frequency audiometry (up to 20 kHz) than with conventional audiologic testing (Fausti et al., 1993; Park, 1996). Fausti et al. (1993) demonstrated that 71% of cisplatin-induced hearing loss was detected first in frequencies of 8000 Hz or above.

The auditory brainstem response (ABR) (Coupland et al., 1991; De Lauretis et al., 1999) and evoked otoacoustic emissions (OAEs) (Ozturan et al., 1996; Allen et al., 1998; Berg et al., 1999; Stavroulaki et al., 2001; Toral-Martinon et al., 2003) can also be used to assess hearing status and to determine the presence of cisplatin ototoxicity in pediatric cancer patients. In a study of a group of eighteen pediatric patients who underwent cisplatin therapy, Coupland et al. (1991) demonstrated that derived-band ABRs were more sensitive than broadband click ABR in detecting early high-frequency hearing loss. In children under three years of age, the study found that the cumulative dose of cisplatin was correlated with the ABR threshold shift. Allen et al. (1998) carried out a study of OEAs in pediatric patients treated with cisplatin chemotherapy. Transient OAEs could be measured in eleven of twelve patients studied. When the middle ear was normal, a significant correlation was found between the transient OAEs and the pure-tone threshold and 90.5% of the patients had a significant sensorineural hearing loss at 8000 Hz. Increased hearing loss was associated with a young age at first dose of cisplatin, a high number of chemotherapy cycles, and a high cumulative dose. In another study, Stavroulaki et al. (2001) reported that a significant high-frequency hearing loss was identified in children even after the first low-dose of cisplatin infusion (50 mg/m²) by audiometry and evoked OAEs. Distortion-product OAEs were extremely sensitive and superior to pure-tone audiometry and/or transient OAEs. Acoustic reflex threshold test can also be used for monitoring cisplatin ototoxicity in the pediatric population (Park, 1996). Although it is not the most sensitive test to ototoxicity, acoustic reflex threshold measurement is one of more objective tests.

Mechanisms of Cisplatin Ototoxicity

The mechanisms of cisplatin ototoxicity are multifactorial. Animal studies indicate that reduced auditory acuity is partially mediated by free radical generation and antioxidant inhibition. The formation of highly reactive oxygen radicals results in glutathione depletion in the cochlea and increased lipid peroxidation (Ravi et al., 1995; Rybak et al., 1999; Rybak & Kelly, 2003). Induction of apoptosis by cisplatin in the hair cells is also implicated in cisplatin ototoxicity (Liu et al., 1998; Wang et al., 2004). The cisplatin-induced permanent hearing loss is linked to the degeneration of cochlear outer hair cells and stria vascularis (Wright & Schaefer, 1982; Comis et al., 1986; Meech et al., 1998; Campbell et al., 1999).

Several animal studies report that following low-dose cisplatin, alterations to the stria vascularis precede changes to the organ of Corti. The strial damage occurs primarily in the marginal cells, with some mild changes in the intermediate cells (Meech et al., 1998; Campbell et al., 1999). Decreases in cell size, which lead to overall thinning of the stria, bulging or ruptured marginal cells, and strial atrophy, are reported. Overall, in the same cochlear region, the strial changes are minor compared with the damage in the organ of Corti.

In the organ of Corti, low-dose cisplatin causes damage primarily to the hair cell stereocilia. The stereocilia abnormalities include a rough surface coat, disruption of the stereocilia cross-links, fused stereocilia, and formation of giant stereocilia (Comis et al., 1986). Higher doses of cisplatin cause hair cell degeneration through sequelae that involve softening of the cuticular plate, aggregation of lysosomes in the supranuclear portion of the hair cell body, and cytoplasmic extrusion from the hair cell (Barron & Daigneault, 1987).

The loss of outer hair cells occurs initially in the most basal region of the cochlea. As the ototoxic damage increases, the loss of outer hair cells progresses more apically (Schweitzer et al., 1984). Outer hair cell loss is most pronounced in the first row and least in the third row. Inner hair cells show damage and degeneration only after all three rows of outer hair cells in the same region have degenerated (Marco-Algarra et al., 1985; Barron & Daigneault, 1987). Focal damage to pillar cells and other supporting cells are noted with high doses of cisplatin (Estrem et al., 1981). A recent study suggests that the initial damage of the supporting cells could be responsible for the late injury of the hair cells (Ramirez-Camacho et al., 2004).

The cochlear histopathology changes in animal studies have been confirmed by examination of human temporal bones (Wright & Schaefer, 1982; Strauss et al., 1983; Hinojosa et al., 1995; Hoistad et al.,

1998). Temporal bones removed from patients with cisplatin-induced hearing loss have demonstrated large, fused stereocilia; damage to the cuticular plate of the outer hair cells; and extensive loss of sensory cells in the vestibular labyrinth in specimens studied with scanning electron microscopy. In addition to noting outer hair cell degeneration in the basal turn of the cochlea, Strauss et al. (1983) reported degeneration of spiral ganglion cells and cochlear neurons in patients with documented cisplatin ototoxicity. However, the vestibular neurons appeared normal. Moreover, Hoistad et al. (1998) reported that the otopathology from cisplatin could be aggravated by a combination of radiation therapy. They noted that temporal bones removed from patients treated with cisplatin, cranial radiation, or a combination of both treatments showed that the spiral ganglion cells and inner and outer hair cells were decreased in number and that the stria vascularis was atrophic. The otopathology identified in these temporal bones also included vascular changes, serum effusion, and fibrosis.

Although cisplatin ototoxicity is considered to be exclusively confined to the cochlea, cisplatin vestibular toxicity has been associated with degeneration of the maculae and cristae (Black et al., 1982; Wright & Schaefer, 1982; Sergi et al., 2003).

Animal studies also showed that the degree of cisplatin-induced ototoxicity was enhanced by coadministration with aminoglycosides (Schweitzer et al., 1984; Comis, et al., 1986; Riggs et al., 1996) or loop diuretics (Brummett, 1981; Komune & Snow, 1981) and was concomitant with excessive noise exposure (Gratton et al., 1990; Laurell, 1992).

CARBOPLATIN

Carboplatin is a second-generation platinum-based chemotherapeutic agent. It is used to treat small cell lung cancer and ovarian and head and neck cancers (Bauer et al., 1992; MacDonald et al., 1994; Cavaletti, et al., 1998; Ettinger, 1998). Carboplatin was introduced into clinical chemotherapy because it was found to cause less nephrotoxicity than cisplatin, while retaining antitumor activity roughly equivalent to that of cisplatin (Wolfgang et al., 1994; Alberts,

1995; DeLauretis et al., 1999). The use of dose escalation has been found to be important in achieving optimal antitumor responses in patients (Bohm et al., 1999; Wandt et al., 1999).

Toxicity Profile

The primary dose-limiting toxicity of carboplatin has been bone marrow toxicity. This toxic effect has been overcome by the use of autologous stem cell rescue. That has allowed medical oncologists to use larger doses of carboplatin in an effort to increase antitumor efficacy.

Initial reports also suggested that carboplatin was less ototoxic than cisplatin. However, the increase in efficacy has come at the expense of greater ototoxicity than that which was initially appreciated (Kennedy et al., 1990; Cavaletti et al., 1998; Neuwelt et al., 1998; Obermair et al., 1998; DeLauretis et al., 1999). Nine of eleven children with neuroblastoma (82%) who were treated with high-dose carboplatin followed by autologous bone marrow transplantation had hearing losses in the speech frequencies that were so severe that hearing aids were recommended. All of those children had had previous treatment with cisplatin, and several patients had also received aminoglycoside antibiotics in the past (Parsons et al., 1998). Another study of Stage 4 pediatric neuroblastoma patients treated with high-dose carboplatin chemotherapy with autologous stem cell reinfusion showed hearing losses in 40% (65/188) of the patients (Simon et al., 2002). A recent study of children with neuroblastoma treated with carboplatin and hematopoietic stem cell transplantation demonstrated hearing loss in 20/45 patients (44%) by routine audiometry or testing of OAEs (Punnett et al., 2004). In combination with osmotic blood-brain barrier disruption using mannitol, carboplatin has been used to successfully treat malignant brain tumors. A large percentage of patients (79%) developed hearing loss with that protocol. When another group of patients was treated with carboplatin, followed by sodium thiosulfate after the blood-brain barrier was allowed to close, very little hearing loss was observed (Neuwelt et al., 1998). Patients with ovarian cancer treated with cisplatin and carboplatin were evaluated for toxicity. Both thrombocytopenia and ototoxicity were associated with high area-under-the-curve (AUC) blood concentrations of carboplatin. No patients in the low AUC group developed ototoxicity, but 12% of the patients in the high AUC group demonstrated ototoxicity and 45% had thrombocytopenia (Obermair et al., 1998). Patients pretreated with up to four cycles of cisplatin chemotherapy followed by three cycles of carboplatin and peripheral blood-derived stem cell support (for cisplatin-resistant tumors) suffered hearing impairment in all nine patients. Three of them required hearing aids, and six complained of tinnitus. Ototoxicity in those patients was strongly related to the cumulative carboplatin AUC (Dubs et al., 2004).

Ototoxicity in Experimental Animals

Carboplatin ototoxicity has been demonstrated in experimental animals, including guinea pig, chinchilla, and rat (Taudy et al., 1992; Mount et al., 1995; Hu et al., 1999; Muldoon et al., 2000). In the guinea pig, systemic administration of carboplatin resulted in elevation of the compound action potential (AP) threshold and damage to the outer hair cells, while the inner hair cells remained intact (Saito et al., 1989).

The morphologic effects of carboplatin appear to be unique in the chinchilla. In this animal, carboplatin ototoxicity has been associated with preferential damage to the inner hair cells regardless of whether the drug was administered systemically (Wake et al., 1993) or directly on the round window membrane (Bauer & Brozoski, 2005).

The mechanisms of ototoxicity of carboplatin may be related to the production of reactive oxygen and reactive nitrogen species. Pretreatment with buthionine sulfoximine (BSO), a drug that inhibits the synthesis of glutathione, enhances the ototoxicity of carboplatin in the chinchilla (Hu et al., 1999). Animals that were given BSO by continuous intracochlear infusion had significantly greater losses of both inner and outer hair cells compared to chinchillas treated with carboplatin alone. Distortion product otoacoustic emissions (DPOAEs) and evoked potentials recorded from the inferior colliculus (IC) were significantly reduced in amplitude in animal subjects receiving BSO in combination with carboplatin compared with those receiving carboplatin alone (Hu et al., 1999). Rats treated with intraperitoneal doses of carboplatin were found to have dose-dependent threshold shifts in ABR. The higher doses of carboplatin were associated with increased lipid peroxidation, glutathione depletion, and reduction in activities of antioxidant enzymes (copper/zinc superoxide dismutase, catalase, glutathione peroxidase, and glutathione S-transferase) in the cochlea (Husain et al., 2001a). In addition, rats treated with carboplatin were found to have significant increases in levels of nitric oxide, malondialdehyde (MDA), and manganese superoxide dismutase activity in the cochlea (Husain et al., 2001b).

Animal experiments have shown that D-methionine pretreated chinchillas have reduced hair cell damage following carboplatin administration (Lockwood et al., 2000). Studies have investigated the effect of carboplatin on the neurochemistry of the IC of rats. Animals were injected with carboplatin (256 mg/kg) or saline by intraperitoneal injection. Auditory brainstem evoked potentials were measured before and four days after treatment. The animals were then sacrificed; and the IC and the cerebellum were removed and analyzed for reduced and oxidized glutathione (GSH and GSSG, respectively), antioxidant enzymes, nitric oxide, lipid peroxidation products (MDA), and xanthine oxidase.

Significant ABR threshold elevations for click and for tone burst stimuli at 2, 4, 8, 16, and 32 kHz were found, with the greatest elevations occurring at the highest frequencies. Carboplatin-treated animals were found to have significant increases in nitric oxide, MDA, xanthine oxidase, and manganese superoxide dismutase activities in the IC, but not in the cerebellum. Those findings suggested a specific increase in free radical production in the IC. Carboplatin-treated rats had significant reductions in the ratio of GSH/GSSG and antioxidant enzyme activities, including copper-zinc superoxide dismutase, catalase, glutathione peroxidase, glutathione reductase and glutathione-S-transferase, and enzyme protein expression in the IC, but not in the cerebellum. Those findings suggest that carboplatin produces oxidative stress specifically in the IC that is correlated with hearing loss (Husain et al., 2003) and perhaps to tinnitus. Those findings contrast with findings reported by Burkard et al. (1997), who found that chinchillas treated with smaller doses of carboplatin (50 mg/kg intraperitoneally) had little or no changes in threshold or peak latencies in the IC potential. In contrast, the amplitude of the IC potential was reduced by an average of one-third. The failure to observe a greater increase in IC potential latency with increasing click rate suggested that the effects of carboplatin in that study were limited to the periphery and had little or no neurotoxic effects on the central auditory system.

However, the study by Husain et al. (2003) employed a five-fold greater dose of carboplatin in the rat. The findings of oxidative stress specific to the IC could indicate that in the rat exposed to higher doses of carboplatin, direct neurotoxic effects to the IC did occur. The differences between that study and the study by Burkard et al. (1997) could be related to species and dosing differences.

VINCA ALKALOIDS

The periwinkle plant, Vinca rosea, is the source from which natural products, vincristine and vinblastine have been extracted. These plant extracts have been found to have significant anti-cancer effects. The pharmacology and toxicity of this family of drugs is discussed below.

Vinblastine

Vinblastine is an active antineoplastic agent extracted from the periwinkle plant. It has greater antimetabolic effects than vincristine. Its pharmacology and toxicology are discusse below.

Pharmacology and Therapeutic Uses

Vinblastine is a vinca alkaloid of high molecular weight (909.07). It blocks mitosis by arresting cells in mitosis and may also interfere with amino acid metabolism. It is cell cycle-specific for the M phase of cell division. It is used to treat a wide variety of tumors, including breast carcinoma, choriocarcinoma, advanced testicular germ cell carcinomas, bladder carcinoma, non-small cell lung carcinoma, carcinomas of the kidney, both Hodgkin's and non-Hodgkin's lymphomas, Kaposi's sarcoma, Letterer-Siwe disease, advanced mycosis fungoides, metastatic malignant melanoma, and germ cell ovarian tumors and is listed as a reasonable treatment for prostatic carcinoma.

Vinblastine is administered by intravenous injection. It is metabolized in the liver by hepatic cytochrome P450 3A isoenzymes and is excreted primarily by the biliary and fecal route. Secondary excretion is by the kidney. Three phases of half-life have been described: an initial rapid phase of 3.7 minutes, a middle phase of 1.6 hours, and a terminal phase of 24.8 hours. This agent does not cross the blood-brain barrier in significant quantities. Side effects include leukopenia, cellulitis at the injection site caused by extravasation, hyperuricemia, uric acid nephropathy, stomatitis, thrombocytopenia, gastrointestinal bleeding, nausea and vomiting, pain in bone or tumor-containing tissues, alopecia, and neurotoxicity (weakness, difficulty walking, mental depression, numbness, pain, drooping eyelids, double vision, and dizziness) (USP-DI, 1999).

Vinblastine has been reported to destroy hair cells in the organ of Corti without adversely affecting either the nerve cells or the fibers of the spiral ganglion in the rabbit (Serafi et al., 1982). The only clinical case of ototoxicity was reported in 1999. A twenty-nine-year-old white male with recurrent Hodgkin's disease was treated with doxorubicin, bleomycin, vinblastine, and dacarbazine chemotherapy. He received the regimen once every two weeks, totaling twelve cycles. He reported tinnitus after each treatment, beginning about 6 hours afterward and lasting 7–10 days. His tinnitus interfered with watching television, reading, and concentrating. Symptoms resolved prior to beginning of each subsequent cycle of treatment. Audiograms obtained before and after several cycles revealed mild high-frequency sensorineural hearing loss, but preservation of speech discrimination scores (Moss et al., 1999).

Vincristine

Vincristine is another alkaloid drug obtained from the periwinkle plant. Fortunately, although both vincristine and vinblastine are related drugs, it appears that no cross-resistance develops between them when they are used to treat various cancers. Its range of activity is similar to vinblastine. The pharmacology and toxicology are discussed below.

Pharmacology and Therapeutic Uses

Like vinblastine, vincristine is a vinca alkaloid of high molecular weight (923.04). It blocks mitosis by arresting cells in metaphase and may also interfere with amino acid metabolism. It is specific for the M phase of cell division. Vinblastine is administered by intravenous injection. Within 15–30 minutes after injection, more than 90% of the drug is distributed from blood into tissue, but it does not cross the blood-brain barrier in appreciable amounts. Vincristine is highly bound to protein (75%) and is extensively bound to tissues. It is metabolized in the liver by the cytochrome P450 3A isoenzymes. Like vinblastine, vincristine has three phases to its half-life: an initial phase of 5 minutes, a middle phase of 2.3 hours, and a terminal phase of 85 hours. It is also excreted predominantly by the biliary/fecal route (about 80%) and secondarily by the kidney (about 10%–20%). Vincristine is used to treat pediatric tumors, including leukemia, neuroblastoma, Wilms' tumor, rhabdomyosarcoma, retinoblastoma, brain tumors, and Ewing's sarcoma. It is also used for a number of adult neoplasms, including carcinomas of the breast and ovary, leukemia, lymphoma (Hodgkin's and non-Hodgkin's), multiple myeloma, hepatoblastoma, osteogenic sarcoma, malignant melanoma, small cell lung carcinoma, colorectal carcinoma, cancer of the cervix, Kaposi's sarcoma, mycosis fungoides, Waldenstrom's macroglobulinemia, and idiopathic thrombocytopenia purpura. Side effects of vincristine therapy include severe constipation, hyperuricemia or uric acid nephropathy, cellulitis at the site of injection, leucopenia, thrombocytopenia, stomatitis, syndrome of inappropriate antidiuretic hormone, bloating, diarrhea, loss of weight, nausea and vomiting, skin rash, and progressive neurotoxicity (blurred or double vision; difficulty in walking; drooping eyelids; pain in the jaw, fingers, and toes; pain in the testicles; weakness; and numbness or tingling in the fingers) (USP-DI, 1999).

Vincristine Ototoxicity

By contrast with vinblastine, vincristine sulfate has been found to destroy not only the sensory cells, but also the spiral ganglion neurons and their fibers in the rabbit (Serafy et al., 1981). There have been a few reported cases of ototoxicity associated with vincristine sulfate. Mahajan (1981) reported one case. A seventy-three-year-old woman suffered two documented episodes of severe bilateral sensorineural hearing loss averaging 60 dB across all frequencies after receiving her sixth and seventh doses of 2 mg of vincristine. The hearing recovered two months later. Lugassy (1990) reported a case of sudden sensorineural hearing loss in a sixty-four-year-old patient after receiving high-dose chemotherapy with vincristine sulfate for multiple myeloma. Yousif et al. (1990) reported a case of partially reversible sensorineural deafness after vincristine. Other patients in a cohort study who received moderate doses of vincristine had no changes on pure tone audiometry or in word recognition score (Lugassy & Shapira, 1996). Additional case reports from Turkey described sudden bilateral hearing loss in a sixty-nine-year-old male patient with multiple myeloma (Aydogdu et al., 2000) and in a sixteen-year-old girl with T-cell lymphoma following vincristine therapy (Kacioglu et al., 2003).

Vinorelbine

Vinorelbine is a semisynthetic vinca alkaloid derived from vinblastine. It differs in structure from other vinca alkaloids in having an eight-member catharanthine ring structure instead of the nine-member catharanthine ring structure that is present in vincristine and vinblastine. Its molecular weight is l079.13. It has been used to treat non-small cell lung carcinoma and breast carcinoma. Vinorelbine appears to have selective activity against mitotic microtubules in a way that may differ somewhat from that of the other vinca alkaloids and, thus, be potentially less toxic. Vinorelbine is administered by intravenous injection. In animal studies, it was found to be widely distributed in the body after injection. In human liver cells, there is rapid uptake; and in human lung tissue, vinorelbine achieves up to a 300-fold greater concentration than in serum. It

is highly bound to proteins in serum, ranging from 80%–91% in cancer patients. It is also highly bound to platelets and lymphocytes. Vinorelbine is metabolized by the liver. The half-life has a prolonged terminal phase due to relatively slow efflux from peripheral compartments. Vinorelbine and its metabolites are excreted in the bile and feces in animal studies, which most likely occurs in humans, as well.

Toxicity

Granulocytopenia is the dose-limiting toxicity. Drug-associated neurotoxicity occurs less often than with other commonly used vinca alkaloids. Anemia, leucopenia, injection site reactions, and asthenia are some of the more frequently encountered side effects. Less frequent side effects include chest pain, peripheral neuropathy (paresthesia and hypesthesia), stomatitis, hemorrhagic cystitis, skin rash, thrombocytopenia, anorexia, constipation, nausea and vomiting, diarrhea, alopecia, shortness of breath, and joint or muscle pain (USP-DI, 1999).

A case of permanent bilateral sensorineural hearing loss and tinnitus was reported following treatment of a fifty-four–year-old woman with metastatic breast cancer with paclitaxel and vinorelbine (Tibaldi et al., 1998). It is unclear whether the ototoxicity should be attributed to paclitaxel, to vinorelbine, or to the combination of the two drugs.

DIFLUOROMETHYLORNITHINE (DFMO)

DFMO is a derivative of the amino acid, ornithine. It has some unusual properties, in that it is useful for prevention and treatment of cancer and certain parasitic diseases. It has a unique profile of pharmacology and toxicology, as discussed below.

Pharmacology and Therapeutic Use

DFMO, also called eflornithine and marketed as Ornidyl, irreversibly inhibits ornithine decarboxylase, which is the first enzyme that controls the rate of polyamine synthesis. DFMO acts by limiting the conversion of the amino acid ornithine to putrescine. Putrescine is actually a diammine but the polyamines spermine and spermidine are formed from putrescine. Consequently, limiting putrescine formation limits spermidine and spermine formation.

The pathway for the synthesis of polyamines is shown in Figure 10-4.

Polyamines promote cell proliferation. Because cancer cells show abnormally high levels of cell proliferation, this drug can help limit certain cancers (see reviews by Russell, 1985; Pegg & McCann, 1988; Wallace & Fraser, 2004). Increased polyamine levels are associated with decreased apoptosis, increased cell proliferation, and expression of genes affecting both metastasis and tumor invasion. Decreased polyamine levels have the opposite effect in each area. DFMO is used both as a chemotherapeutic drug to treat existent cancers and as a chemopreventive drug to keep certain types of cancers from developing or recurring in high-risk patients (see review by Gerner & Meyskens, 2004). DFMO can be given intravenously, by hepatic arterial infusion, or orally with oral bioavailability estimated at about 54% (Burri & Brun, 2003). Interestingly, green tea's anticancer properties may be related to the fact that it reduces ornithine decarboxylase activity (Bachrach & Wang, 2002).

DFMO is not used to treat all cancers, but usually those that arise from epithelial tissues such as the skin and colon because the ornithine decarboxylase and polyamine content are increased for those types of cancers (see review by Gerner & Meyskens, 2004). DFMO is used to treat colon cancer (Ajani 1990) and is being tested to prevent development of colon cancer in patients with colorectal polyps (Love et al., 1998, Doyle et al., 2001) or family history of colon cancer (Love et al., 1998). Ornithine decarboxylase levels are increased in patients with familial adenomatous polyposis, which can lead to hereditary colon cancer; thus, DFMO is being investigated to determine if it can safely prevent the onset of colon cancer in those patients (see review by Gerner & Meyskens, 2004). DFMO reduces the polyamines putrescine and spermidine in rectosigmoid colonic mucosa (Love et al., 1998) and, thus, can specifically act on that tissue.

DFMO is also used to treat metastatic malignant melanoma (Croghan et al., 1991) and is used as an adjuvant agent in the treatment of brain cancers (Levin et al., 2003), although the results are variable (Levin et al., 2000). Additionally, DFMO is continually being studied for potential use in a variety of other cancers either as a primary or adjuvant agent (Horn et al., 1987; O'Shaughnessy et al., 1999).

In addition to cancer treatment, DFMO is used to treat parasitic disorders. DFMO is FDA-approved to treat the meningoencephalitis associated with the protozoan parasites *Trypanosoma brucei* var. *gambiense* (Sjoerdsma et al., 1984; Legros et al., 2002). The resultant disease is commonly referred to as West African sleeping sickness. For this application, DFMO is a fairly slow-acting drug because it is trypanostatic (inhibits the replication of the parasite) rather than trypanocidal (killing the parasite). DFMO has also been used to treat the pneumonia secondary to the parasitic microorganism *Pneumocystis carinii* in AIDS patients (Sjoerdsma et al., 1984; Sahai & Berry, 1989; see review by McCann & Pegg, 1992). Additionally,

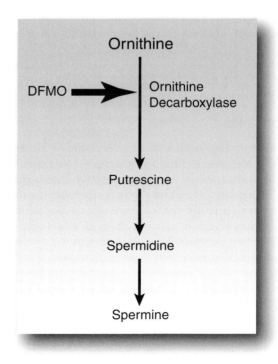

Figure 10-4. Polyamine synthesis

DFMO has been tested for use in treating *Cryptosporidium,* a protozoan parasite that can cause severe gastrointestinal disease in AIDS patients (see review by McCann & Pegg, 1992).

Toxicity Profile

A variety of side effects can occur: convulsions, gastrointestinal symptoms including vomiting and diarrhea, abdominal pain and bloating, mucositis, bone marrow toxicity, thrombocytopenia (reduction in platelet levels, which can lead to hemorrhagic conditions), alopecia, joint pain, rash, insomnia, and ototoxicity (Creaven et al., 1993; Pasic et al., 1997; Meyskens & Gerner, 1999; Levin et al., 2000; Burri & Brun, 2003). Ototoxicity can include both auditory and vestibular effects (Meyskens & Gerner, 1995), but most ototoxicity studies focus on cochleotoxicity. Most side effects, including ototoxicity, are usually, but not always, reversible when treatment is discontinued. Nonetheless, ototoxicity can be dose-limiting and may be the most common dose-limiting toxicity (Horn et al., 1987; Creaven et al., 1993).

Ototoxicity in Experimental Animals

Although the exact mechanism of DFMO ototoxicity is not known, polyamines and ornithine decarboxylase are present both in the cochlea (Schweitzer et al., 1986; Marks et al., 1991; Brock & Henley, 1994; Henley & Rybak, 1995) and in the cochlear nerve (Marks et al., 1991; Brock & Henley, 1994; Henley & Rybak, 1995). Cochlear ornithine decarboxylase activity and the concentration of polyamines are highest in the organ of Corti and stria vascularis (Brock & Henley, 1994; Henley et al., 1995). Cochlear polyamines may interact with hydrophobic environments and thus alter the permeability of membranes regulating inorganic cation flux such as the stria vascularis (Canellakis et al., 1979; Schweitzer et al., 1986).

DFMO reduces both cochlear and cochlear nerve ornithine decarboxylase levels (Marks et al., 1991) and polyamine levels (Schweitzer et al., 1986). Henley et al. (1990) found that high-dose DFMO depleted putrescine and spermidine in the organ of Corti and cochlear nerve in neonatal rats treated with 0.5g/kg/day DFMO for postnatal days 1–10. Those findings correlated with the significant decrements in (DPOAEs) and elevated AP thresholds. However in that animal model, polyamines were not depleted in the stria vascularis nor was the EP reduced after DFMO administration.

Not all animal models reveal the same findings for the stria vascularis and endocochlear potential. In twelve-week-old mice treated with 1mg/g/day for 4 weeks, DFMO markedly reduced the endocochlear potential (Nie et al., 2005) possibly by reduced polyamine levels, altering potassium flux between the stria and scala media. In that animal model, DFMO caused across frequency ABR threshold shift. The authors hypothesized that the across frequency threshold elevation may reflect strial involvement (Nie et al., 2005). Unlike many ototoxins, DFMO can cause hearing loss in animals that is worse at either the midrange or in the high frequencies (McWilliams et al., 2000) or causes threshold elevation across all frequencies (Smith et al., 2004). Although outer and inner hair cell losses tend to be greater in the basal regions of the cochlea, the variable configurations may reflect additional strial involvement secondary to DFMO treatment.

However, most animal models of DFMO ototoxicity assess hair cell rather than strial damage. DFMO administration does cause cochlear outer and inner hair cell loss (Salzer et al., 1990; McWilliams et al., 2000). Unlike most ototoxins, the inner hair cell loss can be greater than the outer hair cell loss, although both inner and outer hair cell loss occur (Salzer et al., 1990; McWilliams et al., 2000). The relative preservation of outer versus inner hair cells may account for the preservation of cochlear microphonics in the presence of elevated AP thresholds at least in the juvenile guinea pig (McWilliams et al., 2000). In addition to the loss of outer hair cells, remaining outer hair cells may be abnormal. The outer hair cell nuclei can degenerate and numerous Hensen bodies may be present in outer hair cells after DFMO administration (Jansen et al., 1989; Salzer et al., 1990). Additionally, outer hair cells may be shorter and Deiters' cell bodies longer following DFMO administration (Salzer et al., 1990).

DFMO ototoxicity, including inner and outer hair cell damage, strial damage, and ABR thresholds, can be reversible after DFMO administration is discontinued. Smith et al. (2004) induced DFMO hearing loss in neonatal gerbils but found that ABR thresholds recovered within 3 weeks after drug discontinuation. Further histologic results for inner and outer hair cells and the basal and apical portions of the stria vascularis showed normal findings after the 3-week recovery period. Doyle (2001) reported that in neonatal gerbils, an 18-day regimen of 1g/kg/day DFMO resulted in click ABR thresholds of 25–65 dB as compared to 5–20 dB in controls. However 3 weeks after drug discontinuation, the animals' ABR thresholds returned to those of the control animals.

Different enantiomers, mirror image molecular structures, of DFMO have different risks of ototoxicity. Juvenile guinea pigs injected with 1g/kg/day ip of D-DFMO for 45 days did not have any hearing loss, while animals given the same dose of L-DFMO had even greater hearing loss than those given the same dose of D,L-DFMO which is the racemate comprising both the D and L mirror image enantiomers (McWilliams et al., 2000). Equivalent studies have not yet been performed in humans, and the relative therapeutic efficacy of the DFMO enantiomers has not been determined. Higher doses of racemic (a mixture of both enantiomers) DFMO of 2 or 3 g/kg/day resulted in high mortality in the animals.

Animal models for DFMO ototoxicity are usually, although not always, in neonatal or juvenile animals because the cochlear ornithine decarboxylase activity and the polyamine biosynthetic pathway are more active in developing animals (Brock & Henley, 1994). For example, cochlear ornithine decarboxylase activity increases in rats during the maturation of hearing (Henley, 1991). In many tissues, not just the cochlea, polyamine synthesis decreases in adulthood (see review by Gerner & Meyskens, 2004).

In adult animals, susceptibility to DFMO ototoxicity appears to vary by species. McWilliams et al. (2000) reported that rats do not demonstrate DFMO ototoxicity even with oral dosing of 0.2–1.2 mg/kg/day for up to 8 weeks. However, because the study used adult rats, it is unclear whether the difference in susceptibility is related to species or age differences. DFMO dosing protocols that cause hearing loss in neonatal rats (Henley et al., 1990) may cause no hearing loss in adult rats (Schweitzer et al., 1986).

Unlike adult rats, adult pigmented guinea pigs are susceptible to DFMO ototoxicity. Salzer et al. (1990) found ABR threshold shifts in pigmented guinea pigs after 8, but not 4, weeks of a 1% DFMO drinking water. Hearing losses were worse at 12 weeks, but high variability was noted. Jansen et al. (1989) did report DFMO ototoxicity in a study of adult pigmented guinea pigs with hearing loss onset occurring between 4 and 8 weeks. Hearing losses ranged from mild to profound. Only the animal with profound loss did not show at least partial recovery within 4 weeks after drug discontinuation. Those findings are similar to findings observed in human clinical studies. Similarly Marks et al. (1991) reported that higher dosing DFMO induced significant ABR threshold shift after 4 weeks in most but not all adult (250–300 g) pigmented guinea pigs, but the degree of hearing loss was highly variable. Additionally, up to a 30 dB asymmetry existed between the two ears in the animals with ototoxic threshold shift. The amount of threshold shift did not correlate with the amount of cochlear polyamine depletion.

Ototoxicity in Humans

Audiologic findings for DFMO can be highly variable. The audiometric configurations for DFMO have been reported as high-frequency (Horn et al., 1987; Creaven et al., 1993; Abeloff et al., 1986; Lipton et al., 1989), flat (Meyskens et al., 1986) and predominantly low-frequency (Croghan et al., 1991; Pasic et al., 1997). Consequently, DFMO patients may not always produce the typical audiogram seen in most other types of ototoxicity. As discussed in the previous section on findings in experimental animals, the variable audiometric configurations may be secondary to strial damage, in addition to the inner and out hair cell damage and perhaps spiral ganglion cell damage.

In some but not all patients, tinnitus can accompany or precede the threshold shifts (Lipton et al., 1989; Creaven et al., 1993). However, tinnitus without hearing loss has also been reported (Prados et al.,

1989; Creaven et al., 1993; Loprinzi et al., 1996; Levin et al., 2000). Even for the same dosing protocol, tinnitus occurrence is variable (Love et al., 1993).

High-dose DFMO has been long reported to cause mild to severe ototoxicity in humans (Horn et al., 1987); but intersubject variability is high in regard to onset time, incidence, degree of hearing loss, and reversibility. Hearing loss onset may be slow, starting 4–9 weeks after onset of DFMO therapy (Jansen et al., 1989; Lipton et al., 1989). The time to onset may be inversely related to the dose (Pasic et al., 1997). Dosing protocols that are 4 weeks or shorter may not yield hearing loss. Meyskens et al. (1994) reported no ototoxicity in any of 111 patients receiving up to 28 days of 0.01–3 g/m^2/day oral DFMO. The treatment duration may have been too short for ototoxicity to develop.

The relationship of DFMO dose to ototoxicity is not always consistent across studies. Some reports find ototoxicity related to daily but not cumulative dosing (Love et al., 1993; Pasic et al., 1997), others reported a correlation of ototoxicity with cumulative dose (Croghan et al., 1991; Meyskens & Gerner, 1999), and still others reported no correlation to dosing (Maddox, 1985). DFMO ototoxicity has been reported in patients with cumulative DFMO dose as low as 45 g/m^2 (Love et al., 1993) or 60 g/m^2 (Croghan et al., 1991). Love et al. (1993) reported that some patients developed ototoxicity at cumulative doses of 92–93g/m^2, while others showed no ototoxicity with cumulative doses of 147.7 g/m^2. Serum levels of DFMO do not appear to correlate with ototoxicity (Pasic et al., 1997). Some patients show no DFMO ototoxicity with cumulative dosing as high as 236/m^2–1000 g/m^2 (Maddox et al., 1985). Some studies have suggested that even reversible DFMO toxicity does not generally occur until doses are at least 2g/m^2/day or cumulatively 250 g/m^2 (Meyskens et al., 1986; Croghan et al., 1988, 1991), but some patients can experience DFMO ototoxicity at lower dosing levels. Part of the differences between study results may be attributable to daily dosing levels, differences in mode of administration, and methods and criteria for ototoxicity detection.

Although the relationship is imperfect, low daily dose DFMO studies tend to show less ototoxicity than high daily dose DFMO studies and most dose escalation studies tend to show a higher incidence of ototoxicity at the higher daily dosing levels. For example, some relatively low-dose DFMO studies have shown little or no ototoxicity. Loprinzi et al. (1996) reported no hearing loss in seventy-six patients receiving up to 1g/day DFMO for up to one year although one or two reported tinnitus. Doyle et al, (2001) reported audiology results for 123 subjects with prior adenomatous colonic polyps in a Phase II clinical trial to assess chemoprevention for colon cancer. The subjects were randomized to either oral DFMO of between 0.075 and 0.4 g/m^2/day or placebo for 12 months. The low doses yielded no significant differences in DPOAE levels and only 2–3 dB differences in hearing thresholds for 250 and 500 Hz, with no changes for 1000–8000 Hz noted for the higher dosing levels. Auditory thresholds above 8000 Hz were not assessed. Although similar dosing levels of 0.075, 0.20 or 0.40 g/m^2/day significantly reduced subjects' polyamine levels in the rectal mucosa (Meyskens et al., 1998), the auditory effects at those dosing levels were minimal (Doyle et al., 2001). However, at only a slightly higher dosing level, Lao et al. (2004) reported that a fifty-seven–year-old patient in a chemoprevention trial for Barrett's esophagus developed a 15 dB threshold shift at 250, 2000, and 3000 Hz in the right ear and an increase of 20 dB or more at 4000 and 6000 Hz in the left ear after taking 0.5g/m^2/day (900 mg daily) DFMO for about 13 weeks for a cumulative dose of 45 g/m^2. Further, those threshold shifts were still present 7 months after drug discontinuation. Word recognition scores were not significantly affected, and the patient reportedly did not notice the threshold shifts. Similarly, Love et al. (1993) reported clinically noticeable and audiologically confirmed hearing loss (threshold shift of 15 dB or greater in two or more frequencies in both ears) within 3 months of 0.5g/m^2/day in three of twenty-four patients and in an additional patient after 12 months. All hearing losses were reversible.

In studies using higher dosing, the incidence of reported hearing loss tends to increase. Lipton et al. (1989) reported ototoxicity in all patients given at least 1.0 g/m^2/day by hepatic arterial infusion. Hearing loss reversed in all but one patient within 1–3 months after

DFMO cessation. That patient also showed poor word recognition, but had previously been treated with cisplatin. Perhaps the prior cisplatin exposure with later DFMO treatment could account for the more severe ototoxicity. Ajani (1990) found reversible hearing loss in some patients receiving $8g/m^2$ in continuous infusion for colon cancer. Croghan et al. (1991) reported that 75% of patients receiving over $250 \, g/m^2$ cumulative dose DFMO, with daily dosing of $2–12 \, g/m^2/day$, experienced threshold shifts exceeding 30dB in the 500 to 8000 Hz range.

DFMO dose escalation studies have reported variable ototoxicity findings, although they generally find that higher dosing increases the risk of DFMO ototoxicity. Pasic et al. (1997) observed ototoxic hearing loss in patients receiving 2, 3, or $5 \, g/m^2/day$ DFMO for 6–12 months with greater threshold shifts noted in low as opposed to high frequencies for high daily dosing levels. Increasing daily dosing increased the incidence and magnitude of hearing threshold shift, while the time to ototoxicity onset decreased. Only three of thirty-two subjects receiving $0.5 \, g/m^2/day$ showed threshold shifts of 15 dB or greater for at least two frequencies, which was similar to the two of nineteen patients in the placebo group with similar findings. At higher dosing, all six of the subjects receiving 2, 3, or $5 \, g/m^2/day$ had significant threshold shift, with an average 16.8 dB threshold shift at 0.5, 1, and 2 kHz. However, high intersubject variability was noted. Similarly, Love et al. (1993), defining ototoxicity as audiometric threshold shift of 15 dB or greater at two or more frequencies, reported that 0.25, 0.5 or $0.75 \, g/m^2$ DFMO administered four times daily caused ototoxicity in one of four subjects at the 0.25 dose and in five of six subjects at the two higher dosing levels. However, no ototoxicity occurred for $0.125 \, g/m^2$ DFMO administered four times daily.

Conversely, Maddox et al. (1985) treated twenty patients with intravenous DFMO with continuous infusion doses of 5.5 to $64g/m^2$. Four of those patients developed ototoxicity, but it did not appear to be related to dosing as the incidence of hearing loss was spread across the dosing levels. However, all patients with hearing loss had been treated for at least 3 weeks.

Additional risk factors for DFMO ototoxicity have not been fully addressed. Risk factors that have been reported include concomitant administration of aminoglycoside antibiotics (Maddox et al., 1985) and prior administration of cisplatin (Lipton et al., 1989). A higher risk of DFMO ototoxicity with increasing patient age has also been reported (Croghan et al., 1991), but Pasic et al. (1997) found no correlation with age. Unlike other ototoxins, renal function does not seem to increase the risk of DFMO ototoxicity (Pasic et al., 1997).

DFMO-induced hearing loss is usually, but not always, reversible after drug discontinuation even for high-dose DFMO protocols (Ajani et al., 1990; Love et al., 1993). Abeloff et al. (1984, 1986) reported that all hearing losses in their studies reversed within 7–61 days, with a median interval of 24 days. Pasic et al. (1997) found that all threshold shifts, even the most severe, were reversible with a median recovery time of 58 days. Although DFMO usually causes reversible ototoxicity, permanent ototoxic hearing loss has been reported (Lipton et al., 1989) even with daily DFMO dosing as low as $0.5 \, g/m^2$ and cumulative dosing as low as $45 \, g/m^2$ (Lao et al., 2004).

Thus, intersubject variability is problematic, and only prospective audiologic monitoring can adequately address the issue for a given patient.

SUMMARY

Dysregulation of normal cell growth and maturation can result in cancer, which is characterized by abnormal growth and invasion of cells. Cancer requires increased cell proliferation, increased cell life span, and a decreased rate of apoptosis. Tumor growth depends on the growth fraction, the cell cycle time, and the rate of cell loss. Most chemotherapeutic agents work by preventing cells from proliferating, invading, and metastasizing. Cancer chemotherapy may act in a variety of ways relative to the cell cycle as phase-specific drugs, cell cycle-specific drugs, or cell cycle-nonspecific drugs.

Cisplatin is used to treat a wide variety of cancers, including germ cell, gynecologic, head and neck, and lung and brain cancers. Cisplatin works by reacting with the cancer cells' DNA, inhibiting replication.

However, cisplatin is also highly ototoxic, causing permanent hearing loss and tinnitus in a high percentage of patients. Hearing loss first starts in the high-frequency region and then progresses to the lower-frequency regions. The ototoxicity is dose-related. The loss may be gradual, progressive, or sudden. Pediatric patients are particularly susceptible to cisplatin ototoxicity. Cisplatin particularly damages cochlear outer cells and the stria vascularis. Spiral ganglion cell damage can also occur. Cisplatin ototoxicity can be exacerbated by concomitant loop diuretic, aminoglycoside, or noise exposure.

Carboplatin is a second-generation platinum-based chemotherapeutic agent. It is used to treat lung, ovarian, brain, and head and neck cancer, among other applications. The primary dose-limiting toxicity is bone marrow toxicity. For equivalent dosing, carboplatin is less ototoxic than cisplatin; but higher dosing of carboplatin is used, and the higher doses can cause ototoxic hearing loss. Carboplatin ototoxicity is dose-dependent. As in cisplatin, carboplatin-induced hearing loss starts at the high frequencies and progresses to the lower frequencies and is generally irreversible. For brain cancer patients, sometimes the blood-brain barrier is disrupted to increase carboplatin delivery to the tumor. However, that procedure can cause a very high incidence of ototoxicity. Consequently, studies of otoprotective agents are being tested to augment those protocols. In the chinchilla (and only in the chinchilla), carboplatin can cause selective inner hair cell loss. However, in other species, carboplatin causes mostly outer hair cell loss.

The vinca alkaloids include vinblastine, vincristine, and vinorelbine. Those agents can be ototoxic, but much less commonly than the platinum-based chemotherapeutics. For vinblastine and vincristine, hearing loss can be sudden, but may reverse when the drug treatment is discontinued. Vinblastine can destroy cochlear hair cells, but it appears to leave spiral ganglion cells intact. Vincristine sulfate destroys not only cochlear hair cells, but also spiral ganglion neurons and fibers. Vinorelbine has been reported to cause permanent hearing loss and tinnitus; but because the patient also received paclitaxel, it is unclear whether vinorelbine is ototoxic as a single agent or only in that combination.

DFMO is used primarily used to treat colon cancer, but it is being tested to treat a number of other cancers. Additionally, it is used to treat a variety of parasitic disorders. DFMO causes sensorineural hearing loss; but unlike most other ototoxins, the configuration of hearing loss can be highly variable. The variability may be related to the fact that DFMO affects the inner hair cells as much as or more than the outer hair cells and clearly affects the stria vascularis, possibly by altering the metabolic exchange into the endolymphatic space. DFMO ototoxicity is generally slow in onset, usually occurring after only 4 weeks of daily administration. The degree of DFMO ototoxicity ranges from mild to severe, but DFMO ototoxicity is usually reversible approximately 1–2 months after drug discontinuation. In animal studies, DFMO is particularly ototoxic in developing animals; but studies in human pediatric patients have not been published. Different enantiomers of DFMO may have different ototoxicity profiles, but further research is needed. Concomitant administration of aminoglycosides or prior cisplatin treatment may increase the risk of DFMO ototoxicity.

REFERENCES

Abeloff, M. D., Rosen, S. T., Luk, G. D., Baylin, S. B., Zeltzman, M., & Sjoerdsma, A. (1986). Phase II trials of alpha-difluoromethylornithine, an inhibitor of polyamine synthesis in advanced small cell lung cancer. *Cancer Treatment Reports, 70,* 843–845.

Ajani, J. A., Ota, D. M., Grosie, V. B., Jr., Abbruzzese, J. L., Faintuch, J. S., Patt, Y. Z., et. al. (1990). Evolution of continuous-infusion alpha-difluoromethylornithine therapy for colorectal carcinoma. *Cancer Chemother Pharmacol, 26,* 223–226.

Alberts, D. S. (1995). Carboplatin versus cisplatin in ovarian cancer. *Semin Oncol, 22,* 188–190.

Allen, G. C., Tiu, C., Koike, K., Ritchey, A. K., KursLasky, M., & Wax, M. K. (1998). Transient-evoked otoacoustic emissions in children after cisplatin chemotherapy. *Otolaryngol Head Neck Surg, 118,* 584–588.

Anniko N., & Sobin, A. (1986). Cisplatin: Evaluation of its ototoxic potential. *Am J Otolaryngol, 7,* 276–293.

Aydogdu, I., Ozturan, O., Kuku, I., Kaya, E., Sevinc, A., & Yildiz, R. (2000). Bilateral transient hearing loss associated with vincristine therapy: Case report. *J Chemother, 12*, 530–532.

Bachrach, U., & Wang, Y. C. (2002). Cancer therapy and prevention by green tea: Role of ornithine decarboxylase. *Amino Acids, 22*, 1–13.

Barron, S. E., & Daigneault, E. A. (1987). Effect of cisplatin on hair cell morphology and lateral wall Na,K-ATPase activity. *Hear Res, 26*, 131–137.

Bauer, C. A., & Brozoski, T. J. (2005). Cochlear structure and function after round window application of ototoxins. *Hear Res, 201*, 121–131.

Bauer, F. P., Westhofen, M., & Kehrl, W. (1992). The ototoxicity of the cytostatic drug carboplatin in patients with head-neck tumors. *Laryngorhinootologie, 71*, 412–415.

Berg, A. L., Spitzer, J. B., & Garvin, J. H., Jr. (1999). Ototoxic impact of cisplatin in pediatric oncology patients. *Laryngoscope, 109*, 1806–1814.

Black, F. O., Myers, E. N., Schramm, V. L., Johnson, J., Sigler, B., Thearle, P. B., et al. (1982). Cisplatin vestibular ototoxicity: Preliminary report. *Laryngoscope, 92*, 1363–1368.

Blakley, B. W., Gupta, A. K., Myers, S. F., & Schwan, S. (1994). Risk factors for ototoxicity due to cisplatin. *Arch Otolaryngol Head Neck Surg, 120*, 541–546.

Blakley, B. W., & Myers, S. F. (1993). Pattern of hearing loss resulting from cisplatinum therapy. *Otolaryngol Head Neck Surg, 109*, 385–391.

Bohm, S., Oriana, S., Satti, G., DiRe, F., Breasciani, G., Pirovano, C., et al. (1999). Dose intensification of platinum compounds with glutathione protection as induction chemotherapy for advanced ovarian carcinoma. *Oncology, 57*, 115–120.

Bokemeyer, C., Berger, C. C., Hartmann, J. T., Kollmannsberger, C., Schmoll, H. J., Kuczyk, M.A., et al. (1998). Analysis of risk factors for cisplatin-induced ototoxicity in patients with testicular cancer. *Br J Cancer, 77*, 1355–1362.

Boulikas, T., & Vougiouka, M. (2003). Cisplatin and platinum drugs at the molecular level [Review]. *Oncol Rep, 10*, 1663–1682.

Boulikas, T., & Vougiouka, M. (2004). Recent clinical trial using cisplatin, carboplatin and their combination chemotherapy drugs [Review]. *Oncol Rep, 11*, 559–595.

Brock, M., & Henley, C. M. (1994). Postnatal changes in cochlear polyamine metabolism in the rat. *Hear Res, 72*, 37–43.

Brummett, R. E. (1981). Ototoxicity resulting from the combined administration of potent diuretics and other agents. *Scand Audiol Suppl, 14* (Suppl.), 215–224.

Burkard, R., Trautwein, P., & Salvi, R. (1997). The effects of click level, click rate, and level of background noise on the inferior colliculus potential (ICP) in the normal and carboplatin-treated chinchilla. *J Acoust Soc Am, 102*, 3620–3627.

Burri, C., & Brun, R. (2003). Eflornithine for the treatment of human African trypanosomiasis. *Parasitol Res, 90* (Suppl. 1), S49–S52.

Campbell, K. C., Meech, R. P., Rybak, L. P., & Hughes, L. F. (1999). D-Methionine protects against cisplatin damage to the stria vascularis. *Hear Res, 138*, 13–28.

Canellakis, E. S., Viceps-Madore, D., Kyriakidis, D. S., & Heller, J. S. (1979). The regulation and function of ornithine decarboxylase and of polyamines. *Curr Top Cell Regul, 15*, 155–202.

Cavaletti, G., Bogliun, G., Zincone, A., Marzorati, L., Melzi, P., Frattola, L., et al. (1998). Neuro and ototoxicity of high dose carboplatin treatment in poor prognosis ovarian cancer patients. *Anticancer Res, 18*, 3797–3802.

Comis, S. D., Rhys-Evans, P. H., Osborne, M. P., Pickles, J. O., Jeffries, D. J., & Pearse, H. A. (1986). Early morphological and chemical changes induced by cisplatin in the guinea pig organ of Corti. *J Laryngol Otol, 100*, 1375–1383.

Coupland, S. G., Ponton, C. W., Eggermont, J. J., Bowen, T. J., & Grant, R. M. (1991). Assessment of cisplatin-induced ototoxicity using derived-band ABRs. *Int J Pediatr Otorhinolaryngo, 22*, 237–248.

Creaven, P. J., Pendyala, L., & Petrelli, N. J. (1993). Evaluation of alpha-difluoromethylornithine as a potential chemopreventive agent: Tolerance to daily oral administration in humans. *Cancer Epidemiology Biomarkers & Prevention, 2*, 243–247.

Croghan, M. K., Aickin, M. G., & Meyskens, F. L. (1991). Dose-related alpha-difluoromethylornithine ototoxicity. *AM J Clin Oncol, 14*, 331–335.

Croghan, M. K., Booth, A., & Meyskens, F. L., Jr. (1988). A phase I trial recombinant interferon-alpha and alpha-difluoromethylornithine in metastatic melanoma. *J Biol Response Mod, 7*(4), 409–415.

de Jongh, F. E., van Veen, R. N., Veltman, S. J., de Wit, R., van der Burg, M. E., van den Bent, M. J., et al. (2003). Weekly high-dose cisplatin is a feasible treatment option: Analysis on prognostic factors for toxicity in 400 patients. *Br J Cancer, 88,* 1199–1206.

DeLauretis, A., DeCapua, B., Barbieri, M. T., Bellussi, L., & Passali, D. (1999). ABR evaluation of ototoxicity in cancer patients receiving cisplatin or carboplatin. *Scand Audiol, 28,* 139–143.

Doyle, K. J., McLaren, C. E., Shanks, J. E., Galus, C. M., & Meyskens, F. L. (2001). Effects of difluoromethylornithine chemoprevention on audiometry thresholds and otoacoustic emissions. *Arch Otolaryngol Head Neck Surg, 127,* 553–558.

Doyle, K. J. (2001). Delayed, reversible hearing loss caused by difluoromethylornithine (DFMO). *Laryngoscope, 111,* 781–785.

Dubs, A., Jacky, E., Stahel, R., & Taverna, C. (2004). Ototoxicity in patients with dose-intensive therapy for cisplatin-resistant germ cell tumors. *J Clin Oncol, 22,* 1158.

Ekborn, A., Hansson, J., Ehrsson, H., Eksborg, S., Wallin, I., Wagenius, G., et al. (2004). High-dose cisplatin with amifostine: Ototoxicity and pharmacokinetics. *Laryngoscope, 114,* 1660–1667.

Estrem, S. A., Babin, R. W., Ryu, J. H., & Moore, K. C. (1981). Cis-diamminedichloroplatinum (II) ototoxicity in the guinea pig. *Otolaryngol Head Neck Surg, 89,* 638–645.

Ettinger, D. S. (1998). The role of carboplatin in the treatment of small-cell lung cancer. *Oncology, 12*(1 Suppl. 2), 36–43.

Fausti, S. A., Henry, J. A., Schaffer, H. I., Olson, D. J., Frey, R. H., & Bagby, G. C., Jr. (1993). High-frequency monitoring for early diction of cisplatin ototoxicity. *Arch Otolaryngol Head Neck Surg, 119,* 661–666.

Fidler, I. J. Biology of cancer metastasis. (2004). In M. D. Abeloff, J. O. Armitage, J. E. Niederhuber, M. B. Kastan, & W. G., McKenna (Eds.), *Clinical Oncology* (3rd ed., pp. 59–80). Philadelphia: Elsevier.

Gerner, E. W., & Meyskens, F. L., Jr. (2004). Polyamines and cancer: Old molecules, new understanding. *Nature Reviews, 4,* 781–792.

Gormley, P. E., Bull, J. M., LeRoy, A. F., & Cysyk, R. (1971). Kinetics of cis-dichlorodiammineplatinum. *Clin Pharmacol Ther, 25,* 351–357.

Granowetter, L., Rosenstock, J. G., & Packer, R. J. (1982). Enhanced cis-platinum neurotoxicity in pediatric patients with brain tumors. *J Neurooncol, 1,* 293–297.

Gratton, M. A., Salvi, R. J., Kamen, B. A., & Saunders, S. S. (1990). Interaction of cisplatin and noise on the peripheral auditory system. *Hear Res, 50,* 211–223.

Hahn, W. C., & Weinberg, R. A. (2002). Rules for making human tumor cells. *N Engl J Med, 347,* 1593–1603.

Hallmark, R. J., Snyder, J. M., Jusenius, K., & Tamimi, H. K. (1992). Factors influencing ototoxicity in ovarian cancer patients treated with Cis-platinum based chemotherapy. *Eur J Gynaecol Oncol, 13,* 35–44.

Hartmann, J. T., & Lipp, H. P. (2003). Toxicity of platinum compounds. *Expert Opin Pharmacother, 4,* 889–901.

Helson, L., Okonkwo, E., Anton, L., et al. (1988). Cis-Platinum ototoxicity. *Clin Toxicol, 13,* 469–478.

Henley, C., Atkins, J., Martin, G., & Lonsbury-Martin, B. (1990). Critical period for alpha-difluoromethylornithine (DFMO) ototoxicity in the developing rat. *J. Cell Biochem* (Suppl. 14F), 22.

Henley, C., Whitworth, C., Rybak, L., & Lonsbury-Martin, B. (1993). Alpha-difluoromethylornithine (DFMO) inhibits cochlear function and polyamine metabolism in developing rats [Abstract] *Society for Neuroscience Abstracts.*

Henley, C. M., & Rybak, L. P. (1995). Ototoxicity in developing mammals. *Brain Research Reviews, 20,* 68–90.

Hill, R. P. (2001). The biology of cancer. In P. Rubin (Ed.), *Clinical Oncology: A Multidisciplinary Approach for Physicians and Students* (8th ed., pp. 32–45). Philadelphia: W. B. Saunders.

Himmelstein, K. J., Patton, T. F., Belt, R. J., Taylor, S., Repta, A. J., & Sternson, L. A. (1981). Clinical kinetics on intact cisplatin and some related species. *Clin Pharmacol Ther, 29,* 658–664.

Hinojosa, R., Riggs, L. C., Strauss, M., & Matz, G. J. (1995). Temporal bone histopathology of cisplatin ototoxicity. *Am J Otol, 16*, 731–740.

Hoistad, D. L., Ondrey, F. G., Mutlu, C., Schachern, P. A., Paparella, M. M., & Adams, G. L. (1998). Histopathology of human temporal bone after cis-platinum, radiation, or both. *Otolaryngol Head Neck Surg, 118*, 825–832.

Horn, Y., Schechter, P. J., & Marton, L. J. (1987). Phase I-II clinical trials with alpha-difluoromethylornithine—an inhibitor of polyamine biosynthesis, *Cancer Clin, Oncol, 23*, 1103–1107.

Hu, B. H., McFadden, S. L., Salvi, R. J., & Henderson, D. (1999). Intracochlear infusion of buthionine sulfoximine potentiates carboplatin ototoxicity in the chinchilla. *Hear Res, 128*, 125–134.

Husain, K., Scott, R. B., Whitworth, C., Somani, S. M., & Rybak, L. P. (2001a). Dose response of carboplatin-induced hearing loss in rats: Antioxidant defense system. *Hear Res, 151*, 71–78.

Husain, K., Whitworth, C., Hazelrigg, S., & Rybak, L. (2003). Carboplatin-induced oxidative injury in rat inferior colliculus. *Int J Toxicol, 22*, 335–342.

Husain, K., Whitworth, C., Somani, S. M., & Rybak, L. P. (2001b). Carboplatin-induced oxidative stress in rat cochlea. *Hear Res, 158*, 14–22.

Jansen, C., Mattox, D. E., Miller, K. D., & Brownell, W. E. (1989). An animal model of hearing loss from alpha-difluoromethylornithine. *Arch Otolaryngol Head Neck Surg, 115*, 1234–1237.

Kalcioglu, M. T., Kuku, I., Kaya, E., Oncel, S., & Aydogdu, I. (2003). Bilateral hearing loss during vincristine therapy: A case report. *J Chemother, 15*, 290–292.

Kartalou, M., & Essigmann, J. M. (2001). Recognition of cisplatin adducts by cellular proteins. *Mutat Res, 478*, 1–21.

Kennedy, I. C., Fitzharris, B. M., Colls, B. M., & Atkinson, C. H. (1990). Carboplatin is ototoxic. *Cancer Chemother Pharmacol, 26*, 232–234.

Klis, S. F., O'Leary, S. J., Wijbenga, J, de Groot, J. C., Hamers, F. P., & Smoorenburg, G. F. (2002). Partial recovery of cisplatin-induced hearing loss in the albino guinea pig in relation to cisplatin dose. *Hear Res, 164*, 138–146.

Komune, S., & Snow, J. B., Jr. (1981). Potentiating effects of cisplatin and ethacrynic acid in ototoxicity. *Arch Otolaryngol, 107*, 594–597.

Kopelman, J., Budnick, A. S., Sessions, R. B., Kramer, M. B., & Wong, G. Y. (1988). Ototoxicity of high-dose cisplatin by bolus administration in patients with advanced cancers and normal hearing. *Laryngoscope, 98*, 858–864.

Lao, C. D., Backoff, P., Shotland, L. I., McCarty, D., Eaton, T., Ondrey, F. G., et al. (2004). Irreversible ototoxicity associated with difluoromethylornithine. *Cancer Epidemiology Biomarkers & Prevention, 13*, 1250–1252.

Laurell, G., & Jungnelius, U. (1990). High-dose cisplatin treatment: Hearing loss and plasma concentrations. *Laryngoscope, 100*, 724–734.

Laurell, G. F. (1992). Combined effects of noise and cisplatin: Short- and long-term follow-up. *Ann Otol Rhino Laryngol, 101*, 969–976.

Legros, D., Ollivier, G., Gastellu-Etchaegorry, M., Paquet, C., Burri, C., & Jannin, J. (2002). Treatment of human African typanosomiasis—present situation and need for research and development. *Lancet Infect Dis, 2*, 437–440.

Levin, V. A., Hess, K. R., Choucair, A., Flynn, P. J., Jaeckle, K. A., Kyritsis, A. P., et al. (2003). Phase III randomized study of postradiotherapy chemotherapy with combination alpha-difluoromethylornithine-PCV versus PCV for anaplastic gliomas. *Clinical Cancer Research, 9*, 981–990.

Levin, V. A., Uhm, J. H., Jaeckle, K. A., Choucair, A., Flynn, P. J., & Yung, W. K. (2000). Phase III randomized study of postradiotherapy chemotherapy with combination alpha-difluoromethylornithine-procarbazine, N-(2-0Choloethyl)-N'-cyclohexyl-N-nitrosurea, vincristine (DFMO-PCV) versus PCV for glioblastoma multiforme. *Clinical Cancer Research, 6*, 3878–3884.

Li, Y., Womer, R. B., & Silber, J. H. (2004). Predicting cisplatin ototoxicity in children: The influence of age and the cumulative dose. *Eur J Cancer, 40*, 2445–2451.

Lipton, A., Harvey, H. A., Glenn, J., Weidner, W., Strauss, M., Miller, S. E., et al. (1989). A phase I study of hepatic arterial infusion using difluoromethylornithine. *Cancer, 63*, 433–437.

Liu, W., Staecker, H., Stupak, H., Malgrange, B., Lefebvre, P., & Van De Water, T. R. (1998). Caspase inhibitors prevent cisplatin-induced apoptosis of auditory sensory cells. *Neuroreport, 9,* 2609–2614.

Lockwood, D. S., Ding, D. L.,Wang, J., & Salvi, R. J. (2000). D-methionine attenuates inner hair cell loss in carboplatin-treated chinchillas. *Audiol Neurootol, 5,* 263–266.

Loprinzi, C. L., Messing, E. M., O'Fallon, J. R., Poon, M. A., Love, R. R., Quella, S. K., et al. (1996). Toxicity evaluation of difluoromethylornithine: Doses for chemoprevention trials. *Cancer Epidemiology Biomarkers & Prevention, 5,* 371–374.

Love, R. R., Carbone, P. P., Verma, A. K., Gilgore, D., Carey, P., Tutsch, K. D., et al. (1993). Randomized phase I chemoprevention dose-seeking study of alpha-difluoromethylornithine, *J Natl Cancer Inst, 85,* 732–737.

Love, R. R., Jacoby, R., Newton, M. A., Tutsch, K. D., Simon, K., Pomplum, M., & Verma, A. K. (1992). A randomized, placebo-controlled trial of low-dose alpha-difluoromethylornithine in individuals at risk for colorectal cancer. *Cancer Epidemiology Biomarkers & Prevention, 7,* 989–992.

Lugassy, G., & Shapira, A. (1990). Sensorineural hearing loss associated with vincristine treatment. *Blut, 61,* 320–321.

Lugassy, G., & Shapira, A. (1996). A prospective cohort study of the effect of vincristine on audition. *Anticancer Drugs, 7,* 525–526.

MacDonald, M. R., Harrison, R. V., Wake, M., Bliss, B., & MacDonald, R. E. (1994). Ototoxicity of carboplatin: Comparing animal and clinical models at the hospital for sick children. *J Otolaryngol, 23,* 151–159.

Maddox, A. M., Keating, M. J., McCredie, K. E., Estey, E., & Freireich E. J. (1985). Phase I evaluation of intravenous difluoromethylornithine—a polyamine inhibitor. *Investigational New Drugs, 3,* 287–292.

Mahajan, S. L. (1981). Acute acoustic nerve palsy associated with vincristine therapy. *Cancer, 47,* 2404.

Marco-Algarra, J., Basterra, J., & Marco, J. (1985). Cis-diaminedichloro platinum ototoxicity. An experimental study. *Acta Otolaryngol, 99,* 343–347.

Marks, S. C., Mattox, D. E., & Casero, R. A. (1991). The effects of DFMO on polyamine metabolism in the inner ear. *Hear Res, 53,* 230–236.

McCann, P. P., & Pegg, A. E. (1992). Ornithine decarboxylase as an enzyme target for therapy. *Pharmac, 54,* 195–215.

McWilliams, M. L., Chen, G. D., & Fetcher, L. D. (2000). Characterization of the ototoxicity of difluoromethylornithine and its enantiomers. *Toxicol Science, 56,* 124–132.

Meech, R. P., Campbell, K. C., Hughes, L. P., & Rybak, L. P. (1998). A semiquantitative analysis of the effects of cisplatin on the rat stria vascularis. *Hear Res, 124,* 44–59.

Melamed, L. B., Selim, M. A., & Schuchman, D. (1985). Cisplatin ototoxicity in gynecologic cancer patients. A preliminary report. *Cancer, 55,* 41–43.

Meyskens, F. L., Jr., Emerson, S. S., Pelot, D., Meshkinpour, H., Shassetz, L. R., & Einspahr, J. (1994). Dose de-escalation chemoprevention trial of alpha-difluoromethylornithine in patients with colon polyps. *Journal of the National Institute, 86,* 1122–1130.

Meyskens, F. L., Jr., & Gerner, E. W. (1995). Development of difluoromethylornithine as a chemoprevention agent for the management of colon cancer. *J Cell Biochem*(Suppl. 22), 126–131.

Meyskens, F. L., Jr., & Gerner, E. W. (1999). Development of difluoromethylornithine (DFMO) as a chemoprevention agent. *Clin Cancer Res, 5,* 945–951.

Meyskens, F. L., Jr., Gerner, E. W., Emerson, S., Pelot, D., Durbin, T., Doyle, K., & Lagerberg, W. (1998). Effect of alpha-difluoromethylornithine on rectal mucosal levels of polyamines in a randomized, double-blinded trial for colon cancer prevention. *Natl Cancer Inst, 19,* 1212–1218.

Meyskens, F. L., Kingsley, E. M., Glattke, T., Loescher, L., & Booth, A. (1986). A phase II study of alpha-difluoromethylornithine (DMFO) for the treatment of metastatic melanoma. *Invest New Drugs, 4*(3), 527–562.

Moroso, M. J., & Blair, R. L. (1983). A review of cisplatinum ototoxicity. *J Otolaryngol, 12,* 365–369.

Moss, P. E., Hickman, S., & Harrison, B. R. (1997). Ototoxicity associated with vinblastine. *Ann Pharmacother, 33,* 423–425.

Mount, R. J., Takeno, S., Wake, M., & Harrison, R. V. (1995). Carboplatin ototoxicity in the chinchilla: Lesions of the vestibular epithelium. *Acta Otolaryngol Suppl, 519*, 60–65.

Muldoon, L. L., Pagel, M. A., Kroll, R. A., Brummett, R. E., Doolittle, N. D., & Zuhowski, E. G. (2000). Delayed administration of sodium thiosulfate in animal models reduces platinum ototoxicity without reduction of antitumor activity. *Clin Cancer Res, 6*, 309–315.

Neuwelt, E. A., Brummett, R. E., Doolittle, N. D., Muldoon, L. L., Kroll, R. A., & Pagel, M. A. (1998). First evidence of otoprotection against carboplatin-induced hearing loss with a two-compartment system in patients with central nervous system malignancy using sodium thiosulfate. *J Pharmacol Exp Ther, 286*, 77–84.

Nie, L., Feng, W., Diaz, R., Gratton, M. A., Doyle, K. J., & Yamoah, E. N. (2005). Functional consequences of polyamine synthesis inhibitions by L-alpha-difluoromethylornithine (DFMO). *J Biol Chem, 280*, 15097–15102.

Obermair, A., Speiser, P., Thoma, M., Kaider, A., Salzer, H., Dittrich, C., et al. (1998). Prediction of toxicity but not of clinical course by determining carboplatin exposure in patients with epithelial ovarian cancer treated with a combination of carboplatin and cisplatin. *Int J Oncol, 13*, 1023–1030.

O'Shaughnessy, J. A., Demers, L. M., Jones, S. E., Arseneau, J., Khandelwal, P, G. (1999). Alpha-difluoromethylornithine as treatment for metastatic breast cancer patients. *Clinical Cancer Research, 5*, 3438–3444.

Ozturan, O., Jerger, J., Lew, H., & Lynch, G. R. (1996). Monitoring of cisplatin ototoxicity by distortion-product otoacoustic emissions. *Auris Nasus Larynx, 23*, 147–151.

Park, K. R. (1996). The utility of acoustic reflex thresholds and other conventional audiologic tests for monitoring cisplatin ototoxicity in the pediatric population. *Ear Hear, 7*, 107–115.

Parsons, S. K., Neault, M. W., Lehmann, L. E., Brennan, L. L., Eickhoff, C. E., Kretachman, C.S., et al. (1998). Severe ototoxicity following carboplatin-containing conditioning regimen for autologous marrow transplantation for neuroblastoma. *Bone Marrow Transplant, 22*, 669–674.

Pasic, T. R., Heisey, D., & Love, R. R. (1997). Alpha-difluoromethylornithine ototoxicity. *Arch Otolaryngol Head Neck Surg, 123*, 1281–1286.

Patton, T. F., Repta, A. J., & Sternson, L. A. (1983). Clinical pharmacology of cisplatin. In M. M. Ames, G. Powis, & J. S. Kovach (Eds.), *Pharmacokinetics of Anticancer Agents in Human*. New York, Elsevier.

Pegg, A. E., & McCann, P. P. (1988). Polyamine metabolism and function in mammalian cells and protozoans. *Atlas of Science and Biochemistry*, 11–18.

Pietenpol, J. A., & Kastan, M. B. (2004). Control of the cell cycle. In M. D. Abeloff, J. O. Armitage, J. E. Niederhuber, M. B. Kastan, & W. G. McKenna (Eds.), *Clinical oncology* (3rd ed., pp. 81–100). Philadelphia: Elsevier.

Pollera, C. F., Marolla, P., Nardi, M., Ameglio, F., Cozzo, L., & Bevere, F. (1988). Very high-dose cisplatin-induced ototoxicity: A preliminary report on early and long-term effects. *Cancer Chemother Pharmacol, 21*, 61–64.

Prados, M., Rodriguez, L., Chamberlain, M., Silver, P., & Levin, V. (1989). Treatment of recurrent gliomas with 1,3-Bis(2-Chloroethyl)-1 nitrosourea and alpha-difluoromethylornithine. *Neurosurgery, 24*, 806–809.

Punnett, A., Bliss, B., Dupuis, L. L., Abdolell, M., Doyle, J., & Sung, L. (2004). Ototoxicity following pediatric hematopoietic stem cell transplantation: A prospective cohort study. *Pediatr Blood Cancer, 42*, 598–603.

Ramirez-Camacho, R., Garcia-Berrocal, J. R., Bujan, J., et al. (2004). Supporting cells as a target of cisplatin-induced inner ear damage: Therapeutic implications. *Laryngoscope, 114*, 533–537.

Ravi, R., Somani, S. M., & Rybak, L. P. (1995). Mechanism of cisplatin ototoxicity: Antioxidant system. *Pharmacology & Toxicology, 76*, 386–394.

Reedijk, J. (1996). New clues for platinum antitumor chemistry: Kinetically controlled metal binding to DNA. *Proc Natl Acad Sci, 100*, 3611–3616.

Riggs, L. C., Brummett, R. E., Guitjens, S. K., & Matz G. J. (1996). Ototoxicity resulting from combined administration of cisplatin and gentamicin. *Laryngoscope, 106*, 401–406.

Russell, D. H. (1985). Ornithine decarboxylase: A key regulatory enzyme in normal and neoplastic growth. *Drug Metabolism Reviews, 16*, 1–88.

Rybak, L. P., & Kelly, T. (2003). Ototoxicity: Bioprotective mechanisms. *Curr Opin Otolaryngol Head Neck Surg, 11,* 328–333.

Rybak, L. P., Whitworth, C., & Somani, S. (1999). Application of antioxidants and other agents to prevent cisplatin otoxicity. *Laryngoscope, 109,* 1740–1744.

Sahai, J., & Berry, A. J. (1989). Eflornithine for the treatment of Pneumocystis carinii pneumonia in patients with the acquired immunodeficiency syndrome: A preliminary review. *Pharmacotherapy, 9,* 29–33.

Saito, T., Saito, H., Saito, K., Wakui, S., Manabe, Y., & Tsuda, G. (1989). Ototoxicity of carboplatin in guinea pigs. *Auris Nasis Larynx, 16,* 13–21.

Salzer, S. J., Mattox, D.E., & Brownnell, W. E. (1990). Cochlear damage and increased threshold in alpha-difluoromethylornithine (DFMO) treated guinea pigs. *Hear Res, 46,* 101–112.

Schaefer, S. D., Post, J. D., Close, L .G., & Wright, C. G. (1985). Ototoxicity of low- and moderate-dose cisplatin. *Cancer, 56,* 1934–1939.

Schell, M. J., McHaney, V. A., Green, A. A., Kun, L. E., Hayes, F. A., & Horowitz, M. (1989). Hearing loss in children and young adults receiving cisplatin with or without prior cranial irradiation. *J Clin Oncol, 7,* 754–760.

Schwietzer, L., Casseday, J. H., Sjoerdsma, A., McCann, P. P., & Bartolomes, J. V. (1986). Identification of polyamines in the cochlea of the rat and their potential role in hearing.
Brain Research Bulletin, 16, 215–218.

Schweitzer, V. G., Hawkins, J. E., Lilly, D. J., Litterst, C. J., Abrams, G., & Davis, J. A. (1984). Ototoxic and nephrotoxic effects of combined treatment with cis-diamminedichloroplatinum and kanamycin in the guinea pig. *Otolaryngol Head Neck Surg, 92,* 38–49.

Serafy, A., & Hashash, M. (1981). The effect of vincristine on the neurological elements of the rabbit cochlea. *J Laryngol Otol, 95,* 49–54.

Serafy, A., Hashash, M., & State, F. (1982). The effect of vinblastine sulfate on the neurological elements of the rabbit cochlea. *J Laryngol Otol, 96,* 975–979.

Sergi, B., Ferraresi, A., Troiani, D., Paludetti, G., & Fetoni, A. R. (2003). Cisplatin ototoxicity in the guinea pig: Vestibular and cochlear damage. *Hear Res, 182,* 56–64.

Simon, T., Hero, B., Dupuis, W., Selle, B., & Berthold, F. (2002). The incidence of hearing impairment after successful treatment of neuroblastoma. *Klin Padiatr, 214,* 149–152.

Sjoerdsma, A., Golden, J. A., Schechter, P. J., Barlow, J. L., & Santi, D. V. (1984). Successful treatment of lethal protozoal infections with the ornithine decarboxylase inhibitors, alpha-difluoromethylornithine. *Trans Assoc AM Physicians, 97,* 70–79.

Skeel, R. T. (1999). Biologic and pharmacologic basis of cancer chemotherapy. In R. T. Skeel (Ed.), *Handbook of Cancer Chemotherapy* (5th ed., pp. 3–19). Philadelphia: Lippincott Williams & Wilkins.

Smith, M. C., Tinling, S., & Doyle, K. J. (2004). Difluoromethylornithine-induced reversible hearing loss across a wide frequency range. *The Laryngoscope, 144,* 1113–1117.

Stavroulaki, P., Apostolopoulos, N., Segas, J., Tsakanikos, M., & Adamopoulos, G. (2001). Evoked otoacoustic emissions—an approach for monitoring cisplatin induced ototoxicity in children. *Int J Pediatr Otorhinolaryngol, 59,* 47–57.

Strauss, M., Towfighi, J., Lord, S., Lipton, A., Harvey, H. A., & Brown, B. (1983). Cis-platinum ototoxicity: Clinical experience and temporal bone histopathology. *Laryngoscope, 93,* 1554–1559.

Sturgeon, J. (2004). Clinical uses of cisplatin. In P. S. Roland & J. A. Rutka (Eds.), *Ototoxicity* (pp. 50–59). Hamilton, Ontario, BC: Decker Inc.

Taudy, M., Syka, J., Popelar, J., & Ulehlova, L. (1992). Carboplatin and cisplatin ototoxicity in guinea pigs. *Audiology, 31,* 293–299.

Tibaldi, C., Pazzagli, I., Berrettini, S., & De Vito, A. (1998). A case of ototoxicity in a patient with metastatic carcinoma of the breast treated with paclitaxel and vinorelbine. *Eur J Cancer, 34,* 1133.

Toral-Martinon, R., Shkurovich-Bialik, P., Collado-Corona, M. A., Mora-Magana, I., Goldgrub-Listopad, S., & Shkurovich-Zaslavsky, M. (2003). Distortion product otoacoustic emissions test is useful in children undergoing cisplatin treatment. *Arch Med Res, 34,* 205–208.

United States Pharmacopeial Convention. (1999). *USP DI: Drug Information for the Health Care Professional* (19th ed., pp. 2946–2958). Taunton, MA: Micromedex, Inc., World Color Book Services.

Vermorken, J. B., Kapteijn, T. S., Hart, A. A., & Pinedo, H. M. (1983). Ototoxicity of cis-diamminedichloroplatinum (II): Influence of dose, schedule and mode of administration. *Eur J Cancer Clin Oncol, 19,* 53–58.

Vermorken, J. B., van der Vijgh, W. J., Klein, I., Hart, A. A., Gall, H. E., & Pinedo, H. M. (1984). Pharmacokinetics of free and total platinum species after short-term infusion of cisplatin. *Can Treat Rep, 68,* 505–513.

Wake, M., Takeno, S., Ibrahim, D., Harrison, R., & Mount, R. (1993). Carboplatin ototoxicity: An animal model. *J Laryngol Otol, 107,* 585-589.

Wallace, H. M., & Fraser, A. V. (2004). Inhibitors of polyamine metabolism: Review article. *Amino Acids, 26,* 353–365.

Wandt, H., Birkmann, J., Denzel, T., Schafer, K., Schwab, G., Pilz, D., et al. (1999). Sequential cycles of high dose chemotherapy with dose escalation of carboplatin with or without paclitaxel supported by G-CSF mobilized blood progenitor cells: A phase I/II study in advanced ovarian cancer. *Bone Marrow Transp, 23,* 763–770.

Wang, J., Ladrech, S., Pujol, R., et al. (2004). Caspase inhibitors, but not c-Jun NH2-terminal kinase inhibitor treatment, prevent cisplatin-induced hearing loss. *Cancer Res, 64,* 9217–9224.

Waters, G. S., Ahmad, M., Katsarkas, A., Stanimir, G., & McKay, J. (1991). Ototoxicity due to cis-diamminedichloroplatinum in the treatment of ovarian cancer: Influence of dosage and schedule of administration. *Ear Hear, 12,* 91–102.

Weinberg, R. A. (1994). Oncogenes and tumor suppressor genes. *CA Cancer J Clin, 44,* 160–170.

Wolfgang, G. H., Dominick, M. A., Walsh, K. M., Hoeschele, J. D., & Pegg, D.G. (1994). Comparative nephrotoxicity of novel platinum compounds, cisplatin, and carboplatin in male Wistar rats. *Fundam Appl Toxicol, 22,* 73–79.

Wright, C. G., & Schaefer, S. D. (1982). Inner ear histopathology in patients treated with cisplatinum. *Laryngoscope, 92,* 1408–1413.

Yousif, H., Richardson, S. G., & Saunders, W. A. (1990). Partially reversible nerve deafness due to vincristine. *Postgrad Med J, 66,* 688–689.

CHAPTER
11

Aminoglycoside Antibiotics

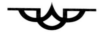

Jochen Schacht, PhD
Professor of Biological Chemistry in Otolaryngology
Director, Kresge Hearing Research Institute
The University of Michigan
Ann Arbor, MI

Acknowledgments: The writing of this review was concluded with the help of Ms. Andra Talaska in April 2005, and some references were updated in May 2006. Dr. Schacht's research on ototoxicity is supported by research grant DC03685 from the National Institute on Deafness and Other Communication Disorders, National Institutes of Health. Additional support has been received from the George and Christine Strumbos Foundation and the Kent and Carol Landsberg Foundation.

INTRODUCTION

Discovered in 1944 by Salman Waksman and collaborators (Schatz et al., 1944), streptomycin was the first of the aminoglycoside antibiotics and the first drug to be effective against tuberculosis[1]. The broad spectrum of its antibacterial efficacy, notably against **gram-negative** bacteria such as **pseudomonas**, made streptomycin and subsequently discovered aminoglycosides indispensable drugs for a number of decades to follow. The adverse side effects on the kidney and the inner ear described shortly after the first introduction of streptomycin (Hinshaw & Feldman, 1945) did not lessen the use of aminoglycosides, but prompted the search for newer compounds and derivatives with lower toxicity. Unfortunately, all aminoglycosides subsequently isolated or synthesized showed at least some potential for ototoxic or nephrotoxic side effects. Only in the last 20 years has the use of aminoglycoside antibiotic steadily declined in industrialized societies, thanks to the introduction of modern drugs with fewer adverse reactions. Nevertheless, the high efficacy of the aminoglycosides, coupled with their low cost, makes them the drug of choice and frequently the drug of necessity in almost all developing countries, where they are frequently available over the counter[2]. Aminoglycoside antibiotics may be the most commonly used antibiotics worldwide today.

STRUCTURE AND ACTIVITY OF AMINOGLYCOSIDES

A wide variety of aminoglycoside antibiotics are currently available (Table 11-1). Their use patterns vary between countries, in part determined by emerging bacterial resistance against individual compounds in this class.

All aminoglycosides share a similar structure of usually three rings that are either **cyclitols** or **five- or six-membered sugars**, linked via a **glycosidic linkage** (Figure 11-1). The presence of **hydroxyl** and **amino** groups gives these drugs their high water solubility and basic character. On the other hand, the high degree of hydrophilicity and polarity prevents these drugs from readily crossing cell membranes. They are poorly absorbed following oral intake (Sande & Mandell, 1990), and the usual methods of administration are **parenteral** or topical by way of eardrops or peritoneal lavage.

The value of aminoglycoside antibiotics lies not only in their broad antibacterial spectrum, but also in the fact that they are bactericidal (i.e., they kill bacteria, not merely inhibit their growth). Aminoglycoside antibiotics are still used today for their original indication, namely, treatment of tuberculosis. In fact, the resurgence of tuberculosis during the last decade (8 million new cases of active tuberculosis annually) and the increasing drug resistance of tuberculosis bacteria to individual drugs have renewed the clinical interest in these drugs. Aminoglycosides (primarily streptomycin and amikacin/kanamycin) are an integral part of the World Health Organization's recommended multidrug regimen (World Health Organization, 2005). Furthermore, the aminoglycosides maintain a leading role in the treatment of **enterococcal**, **mycobacterial**, and severe gram-negative bacterial infections and in

---

1. Waksman and Schatz jointly received the patent for streptomycin while at Rutgers, but a feud over royalties led to a lawsuit. When Selman Waksman received the Nobel prize for his discovery in 1952, Albert Schatz believed that he himself was denied rightful credit for the discovery. A protracted controversy ensued that ended in a belated recognition of Schatz with the Rutgers Medal, the university's highest honor, in 1994.

2. As an example, 10 vials of injectable gentamicin (for a complete 5-day course) cost the equivalent of 20 cents in China (author's inquiries in 2003).

Table 11-1. Aminoglycoside Antibiotics

Generic names of commonly available preparations	
From *Micromonospora*	Gentamicin, Sisomicin
From *Streptomyces*	Kanamycin, Neomycin, Paromomycin, Streptomycin, Tobramycin
Semisynthetic	Amikacin, Dibekacin (from kanamycin), Isepamicin (from gentamicin), Netilmicin (from sisomicin)

Section 1.01 Bacterial strains susceptible to aminoglycosides
Brucella, Enterobacter, Escherichia coli, Klebsiella, Mycobacterium tuberculosis, Proteus, Pseudomonas, Salmonella, Shigella, Staphylococci, Streptococci

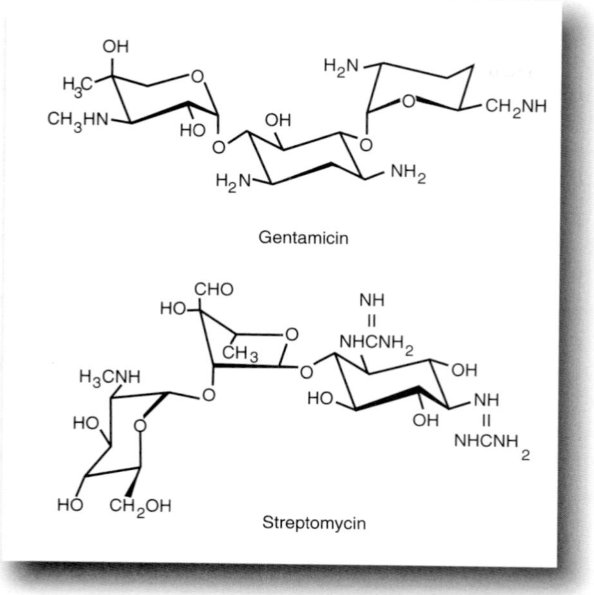

Figure 11-1. Structures of streptomycin and gentamicin C1a. The drawings emphasize the ring structures and the functional groups (hydroxyl, amino, and guanidino). The rings, therefore, are depicted without explicitly labeling their carbon atoms (C) and the hydrogens (H) directly bound to them. Most of the amino and guanidino groups will carry a positive charge at physiological pH. (Adapted from Forge and Schacht (2000), reprinted with permission from S. Karger AG, Basel.)

cystic fibrosis, as patients receive regular treatment with aminoglycosides (primarily tobramycin and amikacin) as prophylaxis against pneumonia primarily caused by *Pseudomonas aeroginosa* (Swan, 1997; Edson & Terrell, 1999).

OTHER "MICIN" DRUGS

The suffix *-mycin* (or *-micin*) is not a chemical or therapeutic classification and does not always indicate an aminoglycoside. It indicates that these compounds are synthesized by different strains of soil **actinomycetes**, "mycins" by *Streptomyces*, and "micins" by *Micromonospora*. Indeed, several prominent "mycins" bear no structural similarity with aminoglycoside

antibiotics. Two of them (namely, vancomycin and erythromycin) are frequently cited in the context of ototoxicity and, therefore, deserve brief mentioning here. Vancomycin is a glycopeptide antibiotic used against both **aerobic** and **anaerobic** gram-positive microorganisms such as **staphylococcus aureus** and **clostridium difficile**. Erythromycin is a **macrolide** antibiotic substituted with one or more **deoxy**-sugars. It has a rather broad spectrum against clinically relevant infections that gained major attention in combating an outbreak of Legionnaires' disease in the United States.

Studies early after the introduction of vancomycin had attributed some ototoxicity to this antibiotic. However, careful analysis of these studies could not confirm that the ototoxicity was indeed due to the antibiotic and was suggested to arise either from impurities in early preparations or from concomitant administration of other drugs (Bailie & Neal, 1988; Cantu et al., 1994; Brummett, 1993). Later prospective studies and screening of newborns receiving vancomycin likewise suggested that it is not associated with ototoxic side effects (de Hoog et al., 2003). Vancomycin may, however, augment the ototoxicity of aminoglycoside antibiotics (Brummett et al., 1990).

Erythromycin does have confirmed effects on the auditory system, which occur mostly at very high doses of the antibiotic. The ototoxic events triggered by erythromycin may include tinnitus or a temporary loss or attenuation of hearing thresholds and may occur in 16% of patients treated at lower doses and up to 53% in patients receiving treatment with 4 grams of erythromycin daily. However, even at high doses, ototoxic effects were completely reversible (Brummett & Fox, 1989; Swanson et al., 1992).

AUDITORY AND VESTIBULAR PATHOLOGY AND PATHOPHYSIOLOGY OF AMINOGLYCOSIDES

From both experimental animals and human temporal bones, it has become clear that the hair cells in the inner ear are the primary targets of aminoglycoside antibiotics. In the cochlea, the outer hair cells are first to be destroyed in a base-to-apex gradient, resulting in a hearing loss starting at high frequencies (Figure 11-2). In the vestibular system, type I hair cells are the first targets, their loss leading to disturbances of vestibular function (Hawkins, 1976). The primary site of the lesion—the vestibular or cochlear structures—varies with the kind of antibiotic given. Gentamicin and streptomycin, for example, are considered more vestibulotoxic than cochleotoxic in the human, while amikacin and neomycin may primarily target the cochlea. Those, however, are not absolute preferences; all aminoglycosides may damage either one or both of the end organs in the inner ear.

Both the vestibular and cochlear deficits generally develop after chronic administration of aminoglycosides, but a precise onset of the side effects cannot be predicted. In the course of a six- to eight-day treatment for an acute infection, not much hearing loss may be noticed. However, adverse effects may progress even after drug administration has ceased, so manifestations of inner ear dysfunctions may become apparent weeks after treatment. The hearing loss is typically bilateral and symmetrical, but may occur unilaterally, as well.

Although the progression of hearing loss is well defined, the clinical detection of early signs of ototoxicity is not routine. In the cochlea, destruction begins at the highest frequencies (16 kHz or higher in the human), which are not covered by most conventional audiometry. By the time the damage has reached the measured frequencies of 8000 Hz and below or even impacts word recognition, much damage to the cochlea has already ensued. Accurate high-frequency audiometry, therefore, is essential for monitoring the progression of ototoxicity. In addition, otoacoustic

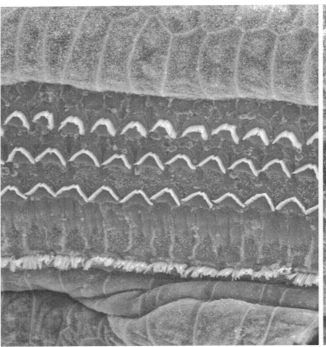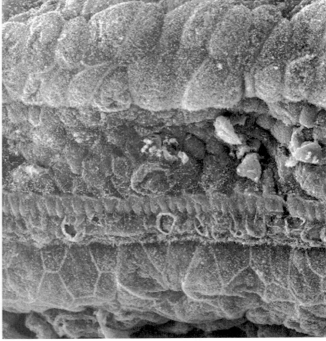

Figure 11-2. Hair cell damage. This scanning electron micrograph shows a surface view of the organ of Corti of a guinea pig. Left: Stereocilia on the three rows of outer hair cells are regularly arranged in the shape of a *W* at the apex of each cell. The single row of inner hair cells is also marked by the stereocilia. Right: Following a traumatic insult such as drug treatment, noise exposure, and even aging, hair cells disappear and the surrounding supporting cells grow into the space to form a "scar." Damage in this experiment was induced by the combined action of kanamycin and ethacrynic acid. (Photos courtesy of Drs. Masahiko Izumikawa and Yehoash Raphael, University of Michigan.)

emissions have emerged as a sensitive tool to determine the integrity of outer hair cells and early signs of drug effects in patients (Probst et al., 1993). Assessment of vestibular damage is also best done by objective testing, because small functional deficits in the end organ can be readily compensated by visual cues and adaptation by the patient.

INCIDENCE OF OTOTOXICITY

It is difficult to give precise numbers on the incidence of ototoxicity. Although criteria for ototoxicity have been defined by the American Speech-Language-Hearing Association ASHA standards (ASHA, 1994), the definition of "hearing loss" is equivocal in the earlier (and even recent) literature, making data from different studies difficult to compare. Individual criteria range from a depression in hearing sensitivity of more than 10 dB at one or more frequencies to more stringent definitions of a loss of 20 dB or more at two or more adjacent test frequencies. Furthermore, most tests are conducted at frequencies of up to 8 kHz and leave the early actions of aminoglycosides undetected. Within those limitations, the majority of studies indicate that the cochleotoxicity of the most commonly used aminoglycoside antibiotics may occur in about 20%–33% of patients, while balance may be affected in about 15% (Fee, 1980; Moore et al., 1984; Lerner et al., 1986; Fausti, 1999). That compares to nephrotoxicity complicating 10%–20% of therapeutic courses (Swan, 1997). Studies in cystic fibrosis patients also show divergent results from no apparent hearing deficits (Ramsey et al., 1999) to an incidence of hearing impairment of 16%–20% (Mulherin et al., 1991; Mulheran et al, 2001).

The long-term treatment required for tuberculosis appears to increase the risk of side effects even further. Again, existing data cannot be compared directly because of varying criteria for hearing loss, duration of treatment (from 2 weeks to more than 10 weeks) and the use of different drugs (mostly streptomycin, kanamycin, amikacin). While earlier studies reported an incidence of 75%–80% (Brouet et al., 1959; Dunaivitser & Davtian, 1989), more recent observations show cochlear toxicity in 18%–37% of the patients (de Jager & van Altena, 2002; Peloquin et al., 2004).

RISK FACTORS

The dosage and the duration of treatment appear to be major determinants of the extent and severity of ototoxic damage as exemplified by the high incidence among tuberculosis patients compared to patients on short-term treatment. The range between therapeutic and toxic serum levels is relatively narrow, and measurement of serum levels and a readjustment of therapeutic dosages is obligatory. The **serum half-life** of the different aminoglycosides varies between 2 and 3 hours if normal renal function is present and the therapeutic efficacy is determined by the peak levels which, in the case of gentamicin, lie in the range of 4–8 micrograms per milliliter.

Over the past decade, attempts to limit aminoglycoside toxicity have included variations in the dosing interval. Aminoglycosides were initially given in multiple daily doses, but recent studies indicate that an "extended interval dosing" may produce more favorable clinical results. The higher loading with a once-daily dose appears to optimize bacterial killing (Freeman et al., 1997; Lacy 1998) and has a predictably lower probability of causing nephrotoxicity than twice daily administration (Rybak et al., 1999). Whether the once-daily dosing also reduces the chances of ototoxicity has not been investigated to the same extent as nephrotoxicity and clinical efficacy. However, once-daily dosing has no greater incidence of ototoxicity than seen in multiple dosing (Barclay et al., 1995).

Other risk factors that have been discussed for aminoglycoside ototoxicity are advanced age, concomitant noise exposure, and preexisting disorders of hearing and balance. While some of those risk factors have been deduced from animal experimentation, it is difficult to confirm any of the factors in prospective studies in humans (Moore et al., 1984). Clearly established risk factors in humans, however, include impaired kidney function and certain drug-drug interactions. In the case of renal dysfunction, the half-life of the drug increases, and patients with reduced creatinine clearance suffer from an increased incidence of toxicity (Gerberding, 1998). Concomitant administration of loop diuretics, particularly ethacrynic acid, can lead to a precipitous and complete hearing loss (Mathog & Klein, 1969).

A genetic predisposition toward aminoglycoside-induced hearing loss is conferred through a mitochondrial mutation commonly referred to as the 1555 mutation, where a guanosine at position 1555 in the mitochondrial ribosomal RNA has been substituted with an adenosine (Prezant et al., 1993; Usami et al., 1998). In these individuals, who are also prone to non-syndromic hearing loss, a single injection of an aminoglycoside may lead to profound deafness. The mutation has a relatively low prevalence in the general population but may account for about 15% of all aminoglycoside-induced cases of deafness in the United States (Fischel-Ghodsian et al., 1997). A rapid mass screening is possible, but not in general use (Usami et al., 1999). A rather enigmatic aspect of the mutation is the fact that these patients suffer from an aggravated toxicity only to the cochlea and not to the vestibular system, although drugs such as gentamicin exert more vestibular toxicity in patients without the mutation (Tono et al., 2001).

PHARMACOKINETICS

Research into the uptake of aminoglycoside antibiotics into the tissues and cells of the inner ear has a long history, but there is still no clear-cut understanding of the underlying mechanisms. Several facts, however, are quite clear. First, the presence of the drug itself is not sufficient to cause pathophysiological effects; the aminoglycosides also penetrate cells and tissues that do not develop signs of toxicity. Consistent with such absence of a direct and predictable effect of the drug is the finding that the distribution pattern of aminoglycoside antibiotics between the cochlea and the vestibular system does not correlate with their preferential toxicity to these structures (Dulon et al., 1986). Even in the outer hair cells, which are the first to be affected, the drugs are present long before the first signs of pathophysiology appear (Hiel et al., 1993). We also cannot invoke an exceptionally high concentration or accumulation of the drugs in the affected tissues. At no time does the concentration in the inner ear exceed the serum concentration; therefore, an "accumulation" of the drug cannot account for the toxic effects (Henley & Schacht, 1988). It is intriguing, however, that the aminoglycosides remain in cochlear tissues for an exceedingly long time. The half-life in the inner ear has been measured to exceed 1 month (Tran Ba Huy et al,, 1986), and traces of the drug may persist for up to 6 months following the end of aminoglycoside treatment (Dulon et al., 1993). That fact may explain delayed drug-drug interactions or enhanced sensitivity that has been claimed to be present in patients receiving a second course of aminoglycoside antibiotics.

Literature data on transport mechanisms of the drugs does not give a clear picture, perhaps because uptake has been measured after different routes of administration in different types of hair cells (cochlear and vestibular) and in different species of amphibians and mammals. A proposed uptake via a **polyamine-like** transport mechanism would be consistent with the polyamine-like properties of aminoglycoside antibiotics (Williams et al., 1987). **Megalin** is considered an aminoglycoside transporter in the kidney (Moestrup et al., 1995), but its involvement in the inner ear has been questioned based on a lack of localization in the sensory and supporting cells of the organ of Corti (Mizuta et al., 1999). Intriguingly, cochleae of mice with mutations in **myosin 7A** do not take up aminoglycosides, and are protected from ototoxicity (Richardson et al., 1997). That finding, however, does not conclusively demonstrate myosin 7A as the transport molecule because mutations in such a critical element of membrane structure may affect a variety of transport systems. In isolated bullfrog saccular hair cells, uptake can be observed at the apical surface, particularly through hair bundles (Steyger et al., 2003), which is consistent with earlier observations that aminoglycoside antibiotics can enter transduction channels (Kroese et al., 1989). Thus, while the precise mechanisms of uptake remain to be elucidated, it is clear that the presence of the drug alone cannot explain the selective toxicity to the hair cells.

MOLECULAR MECHANISMS OF AMINOGLYCOSIDE OTOTOXICITY

In recent years, a cogent hypothesis of aminoglycoside-induced damage has emerged (Figure 11-3). The formation of reactive oxygen species (ROS; free radicals) by aminoglycosides has intermittently been discussed and dismissed for both nephrotoxicity and ototoxicity. The formation of ROS by aminoglycosides had been observed in isolated renal mitochondria (Walker & Shah, 1987), but other experiments failed to link ROS to nephrotoxicity (Ramsammy et al., 1987). Free radical involvement in ototoxicity also remained controversial. Two studies in the 1980s demonstrated the efficacy and the inefficacy of radical scavengers in protecting from aminoglycoside-induced hearing loss, respectively (Pierson & Møller, 1981; Bock et al., 1983). In the intervening years, evidence accumulated from both *in vivo* and *in vitro* experiments that antioxidants could indeed attenuate aminoglycoside toxicity (Garetz et al., 1994a; Garetz et al., 1994b; Song & Schacht, 1996). Subsequently, generation of free radicals in the presence of aminoglycosides was demonstrated in explants of the inner ear (Clerici et al., 1996; Hirose et al., 1997).

A mechanism of such ROS formation was made plausible by the observation that the formation of ROS can be catalyzed by redox-active iron (Fe^{++})-gentamicin complexes (Priuska & Schacht, 1995). *In vitro*, gentamicin can complex with transition metals and abstract electrons from donors, such as unsaturated fatty acids, to produce ROS nonenzymatically (Lesniak et al., 2005). Other aminoglycosides likewise catalyze free radical generation (Sha & Schacht, 1999a) in a reaction in which molecular oxygen is activated and subsequently reduced to the superoxide radical at the expense of an electron donor (Sha & Schacht, 1999b). Iron-catalyzed Fenton reactions can then lead to formation of other radicals, including the highly aggressive hydroxyl radical.

ROS formation by aminoglycosides is strongly supported by several observations *in vivo*. Depletion of the ubiquitous cellular antioxidant glutathione (GSH) in inner ear tissues enhances (and dietary restoration of its levels attenuates) aminoglycoside-induced ototoxicity (Hoffman et al., 1988; Garetz et al., 1994a; Lautermann et al., 1995). Transgenic mice overexpressing the antioxidant enzyme superoxide dismutase (SOD) are protected from kanamycin-induced hearing loss (Sha et al., 2001) as are animals receiving gene therapy with antioxidants (Kawamoto et al., 2004). The involvement of iron is supported by two complementary observations—

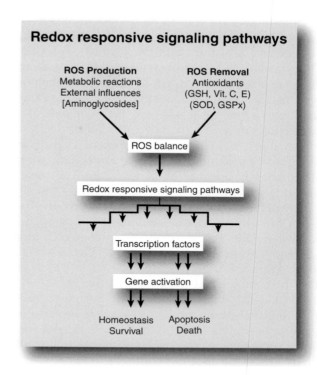

Figure 11-3. Proposed mechanisms of aminoglycoside ototoxicity. An initiating event in the toxic cascade is a shift in the redox balance of the cell. The production of free radicals (ROS), augmented by aminoglycosides, exceeds the capacity of the cell to detoxify them via normal antioxidant mechanisms including but not limited to glutathione (GSH), vitamins E and C, the enzymes superoxide dismutase (SOD), and glutathione peroxidase (GSPx). The ensuing redox imbalance shifts the signaling pathways and gene expression from the homeostatic balance to apoptotic (and necrotic) cell death.

gentamicin-induced ototoxicity in guinea pigs is enhanced by iron supplementation (Conlon & Smith, 1998) and is attenuated by antioxidant and iron chelation treatment (Song et al., 1997; Song et al., 1998). Thus, involvement of ROS in aminoglycoside ototoxicity is most compellingly demonstrated by the prevention of morphological and functional damage by antioxidants.

These initial events triggered by aminoglycosides are followed by downstream pathways of cell death. A considerable body of literature implicates apoptotic pathways in hair cell loss in cochlear and vestibular organ culture (see Forge & Schacht, 2000).

Apoptosis also appears to be the predominant cell fate following chronic drug administration *in vivo*, but necrosis is also evident (Nakagawa et al., 1998; Ylikoski et al., 2002). Pathways of cell death and survival are a complex network of interfacing signaling systems, including the activation of a variety of transcription factors, proteases, and the involvement of intracellular organelles such as mitochondria or lysosomes (Leist & Jäättelä, 2001). Recent years have brought a better understanding of molecular actions of aminoglycosides on homeostatic and cell death signaling pathways.

One of the cell death pathways implicated involves C-jun N-terminal kinase activation. Blocking this pathway results in the rescue of auditory cells from aminoglycoside antibiotics *in vitro* (Pirvola et al., 2000). Mitochondria-associated cell death pathways have been suggested from the fact that in isolated cochlear neurosensory epithelia, mitochondrial permeability transitions can be observed in response to gentamicin (Dehne et al., 2002). Consistent with such pathways is the fact that caspases, the more immediate executors of apoptosis, appear to be activated (Matsui et al., 2004; Shimizu et al., 2003). To what extent such proposed pathways do occur in chronic aminoglycoside ototoxicity in patients remains to be established. One caution in interpreting the literature on those pathways is that results come mostly from *in vitro* experiments using the early postnatal cochlea. Those results may be at variance from chronic toxicity because they are derived from acute toxicity models confounded by the fact that the sensitivity of the inner ear to aminoglycoside insults decreases with the maturation of the auditory system. In the cochlea of the adult mouse, for example, cell death may occur predominantly by caspase-independent pathways (Jiang et al., 2006).

Another signaling pathway has emerged as a rescue pathway in a chronic aminoglycoside model. The **transcription factor NF-κB** is activated by aminoglycoside treatment in those cochlear cells that will eventually survive, but its activation does not occur in outer hair cells that succumb to the treatment (Jiang et al., 2005). When ototoxicity is prevented by the concomitant administration of antioxidants, NF-κB activation is triggered in the outer hair cells, suggesting that this signaling pathway leads to activation of survival mechanisms. The exploitation of such pathways may eventually have clinical implications.

IS PREVENTION OF AMINOGLYCOSIDE OTOTOXICITY POSSIBLE?

Several points of intervention can be delineated from the pathway from noxious stimulus to cell death. Apoptotic processes can be prevented by interfering with specific points in the pathways, such as by blocking **jun-kinase** or **caspase** activity (Pirvola et al., 2000; Forge and Li, 2000). While apoptosis inhibitors (and nerve growth factors) have the potential to block aminoglycoside-induced cell death, a difficulty may arise in the translation to the clinical situation. In fact, inhibitors highly effective *in vitro* (Pirvola et al., 2000) have had limited protective capacity in animals *in vivo* (Ylikoski et al., 2002), perhaps reflecting the inadequacy of acute models to mimic the slow development of ototoxicity in patients.

A currently more feasible approach is a restoration of the redox balance of the cell (i.e., removal of ROS before they can start a noxious cascade). In animal experimentation, a wide variety of antioxidants has been shown to be effective in containing and, in some instances, completely eliminating aminoglycoside-induced cochlear and vestibular damage (Song & Schacht, 1996; Song et al., 1997, 1998; Conlon & Smith, 1999). Antioxidant treatment was effective against deficits induced by gentamicin, kanamycin, streptomycin, neomycin, and amikacin; so it can be assumed that this protection can be extrapolated to other aminoglycosides. It was this prevention by antioxidants that prompted the search for a potential clinical treatment.

Among the medications considered were d-methionine and salicylate, based on their efficacy as antioxidants *in vitro* and their ability to attenuate aminoglycoside-induced hearing loss in animals (Sha & Schacht, 1999c; Sha & Schacht, 2000). In particular, the latter compound was an interesting possibility because salicylate is the active component of aspirin. Approximately 30 minutes after an oral dose of aspirin (acetyl salicylate) is taken, it is hydrolyzed and primarily present in the body as salicylate. It was, therefore, very tempting to propose such a regimen for clinical use since aspirin has been in use for a century and its actions and side effects are well characterized.

However, two major issues need to be resolved before any protective treatment can be considered for a clinical situation. First, effective drug serum concentrations must be maintained. If compounds were to enhance renal clearance of drugs, they might produce a "protective effect" based on lower serum levels of the drugs. That, in turn, would reduce the drug's therapeutic efficacy. Second, the protective drug must not interfere with the antibacterial activity of the aminoglycosides. Those questions were resolved for antioxidants and salicylate in particular—the protective treatments have no negative influence on the therapeutic efficacy of the drugs (Song et al., 1997; Sha & Schacht, 1999c). Data from a recent clinical study (Sha et al., 2006) indicate that a cotherapy of aspirin with aminoglycosides indeed was protective, reducing the incidence of hearing loss by 75% and establishing the principle of antioxidant therapy as a therapeutic prevention against aminoglycoside-induced ototoxicity.

OUTLOOK

The further elucidation of the molecular mechanisms of aminoglycoside ototoxicity will have wide-ranging implications for understanding of auditory pathology. Oxidative stress by ROS is an emerging common mechanism in drug-induced hearing loss (aminoglycosides, cisplatin), noise trauma, and age-related hearing loss. Aminoglycosides, therefore, provide formidable tools to decipher life and death pathways in the dark turns of the labyrinth.

A safe, preventive, pharmacological intervention may have its highest impact in developing countries; but it would benefit industrialized countries alike. Aminoglycosides, as outlined in the introductory paragraphs, are still used in the treatment of enterococcal, mycobacterial, and severe gram-negative bacterial infections and as prophylaxis against *Pseudomonas* infections in cystic fibrosis patients. Furthermore, tuberculosis is of concern in all countries

(World Health Organization, 2005). Although its rise has declined in the United States, case rates remain as high as 37.4/100,000 in certain segments of the population, and Europe has recently (1995–2000) experienced an alarming rise in tuberculosis cases.

SUMMARY

Drug-induced hearing loss accounts for most cases of preventable hearing loss worldwide. Although a number of drugs over the years have been implicated in causing adverse side effects to the cochlea and vestibular system, it is primarily cisplatin and the aminoglycoside antibiotics that are of current clinical concern. Discovered in 1944, streptomycin was the first of the aminoglycosides and the first drug to be effective against tuberculosis. The broad spectrum of their antibacterial efficacy, notably against gram-negative bacteria such as pseudomonas, made streptomycin and subsequently discovered aminoglycosides (such as neomycin, tobramycin, gentamicin, and kanamycin) indispensable drugs for a number of decades to follow. Unfortunately, all aminoglycosides subsequently isolated or synthesized showed at least some potential for ototoxic or nephrotoxic side effects. Only in the last twenty years has the use of aminoglycoside antibiotics steadily declined in industrialized societies, thanks to the introduction of modern drugs with fewer adverse reactions. Nevertheless, the high efficacy of the aminoglycosides, coupled with their low cost, make them the drug of choice and frequently the drug of necessity in most developing countries, where they are frequently available over the counter. Aminoglycoside antibiotics may be the most commonly used antibiotics worldwide today.

Both nephrotoxicity and ototoxicity can be associated with clinical treatment using aminoglycoside antibiotics. While the renal effects are generally reversible, the destruction of hair cells in the inner ear is irreversible, leading to permanent loss of hearing or vestibular function. Risk management is primarily limited to control of dosage and duration of treatment and exclusion of known risk factors. Aside from a genetic predisposition, the nutritional and physiological state of the subject, preexisting disorders of hearing or balance, and impaired kidney function may increase the ototoxic potential of the drugs. Furthermore, drug-drug interactions pose a major threat; for example, the concomitant administration of the loop diuretic ethacrynic acid together with an aminoglycoside poses a greater risk of toxicity.

The pathology and pathophysiology of aminoglycoside ototoxicity has been well characterized for the past fifty years. In the cochlea, the outer hair cells are first being destroyed in a base-to-apex gradient, resulting in a hearing loss starting at the high frequencies that are processed in the base of the cochlea. In the vestibular system, specifically, type 1 hair cells are being attacked, leading to disturbance of vestibular function. Both the vestibular and cochlear deficits develop after chronic administration of aminoglycosides, although a precise onset of the side effects cannot be predicted. Early detection of ototoxic damage is difficult since the cochlear effects begin at frequencies higher than generally tested by routine audiometric procedures and vestibular deficits may be subclinical.

Insights into the molecular mechanisms leading to hair cell death have come during the last decade. ROS are now thought to play a key role in triggering the death of auditory and vestibular sensory cells. That concept places drug-induced hearing loss in the category of pathologies induced by oxidant stress. Following the insult by free radicals, apoptotic and necrotic cell death may ensue. In agreement with those proposed mechanisms, antioxidant treatment and intervention with apoptosis inhibitors have successfully attenuated aminoglycoside-induced loss of vestibular and auditory function in animal models. Furthermore, therapeutic protection against hearing loss in patients has been achieved with aspirin.

REFERENCES

American Speech-Language-Hearing Association (ASHA). (1994, March). *Guidelines for the Audiologic Management of Individuals Receiving Cochleotoxic Drug Therapy* (ASHA 36, Suppl. 12), 11–19.

Bailie, G. R., & Neal, D. (1988). Vancomycin ototoxicity and nephrotoxicity. A review. *Medical Toxicology and Adverse Drug Experience, 3*(5), 376–386.

Barclay, M. L., Duffull, S. B., Begg, E. J., & Buttimore, R. C. (1995). Experience of once-daily aminoglycoside dosing using a target area under the concentration-time curve. *Australian & New Zealand Journal of Medicine, 25*(3), 230–235.

Bock, G. R., Yates, G. K., Miller, J. J., & Moorjani, P. (1983). Effects of N-acetylcysteine on kanamycin ototoxicity in the guinea pig. *Hearing Research, 9,* 255–262.

Brouet, G., Marche, J., Chevallier, J., Liot, F., Le Meur, G., & Bergogne, Mme. (1959). Étude expérimentale et clinique de la kanmycine dans l'infection tuberculeuse. *Re Tub Pneum, 23,* 949–988.

Brummett, R. E. (1993). Ototoxicity of vancomycin and analogues. *Otolaryngologic Clinics of North America, 26*(5), 821–828.

Brummett, R. E., & Fox, K. E. (1989). Vancomycin- and erythromycin-induced hearing loss in humans. *Antimicrobial Agents and Chemotherapy, 33*(6), 791–796.

Brummett, R. E., Fox, K. E., Jacobs, F., Kempton, J. B., Stokes, Z., & Richmond, A. B. (1990). Augmented gentamicin ototoxicity induced by vancomycin in guinea pigs. *Archives of Otolaryngology—Head & Neck Surgery, 11* (1), 61–64.

Cantu, T. G., Yamanaka-Yuen, N. A., & Lietman, P. S. (1994). Serum vancomycin concentrations: Reappraisal of their clinical value. *Clinical Infectious Diseases, 18*(4), 533–543.

Clerici, W. J., Hensley, K., DiMartino, D. L., & Butterfield, D. A. (1996). Direct detection of ototoxicant-induced reactive oxygen species generation in cochlear explants. *Hearing Research, 98,* 116–124.

Conlon, B. J., & Smith, D. W. (1998). Supplemental iron exacerbates aminoglycoside ototoxicity in vivo. *Hearing Research, 155,* 1–5.

Conlon, B. J., Aran, J. M., Erre, J. P., & Smith, D. W. (1999). Attenuation of aminoglycoside-induced cochlear damage with the metabolic antioxidant a-lipoic acid. *Hearing Research 128,* 40–44.

Dehne, N., Rauen, U., de Groot, H., & Lautermann, J. (2002). Involvement of the mitochondrial permeability transition in gentamicin ototoxicity. *Hearing Research, 169,* 47–55.

de Hoog, M., van Zaaten, B. A., Hop, W. C., Overbosch, E., Weisglas-Kuperus, N., & van den Anker, J. N. (2003). New born hearing screening: Tobramycin and vancomycin are not risk factors for hearing loss. *Journal of Pediatrics, 142* (1), 41–46.

de Jager, P., & van Altena, R. (2002). Hearing loss and nephrotoxicity in long-term aminoglycoside treatment in patients with tuberculosis. *International Journal of Tuberculosis and Lung Disease, 6*(7), 622–627.

Dulon, D., Aran, J. M., Zajic, G., & Schacht, J. (1986). Comparative pharmacokinetics of gentamicin, netilmicin and amikacin in the cochlea and the vestibule of the guinea pig. *Antimicrobial Agents and Chemotherapy, 30,* 96–100.

Dulon, D., Hiel, H., Aurousseau, C., Erre, J. P., & Aran, J. M. (1993). Pharmacokinetics of gentamicin in the sensory hair cells of the organ of Corti: Rapid uptake and long term persistence. *Comptes Rendus de L'Academie des Sciences—Serie III, Sciences de la Vie, 316,* 682–687.

Dunaivitser, B. I., & Davtian, M. M. (1989). Prevention of neurosensory hearing disorders in antibiotic-induced ototoxicosis. *Vestnik Ototrinolaringologii, 2,* 3–5.

Edson, R. S., & Terrell, C. L. (1999). The aminoglycosides. *Mayo Clinic Proceedings, 74,* 529–528.

Fausti, S. A., Henry, J. A., Helt, W. J., Phillips, D. S., Frey, R. H., Noffsinger, D., Larson V. D., & Fowler, C. G. (1999, December). An individualized, sensitive frequency range for early detection of ototoxicity. *Ear Hear, 20*(6), 497–505.

Fee, W. E. (1980). Aminoglycoside ototoxicity in the human. *Laryngoscope, 40,* 1–19.

Fischel-Ghodsian, N., Prezant, T. R., Chaltraw, W., Wendt, K. A., Nelson R. A., Arnos, K. S., & Falk, R. E. (1997). Mitochondrial gene mutations: A common predisposing factor in aminoglycoside ototoxicity. *American Journal of Otolaryngology, 18,* 173–178.

Forge, A., & Li, L. (2000). Apoptotic death of hair cells in mammalian vestibular sensory epithelia. *Hearing Research, 139*(1–2), 97–115.

Forge, A., & Schacht, J. (2000). Aminoglycoside antibiotics. *Audiology and Neuro-Otology, 5,* 3–22.

Freeman, C. D., Nicolau, D. P., Belliveau, P. P., & Nightingale, C. H. (1997). Once-daily dosing of aminoglycosides: Review and recommendations for clinical practice. *Journal of Antimicrobial Chemotherapy, 39*(6), 677–686.

Garetz, S. L., Altschuler, R. A., & Schacht, J. (1994a). Attenuation of gentamicin ototoxicity by glutathione in the guinea pig in vivo. *Hearing Research, 77,* 81–87.

Garetz, S. L., Rhee, D. J., & Schacht, J. (1994b). Sulfhydryl compounds and antioxidants inhibit cytotoxicity to outer hair cells of a gentamicin metabolite in vitro. *Hearing Research, 77,* 75–80.

Gerberding, J. L. (1998). Aminoglycoside dosing: Timing is of the essence. *American Journal of Medicine, 105*(3), 256–258.

Hawkins, J. E. (1976). Drug ototoxicity. In W. D. Keidel & W. D. Neff (Eds.), *Handbook of sensory physiology, 5*(3) (pp. 707–748). Berlin: Springer Verlag.

Henley, C. M., & Schacht, J. (1988). Pharmacokinetics of aminoglycoside antibiotics in blood, inner ear fluids and tissues and their relationship to ototoxicity. *Audiology, 27,* 137–146.

Hiel, H., Erre, J., Aurosseau, C., Bouali, R., Dulon, D., & Aran, J. M. (1993). Gentamicin uptake by cochlear hair cells precedes hearing impairment during chronic treatment. *Audiology, 32,* 78–87.

Hinshaw, H. C., & Feldman, W. H. (1945). Streptomycin in treatment of clinical tuberculosis: A preliminary report. *Mayo Clinic Proceedings, 20,* 313–318.

Hirose, K., Hockenberry, D. N., & Rubel, E. W. (1997). Reactive oxygen species in chick hair cells after gentamicin exposure in vitro. *Hearing Research, 104,* 1–14.

Hoffman, D. W., Whitworth, C. A., Jones-King, K. L., & Rybak, L. P. (1988). Potentiation of ototoxicity by glutathione depletion. *Annals of Otology, Rhinology, and Laryngology, 97,* 36–41.

Jiang, H., Sha, S. H., Forge, A., & Schacht, J. (2006). Caspase-independent pathways of hair cell death induced by kanamycin *in vivo. Cell Death and Differentiation, 13,* 20–30.

Jiang, H., Sha, S. H., & Schacht, J. (2005). The NF-κB pathway protects cochlear hair cells from aminoglycoside-induced ototoxicity. *Journal of Neuroscience Research, 79,* 644–651.

Kawamoto, K., Sha, S. H., Minoda, R., Izumikawa, M., Kuriyama, H., Schacht, J., & Raphael, Y. (2004). Antioxidant gene therapy can protect hearing and hair cells from ototoxicity. *Molecular Therapy, 9,* 173–181.

Kroese, A. B., Das, A., & Hudspeth, A. J. (1989). Blockage of the transduction channels of hair cells in the bull frog's sacculus by aminoglycoside antibiotics. *Hearing Research, 37,* 203–218.

Lacy, M. K., Nicolau, D. P., Nightingale, C. H., & Quintiliani, R. (1998). The pharmacodynamics of aminoglycosides. *Clinical Infectious Diseases, 27*(1), 23–27.

Lautermann, J., McLaren, J., & Schacht, J. (1995). Glutathione protection against gentamicin ototoxicity depends on nutritional status. *Hearing Research, 86,* 15–24.

Leist, M., & Jäättelä, M. (2001). Four deaths and a funeral: From caspases to alternative mechanisms. *Nature Reviews, 2,* 1–10.

Lerner, S. A., Schmitt, B. A., & Seligsoh, M. R. (1986). Comparative-study of ototoxicity and nephrotoxicity in patients randomly assigned to treatment with amikacin or gentamicin. *American Journal of Medicine, 80,* 98–104.

Lesniak, W., Pecoraro, V. L., & Schacht, J. (2005). Ternary complexes of gentamicin with iron and lipid catalyze formation of reactive oxygen species. *Chemical Research in Toxicology, 18,* 357–364.

Mathog, R. H., & Klein, W. J., Jr. (1969). Ototoxicity of ethacrynic acid and aminoglycoside antibiotics in uremia. *New England Journal of Medicine, 280,* 1223–1224.

Matsui, J. I., Gale, J. E., & Warhol, M. E. (2004). Critical signaling events during the aminoglycoside-induced death of sensory hair cells in vitro. *Journal of Neurobiology, 61,* 250–266.

Mizuta, K., Siato, A., Watanabe, T., Nagura, M., Arakawa, M., Shimizu, F., & Hoshino, T. (1999). Ultrastructural localization of megalin in the rat cochlear duct. *Hearing Research, 129,* 83–91.

Moestrup, S. K., Cui, S., Vorum, H., Bregengard, C., Bjorn, S. E., Norris, K., Gliemann, J., & Christensen, E. I. (1995). Evidence that epithelial glycoprotein 330/megalin mediates uptake of polybasic drugs. *Journal of Clinical Investigation, 96,* 1404–1413.

Moore, R. D., Smith, C. R., & Lietman, P. S. (1984). Risk factors for the development of auditory toxicity in patients receiving aminoglycosides. *The Journal of Infectious Diseases, 149,* 23–30.

Mulheran, M., Degg, C., Burr, S., Morgan, D. W., & Stableforth, D. E. (2001). Occurrence and risk of cochleotoxicity in cystic fibrosis patients receiving repeated high-dose aminoglycoside therapy. *Antimicrobial Agents and Chemotherapy, 45*(9), 2502–2509.

Mulherin, D., Fahy, J., Grant, W., Keogan, M., Kavanagh, B., & Fitzgerald, M. (1991). Aminoglycoside induced ototoxicity in patients with cystic fibrosis. *Irish Journal of Medical Science, 160,* 173–175.

Nakagawa, T., Yamane, H., Takayama, M., Sunami, K., & Nakai, Y. (1998). Apoptosis of guinea pig cochlear hair cells following aminoglycoside treatment. *European Archives of Otorhinolaryngology, 255,* 127–131.

Peloquin, C. A., Berning, S. E., Nitta, A. T., Simone, P. M., Goble, M., Huitt, G. A., Iseman, M. D., Cook, J. L., & Curran-Everett, D. (2004). Aminoglycoside toxicity: Daily versus thrice-weekly dosing for treatment of mycobacterial diseases. *Clinical Infectious Diseases, 38*(11), 1538–1544.

Pierson, M. G., & Møller, A. R. (1981). Prophylaxis of kanamycin-induced ototoxicity by a radioprotectant. *Hearing Research, 4,* 79–87.

Pirvola, U., Xing-Qun, L., Virkkala, J., Saarma, M., Murakata, C., Camoratto, A.M., Walton K.M.& Ylikoski, J. (2000). Rescue of hearing, auditory hair cells, and neurons by CEP-1347/KT7515, an inhibitor of c-Jun N-terminal kinase activation. *Journal of Neuroscience; 20,* 43–50.

Prezant, T. R., Agapian, J. V., Bohlman, M. C., Bu, X., Oztas, S., Qiu, W. Q., Arnos, K. S., Cortopassi, G. A., Jaber, L., & Rotter, J. I. (1993). Mitochondrial ribosomal RNA mutation associated with both antibiotic-induced and non-syndromic deafness. *Nature Genetics, 4,* 289–294.

Priuska, E. M., & Schacht, J. (1995). Formation of free radicals by gentamicin and iron and evidence for an iron/gentamicin complex. *Biochemical Pharmacology, 50,* 1749–1752.

Probst, R., Harris, F. P., & Hauser, R. (1993). Clinical monitoring using otoacoustic emissions. *British Journal of Audiology, 27*(2), 85–90.

Ramsammy, L. S., Josepovitz, C., Ling, K. Y., Lane, B. P., & Kaloyanides, G. J. (1987). Failure of inhibition of lipid peroxidation by vitamin E to protect against gentamicin nephrotoxicity in the rat. *Biochemical Pharmacology, 36*, 2125–2132.

Ramsey, B. W., Pepe, M. S., Quan, J. M., Otto, K. L., Montgomery, A. B., Williams-Warren, J., Vasiljev-K, M., Borowitz, D., Bowman, C. M., Marshall, B. C., Marshall, S., & Smith, A. L. (1999). Intermittent administration of inhaled tobramycin in patients with cystic fibrosis. *New England Journal of Medicine, 340*, 23–30.

Richardson, G. P., Forge, A., Kros, C. J., Fleming, J., Brown, S. D. M., & Steel, K. P. (1997). Myosin VIIA is required for aminoglycoside accumulation in cochlear hair cells. *Journal of Neuroscience, 17*, 9506–9519.

Rybak, M. J., Abate, B. J., Kang, S. L., Ruffing, M. J., Lerner, S. A., & Drusano, G. L. (1999). Prospective evaluation of the effect of an aminoglycoside dosing regimen on rates of observed nephrotoxicity and ototoxicity. *Antimicrobial Agents and Chemotherapy, 42*(7), 1549–1555.

Sande, M. A., & Mandell, G. L. (1990). Antimicrobial agents. The aminoglycosides. In A. G. Gilman, T. W. Rall, A. S. Nies, & P. Taylor (Eds.), *The Pharmacological Basis of Therapeutics* (p. 1102). New York: Pergamon Press.

Schatz, A., Bugie, E., & Waksman, S. A. (1944). Streptomycin, a substance exhibiting antibiotic activity against gram-positive and gram-negative bacteria. *Proceedings of the Society for Experimental Biology and Medicine, 55*, 66–69.

Sha, S. H., & Schacht, J. (1999a). Formation of free radicals by aminoglycoside antibiotics. *Hearing Research, 128*, 112–118.

Sha, S. H., & Schacht, J. (1999b). Formation of reactive oxygen species following bioactivation of gentamicin. *Free Radical Biology and Medicine, 26*, 341–347.

Sha, S. H., & Schacht, J. (1999c). Salicylate attenuates gentamicin-induced ototoxicity. *Laboratory Investigation, 79*, 807–813.

Sha, S. H., & Schacht, J. (2000). Antioxidants attenuate gentamicin-induced free-radical formation *in vitro* and ototoxicity *in vivo*: D-methionine is a potential protectant. *Hearing Research, 142*, 34–40.

Sha, S. H., Qiu, J. H. & Schacht, J. (2006). Aspirin to prevent gentamicin-induced hearing loss. *New England Journal of Medicine, 354*, 1856–1857.

Sha, S. H., Zajic, G., Epstein, C. J., & Schacht, J. (2001). Overexpression of SOD protects from kanamycin-induced hearing loss. *Audiology and Neuro-Otology, 6*, 117–123.

Shimizu, A., Takumida, M., Anniko, M., & Suzuki, M. (2003). Calpain and caspase inhibitors protect vestibular sensory cells from gentamicin ototoxicity. *Acta Oto-laryngologica, 123*, 459–465.

Song, B. B., Anderson, D. J., & Schacht, J. (1997). Protection from gentamicin ototoxicity by iron chelators in guinea pig in vivo. *Journal of Pharmacology and Experimental Therapeutics, 282*, 369–377.

Song, B. B., & Schacht, J. (1996). Variable efficacy of radical scavengers and iron chelators to attenuate gentamicin ototoxicity in guinea pig in vivo. *Hearing Research, 94*, 87–93.

Song, B. B., Sha, S. H., & Schacht, J. (1998). Iron chelators protect from aminoglycoside-induced cochleo- and vestibulotoxicity in guinea pig. *Free Radical Biology and Medicine, 25*, 189–195.

Steyger, P. S., Peters, S. L., Rehling, J., Hordihok, A., & Dai, C. F. (2003). Uptake of gentamicin by bullfrog saccular hair cells *in vitro*. *Journal of the Association for Research in Otolaryngology, 4*, 565–578.

Swan, S. K. (1997). Aminoglycoside nephrotoxicity. *Seminars in Nephrology, 17*, 27–33.

Swanson, D. J., Sung, R. J., Fine, M. J., Orloff, J. J., Chu, S. Y., & Yu, V. L. (1992). Erythromycin ototoxicity: Prospective assessment with serum concentrations and audiograms in a study of patients with pneumonia. *American Journal of Medicine, 92*(1), 61–68.

Tono, T., Kiyomizu, K., Matsuda, K., Komune, S., Usami, S., Abe, S., & Shinkawa, H. (2001). Different clinical characteristics of aminoglycoside-induced profound deafness with and without the 1555 A--->G mitochondrial mutation. *ORL, 63*(1), 25–30.

Tran Ba Huy, P., Bernard, P., & Schacht, J. (1986). Kinetics of gentamicin uptake and release in the rat: Comparison of inner ear tissues and fluids with other organs. *Journal of Clinical Investigation, 77,* 1492–1500.

Usami, S., Abe, S., Shinkawa, H., Inoue, Y., & Yamaguchi, T. (1999). Rapid mass screening method and counseling for the 1555A -->G mitochondrial mutation. *Journal of Human Genetics, 44*(5), 304–307.

Usami, S., Abe, S., Tono, T., Komune, S., Kimberling, W. J., & Shinkawa, H. (1998). Isepamicin sulfate-induced sensorineural hearing loss in patients with the 1555 A-->G mitochondrial mutation. *ORL, 60,* 164–169.

Walker, P. D., & Shah, S. V. (1987). Gentamicin enhanced production of hydrogen peroxide by renal cortical mitochondria. *American Journal of Physiology, 253,* C495–C499.

Williams, S. E., Smith, D. E., & Schacht, J. (1987). Characteristics of gentamicin uptake in the isolated crista ampullaris of the inner ear of the guinea pig. *Biochemical Pharmacology, 36,* 89–95.

World Health Organization. (2005). WHO Report 2005. *Global tuberculosis control: Surveillance, planning, financing.* Geneva: World Health Organization.

Ylikoski, J., Xing-Qun, L., Virkkala, J., & Pirvola, U. (2002). Blockade of c-Jun N-terminal kinase pathway attenuates gentamicin-induced cochlear and vestibular hair cell death. *Hearing Research, 163,* 71–61.

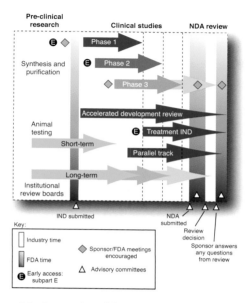

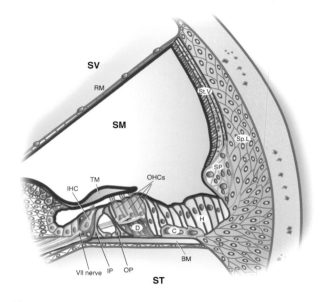

Figure 4-1. An overview of the role of the FDA in the drug development process (page 36).

Figure 15-1. Schematic of a cross section of one turn of the cochlea (see 5-1 for perspective) (page 218).

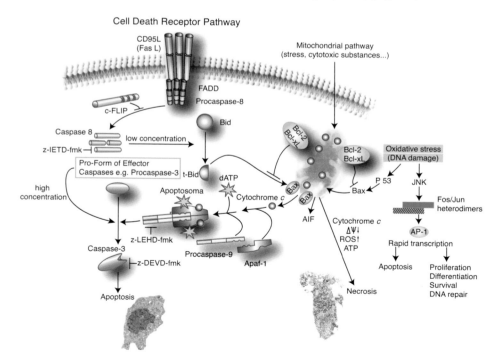

Figure 7-1. A schematic presentation of major apoptotic pathways thought to be active within mammalian hair cells (page 73).

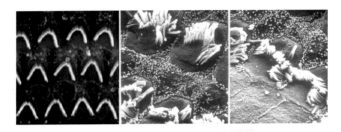

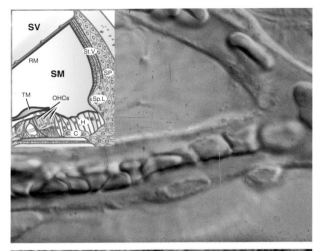

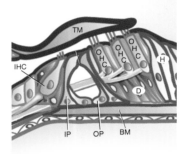

Figure 15-2. (Left) Normal stereocilia. Note that the *V* points toward stria vascularis. (Middle and right) Noise-damaged OHC stereocilia. Note that the orderly organization is disrupted and that individual stereocilia are fused (page 219).

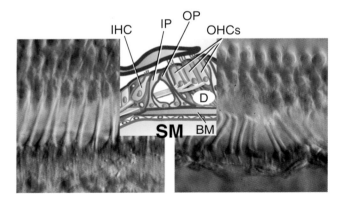

Figure 15-5. Example of structural damage to the cochlea. (Left) The inner pillar cells anchored at the basilar membrane and the top of the organ of Corti. (Right) Pillar anchorage disrupted at the top and bottom (page 221).

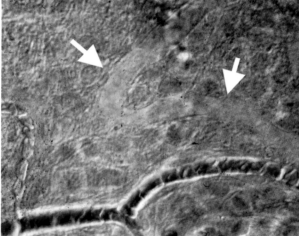

Figure 15-3. (Top) Normal stria vascularis capillary filled with red blood cells. (Bottom) Section of stria adjacent to lesion of OHCs. Note the normal capillary and the avascular channel (arrow), the space in surrounding cells left by a previously existing capillary that has degenerated (page 219).

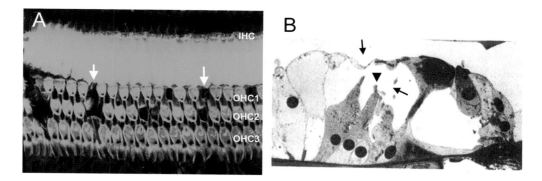

Figure 15-7. (A) Surface preparation showing missing OHCs. (B) Radial section showing missing OHCs and 8th nerve terminals. Arrows indicate the areas of missing OHCs. The arrowhead points to a stretched Deiters' cell (page 222).

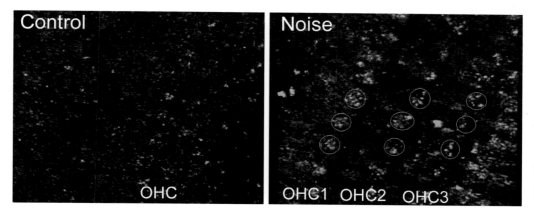

Figure 15-9. Organ of Corti labeled with dichlorofluorescein (DCF), a marker of free radical activity. (Left) In the nonexposed ear, notice a random low level of activity. (Right) A noise-exposed ear shows systematic labeling in the OHC region (page 223).

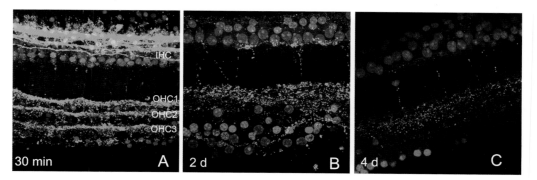

Figure 15-10. (A) DCF-labeled cochleae at 30 minutes, (B) 2 days, and (C) 4 days. Note that even at 4 days, there is still an orderly pattern of free radical labeling (page 224).

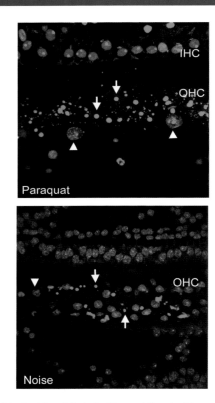

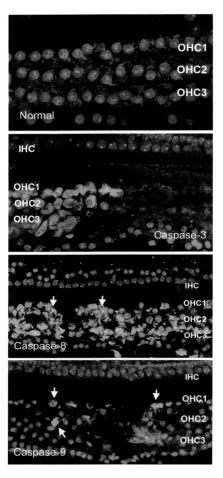

Figure 15-11. Cochleae labeled with propidium iodide, a nucleus dye. (Top) A paraquat-treated ear. (Bottom) A noise-exposed ear. Note that both treatments primarily affect the OHC region. Arrows show apoptotic OHCs. Arrowheads show necrotic OHCs (page 224).

Figure 15-13. Noise-exposed cochlea colabeled with propidium iodide to mark cells in apoptosis and dyes that label either the effector caspases (caspases-3) or the initiator caspases (caspases-8 or caspases-9) (page 225).

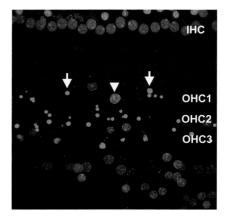

Figure 15-12. Section of organ of Corti 1 hour after exposure to damaging noise. Note the two classes of dying OHCs—apoptotic with a condensed nucleus (arrows) and necrotic with a swollen nucleus (arrowhead) (page 225).

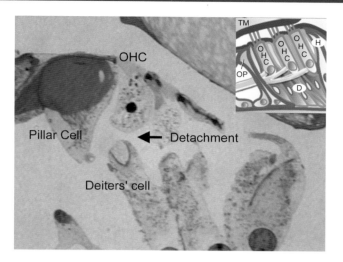

Figure 15-15. A radial section of the organ of Corti 15 minutes after an impulse noise exposure. Notice the separation of Deiters' cell cup and OHCs (page 226).

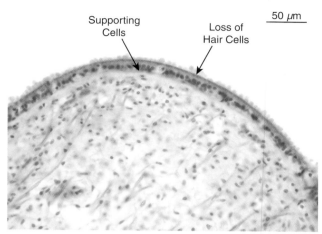

Figure 17-1b. Comparable cross section of a horizontal semicircular canal crista from a fifty-three-year old male who received 1 gm of Streptomycin by systemic administration every day for 10 days at the age of forty-seven. Following this medication, he became ataxic and developed oscillopsia. There was no response to ice water caloric testing in either ear. Histologic studies show a severe loss of hair cells in all cristae of both ears. Postmortem time was 11 hours. (Images courtesy of Saumil N. Merchant, M.D., Otopathology Laboratory, Massachusetts Eye and Ear Infirmary and Harvard Medical School, Boston, MA.) (page 256).

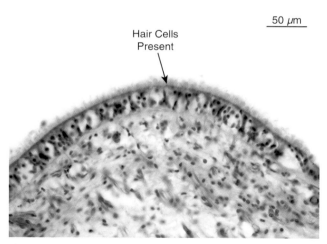

Figure 17-1a. Cross section of the horizontal semicircular canal crista from a patient with no known inner ear disease. Postmortem time was 19 hours (page 256).

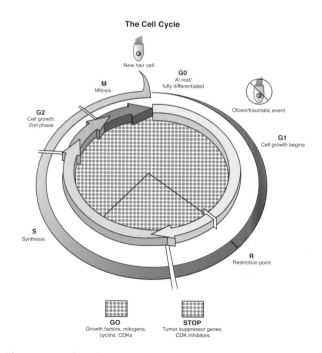

Figure 20-4. The cell cycle (page 306).

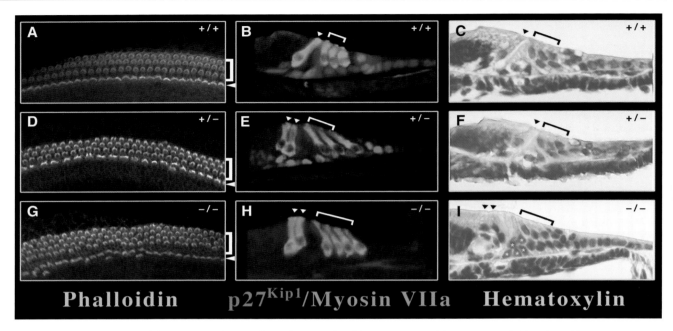

Phalloidin   p27$^{\text{Kip1}}$/Myosin VIIa   Hematoxylin

Figure 20-5. A comparison of the structure of organ of Corti from p27$^{+/+}$ wild-type (A–C), p27$^{+/-}$ heterozygous (D–F) and p27$^{-/-}$ homozygous mutant (G–I) mice, age P6 (page 309).

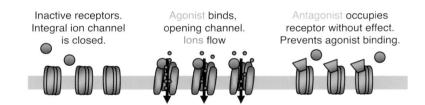

Inactive receptors. Integral ion channel is closed.

Agonist binds, opening channel. Ions flow

Antagonist occupies receptor without effect. Prevents agonist binding.

Figure 21-2. Ionotropic (ligand-gated) receptors (page 323).

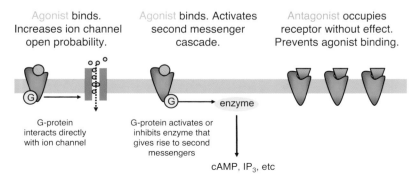

Agonist binds. Increases ion channel open probability.

Agonist binds. Activates second messenger cascade.

Antagonist occupies receptor without effect. Prevents agonist binding.

G-protein interacts directly with ion channel

G-protein activates or inhibits enzyme that gives rise to second messengers

enzyme

cAMP, IP$_3$, etc

Figure 21-3. Metabotropic (G-protein coupled) receptors (page 323).

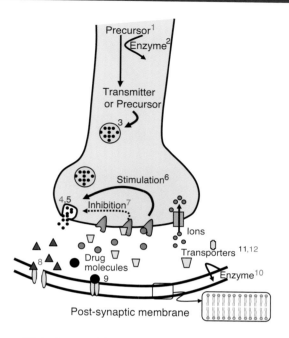

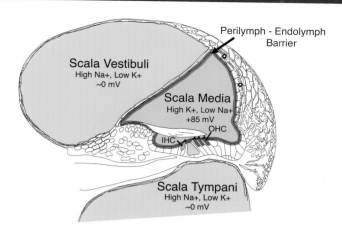

Figure 21-5. Fluid spaces in the cochlea (page 326).

Figure 21-4. Drug modulation of synaptic transmission. This can occur through interference with chemical precursors[1] or enzymes[2] required for transmitter manufacture. interference with packaging and storing transmitter or precursors in vesicles[3], stimulating[4] or inhibiting[5] vesicle fusion and transmitter release, activating[6] or blocking[7] presynaptic autoreceptors, activating[8] or blocking[9] postsynaptic receptors for the transmitter, interfering with enzymes[10] required for breakdown of the released transmitter, or enhancing[11] or interfering[12] with transporters required for reuptake and recycling of the by-products. Drugs that interfere with transmission are coded in **red**; those that facilitate transmission, in **black**. (Adapted from Jackson) (page 324).

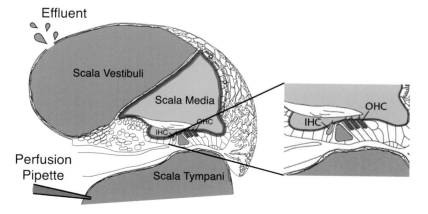

Figure 21-6. Schematic of the cochlear perfusion (page 328).

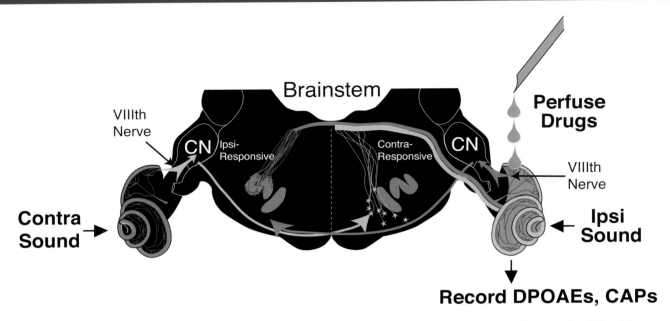

Figure 21-9. Schematic of the medial olivocochlear (MOC) reflex pathway to one ear, showing the afferent inputs (gray arrow) and the origins and projections of ipsilaterally- and contralaterally-responsive MOC units. (Figure after Brown et al. 1998) (page 334).

CHAPTER
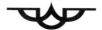
12

Renal Function and Ototoxicity of Loop Diuretics

Leonard P. Rybak, MD, PhD
Southern Illinois University School of Medicine
Springfield, IL

INTRODUCTION

The high-ceiling diuretics have extremely potent effects on the kidney, resulting in excretion of a large volume of water and electrolytes in the urine. Those agents have a distinctive action in that the main site of action is on the thick ascending limb of the loop of Henle of the kidney (Figure 12-1). The members of this class of diuretics include ethacrynic acid, furosemide, bumetanide, and torsemide. Other compounds are in use in other countries. Loop diuretics are the mainstay of the treatment of patients with various disorders associated with fluid overload, such as congestive heart failure and renal failure. The four loop diuretics currently on the market in the United States include ethacrynic acid, furosemide, bumetanide, and torsemide (Wall et al., 2003).

MECHANISM OF DIURETIC ACTION

The diuretics ethacrynic acid, furosemide, bumetanide, and torsemide inhibit the reabsorption of electrolytes in the thick ascending limb of the loop of Henle. The receptor for those diuretics is the Na-K-2Cl transporter on the luminal membrane of the epithelial cells in the loop of Henle. That protein has been cloned and sequenced. It is a protein with a core molecular weight of 121 kDa, consisting of twelve membrane-spanning domains (Obermuller et al., 1996; Haas & Forbush, 2000). Loop diuretics bind to transmembrane domains of the transporter. The loop diuretics vary in their selectivity for this receptor based on three factors:

1. The renal Na-K-2Cl transporter has a greater affinity for bumetanide than does the transporter present in other tissues.

2. Differences are likely to exist in the access of loop diuretics to the site where the transporter is expressed; and since all loop diuretics exhibit a high degree of binding to albumin, active secretion of the drug into the lumen of the kidney must occur to allow access to the Na-K-2Cl transporter.

3. After secretion into the proximal tubule of the kidney, the drug must concentrate at the site of action in the thick ascending limb of the loop of Henle. It is important to note that the expression of the transporter can be influenced by a variety of factors (Shankar & Brater, 2003).

PHARMACOKINETICS

Loop diuretics arrive at the Na-K-2Cl receptor in the luminal membrane of the ascending limb of the loop of Henle after active tubular secretion from blood into urine within the proximal tubule (Odlind & Beermann, 1980). The degree of glomerular filtration is extremely limited because of the extensive binding of the drugs to albumin in serum (>95%). That binding allows delivery of the drug via the plasma to the proximal tubule. There organic secretory sites "strip" the diuretic from albumin and transport it across the cell and deposit it into the lumen, from which it flows downstream to gain access to the receptors in the luminal membrane of the epithelial cells of the ascending limb of the loop of Henle (Shankar & Brater, 2003; Hassanejad et al., 2004).

Ethacrynic acid was the first clinically utilized loop diuretic. It was discovered by rational design (Cragoe, 1983). Limited data are available on the pharmacokinetics of ethacrynic acid (Shankar & Brater, 2003).

Fifty percent of furosemide administered is excreted unchanged into the urine as active drug (Beerman, 1984; Brater, 1998). The other half is conjugated to glucuronic acid in the kidney (Pichette & du Souich, 1996). Patients with renal failure have a prolonged half-life of furosemide because both urinary excretion and renal conjugation are reduced (Beerman, 1984). About one-half of an orally administered dose of furosemide is absorbed (range 10%–100%). The elimination half-life is 1.5–2 hours in healthy individuals, but is prolonged to 2.5 hours in the presence of liver disease and to 2.8 hours in people with liver disease (Shankar & Brater, 2003). Furosemide administered to pregnant women readily crosses the placenta (Beerman et al., 1978).

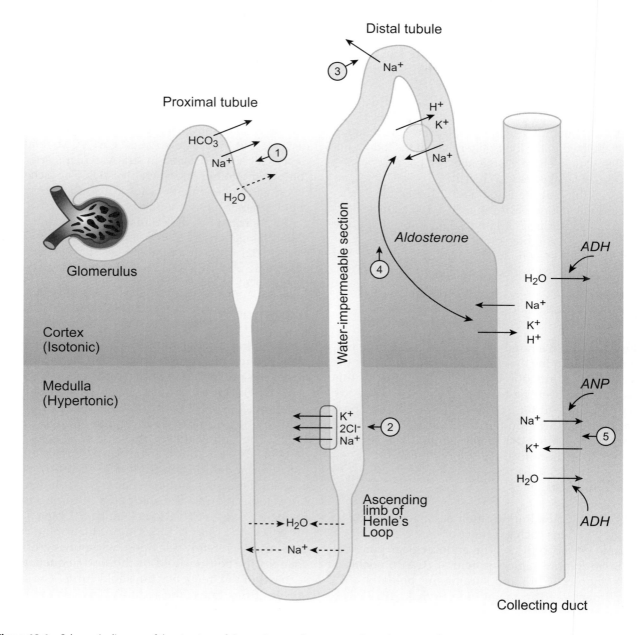

Figure 12-1. Schematic diagram of the structure of the nephron to demonstrate the various sites of action of diuretic agents. The carbonic anhydrase inhibitors (e.g., acetazolamide) and osmotic diuretics act on the proximal tubule (site 1). Loop diuretics such as furosemide act on the ascending limb of the loop of Henle (site 2). The thiazides act on the distal tubule to block absorption of sodium (site 3). Aldosterone antagonists block the actions of the hormone aldosterone in the distal tubule (site 4). Other potassium-sparing diuretics act in the collecting duct to block the entry of potassium from the circulating blood into the lumen of the collecting duct (site 5). ADH is antidiuretic hormone and ANP is atrial natriuretic peptide.

Both bumetanide and torsemide are extensively metabolized. Like furosemide, about 50% of a dose of bumetanide is metabolized. On the other hand, about 80% of a torsemide dose is metabolized. Both of those diuretics are metabolized in the liver rather than in the kidney. Between 80% and 100% of an oral dose of bumetanide is absorbed. Its elimination half-life is short, only 1 hour in healthy people. Since bumetanide is metabolized in the liver rather than in the kidney, its half-life is only slightly prolonged to 1.6 hours in the presence of renal disease. When liver disease is present, however, the half-life is 2.3 hours. Torsemide is also well absorbed after oral dosing (80%–100%). In healthy subjects, the half-life is 3–4 hours. Like bumetanide, the half-life is only slightly prolonged in the presence of renal disease to 4–5 hours; but with liver disease, the half-life is doubled to 8 hours (Shankar & Brater, 2003).

OTOTOXICITY

There have been a number of studies in experimental animals to examine the effects of loop diuretics on the structure and function of the cochlea. Most of this research has been performed in rodents. They are helpful in providing insights into how these drugs could affect hearing in humans. Most of these were short-term studies that demonstrated a reversible effect of loop diuretics on auditory function.

Ethacrynic Acid

After parenteral administration of ethacrynic acid to animals, various cochlear functions are reduced for a variable period of time. The endocochlear potential (EP), compound action potential (CAP), cochlear microphonics (CM), and summating potential (SP) are all decreased in magnitude (Rybak, 1993). The recovery of the cochlear potentials appears to follow a very gradual time course, which parallels the persistent edema of the stria vascularis that is observed (Brummett et al., 1977). Although CM and EP decrease in parallel in experimental animals receiving ethacrynic acid, the CM may recover more rapidly (Komune & Morimitsu, 1985). Ototoxic doses of ethacrynic acid have been shown to reduce the

potassium gradient between endolymph and perilymph (Melichar & Syka, 1978).

The effects of intravenous ethacrynic acid on the blood flow in the chinchilla cochlea have been studied. Microcirculation changes in the lateral wall blood vessels were seen. Vessels in the spiral ligament and stria vascularis were devoid of red blood cells at 30 minutes after injection. Those changes were accompanied by decline, but not recovery, of CAP, CM, and SP. Reperfusion was delayed in stria vascularis arterioles compared to other lateral wall vessels. The ischemia-reperfusion phenomenon caused by ethacrynic acid could generate large amounts of free radicals that trigger or contribute to the cellular pathologic and functional changes observed in this study and others (Ding et al., 2002). Ultrastructural studies have shown that ethacrynic acid causes edema of the stria vascularis (Matz, 1976).

Furosemide

Systemic injection of furosemide in the guinea pig was found to reduce the EP (Chodynicki & Kostrzewska, 1974) in a dose-related manner (Green et al., 1981). This effect was typically a reversible phenomenon. CM were found to be reduced in the cat following furosemide administration (Mathog et al., 1970). The amplitude of the eighth nerve action potential (N_1) is reduced in various mammals following furosemide injection (Brown et al., 1979). Single unit studies of the auditory nerve have shown that furosemide reduces the sharpness of tuning in the frequency range of 7–30 kHz (Klinke & Evans, 1974). In the cat, the sharply tuned tip of the tuning curve was also reversibly elevated without significant changes in the threshold of the low-frequency tail segment of the frequency threshold curve. The spontaneous firing rate of the auditory nerve was reduced in proportion to the degree of reduction of EP. The threshold was elevated about 1 dB for every millivolt reduction in EP (Sewell, 1984). However, suppression tuning curves of distortion-product otoacoustic emissions in rabbits behaved differently following diuretic treatment compared to their neural counterparts (Martin et al., 1998). Furosemide was found to reversibly alter the response of the chinchilla basilar membrane to tones and clicks. The response-magnitude reductions were largest at low stimulus intensities at the characteristic frequency and small to negligible at high intensities and at frequencies far removed from the characteristic frequency. Furosemide also caused response-phase lags that were largest at low stimulus intensities and were limited to frequencies close to the characteristic frequency (Ruggero & Rich, 1991). Furosemide can also directly alter the motility of outer hair cells by affecting their nonlinear capacitance (Santos-Sacchi et al., 2001).

Chronic reductions of the EP in gerbils by application of continuous doses of furosemide to the round window were used to produce a model for metabolic presbycusis (Schmiedt et al., 2002; Mills & Schmiedt, 2004). In comparing the threshold for distortion product otoacoustic emissions (DPOAEs) with the ABR threshold, the following observations were made:

1. The mean increase in DPOAE threshold was about 55% of the increase in ABR threshold.

2. The primary dysfunction in metabolic presbycusis appears to be a decrease in the gain of the cochlear amplifier, combined with an additional smaller increase in neural threshold, both caused by a chronically reduced EP.

3. For ABR threshold increases above 20 dB, the points for the chronically low EP condition were largely separate from those previously reported for acoustic trauma (Mills & Schmiedt, 2004).

Morphologic studies in animals have shown a good correlation between edema of the stria vascularis and reductions in EP (Pike & Bosher, 1980; Rybak, 1993). Most studies have not shown hair cell damage in furosemide-treated animals. Recovery of the EP following chronic furosemide application to the round window was accompanied by an increase in fibrocyte turnover in the spiral ligament. Thus, fibrocyte proliferation may maintain the EP and cochlear function in normal and damaged cochleas (Lang, et al., 2003).

Neonatal rats appear to be more sensitive to furosemide than do their adult counterparts. Rat pups from 9–28 days were found to have a greater reduction of EP and elevation of CAP thresholds than rats older than 30 days. Animals with substantial reductions of

EP also had significant edema of the stria vascularis. On the other hand, rats with little or no changes in EP after furosemide had no significant alteration of the ultrastructure of the stria vascularis (Rybak et al., 1991). The administration of furosemide at the recommended dosing intervals of 12 hours in premature infants could lead to the accumulation of furosemide to potentially ototoxic plasma concentrations (Chemtob, et al., 1987; Mirochnick et al., 1990).

Bumetanide

Bumetanide causes a reduction of the EP in experimental animals with a very steep dose-response curve (Kusakari et al., 1978; Rybak et al., 1991). The CAP is correspondingly elevated (Gottl et al., 1985). Ultrastructural studies show edema of the stria vascularis (Santi & Duvall, 1979), which may result from an imbalance between the activities of the Na-K-2Cl cotransporter and Na-K-ATPase activity in the stria vascularis (Azuma et al., 2002).

Torsemide

Torsemide was tested for ototoxicity in cats. The dose that caused a hearing loss in 50% of animals (TD 50) was determined. The TD 50 was calculated at 20.8 mg/kg, which was slightly higher than that determined for furosemide (18.37 mg/kg). Hearing function tended to recover after the acute effect. The main metabolite of torsemide in humans (1-isopropyl-3-([[(3-carboxy-anilino)-3-pyridyl] sulfonyl) urea, M5) showed no ototoxic effect even in very high doses. Even in animals pretreated with doses higher than the TD 50, there was no sign of permanent hearing impairment (Klinke & Mertens, 1988).

MECHANISMS OF OTOTOXICITY

The strial marginal cells possess the Na-K-2Cl cotransporter in the basolateral membrane that is an isoform (SLC12A2) of the transporter expressed exclusively in the apical membrane of the thick ascending limb of the loop of Henle in the kidney (SLC12A1). This transporter has been linked to potassium secretion in the marginal cells of the stria vascularis (Wangemann, 2002). Immunohistochemical studies have confirmed the localization of this transporter (Crouch et al., 1997; Goto et al., 1997; Mizuta et al., 1997). The findings were confirmed using reverse transcriptase-polymerase chain reaction of the messenger RNA from the rat cochlear lateral wall (Ikeda et al., 1997). Mice lacking this transporter were found to have collapse of the endolymphatic spaces because of the inability of strial marginal cells and dark cells in the vestibular system to secrete potassium and reabsorptive processes continuing unchecked. That results in deafness in the mice (Flagella et al., 1999). The mice exhibit classic shaker-waltzer behavior (deafness and imbalance), indicating inner ear defects (Delpire et al., 1999). Temporary inhibition of this transporter in the inner ear by loop diuretics can cause transient deafness by reducing the EP generated by the stria vascularis (Ikeda et al., 1997; Delpire et al., 1999; Flagella et al., 1999; Wangemann, 2002). Studies with cochlear explants to which furosemide was added demonstrated the production of hydroxyl free radicals that can damage cochlear membranes and tissues (Clerici et al., 1996).

CLINICAL STUDIES OF OTOTOXICITY

A number of clinical reports about the ototoxicity of loop diuretics have appeared in the literature. These publications have demonstrated that each of the loop diuretics except for torsemide have been shown to cause hearing loss in humans. Newborn infants are particularly sensitive to the ototoxic effects of loop diuretics. Both temporary and permanent hearing loss have been reported in patients, as described below.

Ethacrynic Acid

Soon after the introduction of ethacrynic acid into clinical medicine, numerous reports of acute transient deafness appeared in the literature (Rybak, 1993). Later, cases of permanent deafness were published (Mathog & Klein, 1969; Pillay et al., 1969; Meriwether et al., 1971; Matz, 1976; Rybak, 1988). Most of those incidents occurred in the presence of renal failure. A cooperative study reported that the incidence of deafness associated with ethacrynic acid administration was 7 patients per 1,000 (Boston, 1973).

Human temporal bone studies demonstrated edematous changes in the stria vascularis (Matz, 1976). An ultrastructural study of the temporal bones of a patient experiencing ototoxicity from ethacrynic acid and furosemide also revealed marked edema in the stria vascularis (Arnold et al., 1981). Loss of outer hair cells in the basal turn of the cochlea has been demonstrated in human temporal bone histopathologic studies (Federspil & Mausen, 1973; Matz, 1976).

Furosemide

As with ethacrynic acid, furosemide was found to cause reversible sensorineural hearing loss soon after it was introduced into clinical practice (Rybak, 1993). Infusion of furosemide at a constant rate of 25 mg/min resulted in marked hearing loss in two-thirds of patients. When the infusion rate was slowed to 15 mg/min in patients with severe renal failure, only minor hearing losses were observed. The authors recommended that furosemide should be administered intravenously at a rate not exceeding 4 mg/min to avoid hearing loss (Heidland & Wigand, 1970). Audiometric studies of patients receiving high doses of furosemide by rapid intravenous infusion (1000 mg in 40 minutes) demonstrated reversible hearing loss in half of the patients, with greatest losses measured in the middle frequency range (Wigand & Heidland, 1971). A comparison of the incidence of hearing loss (audiometric changes) in patients receiving furosemide to those receiving bumetanide was carried out. Pure-tone thresholds were elevated at least 15 dB in 6.4% of furosemide-treated patients, as opposed to 1.1% of those receiving bumetanide (Tuzel, 1981). A database of random-controlled trials of bolus injection versus continuous infusion in patients with congestive heart failure revealed greater diuresis and a statistically significant reduction or risk of tinnitus and hearing loss in patients receiving continuous infusion of loop diuretics (Salvador et al., 2004).

Permanent deafness after furosemide administration has been reported in several publications (Lloyd-Mostyn & Lord, 1971; Brown et al., 1974; Quick & Hoppe, 1975; Keefe, 1978; Rifkin et al., 1978; Gallagher & Jones, 1979).

The administration of furosemide at the recommended dosing intervals of 12 hours in premature infants could lead to the accumulation of furosemide to potentially ototoxic plasma concentrations (Chemtob et al., 1987; Mirochnick et al., 1990). Sensorineural hearing loss in neonates followed long-term with serial ABR testing and confirmed by behavioral testing was found to be statistically associated with greater amounts of furosemide administered for longer periods and in combination with aminoglycoside antibiotics (Salamy et al., 1989). A multivariate analysis of human neonates treated with ototoxic drugs and tested with serial ABR revealed that exposure only to furosemide was a significant risk factor for hearing loss (Brown et al., 1991).

Bumetanide

Bumetanide has been reported to be 40–60 times as potent as furosemide (Friedman & Roch-Ramel, 1977). Hearing loss was reported in a patient who was treated with 1 mg of bumetanide daily for 2 weeks (Asano et al., 1974). However, another patient who complained of hearing loss after furosemide administration recovered hearing when bumetanide was substituted for furosemide (Bourke, 1976). A prospective study of patients receiving bumetanide looked at their high-frequency audiograms (8–20 kHz) before and after treatment with fixed low doses of bumetanide. No change in hearing was detected (Fausti et al., 1979). Two of 179 patients treated with bumetanide had at least a 15 dB elevation of pure-tone audiometric thresholds (Tuzel, 1981).

Torsemide

No evidence of ototoxicity has been demonstrated with the use of torsemide in humans (Dunn, et al., 1995).

SUMMARY

Each of the loop diuretics, with the exception of torsemide, has been associated with experimental and clinical evidence of hearing loss. In most cases, the ototoxicity is temporary and recovers within a short time.

However, many cases of permanent hearing loss have been reported in the literature. The ototoxicity may be associated with binding of the diuretic drug to a receptor in the stria vascularis that is similar to the receptor in the loop of Henle of the kidney that mediates the diuretic effect, namely, the Na-K-2Cl co-transporter. Inhibition of this transporter in the cochlea may cause edema to develop within the stria vascularis, which is a typical finding in experimental studies of loop diuretic ototoxicity and has been confirmed in human temporal bone studies of tissues from patients who experienced ototoxicity from loop diuretics just before death. Most of the permanent cases of loop diuretic ototoxicity occurred in patients with advanced kidney failure. In those patients, the blood levels of the diuretic could have reached ototoxic levels. The ototoxicity of loop diuretics may be reduced by administering the drug more slowly, rather than by rapid injection. Future studies should be done to confirm the lack of ototoxicity of the loop diuretic torsemide.

REFERENCES

Arnold, W., Nadol, J. B., Jr., & Geidauer, H. (1981). Ultrastructural histopathology in a case of human ototoxicity due to loop diuretics. *Acta Otolaryngol, 91*, 391–414.

Asano, Y., Masuzawa, H., Tabata, Y., et al. (1974). Clinical trial of bumetanide. *Basic Pharmacol Ther, 2*, 47–54.

Azuma, H., Takeuchi, S., Higashiyama, K., Ando, M., Kakigi, A., Nakahira, M., Yamakawa, K., & Takeda, T. (2002). Bumetanide-induced enlargement of the intercellular space in the stria vascularis requires an active Na+-K+-ATPase. *Acta Otolaryngol, 122*, 816–821.

Beerman, B., Groschinsky-Grind, M., Fahraeus, I., & Lindstrom, B. (1978). Placental transfer of furosemide. *Clin Pharmacol Ther, 24*, 560–562.

Beerman, B. (1984). Aspects on pharmacokinetics of some diuretics. *Acta Pharmacol Toxicol, 54*, 17–32.

Boston Collaborative Drug Surveillance Program. (1973). Drug-induced deafness: A cooperative study. *JAMA, 224*, 516–517.

Bourke, E. (1976). Furosemide, bumetanide and ototoxicity. *Lancet, 1,* 917–918.

Brater, D. C. (1998). Diuretic therapy. *N Engl J Med, 339,* 387–395.

Brown, C. G., Ogg, C. S., Cameron, J. S., et al. (1974). High dose furosemide in acute reversible intrinsic renal failure. *Scott Med J, 19*(Suppl), 35–38.

Brown, D. R., Watchko, J. F., & Sabo, D. (1991). Neonatal sensorineural hearing loss associated with furosemide: A case control study. *Dev Med Child Neurol, 33,* 816–823.

Brown, R. D., Manno, J. E., Daigneault, E. A., et al. (1979). Comparative acute ototoxicity of intravenous bumetanide and furosemide in the purebred beagle. *Toxicol Appl Pharmacol, 48,* 157–169.

Brummett, R., Smith, C. A., Ueno, Y., et al. (1977). The delayed effects of ethacrynic acid on the stria vascularis of the guinea pig. *Acta Otolaryngol, 83,* 98–112.

Chemtob, S., Papageorgiou, A., DuSouich, P., & Aranda, J. V. (1987). Cumulative increase in serum furosemide concentration following repeated doses in the newborn. *Am J Perinatol, 4,* 203–205.

Chodynicki, S., & Kostrzewska, A. (1974). Effects of furosemide and ethacrynic acid on endolymph potential in guinea pigs. *Otolaryngol Pol, 28,* 5–8.

Clerici, W. J., Hensley, K., DiMartino, D. L., & Butterfield, D. A. (1996). Direct detection of ototoxicant-induced reactive oxygen species generation in cochlear explants. *Hear Res, 98,* 116–124.

Cragoe, E. J., Jr. (1983). *Diuretics: Chemistry, Pharmacology, and Medicine* (pp. 201–266). New York: John Wiley and Sons.

Crouch, J. J., Sakaguchi, N., Lytle, C., & Schulte, B. A. (1997). Immunohistochemical localization of the Na-K-Cl co-transporter (NKCCl) in the gerbil inner ear. *J Histochem Cytochem, 45,* 773–778.

Delpire, E., Lu, J., England, R., Dull, C., & Thorne, T. (1999). Deafness and imbalance associated with inactivation of the secretory Na-K-2Cl-cotransporter. *Nature Genetics, 22,* 192–195.

Ding, D., McFadden, S. L., Woo, J. M., & Salvi, R. J. (2002). Ethacrynic acid rapidly and selectively abolishes blood flow in vessels supplying the lateral wall of the cochlea. *Hear Res, 173,* 1–9.

Dunn, C. J., Fitton, A., & Brogden, R. N. (1995). Torasemide. An update of its pharmacological properties and therapeutic efficacy. *Drugs, 49,* 121–142.

Fausti, S. A., Frey, R. H., Rappaport, B. Z., et al. (1979). An investigation of the effect of bumetanide on high frequency (8-20 kHz) hearing in humans. *J Aud Res, 19,* 243–250.

Federspil, P., & Mausen, H. (1973). Experimentelle Untersuchungen zur Ototoxicität des Furosemids. *Res Exp Med, 161,* 175–184.

Flagella, M., Clarke, L. L., Miller, M. L., Erway, L. C., Giannella, R. A., Andringa, A., Gawenis, L. R., Kramer, J., Duffy, J. J., Doetschman, T., Lorenz, J. N., Yamoah, E., Cardell, E. L., & Shull, G. E. (1999). Mice lacking the basolateral Na-K-2Cl cotransporter have impaired epithelial chloride secretion and are profoundly deaf. *J Biol Chem, 274,* 26946–26955.

Friedman, P. A., & Roch-Ramel, F. (1977). Hemodynamic and natriuretic effects of bumetanide in the cat. *J Pharmacol Exp Ther, 203,* 82–91.

Gallagher, K. L., & Jones, J. K. (1979). Furosemide-induced ototoxicity. *Ann Intern Med, 91,* 744–745.

Goettl, K. H., Roesch, A., & Klinke, R. (1985). Quantitative evaluation of ototoxic side effects of furosemide, piretanide, bumetanide, azosemide and ozolinone in the cat—a new approach to the problem of ototoxicity. *Naunyn Schmiedebergs Arch Pharmacol, 331,* 275–282.

Goto, S., Oshima, T., Ikeda, K., Ueda, N., & Takasaka, T. (1997). Expression and localization of the Na-K-2Cl cotransporter in the rat cochlea. *Brain Res, 765,* 324–326.

Green, T. P., Rybak, L. P., Mirkin, B. L., et al. (1981). Pharmacologic determinants of ototoxicity of furosemide in the chinchilla. *J Pharmacol Exp Ther, 216,* 537–542.

Haas, M., & Forbush, B. III. (2000). The Na-K-Cl cotransporter of secretory epithelia. *Annu Rev Physiol, 62,* 515–534.

Hasannejad, H., Takeda, M., Taki, K., Shin, H. J., Babu, E., Jutabha, P., et al. (2004). Interactions of human organic anion transporters with diuretics. *J Pharmacol Exp Ther, 308,* 1021–1029.

Heidland, H., & Wigand, M. E. (1970). The effect of furosemide at high doses on auditory sensitivity in patients with uremia. *Klin Wochenschr, 48,* 1052–1056.

Ikeda, K., Oshima, T., Hidaka, H., & Takasaka, T. (1997). Molecular and clinical implications of loop diuretic ototoxicity. *Hear Res, 107,* 1–8.

Keefe, P. E. (1978). Ototoxicity from oral furosemide. *Drug Intell Clin Pharm, 12,* 428.

Klinke, R., & Evans, E. F. (1974). The effects of drugs on the sharpness of tuning of single cochlear nerve fibers. *Pflugers Arch, 347*(Suppl.), R53.

Klinke, R, & Mertens, M. (1988). Quantitative assessment of torasemide ototoxicity. *Arzneimittelforsch, 38,* 153–155.

Komune, S., & Morimitsu, T. (1985). Dissociation of the cochlear microphonics and endocochlear potential after ethacrynic acid injection. *Arch Otorhinolaryngol, 241,* 149–156.

Kusakari, J., Kambayashi, J., Ise, I., et al. (1978). Reduction of the endocochlear potential by the new "loop" diuretic bumetanide. *Acta Otolaryngol, 86,* 336–342.

Lang, H., Schulte, B. A., & Schmiedt, R. A. (2003). Effects of chronic furosemide treatment and age on cell division in the adult gerbil inner ear. *J Assoc Res Otolaryngol, 4,* 164–175.

Lloyd-Mostyn, R. M., & Lord, I. J. (1971). Ototoxicity of intravenous furosemide. *Lancet, 2,* 1156.

Martin, G. K., Jassir, D., Stagner, B. B., & Lonsbury-Martin, B. L. (1998). Effects of loop diuretics on the suppression tuning of distortion-product otoacoustic emissions in rabbits. *J Acoust Soc Am, 104,* 972–983.

Mathog, R. H., & Klein, W. J. (1969). Ototoxicity of ethacrynic acid and aminoglycoside antibiotics in uremia. *N Engl J Med, 280,* 1223–1224.

Mathog, R. H., Thomas, W. G., & Hudson, W. R. (1970). Ototoxicity of new and potent diuretics. *Arch Otolaryngol, 92,* 7–13.

Matz, G. J. (1976). The ototoxic effects of ethacrynic acid in man and animals. *Laryngoscope, 86,* 1065–1086.

Melichar, I., & Syka, J. (1978). The effects of ethacrynic acid upon the potassium concentration in guinea pig inner ear fluids. *Hear Res, 1,* 35–42.

Meriwether, W. D., Mangi, R. I., & Serpick, A. A. (1971). Deafness following standard intravenouse dose of ethacrynic acid. *JAMA, 216,* 795–798.

Mills, D. M., & Schmiedt, R. A. (2004). Metabolic presbycusis: Differential changes in auditory brainstem and otoacoustic emission responses with chronic furosemide application in the gerbil. *J Assoc Res Otolaryngol, 5,* 1–10.

Mirochnick, M. H., Micelli, J. J., Kramer, P. A., et al. (1990). Decreased renal response to furosemide in very low birth weight infants during chronic administration. *Dev Pharmacol Ther, 15,* 1–8.

Mizuta, K., Adachi, M., & Iwasa, K. H. (1997). Ultrastructural localization of the Na-K-Cl-cotransporter in the lateral wall of the cochlear duct. *Hear Res, 106,* 154–162.

Obermuller, N., Kunchaparty, S., Ellison, D. H., & Bachmann, S. (1996). Expression of the Na-K-2Cl cotransporter by macula densa and thick ascending limb cells of rat and rabbit nephron. *J Clin Invest, 98,* 635–640.

Odlind, B., & Beermann, B. (1980). Renal tubular secretion and effects of furosemide. *Clin Pharmacol Ther, 27,* 784–790.

Pichette, V., & du Souich, P. (1996). Role of the kidneys in the metabolism of furosemide: Its inhibition by probenecid. *J Am Soc Nephrol, 7,* 345–349.

Pike, D., & Bosher, S. K. (1980). The time course of the strial changes produced by intravenous furosemide. *Hear Res, 3,* 79–89.

Pillay, V. K., Schwartz, F. D., Aimi, K., et al. (1969). Transient and permanent deafness following treatment with ethacrynic acid in renal failure. *Lancet, 1,* 77–79.

Quick, C. A., & Hoppe, W. (1975). Permanent deafness associated with furosemide administration. *Ann Otol Rhinol Laryngol, 84,* 94–101.

Rifkin, S. I., DeQuesada, A. M., Pickering, M. J., et al. (1978). Deafness associated with oral furosemide. *South Med J, 71,* 86–88.

Ruggero, M. A., & Rich, N. C. (1991). Furosemide alters the organ of Corti mechanics: Evidence for feedback of outer hair cells upon the basilar membrane. *J Neurosci, 11,* 1057–1067.

Rybak, L. P. (1988). Ototoxicity of ethacrynic acid (a persistent clinical problem). *J Laryngol Otol, 102,* 518–520.

Rybak, L. P. (1993). Ototoxicity of loop diuretics. *Otolaryngol Clin N Am, 26,* 829–844.

Rybak, L. P., Whitworth, C., & Scott, V. (1991). Comparative acute ototoxicity of loop diuretic compounds. *Eur Arch Oto-Rhino-Laryngol, 248,* 353–357.

Rybak, L. P., Whitworth, C., Scott, V., et al. (1991). Ototoxicity of furosemide during development. *Laryngoscope, 101,* 1167–1174.

Salamy, A., Eldredge, L., & Tooley, W. H. (1989). Neonatal status and hearing loss in high risk infants. *J Pediatr, 114,* 847–852.

Salvador, D. R., Rey, N. R., Ramos, G. C., & Punzlan, F. E. (2004). Continuous infusion versus bolus injection of loop diuretics in congestive heart failure. *Cochrane Database Syst Rev* (1): CD003178.

Santi, P. A., & Duvall, A. J. III. (1979). Morphological alteration of the stria vascularis after administration of the diuretic bumetanide. *Acta Otolaryngol, 88,* 1–12.

Santos-Sacchi, J., Wu, M., & Kakehata, S. (2001). Furosemide alters nonlinear capacitance in isolated outer hair cells. *Hear Res, 159,* 69 –73.

Schmiedt, R. A., Lang, H., Okamura, H., & Schulte, B. A. (2002). Effects of furosemide applied chronically to the round window: A model of metabolic presbycusis. *J Neurosci, 22,* 9643–9650.

Sewell, W. F. (1984). The relation between the endocochlear potential and spontaneous activity in the auditory nerve fibers in the cat. *J Physiol, 347,* 685–696.

Shankar, S. S., & Brater, D. C. (2003). Loop diuretics: From the Na-K-2Cl transporter to clinical use. *Am J Physiol Renal Physiol, 284,* F11–F21.

Tuzel, I. H. (1981). Comparison of adverse reactions to bumetanide and furosemide. *J Clin Pharmacol, 21,* 615–619.

Wall, G. C., Bigner, D., & Craig, S. (2003). Ethacrynic acid and the sulfa sensitive patient. *Arch Intern Med, 163,* 116–117.

Wangemann, P. (2002). K+ cycling and the endocochlear potential. *Hear Res, 165,* 1–9.

Wigand, M. D., & Heidland, A. (1971). Ototoxic side effects of high doses of furosemide in patients with uremia. *Postgrad Med J, 47*(Suppl.), 54–56.

CHAPTER
13

Other Ototoxins: Aspirin and Other Nonsteroidal Anti-inflammatory Drugs, Quinine, and Macrolides

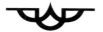

Brenda L. Lonsbury-Martin, PhD
Division of Otolaryngology, Department of Surgery
Loma Linda University School of Medicine
Loma Linda, CA

Glen K. Martin, PhD
Division of Otolaryngology, Department of Surgery
Loma Linda University School of Medicine
Loma Linda, CA
and
Jerry Pettis Memorial Veterans Medical Center
Loma Linda, CA

Acknowledgments: This work was supported in part by funds from the National Institutes of Health (DC00613, DC03114).

INTRODUCTION

Previous chapters in this text have shown that a number of drugs taken for life-threatening infections or chemotherapy can cause ototoxic reactions that are primarily irreversible. Certain common pharmaceutical agents taken mostly for relatively minor disorders, including the aspirin and nonaspirin types of nonsteroidal anti-inflammatory drugs (NSAIDs), quinine, and the macrolide antibiotics, can result in ototoxic effects, too. Like the aminoglycoside antibiotics and some antitumor agents that typically cause irreversible ototoxicity, the NSAIDs, quinine, and the macrolides result in ototoxic side effects that usually include a bilateral high-frequency sensorineural hearing loss and tinnitus. However, the hearing problems caused by these latter types of ototoxic agents are generally temporary in that patients recover following cessation of the pharmacologic treatment. Most importantly, consistent with their reversible actions, they do not typically produce permanent structural damage to inner ear elements.

Given their reversible effects, it is not too surprising that aspirin or the salicylate category of NSAIDs, in particular, has a historical association in the investigation of the site(s) and mechanism(s) of both tinnitus and ototoxicity, using behavioral, anatomic, and physiological approaches in either humans (Wier et al., 1988) or animal subjects (Stypulkowsi, 1990). The specific research application of salicylates to the study of the fundamental basis of tinnitus is clearly based on their ability to mimic one of the classical symptoms related to reduced hearing sensitivity (Cazals, 2000). Moreover, salicylates have an appreciable history, too, in the study of the basic mechanisms of hearing in general because of their well-documented transitory effects on the sensory, neural, and mechanical aspects of cochlear transduction (Boettcher & Salvi, 1991).

In the following review, the ototoxic side effects of the aspirin and nonaspirin NSAIDs, including acetaminophen, are addressed. In addition, the related adverse effects of quinine and macrolide antibiotic treatments on inner ear function are also discussed. Finally, what is currently known about the underlying fundamental mechanisms of action that bring about such transitory ototoxic effects is considered. See Table 13-1 for a list of common abbreviations and acronyms that are used throughout this chapter.

SALICYLATES AND NONASPIRIN NSAIDS AND ACETAMINOPHEN

The salicylates and nonaspirin NSAIDs, including acetaminophen, make up a class of pharmacological therapeutics called non-narcotic analgesics. These over-the-counter medications are among the most commonly used medicines in the world. Although many ototoxic drugs can affect the inner ear generally (i.e., be associated with both hearing and balance problems), the salicylates and other NSAIDs, unless otherwise noted, predominantly produce a hearing-related dysfunction.

Table 13-1 Abbreviations and Acronyms

ASA	acetylsalicyclic acid
AZ	azithromycin
CL	clarithromycin
COX	cyclooxygenase
COX-1	cyclooxygenases-1
COX-2	cyclooxygenases-2
dB	decibel
ER	erythomycin
FDA	Food and Drug Administration
g	gram
HIV	human immunodeficiency virus
HL	hearing level
kHz	kilohertz
L	liter
mg	milligram
NSAID	nonsteroidal anti-inflammatory drug
OHC	outer hair cell
q.i.d.	prescriptive instruction to take medication 4 times a day

Salicylates

The salicylates are a group of pain-relieving drugs that are derivatives of salicylic acid, with aspirin or ASA being the prototypical salicylate. They come in many forms besides aspirin (e.g., Bayer Aspirin, Anacin, Bufferin, and Excedrin), including choline salicylate, magnesium salicylate, and sodium salicylate. Salicylates, like aspirin, are often used as (1) an analgesic against minor pains and aches, (2) an antipyretic against fever, (3) an anti-inflammatory against many forms of arthritis as well as soft tissue injuries (e.g., tendonitis and bursitis), and (4) an anticoagulant to prophylactically reduce the risk of strokes or heart attacks.

The dominant ototoxic effect of the chronic use of large doses of salicylates is the production of tinnitus. However, in subjects with normal hearing, either acute intoxication or long-term administration of salicylates can cause an additional ototoxic side effect in the form of a mild to moderate sensorineural hearing loss. This bilaterally symmetric hearing loss often exhibits a predominance at the high frequencies; but it can be relatively flat, too, thus affecting all frequencies about equally. Other salicylate-induced modifications of perceived sounds can include broadening of frequency filtering, alterations in temporal detection, deterioration of the ability to understand speech, and hypersensitivity to noise (Cazals, 2000). Notably, recovery from a salicylate-induced ototoxicity usually occurs within 24–72 hours after cessation of the drug.

In a classic study of salicylate toxicity by McCabe and Dey (1965), serum salicylate levels were correlated with the development of a temporary high-frequency hearing loss and tinnitus. After administering almost a gram (925 mg) of aspirin to volunteer subjects q.i.d., the subjects' hearing loss became worse in that it steadily progressed over a 5-day interval from about 4 dB after 24 hours to an average of almost 30 dB after 4 days. Moreover, increasing the dosage and duration of treatment increased the related hearing loss, although all subjects returned to baseline thresholds within 72 hours after aspirin dosing was terminated.

Other observations in rheumatoid arthritis patients, in particular, who take large doses of salicylates chronically, indicate that the onset of tinnitus typically is the initial sign of ototoxicity. However, in general, according to the results of a number of studies summarized by Jung et al. (1993), the onset of tinnitus should not be used as a predictor of serum salicylate level as ototoxic symptoms can be present in some patients at extremely low blood levels.

The acoustical characteristics of the percept of salicylate-induced tinnitus have been described as tonal and high-frequency and of mild loudness. For example, pitch matching between the tinnitus and a pure tone, which forms an important part of the standard clinical assessment of a tinnitus complaint, identified salicylate-related tinnitus at frequencies of 7–9 kHz, on average (McCabe & Dey, 1965). Other studies have indicated that loudness matching between the tinnitus and a tone at a frequency related to the tinnitus frequency, also a customary part of the tinnitus assessment battery of tests, results in a fairly homogenous distribution for levels around 8 dB HL (and seldom over 15 dB HL) in the absence of any correspondence to the subjective judgment of tinnitus intensity (Day et al., 1989). In other words, tinnitus induced by salicylates presents with the same frequency and magnitude features as does general subjective tinnitus.

It is important to note, too, that despite the fact that most reports of salicylate toxicity document reversible ototoxic effects, some cases of permanent aspirin-induced hearing loss have also been reported (Kapur, 1965; Jarvis, 1966).

Nonaspirin NSAIDs

The NSAIDs are widely used for the treatment of edema and tissue damage resulting from chronic inflammatory joint diseases such as rheumatoid arthritis, osteoarthritis, and ankylosing spondylitis. In addition to their analgesic and anti-inflammatory actions, a number of the NSAIDs have antipyretic activity and, consequently, have utility in the treatment of fever. The efficacy of the NSAIDs as anti-inflammatory, analgesic, and antipyretic agents is based on their ability to reduce the synthesis of a group of localized hormonelike lipid compounds called **prostaglandins,** which are associated with homeostatic regulation along with tissue inflammation processes and the resulting pain. The NSAIDs diminish the production of prostaglandins through their inhibition of the biosynthesizing enzyme COX.

Based on their ability to inhibit one or both isoforms of the COX enzyme (i.e., COX-1 and COX-2), the nonaspirin NSAIDs are divided into several general categories that include the traditional or nonselective and the selective agents. The nonselective NSAIDs, along with the salicylates, are referred to as dual inhibitors because they inhibit both COX enzymes (i.e., COX-1) responsible for maintaining baseline levels of prostaglandins and COX-2, which produces prostaglandins through localized cellular response mechanisms. There are a number of subclasses of the conventional NSAIDs; but the primary ones include ibuprofen (e.g., Advil and Motrin), indomethacin (e.g., Indocin), and naproxen (e.g., Aleve).

The selective nonaspirin NSAIDs, which are referred to as coxibs, uniquely block the COX-2 enzyme that is associated mainly with inflammation processes. The COX-2 inhibitors, including celecoxib (e.g., Celebrex) and the recently withdrawn rofecoxib (e.g., Vioxx), have enjoyed great popularity, particularly with patients suffering from arthritis and a variety of other chronic painful musculoskeletal conditions. The attractiveness of COX-2 inhibitors by users of high-dose painkillers is based on their ability to reduce the gastrointestinal complications primarily involving abdominal pain, heartburn, and dyspepsia that represent the significant major side effects of the standard NSAIDs. However, as hinted at above, despite the less toxic gastrointestinal effects of the COX-2 inhibitors, their overall safety profile has recently become questionable because of emerging evidence that coxibs may be associated with an increased risk of serious cardiovascular problems such as heart attack and stroke (Pham & Hirschberg, 2005).

Like the salicylates, when high doses are administered, the nonaspirin NSAIDs tend to, in general, be only reversibly ototoxic to hearing in that they can be associated with a transitory tinnitus and a reduction in hearing that recovers once drug treatment is terminated. However, although extremely rare, it is possible that reasonably healthy patients can experience a permanent sensorineural hearing loss after a brief course of a NSAID such as naproxen (McKinnon & Lassen, 1998). Conversely, unlike salicylates, a reversible dizziness can also result, which is more common with the indomethacin class of these agents (Forderreuther & Straube, 2000).

Acetaminophen

Acetaminophen (e.g., Tylenol) is a type of nonaspirin NSAID that is used mainly for the relief of fever and the mild pain associated with headaches. However, although acetaminophen is considered an antipyretic and analgesic, unlike aspirin, it is not an anti-inflammatory agent. Notably, there does not appear to be any published evidence of acetaminophen-induced ototoxicity of either a temporary or permanent nature. However, its overuse or abuse in the form of a multi-ingredient controlled substance such as Vicodin (i.e., acetaminophen plus a codeine-derived opioid, hydrocodone, which is a narcotic analgesic and antitussive) can be associated with a rapidly progressive profound hearing loss that is permanent (Friedman et al., 2000; Oh et al., 2000).

QUININE

Quinine is available therapeutically as sulfate or hydrochloride salts and is widely used in tonic water. Therapeutically, it is used primarily to treat malaria, particularly the drug-resistant type. In addition, it has a long history as a remedy for benign nocturnal muscle spasms of the legs, which is a common complaint of the elderly (Woodfield et al., 2005). Like salicylates, the ototoxic side effects of quinine and its products (such as chloroquine, quinidine, and tonic water) include reversible hearing loss and tinnitus. However, unlike salicylates and most of the other NSAIDs, quinine products can also temporarily cause balance problems such as dizziness (i.e., quinine can be both cochleotoxic and vestibulotoxic). In fact, the hallmark set of symptoms of acute quinine toxicity, which is referred to as **cinchonism,** includes tinnitus along with hearing loss, dizziness, headache, nausea, and vision changes (Wolf et al., 1992).

The clinical manifestations of quinine ototoxication include tinnitus, a transient sensorineural hearing loss, and vertigo (Jung et al., 1993). An early side effect, which occurs a few hours after initiation of high-dose drug therapy, is typically a reversible, bilateral, and symmetric sensorineural hearing loss. The hearing loss affects the high frequencies first with a characteristic 4-kHz notch. Moreover, the acoustical features of the perceptual tinnitus, like that caused by salicylates, are frequently described as being high-pitched and tonal.

As noted above, vertigo can also occur (Balfour, 1989). For example, Zajtchuk et al. (1984) showed in humans who drank 1.6 L of tonic water daily for 2 weeks that testing with electronystagmography uncovered clear positional abnormalities that were reversible. Together the hearing and balance problems noted for quinine intoxication suggest that this drug produces biochemical alterations throughout the inner ear.

Utilization of quinine as an antimalarial agent has decreased, other than for treating certain types of drug-resistant malaria, as indicated previously, because of the more recent use of less toxic synthetic derivatives. In addition, based on the negative outcomes of several clinical investigations on the use of quinine for treating nocturnal leg cramps using the randomized-controlled trials approach, the FDA imposed regulatory actions on its prescribed used. However, quinine remains available in the United States by prescription and in food and beverage products, as well as in dietary supplements. Thus, practitioners should maintain a clinical vigilance for ingestion of quinine in patients exhibiting tinnitus, hearing loss, and vertigo in the absence of other ototoxic-related medications.

MACROLIDE ANTIBIOTICS

Macrolides are a group of antibacterial antibiotics widely used in clinical medicine; they are generally considered to be safe drugs. Since its introduction during the mid-twentieth century, the common macrolide antibiotic ER has seen widespread use in clinical medicine, particularly in penicillin-sensitive individuals, because of the mild nature of its side effects. Moreover, ER, which is sometimes referred to as the "last option" antibiotic, is the drug of choice to treat atypical pneumonias such as *Legionella pneumonia*, probably because it has an antimicrobial spectrum that is slightly wider than that of penicillin. It took some twenty years of usage before the first reports of ER ototoxicity were noted in several patients (Mintz et al., 1973). That ototoxicity was described as a bilateral sensorineural hearing loss of 20–30 dB across all frequencies after the administration of the drug intravenously. In both cases, hearing returned to normal after the drug was discontinued. Since then, however, periodic cases of ototoxicity have been reported in which a similar pattern of hearing loss was noted; and, again, those effects have generally been reversible (Brummett, 1993a; Swanson et al., 1993).

Characteristically, ER ototoxicity usually appears within 3 days of starting treatment and is apparent as a relatively flat threshold shift with or without tinnitus, but with good speech discrimination. Based on a single pathological case report, it is likely that the flat hearing loss is caused by strial edema throughout all cochlear turns (McGhan & Merchant, 2003). In addition, significant recovery occurs within a day of stopping the drug and is typically complete at 1 month post-treatment. Patients who are susceptible to ER ototoxicity tend to have other risk factors including renal or hepatic failure and typically have received high doses of about 4 g/day that were administered intravenously (Vasquez et al., 1993).

Newer second-generation macrolide antibiotics such as AZ and CL are semisynthetic drugs that are derived from ER. AZ, which was introduced about fifteen years ago, has seen widespread clinical use, particularly for treatment of hospitalized patients with community-acquired pneumonia. Although initially only a few adverse side effects were reported for AZ (e.g., minor gastrointestinal irritation), more recently, some sporadic reports have appeared regarding possible ototoxic effects (Tseng et al., 1997; Bizjak et al., 1999; Ress & Gross, 2000). Moreover, CL, which is also used for the treatment of respiratory infections, has been reported to cause an irreversible sensorineural hearing loss (Coulston & Balaratnam, 2005). In contrast, though, experimental findings in a guinea pig model, which are in accordance with the clinical picture of AZ and CL, showed that intravenous doses produced only a temporary ototoxic effect in that they reversibly reduced transiently evoked otoacoustic emissions (Uzun et al., 2001). Although irreversible ototoxicity has rarely been observed for either AZ or CL, the relatively recent availability of intravenous forms of AZ, which allow for increased tissue penetration and higher concentrations, suggests that such cases may occur more frequently in the future. In general, though, instances of ototoxicity in patients treated with macrolide antibiotics are reported only occasionally. Clearly, further systematic investigation is needed to provide solid scientific proof of their adverse effects on hearing.

VANCOMYCIN AND NEWER COMPOUNDS

Because of its *mycin* suffix, **vancomycin**, a glycopeptide antibiotic that is unrelated to the aminoglycosides, is often believed to be irreversibly ototoxic. In fact, many cases of vancomycin ototoxicity associated with changes in hearing, tinnitus, and dizziness have been reported in the literature. However, in the majority of those instances, such adverse effects were only transitory in that patients fully recovered once the vancomycin therapy was complete. In other cases in which a permanent ototoxicity was attributed to vancomycin, other confounding variables such as concomitant treatment either before or after therapy with an aminoglycoside antibiotic also occurred. And, clearly, experimental animal studies have shown no convincing evidence of ototoxicity from vancomycin (Brummett, 1993b) even when very large doses were administered.

The FDA does not require either the testing of inner ear function or the examination of the cochlea's organ of Corti when determining the safety of a new drug before it is released into the marketplace. Thus, clinicians must be alert to a potential connection between ototoxic symptoms and a new drug by closely monitoring hearing and balance function in patients who are prescribed recently developed pharmacological agents. For example, some of the novel antiretroviral therapeutic compounds developed to treat conditions such as HIV infection have been implicated as a cause of ototoxic symptoms. In fact, Simdon et al. (2001) recently reported that nucleoside analog reverse transcriptase inhibitors likely caused the tinnitus and hearing impairment observed in three HIV type 1 patients who were administered those drugs. Clearly, prospective studies in humans and experimental animals are necessary to determine definite ototoxicity before any of the compounds just discussed can be labeled as being ototoxic.

MECHANISM OF OTOTOXICITY

The site and mechanism of salicylate ototoxicity have long been sought (Stypulkowski, 1990). Histopathological examinations of temporal bones of patients who had taken large amounts of salicylates prior to death have consistently revealed normal organs of Corti with no significant hair cell loss. Thus, reversible biochemical or metabolic changes in the cochlea rather than structural morphologic abnormalities, at least at the light microscopic level, are thought to induce this temporary ototoxicity. In fact, it has long been thought that the fundamental basis of salicylate ototoxicity is multifactorial, with decreased blood flow and biochemical abnormalities being the clearest causes (Jung et al., 1993). Likely, many of the aspirin and nonaspirin-related NSAIDs as well as quinine affect portions of the peripheral and perhaps, indirectly, some early stages of the central auditory pathway as well, which all contribute toward causing the reversible hearing losses and tinnitus. In fact, Zheng et al. (2001) used electrically evoked otoacoustic emissions and cochlear potentials to examine the effects of quinine on the electromotility of OHCs and the mechanical response of the basilar membrane. After infusing quinine directly into the cochlea, they showed adverse changes in the electromechanical transduction process as well as in the electrical potentials of other cochlear structures including spiral ganglion neurons. Those findings indicate the potential contributions of more central auditory structures to the hearing impairment produced by quinine.

Findings from several other studies indicate that aspirin at high concentrations can act directly on OHCs to affect their electromotility, which is the mechanical force provided by the OHCs that amplifies the vibration pattern of the organ of Corti's basilar membrane. For example, it has been known for some time that salicylates can diminish OHC electromotility (Dieler et al., 1991; Shehata et al., 1991) along with otoacoustic emissions (Wier et al., 1988; Long & Tubis, 1988). Such adverse effects infer that salicylates are capable of directly interfering with the ability of active cochlear mechanics to enhance basilar membrane vibration, thus causing a reversible reduction in the gain of the organ of Corti's cochlear amplifier.

More recent findings supporting the ability of salicylates to act directly on the cochlear amplifier come from the studies in awake guinea pigs by Huang et al. (2005). The experiments showed that long-term administration of salicylates paradoxically enhanced active cochlear mechanics by gradually increasing the levels of DPOAEs over a period of 4 weeks during which salicylates were regularly administered. Such observations also suggest that salicylate-induced tinnitus might be generated at the OHC level, which may help explain why, in a small percentage of patients who have normal to near normal hearing and spontaneous otoacoustic emission-induced tinnitus, the annoying tinnitus condition is relieved ironically by medicating with high doses of aspirin (Penner & Coles, 1992).

Current research by Santos-Sacchi and his colleagues (Rybalchenko & Santos-Sacchi, 2003; Song et al., 2005) suggests that salicylates may act as competitive inhibitors of chloride anions at the anion-binding site of prestin, the motor molecule of the OHC that is believed to support its motile properties. Such a molecular mechanism embedded as a protein within the membrane layers of the basolateral region of the OHC correlates well with the clinical audiological manifestations of a reversible aspirin-induced hearing impairment that includes hearing loss.

It is also known that ototoxic doses of quinine cause a diminution of the evoked rapid motile responses of isolated OHCs, which is more apparent in response to hyperpolarizing than to depolarizing electrical pulses (Dieler et al., 2002). Similar to the salicylates, quinine also is associated with a reduction or elimination of various forms of otoacoustic emissions (McFadden & Pasanen, 1994). However, *in vitro*, in contrast to what has been observed for salicylate-bathed OHCs, no changes were observed in turgor or shape or in the fine ultrastructure of isolated OHCs when superfused with quinine (Dieler et al., 2002), although such cells tended to change shape by elongating and dilating in diameter (Jarboe & Hallworth, 1999). Clearly, the combined *in vitro* findings for OHCs indicate that both salicylates and quinine directly and reversibly affect the electromechanical transduction processes in this class of cochlear receptor. However, the distinct morphological changes observed for quinine- versus salicylate-immersed OHCs also indicates that the underlying cellular and subcellular mechanisms of quinine ototoxicity are considerably different from those of salicylate ototoxicity, despite the knowledge that both substances lead to almost identical clinical symptoms, at least with respect to hearing.

Like that for aminoglycosides, the mechanism of action at the molecular level for the macrolide-related ototoxicity remains unknown. In fact, in contrast to the steady progress made with respect to the basis of aminoglycoside ototoxicity, there is a dearth of mechanistic research with respect to the macrolides. Clearly, though, except in very rare cases of permanent hearing dysfunction, for the macrolides, which in general, typically cause reversible impairment, such underlying dysfunctional molecular processes would only be temporary in that they would vanish following cessation of the drug treatment.

SUMMARY

A number of drugs used in the pharmacological management of chronic pain have been associated with reversible alterations to inner ear function in the form of hearing loss, tinnitus, and sometimes vertigo. Those drugs include the salicylates and other nonaspirin NSAIDs along with the macrolide antibiotics. In general, they have similar dose-related ototoxic effects in that they can produce a temporary loss of hearing with tinnitus and sometimes, depending on the agent, dizziness or vertigo.

Given the continuous search for novel compounds designed to offer the patient not only enhanced bioavailability and biochemical selectivity, but also a reduced incidence of adverse effects, new pharmacological products with improved features are continually being discovered and developed. Thus, the audiologist needs to be persistently vigilant with respect to signs of ototoxicity in patients. This careful watchfulness is particularly important when high doses are administered rapidly by intravenous infusion over long periods of time, especially to patients who are very young or to patients with renal and hepatic impairment. In addition, special vigilance needs to be given to patients receiving the NSAIDs and any of the other miscellaneous agents discussed, particularly when they are combined with drugs such as the aminoglycosides, which are known to have the potential for producing irreversible ototoxicity.

The concept of potentiation of ototoxicity through synergistic mechanisms is common and has been shown for medications that combine, for example, with vancomycin and gentamcin (Triggs & Charles, 1999). In addition, the audiologist should be aware that some individuals exhibit a sensitivity to a synergistic combination of aspirin ingestion with exposure to loud sounds that eventually produce a noise-induced hearing loss (McFadden et al., 1984), even though such noises were within the safe boundaries demanded by hearing-conservation limits. Although ongoing audiologic monitoring for possible ototoxicity would be ideal for patients receiving any potentially ototoxic medication, it is not practical in most cases, given the scarcity of sufficient financial resources to cover the necessary personnel and instrumentation costs involved in such surveillance programs. Thus, in the case of adults in particular, the audiologist should counsel the patient to be aware of changes in hearing status and to report them to the medical staff so that adequate tests for detecting an ototoxic reaction can be conducted.

REFERENCES

Balfour, A. J. (1989). The bite of Jesuits' bark. *Aviat Space Environ Med, 60,* A4–A5.

Bizjak, E. D., Haug, M. T. III, Schilz, R. J., Sarodia, B. D., & Dresing, J. M. (1999). Intravenous azithromycin-induced ototoxicity. *Pharmacotherapy, 19,* 245–248.

Boettcher, F. A., & Salvi, R. J. (1991). Salicylate ototoxicity: Review and synthesis. *Am J Otolaryngol, 12,* 33–47.

Brummett, R. E. (1993a). Ototoxicity liability of erythromycin and analogues. *Otolaryngol Clin North Am, 26,* 811–819.

Brummett, R. E. (1993b). Ototoxicity of vancomycin and analogues. *Otolaryngol Clin North Am, 26,* 821–828.

Cazals, Y. (2000). Auditory sensori-neural alterations induced by salicylate. *Progr Neurobiol, 62,* 583–631.

Coulston, J., & Balaratnam, N. (2005). Irreversible sensorineural hearing loss due to clarithromycin. *Postgrad Med J, 81,* 58–59.

Day, R. O., Graham, G. G., Bieri, D., Brown, M., Cairns, D., Harris, G., Hounsell, J., Platt-Hepworth, S., Reeve, R., & Sambrook, P. N. (1989). Concentration-response relationships for salicylate-induced ototoxicity in normal volunteers. *Br J Clin Pharmacol, 28,* 695–702.

Dieler, R., Davies, C., & Shehata-Dieler, W. E. (2002). The effects of quinine on active motile responses and fine structure of isolated outer hair cells from the guinea pig cochlea. *Laryngorhinootologie, 81,* 196–203.

Dieler, R., Shehata-Dieler, W. E., & Brownell, W. E. (1991). Concomitant salicylate-induced alterations of outer hair cell subsurface cisternae and electromotility. *J Neurocytol, 20,* 637–653.

Forderreuther, S., & Straube, A. (2000). Indomethacin reduces CSF pressure in intracranial hypertension. *Neurology, 55,* 1043–1045.

Friedman, R. A., House, J. W., Luxford, W. M., Gherini, S., & Mills, D. (2000). Profound hearing loss associated with hydrocodone/acetaminophen abuse. *Am J Otol, 21,* 188–191.

Jarboe, J. K., & Hallworth, R. (1999). The effect of quinine on outer hair cell shape, compliance and force. *Hear Res, 132,* 43–50.

Jarvis, J. F. (1966). A case of unilateral permanent deafness following acetylsalicylic acid. *J Laryngol Otol, 80,* 318–320.

Jung, T. T., Rhee, C. K., Lee, C. S., Park, Y. S., & Choi, D. C. (1993). Ototoxicity of salicylate, nonsteroidal anti-inflammatory drugs, and quinine. *Otolaryngol Clin North Am, 26,* 791–810.

Kapur, Y. P. (1965). Ototoxicity of acetylsalicylic acid. *Arch Otolaryngol, 81,* 134–138.

Long, G. R., & Tubis, A. (1988). Modification of spontaneous and evoked otoacoustic emissions and associated psychoacoustic microstructure by aspirin consumption. *J Acoust Soc Am 84,* 1343–1353.

McCabe, P. A., & Dey, F. L. (1965). The effect of aspirin upon auditory sensitivity. *Ann Otol Rhinol Laryngol, 74,* 312–325.

McFadden, D., & Pasanen, E. G. (1994). Otoacoustic emissions and quinine sulfate. *J Acoust Soc Am, 95,* 3460–3474.

McFadden, D., Plattsmier, H. S., & Pasanen, E. G. (1984). Temporary hearing loss induced by combinations of intense sounds and nonsteroidal anti-inflammatory drugs. *Am J Otolaryngol, 5,* 235–241.

McGhan, L. J., & Merchant, S. N. (2003). Erythromycin ototoxicity. *Otol Neurotol, 24,* 701–702.

McKinnon, B. J., & Lassen, L. F. (1998). Naproxen-associated sudden sensorineural hearing loss. *Mil Med, 163,* 792–793.

Mintz, U., Amir, J., Pinkhas, J., & de Vries, A. (1973). Transient perceptive deafness due to erythromycin lactobionate. *J Am Med Assn, 226,* 1122–1123.

Oh, A. K., Ishiyama, A., & Baloh, R. W. (2000). Deafness associated with abuse of hydrocodone/acetaminophen. *Neurology, 54,* 2345.

Penner, M. J., & Coles, R. R. (1992). Indications for aspirin as a palliative for tinnitus caused by SOAEs: A case study. *Br J Audiol, 26,* 91–96.

Pham, K., & Hirschberg, R. (2005). Global safety of coxibs and NSAIDs. *Curr Top Med Chem, 5,* 465–473.

Ress, B. D., & Gross, E. M. (2000). Irreversible sensorineural hearing loss as a result of azithromycin ototoxicity. A case report. *Ann Otol Rhnol Laryngol, 109,* 435–437.

Roland, P. S. (2003). Characteristics of systemic and topical agents implicated in toxicity of the middle and inner ear. *Ear Nose Throat J, 82*(Suppl. 1), 3–8.

Rybalchenko, V., & Santos-Sacchi, J. (2003). Cl- flux through a non-selective, stretch-sensitive conductance influences the outer hair cell motor of the guinea-pig. *J Physiol, 547,* 873–891.

Shehata, W. E., Brownell, W. E., & Dieler, R. (1991). Effects of salicylate on shape, electromotility and membrane characteristics of isolated outer hair cells from guinea pig cochlea. *Acta Otolaryngol, 111,* 707–718.

Simdon, J., Watters, D., Bartlett, S., & Connick, E. (2001). Ototoxicity associated with use of nucleoside analog reverse transcriptase inhibitors: A report of 3 possible cases and review of the literature. *Clin Infect Dis, 32,* 1623–1627.

Song, L., Seeger, A., & Santos-Sacchi, J. (2005). On membrane motor activity and chloride flux in the outer hair cell: lessons learned from the environmental toxin tributyltin. *Biophys J, 88,* 2350–2362.

Stypulkowski, P. H. (1990). Mechanisms of salicylate ototoxicity. *Hear Res, 46,* 113–145.

Swanson, D. J., Sung, R. J., Fine, M. J., Orloff, J. J., Chu, S. Y., & Yu, V. L. (1993). Erythromycin ototoxicity: Prospective assessment with serum concentrations and audiograms in a study of patients with pneumonia. *Am J Med, 92,* 61–68.

Triggs, E., & Charles, B. (1999). Pharmacokinetics and therapeutic drug monitoring of gentamicin in the elderly. *Clin Pharmacokinet, 37,* 331–341.

Tseng, A. L., Dolovich, L., & Salit, I. E. (1997). Azithromycin-related ototoxicity in patients infected with human immunodeficiency virus. *Clin Infect Dis, 24,* 76–77.

Uzun, C., Koten, M., Adali, M. K., Yorulmaz, F., Yagiz, R., & Karasalihoglu, A. R. (2001). Reversible ototoxic effect of azithromycin and clarithromycin on transiently evoked otoacoustic emissions in guinea pigs. *J Laryngol Otol, 115,* 622–628.

Vasquez, E. M., Maddux, M. S., Sanchez, J., & Pollak, R. (1993). Clinical significant hearing loss in renal allograft recipients treated with intravenous erythromycin. *Arch Inter Med, 153,* 879–882.

Wier, C. C., Pasanen, E. G., & McFadden, D. (1988). Partial dissociation of spontaneous otoacoustic emissions and distortion products during aspirin use in humans. *J Acoust Soc Am, 84,* 230–237.

Wolf, L. R., Otten, E. J., & Spadafora, M. P. (1992). Cinchonism: Two case reports and review of acute quinine toxicity and treatment. *J Emerg Med, 10,* 295–301.

Woodfield, R., Goodyear-Smith, F., & Arroll, B. (2005). N-of-1 trials of quinine efficacy in skeletal muscle cramps of the leg. *Br J Gen Pract, 55,* 181–185.

Zajtchuk, J. T., Mihail, R., Jewell, J. S., Dunne, M. J., & Chadwick, S. G. (1984). Electronystagmographic findings in long-term low-dose quinine ingestion. *Arch Otolaryngol, 110,* 788–791.

Zheng, J., Ren, T., Parthasarathi, A., & Nuttall, A. L. (2001). Quinine-induced alterations of electrically evoked otoacoustic emissions and cochlear potentials in guinea pigs. *Hear Res, 154,* 124–134.

Industrial Chemicals and Solvents Affecting the Auditory System

Benoit Pouyatos, PhD, and Laurence D. Fechter, PhD
Research Service (151)
Jerry Pettis Memorial Veterans Medical Center
Loma Linda, CA

INTRODUCTION

The concept that chemical contaminants might be ototoxic themselves or might potentiate noise-induced hearing loss (NIHL) may seem strange at first. It is well known that certain chemicals released into the environment or encountered in the workplace can cause cancer. Contaminants such as lead can cause mental retardation in children. Additionally excessive consumption of fish containing high mercury levels can be dangerous in pregnant women because of the risk for neurological damage to their babies. Chemicals such as hydrogen cyanide and carbon monoxide can be lethal in high concentrations. Yet most people (including most scientists) have never considered that chemical contaminants can target the auditory system, producing permanent impairment of function. Nonetheless, when one considers how well established the relationship is between exposure to specific drugs like the aminoglycoside antibiotics (see Chapter 11) and platinum-containing antitumor agents (see Chapter 10), the notion of ototoxicity stemming from chemical agents seems far more credible.

As audiologists, it is important to be aware of the fact that certain chemicals can be ototoxic and/or can promote NIHL, especially with regard to potential workplace exposures. If audiologists recognize that specific chemical agents can increase susceptibility to NIHL, they will be able to exercise greater care in evaluating records of workers who are being exposed to noise and who are working in job categories with risks of chemical exposure.

The development of regulations for permissible workplace exposure to noise and permissible workplace exposure to chemicals are commonly performed in isolation from each other. It is the exceptional case where chemical ototoxicity has been considered in recommending permissible exposure standards for noise. The **Occupational Safety & Health Administration (OSHA)** sets permissible exposures for noise in the workplace—the current standards being 90 dBA$_\text{leq}$ based on an 8-hour time-weighted average, with a trade-off of 5 dB for doubling noise duration. That is, 95 dBA noise exposure for 2 hours is considered to be equivalent to 90 dBA noise exposure for 4 hours and to 85 dBA noise exposure for 8 hours, all of those

exposures being currently permissible under the law. The **American Conference of Governmental Industrial Hygienists (ACGIH)** also recommends noise exposure standards.

Both OSHA and the ACGIH have committees that establish **permissible exposure levels (PELs)** and **threshold limit values (TLVs),** respectively, for exposure to chemicals in the workplace. Those published values can be found in the handbook *Threshold Limit Values and Biological Exposure Indices (TLVs and BEIs),* published by the ACGIH (2006). In addition, the ACGIH has recommended that increased audiometric surveillance be used in instances where workers are exposed to noise and a select list of chemical contaminants that have been shown to produce hearing loss by themselves or to promote NIHL. Those agents are carbon monoxide, lead, manganese, **styrene, toluene,** and **xylene.**

This chapter presents information concerning chemicals that are known to produce hearing loss directly (ototoxicants) as well as those that promote or potentiate NIHL. These ototoxic agents are grouped by their chemical "class" when one can be identified and as individual agents for those that do not readily fit an established class of compounds. Information is presented concerning the uses of the chemical agents; the types of occupational settings or other settings in which they might be encountered; and when known, the possible reasons for their ototoxicity and doses at which ototoxicity is observed. Note that the usage of the term *threshold* refers to the lowest dose of a chemical agent that produces an effect, and must be distinguished from the audiological *threshold*—the lowest sound level at which the sound is detected. Finally, general guidelines are offered concerning other agents that might be ototoxic, as well as approaches to confirming ototoxicity in human populations.

The authors' hope is that audiologists might be motivated to investigate the relationship between chemical exposure and hearing loss. Such studies would benefit from professional expertise in the fields of audiology, **industrial hygiene** (especially the measurement of noise and chemical exposure levels), and **epidemiology** (especially the selection of subjects into population classifications that represent different exposure conditions).

CHEMICAL ASPHYXIANTS AND HYPOXIA

The **chemical asphyxiants** as a class of agents reduce the delivery of oxygen to tissue or the utilization of oxygen by tissues. Clearly, they are chemical contaminants, not agents that have direct commercial benefit. **Hypoxia** is a state of reduced oxygen delivery that occurs when chemical asphyxiants are applied, but it can also occur under conditions of reduced oxygen delivery *per se*. For example, living at high altitudes can actually be considered a form of mild hypoxia. Two especially important chemical asphyxiants with respect to frequency of exposure are carbon monoxide and hydrogen cyanide gas.

Carbon Monoxide

Carbon monoxide is a product of all combustion. The most common sources of potential exposure include cigarette smoke; exhaust from vehicles; and fireplaces, hot water heaters, and furnaces. Carbon monoxide is the chemical contaminant that causes the most deaths worldwide. In the workplace, firefighters, foundry workers, toll and tunnel workers, and auto/truck mechanics are some of the occupations in which carbon monoxide exposure can potentially occur. Carbon monoxide can also be encountered in homes from faulty stoves, furnaces, and hot water heaters. It can be produced when **methylene chloride** paint strippers are used.

Most of the human data relating hypoxia and hearing loss are anecdotal, relying on case reports. Sato (1966), Morris (1969), and Goto et al. (1972) all reported evidence of hearing loss in individuals exposed to carbon monoxide at levels severe enough to produce unconsciousness. Baker and Lilly (1977) reported a case of fluctuating sensorineural hearing loss following acute high-level carbon monoxide exposure. The audiogram was described as being U-shaped. Zelman (1973) also suggested an association between human cigarette smoking and hearing loss by audiometric testing between 125 and 12,000 Hz. Whether that effect was due to carbon monoxide, to nicotine, or to some other component of tobacco smoke remains unclear. A recent review of fifteen reports concerning smoking and hearing ability was recently undertaken by Nomura et al. (2005). Their **meta-analysis** attempted to determine the **relative risk** between smoking and impaired hearing as measured by pure-tone audiometry. By reviewing a series of reports, the meta-analysis attempted to overcome the weakness of any given report and thus provide an overarching conclusion from a number of reports. It showed a weak association between smoking and hearing loss. In general, the relative risk of hearing loss as measured by pure-tone audiometry was below 2 as compared to nonsmokers. In terms of epidemiological studies, such a small relative risk should be interpreted with caution. For example, there may be other characteristics of individuals who smoke that might be the actual basis for a chance association between smoking and hearing impairment (e.g., perhaps smokers have different cardiovascular characteristics that affect hearing or perhaps smokers have a different risk of noise exposure). Perhaps future studies will clarify the nature of the relationship between smoking and hearing. In any event, the fact that cigarette smokers continue to smoke despite health warnings is not likely to be due to a hearing loss. It has also been hypothesized that interaction of carbon monoxide exposure with noise might account for the high rate of hearing loss among firefighters, but that relationship has yet to be established.

Despite the lack of strong evidence in humans that carbon monoxide can cause hearing loss directly, there is clear evidence from laboratory animal studies that carbon monoxide can make the cochlea more vulnerable to noise exposure. Furthermore, there are strong data implicating oxidative stress as the underlying cause. (The role of oxidative stress in ototoxicity is a recurrent theme that is discussed in Chapters 7, 10, 11, 15, and 19). Basically, **oxidative stress** refers to the overproduction of unstable and highly reactive forms of oxygen that can damage cells.

Young, Upchurch, Kaufman, and Fechter (1987) were the first to show that carbon monoxide could potentiate NIHL in rats. In their study, subjects received either carbon monoxide alone, noise alone, carbon monoxide and noise presented together, or no experimental treatment. While carbon monoxide alone yielded no impairment in pure-tone auditory thresholds, combined exposure yielded profound high-frequency hearing loss, which greatly surpassed the effect of noise by itself. The finding that carbon monoxide can potentiate NIHL in laboratory animals has been replicated several times. Scientists have learned that combined exposure to noise and carbon monoxide produces a loss of outer hair cells (OHCs), especially in the basal or high-frequency end of the cochlea (Fechter, Young, & Carlisle, 1988). In addition, scientists have discovered that agents that reduce free radical formation can protect against the effects of noise and carbon monoxide (Rao & Fechter, 2000a). Finally, dose effect studies have been performed to estimate how much carbon monoxide is necessary before potentiation of NIHL occurs (Fechter, Chen, Rao, & Larabee, 2000; Rao & Fechter, 2000b). Those studies suggest that exposure levels of 200 **parts per million** approach the level at which slight exacerbation of hearing loss occurs beyond that which can be accounted for by noise. Such an exposure level is far higher than what is experienced even in highly polluted environments. However, such levels may occur for short time periods in specific industrial settings (e.g., fires and foundries) and may pose some additional hazard for workers.

Cyanide

Cyanide is present not only as a poisonous gas (hydrogen cyanide), but also as a combustion product of many plastics and some fabrics, such as wool. In fact, cyanide poisoning is identified as an important cause of death in many fires. Cyanide is used in the production of certain chemicals, as a fumigant of grains, in the refining of low-grade metals, and in electroplating.

Unlike the case for **hypoxic hypoxia** (reduction of oxygen concentration in inspired air typically by the dilution of air with nitrogen), carbon monoxide, and **ischemia**, the effect of cyanide on auditory function has not been as well studied. van Heijst, Maes, Mtanda, Chuwa, Rwiza et al. (1994) studied twenty patients in Tanzania with sudden onset **polyneuropathies** correlated with elevated blood cyanide. Hearing loss was identified in nearly half of those cases. The source of cyanide exposure was believed to be increased dietary intake of **cassava** due to food shortages.

Direct experimental evidence that cyanide can produce cochlear impairment is limited to a handful of studies. Konishi and Kelsey (1968) and Evans and Klinke (1982) showed acute impairments in cochlear function due to cochlear perfusion with cyanide salts in experimental animals. Tawackoli, Chen, and Fechter (2001) showed that injection with cyanide salts could also acutely disrupt pure-tone thresholds in rats. This transient auditory threshold loss, seen particularly for high-frequency stimuli, correlated well with an abrupt drop in the **endocochlear potential** generated by the **stria vascularis**. Fechter, Chen, and Johnson (2002) investigated the permanent effects of hydrogen cyanide exposure on permanent NIHL. They showed that even low doses of hydrogen cyanide were able to potentiate NIHL in rats.

METALS

Limited published data show that certain metals having toxic potential can also disrupt auditory function. As noted earlier, the ACGIH has recommended that for several of these metals, increased surveillance of hearing be conducted if noise also is present in the workplace. The following sections present the data available concerning the ototoxic and neurotoxic consequences of overexposure to lead, mercury, and manganese.

Lead

Lead exposure not only impairs cognitive development in children, but also produces auditory impairments. Lead neurotoxicity is thought to represent a particular risk in children because it is able to pass more easily into the developing brain than into the fully developed brain. Schwartz and Otto (1987, 1991) showed significant elevations in pure-tone auditory thresholds in children that were correlated with blood lead levels. Even **blood lead levels** in the range of $10 \mu g/dl$ were associated with small losses in auditory function. Such levels of blood lead have been reported in young children exposed to lead through ingestion of paint chips and from other sources. Discalzi, Fabbro, Meliga, Mocellini, and

Capellaro (1993) also reported modest impairment in auditory brainstem responses (ABRs) among adult lead workers when blood levels reached into the range of $50\mu g/dl$. Both a delay in wave I and a shift in later peak latencies were observed. Such effects suggest alteration in **nerve conduction time;** the increased peak latency for later peaks is suggestive of a central auditory effect.

Mercury

Most people are familiar with pure metallic mercury in thermometers, but mercury is found in a variety of other places. For example, it has been used in the separation of gold from river sediments, in the production of papers, and as a fumigant; it is also a contaminant released into the atmosphere during the burning of coal. Once liberated into water, metallic mercury and mercury salts can be metabolized by bacteria, resulting in the production of organic or "methyl" mercury. This contaminant is taken up by fish, where it concentrates in the muscle of large fish such as swordfish, tuna, and halibut. Consequently, the **Food and Drug Administration (FDA)** recommends that pregnant women limit their fish consumption. Accidental high-dose overexposures to mercury are associated with abnormalities in brain development.

Methylmercury is also known to produce auditory impairments in both humans and laboratory animals, with clear effects on central auditory pathways and more questionable effects on the cochlea. Amin-zaki, Majeed, Clarkson, and Greenwood (1978) and Mizukoshi, Watanabe, Kobayashi, Nakano, Koide, Inomata et al. (1989) identified audiological impairments in humans who were accidentally exposed to high levels of methylmercury. In the first instance, Iraqi children were mistakenly fed bread that had been made from seeds coated with mercury as a fungicide. The seeds were intended to be planted and not eaten. In the second instance, a report is given of people in the town of Minimata, Japan, who ate fish caught in a bay having high mercury content. In both instances, hearing loss was just one of many serious neurological effects of exposure, including profound birth defects, mental retardation, and severe neuromotor defects.

Controlled laboratory experiments conducted in several species show more clearly how methylmercury disrupts hearing. For example, Rice and Gilbert (1992) conducted a study to determine the neurotoxic effect of methylmercury in developing monkeys. They showed a permanent, preferential high-frequency auditory impairment in the mercury-exposed subjects. Similar outcomes have been observed in rats (Wu, Ison, Wecker, & Lapham, 1985) and in guinea pigs (Falk, Klein, Haseman, Sanders, Talley et al., 1974; Konishi & Hamrick, 1979).

Manganese

Nikolov (1974) studied battery workers who were exposed to **manganese dioxide** and to noise. He reported that manganese exposure potentiated NIHL in workers exposed to noise intensities of 97–102 dB and suggested that the combined effect was secondary to cochlear as well as retrocochlear damage. Only three cases were presented in that paper; thus, conclusions must be considered tentative in the absence of better documentation of exposure conditions and of full epidemiological study.

ORGANIC SOLVENTS

Volatile organic solvents are encountered in many contexts in industrialized societies, often as mixtures or blends. They are used extensively in home-cleaning products; in paints, thinners, and glues; and in some industries. Solvents have also been voluntarily inhaled at very high levels for "recreational" purposes. In fact, the neurotoxic effects observed in solvent abusers were incidentally the first clues that motivated subsequent research on the potential ototoxicity of organic solvents. Because the levels of exposure encountered by the general population is generally low, this section will focus primarily on the industry, where the potential risk of exposure to a solvent or a mixture of solvents at high levels is significant. Additionally, industrial settings commonly engender high noise levels, which can increase the deleterious effect of solvents on the hearing function, as delineated later in this chapter.

Organic solvents are one of the most widely used groups of chemicals in the workplace. The **National Institute for Occupational Safety and Health (NIOSH)** has identified 335 different occupations that have the potential to expose workers to solvents. NIOSH estimates that in the United States, 3 million women and 6 million men are occupationally exposed to solvents. Occupations with the greatest number of exposed workers are janitors and cleaners, metal precision assemblers, textile sewing machine operators, and printing machine operators. Also at risk of exposure are any workers who handle solvent-containing products such as inks, cleaning products, degreasers, paints and paint thinners, enamels and lacquers, adhesives, resins, and marking fluids.

Because organic solvents are so volatile, the major route of exposure is through the respiratory system. Once vapors enter the lungs, they diffuse across the respiratory membranes and enter the blood flow. Liquid solvents are also rapidly absorbed through the skin due to their highly **lipophilic** nature. Solvents are so prone to penetrating the human body that the solvent uptake into the peripheral blood can begin within minutes of the onset of exposure (WHO, 1985; Engstrom, Astrand, & Wigaeus, 1978). Following absorption, **organic solvents** are metabolized (primarily in the liver) or they accumulate in lipid-rich tissues such as those of the nervous system (WHO, 1985; Bergman, 1983). The cochlea represents a preferential target for solvents because it is a highly vascularized organ containing a significant proportion of lipid-rich tissues. Actually, solvents are believed to migrate from the blood vessels of the stria vascularis to the sensory cells of the organ of Corti through these lipid-rich tissues—in particular, the Hensen's cells and the Deiters' cells of the outer sulcus (Figure 14-1). To make matters worse, the number of cochlear sensory cells (inner and outer hair cells) in the organ of Corti is very small, which makes the cochlea particularly susceptible to chemical attack because of a limited functional redundancy.

The ototoxicity of organic solvents has been studied during the last twenty years in both laboratory animals and workers in the workplace. The results of those studies suggest that at least six chemicals belonging to the **aromatic** and **aliphatic solvent** families are ototoxic in laboratory animals and *probably* ototoxic in humans at some exposure levels: styrene, toluene, ethyl benzene, xylene, trichloroethylene, and *n*-hexane (Figure 14-2 shows the chemical structure).

Styrene

Styrene (Figure 14-2) is an aromatic solvent widely used in the manufacturing of reinforced plastics, resins, synthetic rubbers, protective coatings, and insulating materials. The highest occupational exposures to styrene occur during the manufacturing of glass-reinforced polyester products, especially of large items such as boats (Miller, Newhook, & Poole, 1994). It was estimated by NIOSH (1988, 1990) that approximately 500,000 American workers are exposed to styrene as a regular part of their jobs. The permissible limit for an 8-hour time-weighted average is 100 ppm in the United States, while it is between 20 and 50 ppm in several European countries.

The pioneer animal studies on the ototoxicity of styrene were carried out by Pryor, Rebert, and Howd in the late 1980s. They showed that styrene (3-week exposure at 800 ppm for 14 hours/day) caused marked hearing loss in the rat as assessed by behavioral and electrophysiologic methods (Pryor et al., 1987). Subsequent studies by other research teams have demonstrated that styrene causes a selective mid-frequency hearing loss (Crofton, Rebert, & Lassiter, 1994) by specifically destroying the OHCs of the organ of Corti. As shown in Figure 14-3, hair cell loss induced by styrene in the rat cochlea is gradually decreasing from the third to the first OHC row (Lataye, Campo, Barthelemy, Loquet, & Bonnet, 2001). This histopathological pattern, which is typical of aromatic solvents, suggested an intoxication route through the outer edge of the cochlea (Figure 14-1), more precisely through the lipid-rich cells of the outer sulcus (Campo, Loquet, Blachere, & Roure, 1999). A hypothesis proposed by Campo, Lataye, Loquet, and Bonnet (2001) suggests that the disorganization of the membranous structures of both supporting cells and OHCs could be the starting point for the cochlear injury induced by styrene. However, the precise mechanism is still unknown.

In the rat, styrene is not only ototoxic by itself; it also can interact with noise. Two studies have shown

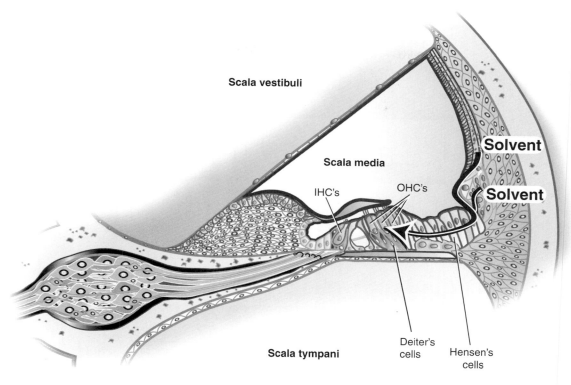

Figure 14-1. Hypothetical route of intoxication of the organ of Corti by organic solvents. Adapted from Campo et al. (1999).

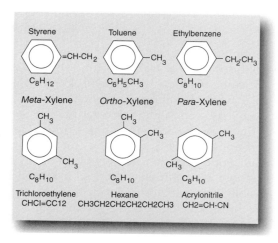

Figure 14-2. Chemical formula of the organic compounds cited in this chapter.

increased permanent hearing loss in animals exposed to styrene and noise compared to animals exposed to noise alone (Lataye, Campo, & Loquet, 2000; Makitie, Pirvola, Pyykko, Sakakibara, Riihimaki et al., 2003). Both investigations determined a synergistic mechanism between styrene and noise, the hearing loss caused by the combined exposure to styrene and noise exceeding the sum of the loss induced by the individual factors.

A surprising characteristic of styrene ototoxicity is that it is strongly species-dependent. While the rat is sensitive to styrene, the guinea pig seems to be resistant to permanent impairment (Fechter, 1993). In a recent study, Lataye, Campo, Pouyatos, Cossec, Blachere et al. (2003) evaluated the effect of styrene exposure (1000 ppm) in both rats and guinea pigs exposed 6 hours/day for 5 consecutive days.

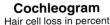

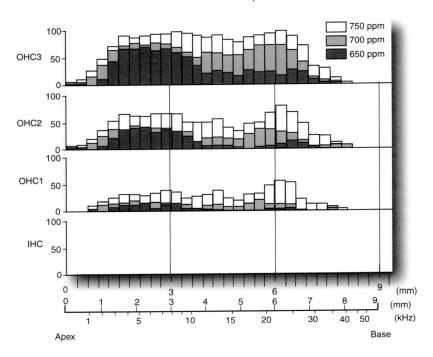

Figure 14-3. Average hair cell loss obtained in rats exposed to 650, 700, or 750 ppm styrene (6 hours/day, 5 days/week, 4 weeks). Abscissa: upper trace: length (mm) of the entire spiral course of the organ of Corti including the bottom of the hook; lower trace: frequency map according to Müller (1991). Ordinate: hair cell loss in percent.

Cochlear function was tested by using distortion product otoacoustic emissions (DPOAE). The rat showed severe disruption of auditory function and cochlear pathology, whereas the guinea pig had no disruption of DPOAE or cochlear pathological alterations. An important difference in the styrene concentration in blood was also observed: the solvent concentrations were four times higher in the rat than in the guinea pig. Therefore, a pharmacokinetic or an uptake difference might explain the difference in susceptibility observed between the two species. This species specificity raises the question of the human sensitivity to styrene: are we more like the rat or the guinea pig model? Unfortunately, styrene metabolism in human is closer to the rat than that of the guinea pig.

In summary, styrene is ototoxic in the rat above a threshold dose of 300–600 ppm for a 4-week exposure (Loquet, Campo, & Lataye, 1999; Makitie, Pirvola, Pyykko, Sakakibara, Riihimaki et al., 2002). That dose may seem high with regard to the occupational limits in the industry; but workers can be exposed not only for 4 weeks, but for their whole active life. For that reason, a safety factor of ten times the threshold dose is frequently used in establishing permissible human exposure levels. In that case, the ototoxic threshold cited above is not that high.

The human data on occupational hearing loss caused by styrene are scarce and quite equivocal when compared to the clear results obtained in laboratory animals. Several case reports on the neurotoxic and ototoxic effects of styrene can be found in the literature published since the 1960s (Lehnhardt, 1965). Those effects have been generally observed in the case of short-term exposure to high concentrations (see review by Arlien-Soborg, 1992).

Since 1988, only a handful of large-scale occupational studies have been carried out in order to investigate whether the effect of styrene on the rat's hearing system can be observed in workers in industry at moderate concentrations. The older investigations on occupational hearing loss, which relied on pure-tone audiometric thresholds, have identified only minimal effects of styrene at levels below 50 ppm (Muijser, Hoogendijk, & Hooisma, 1988; Möller, Odkvist, Larsby, Tham, Ledin et al., 1990; Sass-Kortsak, Corey, & Robertson, 1995). More recent studies in which a battery of audiometric tests was used in conjunction with monitoring of solvent concentrations in body fluids showed significant effects of styrene (Sliwinska-Kowalska, Zamyslowska-Szmytke, Szymczak, Kotylo, Fiszer et al., 1999, 2003; Morioka, Miyai, Yamamoto, & Miyashita, 2000; Morata, Johnson, Nylen, Svensson, Cheng et al., 2002).

In Poland, Sliwinska-Kowalska et al. (1999) conducted a large investigation on the auditory effects of several solvents and noise. A group of workers specifically exposed to styrene was included in the study. The authors observed that hearing loss (>25dB at more than one frequency above 2 kHz) was measured in 70% of the workers exposed to styrene and noise compared to 20% of the workers exposed to noise only. The risk for developing a hearing loss was twelve times greater in the styrene-exposed workers when compared to the unexposed group. Morioka et al. (2000) carried out a study on workers exposed to low levels of styrene (2.9–28.9 ppm) and noise ranging from 69–79 dB(A) compared to workers exposed to noise alone and unexposed individuals: despite the fact that both styrene and noise levels were within permissible occupational limits, high-frequency hearing thresholds were reduced in workers exposed for 5 years or more. Morata et al. (2002) conducted audiometric and exposure measurements on 313 workers from fiberglass and metal products manufacturing plants and a mail distribution terminal. Workers exposed to noise and styrene had significantly worse pure-tone thresholds at 2, 3, 4, and 6 kHz when compared with noise-exposed or nonexposed workers.

Finally, the most recent study carried out by Sliwinska-Kowalska et al. (2003) investigated the auditory effect of a mixture of solvents, having styrene as the main component, in 290 yacht yard and plastic factory workers. They demonstrated almost a fourfold increase in the odds (risk) of developing hearing loss related to styrene exposure as compared to nonexposed workers. In cases of combined exposures to styrene and noise, the odds ratios were two to three times higher than the respective values for styrene-only and noise-only exposed subjects.

The above-mentioned studies provide the epidemiological evidence that occupational exposure to styrene is related to an increased risk of hearing loss and that combined exposures to noise and styrene seem to be more ototoxic than exposure to noise alone. However, despite the positive results, controversy still remains about the risk of hearing loss in workers when the styrene concentrations are within the recommended limits (Rebert & Hall, 1994). Clearly, continuing audiological monitoring of workers exposed to styrene is essential to determine whether exposure limits are adequate or whether they should be lowered, especially when noise is present.

Toluene

Toluene (Figure 14-2) is one of the most commonly used industrial solvents in the world; it is used in making paints, paint thinners, fingernail polish, lacquers, adhesives, and rubber and is used in some printing and leather tanning processes. Toluene exposure may occur in the workplace, especially in the printing industry where toluene is used as a solvent for inks and dyes. Personnel working with various types of fuel are also at risk of toluene exposure, as are industrial painters (Vincent, Poirot, Subra, Rieger, & Cicolella, 1994). Concentrations of 5–50 ppm are actually common in the workplace with some reported values as high as 250 ppm (NCI, 1985). OSHA has set a limit of 200 ppm of toluene for air in the workplace, averaged for an 8-hour exposure per day. The ACGIH and NIOSH recommend that toluene not exceed 50 ppm and 100 ppm, respectively.

The early reports of adverse health effects of toluene in humans were made on solvent abusers, mainly "glue or paint sniffers." They were diagnosed with sensorineural hearing loss, the cortical evoked potential being generally more affected than brainstem evoked potential, indicating a probable disruption of central auditory pathways (Metrick & Brenner, 1982; Ehyai & Freemon, 1983; Poulsen & Jensen, 1986). Accurate exposure levels are not available, but the concentrations inhaled by chronic abusers have been estimated to range from 4,000–12,000 ppm (Gospe, Saeed, Zhou, & Zeman, 1994). Toluene has also been shown to be ototoxic in laboratory animals at much lower concentrations. Much of the early work was conducted by Pryor, Dickinson, Howd, and Rebert (1983a, 1983b 1991). Rebert, Sorenson, Howd, and Pryor (1983) demonstrated that toluene exposure induces marked sensorineural hearing loss on adult and weanling rats exposed to toluene vapors between 1200 and 2000 ppm for a duration of 1 or 2 weeks. Subsequent research determined that the functional threshold of toluene-induced hearing loss is close to 1300 ppm for a 4-week-long exposure (Loquet, 1999). The ototoxic "power" of toluene is 2.4 times lower than styrene's. In other words, toluene exposure levels have to be 2.4 times higher than styrene levels to induce the same permanent auditory dysfunction. However, styrene and toluene ototoxic profiles are fairly similar: both solvents disrupt, specifically, OHCs (Figure 14-4b: toluene; Figure 14-4a: control), and the route of intoxication is believed to be similar (Figure 14-1) (Campo et al., 1999). In addition, Lataye and Campo (1997) demonstrated that combined exposure to toluene and noise produced a greater hearing loss in rats than separate exposure to toluene or noise.

The results obtained in laboratory animals and solvent abusers logically raised the question of the potential ototoxicity of toluene in occupational settings. One again, the amount of human data is extremely limited despite the widespread use of toluene in industry.

Low-level occupational exposure to an averaging 97 ppm toluene for 12–14 years had an apparent effect on hearing in forty rotogravure workers when ABR results were compared to a group of forty nonexposed workers (Abbate, Giorgianni, Munao, & Brecciaroli,

1993). In two other studies by Vrca, Bozicevic, Bozikov, Fuchs, and Malinar (1996, 1997), ABRs in workers exposed to average concentrations of about 50 ppm for an average of 21.4 years were found to be affected, with a significant decrease in all wave amplitudes. Additionally, a cross-sectional study of 124 Brazilian workers exposed to various levels of noise and a variety of organic solvents, including toluene at concentrations ranging from 0.037–244 ppm (midpoint = 122 ppm), showed hearing loss in nearly half of the exposed workers (Morata, Fiorini, Fischer, Colacioppos, Wallingford et al., 1997). Toluene exposure was estimated by personal monitoring and measurement of the main toluene metabolite, hippuric acid, in urine samples. Logistic regression analysis showed hippuric acid concentration to be associated significantly with hearing loss.

The findings of those few studies show that, at concentrations below or slightly above the occupational permitted levels, long-term exposure to toluene can have deleterious effects on hearing in workers. Therefore, additional follow-up studies need to be conducted to determine dose/effect relationship at low levels to determine whether the 200 ppm limit is adequate or if the 50 ppm level recommended by the ACGIH should be applied. In any case, when monitoring workers exposed to toluene and noise in the workplace, audiologists must consider both noise and toluene levels.

Ethyl Benzene

Ethyl benzene (Figure 14-2) is a colorless liquid that smells like gasoline. More than 99% of the ethyl benzene is used in the production of styrene, the remaining being used as a solvent in asphalt and fuels. It is also found in many products, including paints, inks, and insecticides. Gasoline contains about 2% (by weight) ethyl benzene.

In 1994, approximately 12 billion pounds were produced in the United States. Gas and oil workers may be exposed to ethyl benzene either by skin contact or inhalation of vapors. Varnish workers, spray painters, and people involved in gluing operations may also be exposed to high levels of ethyl benzene. Exposures may occur in factories that use ethyl benzene to

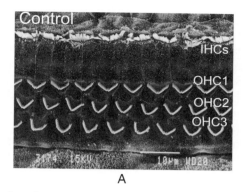 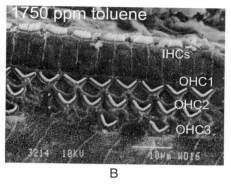

A   B

Figures 14-4a and 14-4b.   High-power scanning electron micrographs of portions of organ of Corti corresponding to the 20-kHz region from (A) control rat and (B) toluene-exposed rat (1750 ppm, 6 hours/day, 5 days/week, 4 weeks). Photos: Pierre Campo (INRS), with permission.

produce other chemicals. In the workplace, OSHA set a legal limit of 100 ppm in air for an 8-hour period. NIOSH also recommends an exposure limit for ethyl benzene of 100 ppm.

Laboratory animal data on the auditory effect of ethyl benzene come from the work conducted by Cappaert et al. between 1999 and 2002 in rats. Results are clear: ethyl benzene is the most potent ototoxic organic solvent known today. The functional and histologic patterns of the hearing loss induced by ethyl benzene are very similar to the effects of toluene and styrene (i.e., mid-frequency hearing loss; selective outer cell damage; potentiation of NIHL; sensitivity of rats but not guinea pigs), suggesting a common ototoxic mechanism (Cappaert et al., 1999, 2001, 2002); but the threshold ototoxic dose is very low— 300–400 ppm for 5 days (Cappaert et al., 2000).

Despite the fact that ethyl benzene has been shown to be a very potent ototoxicant in the rat and that it is widely used in the industry, no human exposure data are available. That is unfortunate because the small difference between the occupational limits and the threshold ototoxic dose in rats raises some questions on the adequacy of human exposure regulations.

Xylene

Xylene (Figure 14-2) is one of the top thirty chemicals produced in the United States, with approximately 12 billion pounds produced annually (Reisch, 1992; US EPA, 1993). In 1976, a survey conducted by NIOSH (1976) found that based on average concentrations in the workplace air, xylene ranked thirteenth out of approximately 7,000 chemicals. In 1984, more than 1 million workers were potentially exposed to xylene (NIOSH, 1984). Xylene is used as a solvent in the printing, rubber, and leather industries. Along with other solvents, xylene is also used as a thinner for paint and in varnishes. Occupational exposures to xylene vapors are possible in chemical, plastic, textile and paper industries. It is also found in small amounts in airplane fuel and gasoline. The chemical structure of xylene is a benzene ring with two methyl groups. Therefore, xylene exists as three different isomers: *meta-*, *ortho-*, and *para-*xylene (Figure 14-2). Generally, the industrial xylene is used as a blend of those three isomers, commonly referred to as mixed-xylene. OSHA has set an occupational exposure limit of 100 ppm time-weighted average, which matches the recommendation of the ACGIH and NIOSH.

While the neurotoxic effects of xylene in human and animal models have been studied extensively, the literature concerning its ototoxicity is very limited. Pryor et al. (1987) measured a severe permanent hearing loss in rats exposed for 14 hours/day for 6 weeks to 800 ppm of xylene by inhalation. Crofton et al. (1994) showed a mid-frequency hearing loss after 5 days of exposure to xylene vapors at 1800 ppm.

Both investigations determined that at equal doses, xylene was less ototoxic than styrene but more ototoxic than toluene. A few years later Gagnaire, Marignac, Langlais, and Bonnet (2001) exposed groups of rats to individual xylene isomers for 13 weeks and observed that only *para*-xylene induced severe hearing loss and OHC loss for concentrations of 900 ppm or more. *Meta*- and *ortho*-xylene did not induce any hearing loss even at the highest dose. Unfortunately, more than 70% of the xylene used in the United States is *para*-xylene.

The literature contains no human data on occupational exposure to pure xylene. However, two recent epidemiological studies conducted in Poland on workers in paint and varnish production plants showed that exposure to low doses of solvent mixtures, including mixed xylene, significantly increased the risk of developing hearing loss (Sliwinska-Kowalska, Zamyslowska-Szmytke, Szymczak, Kotylo, Fiszer et al., 2001; Sulkowski, Kowalska, Matyja, Guzek, Wesolowski et al., 2002).

Trichloroethylene

Unlike the organic solvents cited above, trichloroethylene (TCE) is not an aromatic solvent, meaning that it does not have a benzene ring in its chemical formula (Figure 14-2). However, its physical properties are quite similar: it is volatile, and it is used to dissolve grease.

About 400,000 workers are routinely exposed to TCE in the United States either by inhalation of vapors or by skin contact (NIOSH, 1990). The most important use of TCE, vapor degreasing of metal parts, is closely associated with the automotive and metal industries (CMR, 1983). A person may also be exposed to TCE at home when using typewriter correction fluids, paint removers/strippers, adhesives, spot removers, and rug-cleaning fluids (Frankenberry, Kent, & Stroup, 1987). At one time, TCE was used extensively in dry cleaning although it has been replaced by perchloroethylene, which appears to be less toxic.

TCE has been identified as an auditory toxicant in laboratory animals (Rebert, Day, Matteucci, & Pryor, 1991; Jaspers, Muijser, Lammers, & Kulig 1993;

Crofton & Zhao, 1993, 1997; Crofton et al., 1994). However, the ototoxic mechanism, which is still not fully understood, seems different from the way aromatic solvents act. Early published reports on the auditory effects of TCE do not clearly address the involvement of the cochlea in the auditory impairment. Behavioral studies demonstrated a clear pattern of mid-frequency hearing impairment, but were not able to determine the site within the auditory system where this impairment occurs (Jaspers et al., 1993; Crofton & Zhao, 1993, 1997; Crofton et al., 1994). Electrophysiologic studies showed a drop in the amplitude of all components of the ABRs following TCE exposure (Rebert et al., 1983, 1991). Those data were therefore consistent with, but did not firmly establish, a cochlear locus of dysfunction.

More recently Fechter, Liu, Herr, and Crofton (1998) demonstrated that exposure to TCE (4000 ppm for 5 days) induced compound action potential threshold elevation in rats, indicating cochlear impairment. However, cochlear microphonics, a nonpropagated AC potential generated largely by the OHCs, was not affected by the TCE treatment. Cochlear histopathology revealed a loss of spiral ganglion cells that was significant in the middle turn but not in the basal turn, suggesting that the spiral ganglion cells coding for the midfrequencies are the preferential target of TCE toxicity. However, no surface preparation was made to determine the extent of hair cell loss.

n-Hexane

n-hexane (Figure 14-2) is a widely used aliphatic hydrocarbon. Several hundred million pounds of *n*-hexane are produced each year in the United States. Most of the *n*-hexane used in the industry is mixed with other solvents. Pure *n*-hexane is used only in laboratories. The major use for solvents containing *n*-hexane is to extract vegetable oil from crops such as soybeans. The solvents are also used as cleaning agents in the printing, textile, furniture, and shoe-making industries. *N*-hexane is also present in gasoline (1%–3%). Since *n*-hexane is very volatile, the main route of exposure is through the respiratory system, but exposure by skin contact is also possible.

Current empirically based estimates of exposures to *n*-hexane in various occupations are lacking; but based on the conditions typical of the mid-1970s, it was estimated that more than 600,000 workers had potential exposure to this compound (NIOSH, 1991). OSHA has set a permissible exposure limit of 500 ppm for *n*-hexane in workplace air; but because nerve damage has been found in workers exposed to 500 ppm, a court decision struck down a proposed PEL of 50 ppm (which is the level recommended by both the ACGIH and NIOSH). The major public health concern regarding *n*-hexane is the potential for development of neurotoxicity. Occupational studies have documented that human exposure to *n*-hexane can result in a peripheral neuropathy that, in severe cases, can lead to paralysis (Altenkirch, Wagner, Stoltenburg, & Spencer, 1982; Yamamura, 1969; Wang, Chang, Kao, Huang, Lin et al., 1986). The dose-duration relationship has not been well characterized in humans. Concentrations of 500 ppm and above and exposure for 6 months or more have been associated with human neurotoxicity.

As far as the ototoxicity of *n*-hexane is concerned, only an old experimental study investigated the auditory effects of pure *n*-hexane in rats. Rebert, Houghton, Howd, and Pryor (1982) showed that the fifth component of the brainstem auditory evoked response (BAER) increased in latency and decreased in amplitude in rats exposed to 1,000 ppm of hexane 24 hours per day 5 days per week for 11 weeks; the first component of the BAER was only slightly affected. That suggests a brainstem dysfunction with no involvement of the cochlea. Therefore, the probable risk from hexane is peripheral neuropathy with hearing loss being simply one aspect of such neurotoxicity. Clearly, further studies in the rat model to assess the adequacy of occupational PEL for *n*-hexane would be helpful.

ACRYLONITRILE

There is strong evidence that intense noise can initiate reactive oxygen species (ROS) in the cochlea and that antioxidants may be effective in reducing or blocking NIHL (see Chapters 7, 15, and 19). First, pharmacological studies have documented the ability of antioxidant drugs or prodrugs to block or reduce NIHL (Seidman, Shivapuja, & Quirk, 1993; Yamasoba, Schacht, Shoji, & Miller, 1999; Henderson, McFadden, Liu, Hight, & Zheng, 1999). Second, genetic studies have demonstrated that laboratory animal models with reduced antioxidant buffering capacity are more vulnerable to NIHL than are wild-type subjects (Ohlemiller, McFadden, Ding, Flood, Reaume, Hoffman et al., 1999a; Ohlemiller, McFadden, Ding, Lear, & Ho, 2000). Finally, there are a limited number of reports with direct evidence of oxidative stress or of increased ROS in subjects who have been exposed to noise (Yamane, Nakai, Takayama, Iguchi, Nakagawa et al., 1995; Ohlemiller, Wright, & Dugan, 1999b, 2000; Ohinata et al., 2000a, b). Those observations led to the prediction that chemicals that disrupt intrinsic antioxidant defenses hold significant risk for potentiating NIHL. Acrylonitrile (ACN; Figure 14-2) is one of those chemical compounds.

ACN ranks forty-second on the list of chemicals used in the United States (Anonymous, 1980). Some 3.21 billion pounds of ACN were produced in the United States alone in 1995, with estimated exposure to approximately 125,000 workers (Kirshner, 1995). ACN is used to make synthetic fibers (acrylic and nylon), nitrile rubbers, and plastics and is used as a chemical intermediate in the synthesis of a variety of products including dyes and pharmaceuticals. While NIOSH-recommended permissible exposure level to ACN is quite low (1 ppm), exposure can reach high levels via skin contact in case of accidental exposure (Kirschner, 1995).

The metabolism of ACN is associated with significant potential for oxidative stress. ACN conjugates glutathione (Benz, Nerland, Li, & Corbett, 1997), depleting this important antioxidant rapidly. A second pathway involves the formation of cyanide as a by-product (Langvardt, Putzig, Braun, & Young, 1980; van Bladeren, Delbressine, Hoogeterp, Beaumont, Breimer et al., 1981). Cyanide, in turn, can inhibit superoxide dismutase and produce oxidative stress through other pathways as well.

Fechter, Klis, Shirwany, Moore, and Rao (2003) and Fechter, Gearhart, and Shirwany (2004) have shown recently that ACN (50 mg/kg sc/day) can potentiate permanent NIHL for noise levels ranging from 105 dB for 5 days (4 hours/day) to 108 dB for 8 hours and that this potentiation can be prevented by the administration of phenyl-N-tert-butylnitrone, a spin-trap agent that sequesters ROS. Pouyatos, Gearhart, and Fechter (2005) also showed that combined exposure to ACN and noise yielded pronounced loss of threshold, even for noise levels that did not cause any hearing loss by themselves (95 and 97 dB SPL for 5 days, 4 hours/day). The mechanism of this potentiation is not fully understood, but it is likely that the disruption of anti-oxidant functions in the cochlea are involved.

SUMMARY

Audiologists are acutely aware of the ability of noise to damage hearing; indeed, NIHL is recognized as one of the leading occupational injuries. Recognition that exposure to chemicals in the workplace can also damage hearing directly and make people more vulnerable to the adverse effects of noise is less understood and less recognized. This chapter focuses attention on a group of specific chemical agents that can impair hearing and has sought to identify both potential mechanisms by which such hearing loss occurs, as well as the cells that are targets for toxic insult. Understanding how chemicals can affect hearing helps audiologists predict other potentially ototoxic agents and to develop therapeutic strategies for increasing recovery from such hearing loss.

A review of the literature shows that ototoxic chemicals often are agents that can produce central nervous system injury. They include chemical asphyxiants, specific metals, and several organic solvents. While those agents have very different chemical structures and may produce toxicity via different mechanisms, it is remarkable that most of them produce injury at the level of the cochlea and that hearing loss is often accompanied by OHC loss. While that is also a pattern of injury that is observed for ototoxic drugs such as aminoglycoside antibiotics, it turns out that the ototoxic organic solvents tend to damage hearing and hair cells primarily for mid-frequency tones and their associated hair cells. By contrast, ototoxic drugs tend to impair high-frequency hearing preferentially.

While several mechanisms are likely responsible for chemical ototoxicity, one mechanism that has received substantial investigation is that of oxidative stress. One can, in fact, hypothesize that chemicals that impair antioxidant pathways in the ear will predispose the hearing organ to injury from subsequent noise exposure. Consequently, using laboratory animal models, it is possible to block or greatly reduce hearing loss from chemicals and noise by administration of antioxidant drugs. Such strategies have also been applied in the case of aminoglycoside antibiotic and cisplatin treatment and in the case of noise exposure alone. It remains uncertain whether antioxidant foods or food supplements actually increase cochlear antioxidant capacity and whether such agents might be protective in advance of noise or noise and chemical exposure.

Future epidemiological research in which workplace exposure to chemicals and noise is evaluated for ototoxicity is essential to develop an understanding of the dosing regimens under which chemicals produce hearing loss. Among the important questions is whether peak exposure for short time periods or whether duration of chemical exposure is more important as a predictor of hearing loss.

REFERENCES

Abbate, C., Giorgianni, C., Munao, F., & Brecciaroli, R. (1993). Neurotoxicity induced by exposure to toluene. An electrophysiologic study. *Int Arch Occup Environmental Health, 64*(6), 389–392.

ACGIH (American Conference of Government Industrial Hygenists) Worldwide. (2006). *Threshold Limit Values for Chemical Substances and Physical Agents and Biological Exposure Indices (TLVs and BEIs).* Cincinnati, OH.

Altenkirch, H., Wagner, H. M., Stoltenburg, G., & Spencer, P. S. (1982). Nervous system responses of rats to subchronic inhalation of *n*-hexane and *n*-hexane + methyl-ethyl-ketone mixtures. *Journal of the Neurological Sciences, 57*(2–3), 209–219.

Amin-zaki, L., Majeed, M. A., Clarkson, T. W., & Greenwood, M. R. (1978). Methylmercury poisoning in Iraqi children: Clinical observations over two years. *British Medical Journal, 1*(6113), 613–616.

Anonymous. (1980). Chemical engineering news. *Chemical Engineering News, 58*(18), 35.

Arlien-Soborg, P. (1992). *Solvent Neurotoxicity*. Boca Raton, FL: CRC Press.

Baker, S. R., & Lilly, D. J. (1977). Hearing loss from acute carbon monoxide intoxication. *Annals of Otology, Rhinology, and Laryngology, 86*(3 Pt 1), 323–328.

Benz, F. W., Nerland, D. E., Li, J., & Corbett, D. (1997). Dose dependence of covalent binding of acrylonitrile to tissue protein and globin in rats. *Fundamental and Applied Toxicology, 36*, 149–156.

Bergman, K. (1983). Application and results of whole-body autoradiography in distribution studies of organic solvents. *Critical Reviews in Toxicology, 12*(1), 59–118.

Campo, P., Lataye, R., Loquet, G., & Bonnet, P. (2001). Styrene-induced hearing loss: A membrane insult. *Hearing Research, 154*(1–2), 170–180.

Campo, P., Loquet, G., Blachere, V., & Roure, M. (1999). Toluene and styrene intoxication route in the rat cochlea. *Neurotoxicology and Teratology, 21*(4), 427–434.

Cappaert, N. L., Klis, S. F., Baretta, A. B., Muijser, H., & Smoorenburg, G. F. (2000). Ethyl benzene-induced ototoxicity in rats: A dose-dependent mid-frequency hearing loss. *Journal of the Association for Research in Otolaryngology, 1*(4), 292–299.

Cappaert, N. L., Klis, S. F., Muijser, H., deGroot, J. C., Kulig, B. M., & Smoorenburg, G. F. (1999). The ototoxic effects of ethyl benzene in rats. *Hearing Research, 137*(1–2), 91–102.

Cappaert, N. L., Klis, S. F., Muijser, H., Kulig, B. M., Ravensberg, L. C., & Smoorenburg, G. F. (2002). Differential susceptibility of rats and guinea pigs to the ototoxic effects of ethyl benzene. *Neurotoxicology and Teratology, 24*(4), 503–510.

Cappaert, N. L., Klis, S. F., Muijser, H., Kulig, B. M., & Smoorenburg, G. F. (2001). Simultaneous exposure to ethyl benzene and noise: Synergistic effects on outer hair cells. *Hearing Research, 162*(1–2), 67–79.

CMR (Chemical Marketing Reporter). (1983). *Chemical profile - Trichloroethylene*. New York: Schnell Publishing Co.

Crofton, K. M., Rebert, C. S., & Lassiter, T. L. (1994). Solvent-induced ototoxicity in rats: An atypical selective mid-frequency hearing deficit. *Hearing Research, 80*(1), 25–30.

Crofton, K. M., & Zhao, X. (1993). Mid-frequency hearing loss in rats following inhalation exposure to trichloroethylene: Evidence from reflex modification audiometry. *Neurotoxicology and Teratology, 15*(6), 413–423.

Crofton, K. M., & Zhao, X. (1997). The ototoxicity of trichloroethylene: Extrapolation and relevance of high-concentration, short-duration animal exposure data. *Fundamental and Applied Toxicology, 38*(1), 101–106.

Discalzi, G., Fabbro, D., Meliga, F., Mocellini, A., & Capellaro, F. (1993). Effects of occupational exposure to mercury and lead on brainstem auditory evoked potentials. *International Journal of Psychophysiology, 14*(1), 21–25.

Ehyai, A., & Freemon, F. R. (1983). Progressive optic neuropathy and sensorineural hearing loss due to chronic glue sniffing. *Journal of Neurology, Neurosurgery, and Psychiatry, 46*(4), 349–351.

Engstrom, J., Astrand, I., & Wigaeus, E. (1978, December). Exposure to styrene in a polymerization plant. Uptake in the organism and concentration in subcutaneous adipose tissue. *Scand J Work Environ Health, 4*(4), 324–329.

Evans, E. F., & Klinke, R. (1982). The effects of intra-cochlear cyanide and tetrodotoxin on the properties of single cochlear nerve fibres in the cat. *Journal of Physiology, 331*, 385–408.

Falk, S. A., Klein, R., Haseman, J. K., Sanders, G. M., Talley, F. A., & Lim, D. J. (1974). Acute methyl mercury intoxication and ototoxicity in guinea pigs. *Archives of Pathology, 97*(5), 297–305.

Fechter, L. D. (1993). Effects of acute styrene and simultaneous noise exposure on auditory function in the guinea pig. *Neurotoxicology and Teratology, 15*(3), 151–155.

Fechter, L. D., Chen, G. D., & Johnson, D. L. (2002). Potentiation of noise-induced hearing loss by low concentrations of hydrogen cyanide in rats. *Toxicological Sciences, 66*(1), 131–138.

Fechter, L. D., Chen, G. D., Rao, D., & Larabee, J. (2000). Predicting exposure conditions that facilitate the potentiation of noise-induced hearing loss by carbon monoxide. *Toxicological Sciences, 58*(2), 315–323.

Fechter, L. D., Gearhart, C., & Shirwany, N. A. (2004). Acrylonitrile potentiates noise-induced hearing loss in rat. *Journal of the Association for Research in Otolaryngology, 5*(1), 90–98.

Fechter, L. D., Klis, S. F. L., Shirwany, N. A., Moore, T. G., & Rao, D. (2003). Acrylonitrile produces transient cochlear function loss and potentiates permanent noise-induced hearing loss. *Toxicological Sciences, 75*(1), 117–123.

Fechter, L. D., Liu, Y., Herr, D. W., & Crofton, K. M. (1998). Trichloroethylene ototoxicity: Evidence for a cochlear origin. *Toxicological Sciences, 42*(1), 28–35.

Fechter, L. D., Young, J. S., & Carlisle, L. (1988). Potentiation of noise induced threshold shifts and hair cell loss by carbon monoxide. *Hearing Research, 34*(1), 39–47.

Frankenberry, M., Kent, R., & Stroup, C. (1987). *Household Products Containing Methylene Chloride and other Chlorinated Solvents: A Shelf Survey* (pp. 1–29). Rockville, MD: Westat, Inc.

Gagnaire, F., Marignac, B., Langlais, C., & Bonnet, P. (2001). Ototoxicity in rats exposed to ortho-, meta- and para-xylene vapours for 13 weeks. *Pharmacology & Toxicology, 89*(1), 6–14.

Gospe, S. M., Jr., Saeed, D. B., Zhou, S. S., & Zeman, F. J. (1994). The effects of high-dose toluene on embryonic development in the rat. *Pediatric Research, 36*(6), 811–815.

Goto, I., Miyoshi, T., & Ooya, Y. (1972). Deafness and peripheral neuropathy following carbon monoxide intoxication—report of a case. *Folia Psychiatrica et Neurologica Japonica, 26*(1), 35–38.

Henderson, D., McFadden, S. L., Liu, C. C., Hight, N., & Zheng, X. Y. (1999). The role of antioxidants in protection from impulse noise. *Annals of the New York Academy of Sciences, 884*, 368–380.

Jaspers, R. M., Muijser, H., Lammers, J. H., & Kulig, B. M. (1993). Mid-frequency hearing loss and reduction of acoustic startle responding in rats following trichloroethylene exposure. *Neurotoxicology and Teratology, 15*(6), 407–412.

Kirschner, E. M. (1995). Production of top 50 chemicals increased substantially in 1994. *Chemical Engineering News*, 10–22.

Konishi, T., & Hamrick, P. E. (1979). The uptake of methyl mercury in guinea pig cochlea in relation to its ototoxic effect. *Acta Oto-Laryngologica, 88*(3–4), 203–210.

Konishi, T., & Kelsey, E. (1968). Effect of cyanide on cochlear potentials. *Acta Oto-Laryngologica, 65*(4), 381–390.

Langvardt, P. W., Putzig, C. L., Braun, W. H., & Young, J. D. (1980). Identification of the major urinary metabolites of acrylonitrile in the rat. *Journal of Toxicology and Environmental Health, 6*(2), 273–282.

Lataye, R., & Campo, P. (1997). Combined effects of a simultaneous exposure to noise and toluene on hearing function. *Neurotoxicology and Teratology, 19*(5), 373–382.

Lataye, R., Campo, P., Barthelemy, C., Loquet, G., & Bonnet, P. (2001). Cochlear pathology induced by styrene. *Neurotoxicology and Teratology, 23*(1), 71–79.

Lataye, R., Campo, P., & Loquet, G. (2000). Combined effects of noise and styrene exposure on hearing function in the rat. *Hearing Research, 139*(1–2), 86–96.

Lataye, R., Campo, P., Pouyatos, B., Cossec, B., Blachere, V., & Morel, G. (2003). Solvent ototoxicity in the rat and guinea pig. *Neurotoxicology and Teratology, 25*(1), 39–50.

Lehnhardt, E. (1965). [Occupational injuries to the ear]. *Archiv fur Ohren-, Nasen- und Kehlkopfheilkunde, 185*, 1–242.

Loquet, G., Campo, P., & Lataye, R. (1999). Comparison to toluene-induced and styrene-induced hearing losses. *Neurotoxicology and Teratology, 21*(6), 689–697.

Makitie, A. A., Pirvola, U., Pyykko, I., Sakakibara, H., Riihimaki, V., & Ylikoski, J. (2002). Functional and morphological effects of styrene on the auditory system of the rat. *Archives of Toxicology, 76*(1), 40–47.

Makitie, A. A., Pirvola, U., Pyykko, I., Sakakibara, H., Riihimaki, V., & Ylikoski, J. (2003). The ototoxic interaction of styrene and noise. *Hearing Research,* 179(1–2), 9–20.

Metrick, S. A., & Brenner, R. P. (1982). Abnormal brainstem auditory evoked potentials in chronic paint sniffers. *Annals of Neurology,* 12(6), 553–556.

Miller, R. R., Newhook, R., & Poole, A. (1994). Styrene production, use, and human exposure. *Critical Reviews in Toxicology,* 24(Suppl.), S1–S10.

Mizukoshi, K., Watanabe, Y., Kobayashi, H., Nakano, Y., Koide, C., Inomata, S., & Saitoh, H. (1989). Neurotological follow-up studies upon Minamata disease. *Acta Oto-Laryngologica. Supplementum,* 468, 353–357.

Moller, C., Odkvist, L. M., Larsby, B., Tham, R., Ledin, T., & Bergholtz, L. (1990). Otoneurological findings in workers exposed to styrene. *Scandinavian Journal of Work, Environment & Health,* 16(3), 189–194.

Morata, T. C., Fiorini, A. C., Fischer, F. M., Colacioppo, S., Wallingford, K. M. M., Krieg, E. F., Dunn, D. E., Gozzoli, L., Padrao, M. A., & Cesar, C. L. (1997). Toluene-induced hearing loss among rotogravure printing workers. *Scandinavian Journal of Work, Environment & Health,* 23(4), 289–298.

Morata, T. C., Johnson, A., Nylen, P., Svensson, E. B., Cheng, J., Krieg, E. F., Lindblad, A., Ernstgard, L., & Franks, J. (2002). Audiometric findings in workers exposed to low levels of styrene and noise. *Journal of Occupational and Environmental Medicine,* 44(9), 806–814.

Morioka, I., Miyai, N., Yamamoto, H., & Miyashita, K. (2000). Evaluation of combined effect of organic solvents and noise by the upper limit of hearing. *Industrial Health,* 38(2), 252–257.

Morris, T. M. (1969). Deafness following acute carbon monoxide poisoning. *Journal of Laryngology and Otology,* 83(12), 1219–1225.

Muijser, H., Hoogendijk, E. M. G., & Hooisma, J. (1988). The effects of occupational exposure to styrene on high-frequency hearing thresholds. *Toxicology,* 49(2–3), 331–340.

NCI (National Cancer Institute). (1985). NCI 1985 Monograph on human exposure to chemicals in the workplace: Toluene (PB86-144698). Bethesda, MD: Author.

Nikolov, Z. (1974). [Hearing reduction caused by manganese and noise]. *Journal Français d'Oto-Rhino-Laryngologie; Audiophonologie et Chirurgie Maxillo-Faciale,* 23(3), 231–234.

NIOSH (National Institute for Occupational Safety and Health). (1976). National Occupational Hazard Survey (1970). Cincinnati: U.S. Department of Health & Human Services.

NIOSH (National Institute for Occupational Safety and Health). (1984). National Occupational Hazard Survey (1980–83). Cincinnati: U.S. Department of Health & Human Services.

NIOSH (National Institute for Occupational Safety and Health). (1988). National Exposure Survey (PB88-106, 89-102, 89-103). Washington, DC: U.S. Department of Health & Human Services.

NIOSH (National Institute for Occupational Safety and Health). (1990). National Occupational Exposure Survey (NOES) (1981–1983). Cincinnati: U.S. Department of Health & Human Services.

NIOSH (National Institute for Occupational Safety and Health). (1991). National Occupational Exposure Survey (NOES): *n*-hexane: numbers of potentially exposed employees for the national occupational exposure database. Cincinnati: U.S. Department of Health & Human Services.

Nomura, K., Nakao, M., & Morimoto, T. (2005). Effect of smoking on hearing loss: Quality assessment and meta-analysis. *Preventive Medicine,* 40, 138–144.

Ohinata, Y., Miller, J. M., Altschuler, R. A., & Schacht, J. (2000a). Intense noise induces formation of vasoactive lipid peroxidation products in the cochlea. *Brain Research,* 878(1–2), 163–173.

Ohinata, Y., Yamasoba, T., Schacht, J., & Miller, J. M. (2000b). Glutathione limits noise-induced hearing loss. *Hearing Research,* 146(1–2), 28–34.

Ohlemiller, K. K., McFadden, S. L., Ding, D. L., Flood, D. G., Reaume, A. G., Hoffman, E. K., Scott, R. W., Wright, J. S., Putcha, G. V., & Salvi, R. J. (1999a). Targeted deletion of the cytosolic Cu/Zn-superoxide dismutase gene (Sod1) increases susceptibility to noise-induced hearing loss. *Audiology & Neuro-Otology,* 4(5), 237–246.

Ohlemiller, K. K., McFadden, S. L., Ding, D. L., Lear, P. M., & Ho, Y. S. (2000). Targeted mutation of the gene for cellular glutathione peroxidase (Gpx1) increases noise-induced hearing loss in mice. *Journal of the Association for Research in Otolaryngology, 1*(3), 243–254.

Ohlemiller, K. K., Wright, J. S., & Dugan, L. L. (1999b). Early elevation of cochlear reactive oxygen species following noise exposure. *Audiology & Neuro-Otology, 4*(5), 229–236.

Poulsen, P., & Jensen, J. H. (1986). Brain-stem response audiometry and electronystagmographic findings in chronic toxic encephalopathy (chronic painter's syndrome). *Journal of Laryngology and Otology, 100*(2), 155–156.

Pouyatos, B., Gearhart, C., & Fechter, L. D. (in press). Acrylonitrile potentiates hearing loss and cochlear damage induced by moderate noise exposure in rats. *Toxicology and Applied Pharmacology.*

Pryor, G., Rebert, C., Kassay, K., Kuiper, H., & Gordon, R. (1991). The hearing loss associated with exposure to toluene is not caused by a metabolite. *Brain Research Bulletin, 27*(1), 109–113.

Pryor, G. T., Dickinson, J., Howd, R. A., & Rebert, C. S. (1983a). Neurobehavioral effects of subchronic exposure of weanling rats to toluene or hexane. *Neurobehavioral Toxicology and Teratology, 5*(1), 47–52.

Pryor, G. T., Dickinson, J., Howd, R. A., & Rebert, C. S. (1983b). Transient cognitive deficits and high-frequency hearing loss in weanling rats exposed to toluene. *Neurobehavioral Toxicology and Teratology, 5*(1), 53–57.

Pryor, G. T., Rebert, C. S., & Howd, R. A. (1987). Hearing loss in rats caused by inhalation of mixed xylenes and styrene. *Journal of Applied Toxicology, 7*(1), 55–61.

Rao, D. B., & Fechter, L. D. (2000a). Protective effects of phenyl-N-tert-butylnitrone on the potentiation of noise-induced hearing loss by carbon monoxide. *Toxicology & Applied Pharmacology, 167*(2), 125–131.

Rao, D. B., & Fechter, L. D. (2000b). Increased noise severity limits potentiation of noise induced hearing loss by carbon monoxide. *Hearing Research, 150*(1–2), 206–214.

Rebert, C. S., Day, V. L., Matteucci, M. J., & Pryor, G. T. (1991). Sensory-evoked potentials in rats chronically exposed to trichloroethylene: Predominant auditory dysfunction. *Neurotoxicology and Teratology, 13*(1), 83–90.

Rebert, C. S., & Hall, T. A. (1994). The neuroepidemiology of styrene: A critical review of representative literature. *Critical Reviews in Toxicology, 24*(Suppl.), S57–S106.

Rebert, C. S., Houghton, P. W., Howd, R. A., & Pryor, G. T. (1982). Effects of hexane on the brainstem auditory response and caudal nerve action potential. *Neurobehavioral Toxicology and Teratology, 4*(1), 79–85.

Rebert, C. S., Sorenson, S. S., Howd, R. A., & Pryor, G. T. (1983). Toluene-induced hearing loss in rats evidenced by the brainstem auditory-evoked response. *Neurobehavioral Toxicology and Teratology, 5*(1), 59–62.

Reisch, M. S. (1992). Top 50 chemical production stagnated last year. *Chemical Engineering News, 70,* 16–22.

Rice, D. C., & Gilbert, S. G. (1992). Exposure to methyl mercury from birth to adulthood impairs high-frequency hearing in monkeys. *Toxicology and Applied Pharmacology, 115*(1), 6–10.

Sass-Kortsak, A. M., Corey, P. N., & Robertson, J. M. D. (1995). An investigation of the association between exposure to styrene and hearing loss. *Annals of Epidemiology, 5*(1), 15–24.

Sato, T. (1966). [Hearing disturbances in monoxide-gas toxicosis]. *Jibi inkoka Otolaryngology, 38*(8), 805–816.

Schwartz, J., & Otto, D. (1987). Blood lead, hearing thresholds, and neurobehavioral development in children and youth. *Archives of Environmental Health, 42*(3), 153–160.

Schwartz, J. & Otto, D. (1991). Lead and minor hearing impairment. *Archives of Environmental Health, 46*(5), 300–305.

Seidman, M. D., Shivapuja, B. G., & Quirk, W. S. (1993). The protective effects of allopurinol and superoxide dismutase on noise-induced cochlear damage. *Otolaryngology and Head and Neck Surgery, 109*(6), 1052–1056.

Sliwinska-Kowalska, M., Zamyslowska-Szmytke, E., Kotylo, P., Wesolowski, W., Durdarewitcz, A., Fiszer, M., Pawlaczyk-Luszczynska, M., & Politanski, B. B. (1999). Effects of occupational exposure to noise and organic solvents on hearing. Abstract presented at the PAN 99 Conference, Zakopane, Poland.

Sliwinska-Kowalska, M., Zamyslowska-Szmytke, E., Szymczak, W., Kotylo, P., Fiszer, M., Dudarewicz, A., Wesolowski, W., Pawlaczyk-Luszczynska, M., & Stolarek, R. (2001). Hearing loss among workers exposed to moderate concentrations of solvents. *Scandinavian Journal of Work, Environment & Health, 27*(5), 335–342.

Sliwinska-Kowalska, M., Zamyslowska-Szmytke, E., Szymczak, W., Kotylo, P., Fiszer, M., Wesolowski, W., & Pawlaczyk-Luszczynska, M. (2003). Oto-toxic effects of occupational exposure to styrene and co-exposure to styrene and noise. *Journal of Occupational and Environmental Medicine, 45*(1), 15–24.

Sulkowski, W. J., Kowalska, S., Matyja, W., Guzek, W., Wesolowski, W., Szymczak, W., & Kostrzewski, P. (2002). Effects of occupational exposure to a mixture of solvents on the inner ear: A field study. *International Journal of Occupational Medicine and Environmental Health, 15*(3), 247–256.

Tawackoli, W., Chen G. D., & Fechter, L. D. (2001). Disruption of cochlear potentials by chemical asphyxiants. Cyanide and carbon monoxide. *Neurotoxicology and Teratology, 23*(2), 157–165.

U.S. EPA (U.S. Environmental Protection Agency). (1993). Chemical Update System (CUS). Washington, D.C.: Information Management Division.

van Bladeren, P. J., Delbressine, L. P., Hoogeterp, J. J., Beaumont, A. H., Breimer, D. D., Seutter-Berlage, F., & van der Gen, A. (1981). Formation of mercapturic acids from acrylonitrile, crotononitrile, and cinnamonitrile by direct conjugation and via an intermediate oxidation process. *Drug Metabolism and Disposition: The Biological Fate of Chemicals, 9*(3), 246–249.

van Heijst, A. N., Maes, R. A., Mtanda, A. T., Chuwa, L. M., Rwiza, H. T., & Moshi, N. H. (1994). Chronic cyanide poisoning in relation to blindness and tropical neuropathy. *J Journal of Toxicology. Clinical Toxicology, 32*(5), 549–556.

Vincent, R., Poirot, P., Subra, I., Rieger, B., & Cicolella, A. (1994). Occupational exposure to organic solvents during paint stripping and painting operations in the aeronautical industry. *International Archives of Occupational and Environmental Health, 65*(6), 377–380.

Vrca, A., Bozicevic, D., Bozikov, V., Fuchs, R., & Malinar, M. (1997a). Brain stem evoked potentials and visual evoked potentials in relation to the length of occupational exposure to low levels of toluene. *Acta Medica Croatica, 51*(4–5), 215–219.

Vrca, A., Karacic, V., Bozicevic, D., Bozikov, V., & Malinar, M. (1996). Brainstem auditory evoked potentials in individuals exposed to long-term low concentrations of toluene. *American Journal of Industrial Medicine, 30*(1), 62–66.

Wang, J. D., Chang, Y. C., Kao, K. P., Huang, C. C., Lin, C. C., & Yeh, W. Y. (1986). An outbreak of N-hexane induced polyneuropathy among press proofing workers in Taipei. *American Journal of Industrial Medicine, 10*(2), 111–118.

WHO (World Health Organization). (1985). Environmental Health Criteria 52: Toluene. Geneva: Author.

Wu, M. F., Ison, J. R., Wecker, J. R., & Lapham, L. W. (1985). Cutaneous and auditory function in rats following methyl mercury poisoning. *Toxicology and Applied Pharmacology, 79*(3), 377–388.

Yamamura, Y. (1969). n-Hexane polyneuropathy. *Folia Psychiatrica et Neurologica Japonica, 23*(1), 45–57.

Yamane, H., Nakai, Y., Takayama, M., Iguchi, H., Nakagawa, T., & Kojima, A. (1995). Appearance of free radicals in the guinea pig inner ear after noise-induced acoustic trauma. *European Archives of Oto-Rhino-Laryngology, 252*(8), 504–508.

Yamasoba, T., Schacht, J., Shoji, F., & Miller, J. M. (1999). Attenuation of cochlear damage from noise trauma by an iron chelator, a free radical scavenger and glial cell line-derived neurotrophic factor in vivo. *Brain Research, 815*(2), 317–325.

Young, J. S., Upchurch, M. B., Kaufman, M. J., & Fechter, L. D. (1987). Carbon monoxide exposure potentiates high-frequency auditory threshold shifts induced by noise. *Hearing Research, 26*(1), 37–43.

Zelman, S. (1973). Correlation of smoking history with hearing. *Journal of the American Medical Association, 223*(8), 920.

CHAPTER
15

Cellular Mechanisms of Noise-Induced Hearing Loss

Donald Henderson, PhD, Professor
Center for Hearing and Deafness
Department of Communicative Disorders and Sciences
University at Buffalo
Buffalo, NY

Bohua Hu, PhD
Center for Hearing and Deafness
Department of Communicative Disorders and Sciences
University at Buffalo
Buffalo, NY

Eric Bielefeld, PhD
Center for Hearing and Deafness
Department of Communicative Disorders and Sciences
University at Buffalo
Buffalo, NY

Thomas Nicotera, PhD
Center for Hearing and Deafness
Department of Communicative Disorders and Sciences
University at Buffalo
Buffalo, NY

INTRODUCTION

Exposure to high-level noise is the most common cause of hearing loss in the working population. It is recognized that noises above 85–90 dBA have the potential for damaging the ear after years of exposure. Gunfire, firecrackers, explosions (>140 dB peak), etc., can irrevocably damage the ear with a single exposure (Henderson & Hamernik, 1986). The clinical description of noise-induced hearing loss (NIHL) is that of a high-frequency-based hearing loss with a notch in the audiogram in the 3–6 kHz region (Cooper & Owen, 1976), loudness recruitment, and often tinnitus (Ward, 1979). Those sequela of audiometric symptoms are the consequence of a number of pathological changes in the cochlea, including stereocilia damage, loss of capillaries and fibrocytes in the outer sulcus, impaired or damaged supporting cells (Deiters' or pillars), loss of VIII nerve neurons and inner hair cells (IHCs), and (most commonly) loss of outer hair cells (OHCs) (McGill & Schuknecht, 1976). This chapter reviews the pathology of NIHL and introduces new information on the causes and pathways of cell death.

PATHOLOGY OF NIHL

While it is true that the OHCs are most vulnerable to noise, most of the cellular systems of the cochlea can be damaged by exposure to noise. Figure 15-1 shows some of the most vulnerable points in the cochlea highlighted in red.

The OHC stereocilia are connected by a network of mucopolysaccharide fibrilla, and the tallest stereocilia are attached to the tectorial membrane (Soudijn et al., 1976). The stereocilia serve as the mechanical link to the OHCs, and channels in the tips of the stereocilia transduce the frequency of vibration into an electrochemical response (Hudspeth & Jacobs, 1979), leading to movement of the OHCs (see Chapter 8). High-level noise exposure can play havoc with the OHCs by breaking the cross links between stereocilia (Mulroy & Curley, 1982) and decoupling the connections to the tectorial membrane (Nordmann et al., 2000); and at more extreme exposures, the stereocilia may fuse into a single large stereocilia (Slepecky et al., 1981) (Figure 15-2).

The IHC stereocilia do not connect with the tectorial membrane, but are stimulated by the viscous drag created when the organ of Corti is mechanically stimulated with the traveling wave (Zwislocki, 1974). That causes the endolymph to move across the plane of the cuticular plate. The IHC stereocilia can be damaged by noise, and that damage causes changes primarily in the 8th nerve firing pattern for the neurons attached to the damaged IHCs (Liberman & Beil, 1979; Liberman & Kiang, 1984).

The cochlea has three major capillary systems: the spiral ligament, stria vascularis, and spiral ganglion (Axelsson, 1988). With a high-level noise exposure, the transient response of the cochlea vascular system is complicated and there can be both increased and decreased blood flow (Perlman & Kimura, 1962; Hultcrantz, 1979; Prazma et al., 1987; Thorne & Nuttall, 1987; Lamm & Arnold, 2000). There are, however, permanent changes in the capillaries and the stria vascular system in cases of NIHL. In the region with maximal damage to the organ of Corti, there can be a loss a loss of capillaries in the stria vascularis (Wang et al., 2002) (Figure 15-3).

Stria vascularis is highly energy-consumptive because it generates the +80mv endolymphatic potential and the high concentration of K^+ ions in the endolymph. Spicer and Schulte (1998) have described a circuit for recycling K^+ ions that includes stria vascularis and scala media. The K^+ ions are cycled through the hair cells and then actually transmitted through fibrocytes in the outer sulcus region of the cochlea back to the stria vascularis. With noise damage to the organ of Corti, there is often associated damage to the fibrocytes in the outer sulcus (Wang et al., 2002) (Figure 15-4), potentially disrupting the ion cycling pathway.

Exposure to high-level noise (i.e., continuous noise over 115 dBA), gunfire, or high-level impact noise (>115 dB peak) can cause direct mechanical damage to the cochlea. Figure 15-5 shows a chinchilla cochlea after exposure to impulse noise (150 dB peak SPL). There is a detachment of the inner pillar cells from the basilar membrane. The inner pillar cells together with the outer pillar cells are structural elements that provide mechanical support and an anchor for the organ of Corti. Loss of the pillar cell support leads to

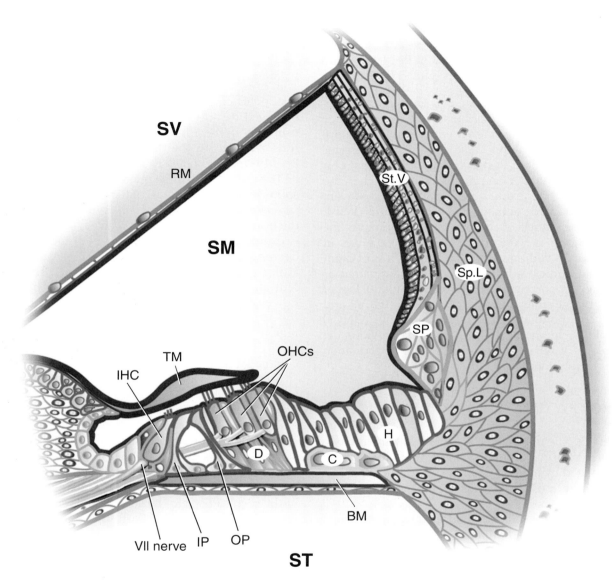

Figure 15-1. Schematic of a cross section of one turn of the cochlea (see 5-1 for perspective). SV: scala vestibuli; SM : scala media; ST: scala tympani; StV: stria vascularis; TM: tectorial membrane; D: Deiters' cells; OHCs: outer hair cells; IPs: inner pillar cells; OPs: outer pillar cells; IHCs: inner hair cells

a local change in the impedance of the basilar membrane complex, thereby interfering with the mechanical spatial code of the traveling wave.

Figure 15-6 shows more severe damage to the organ of Corti 15 minutes after exposure to simulated cannon fire (>165 dB peSPL). The organ of Corti is

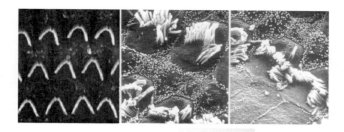

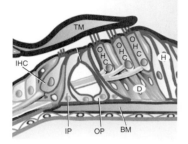

Figure 15-2. (Left) Normal stereocilia. Note that the *V* points toward stria vascularis. (Middle and right) Noise-damaged OHC stereocilia. Note that the orderly organization is disrupted and that individual stereocilia are fused.

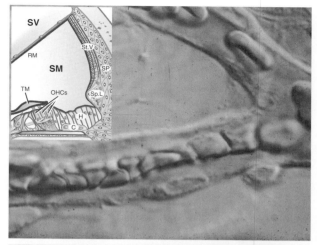

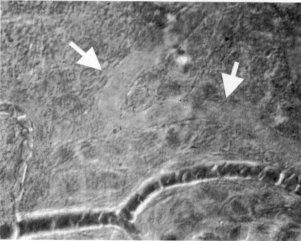

Figure 15-3. (Top) Normal stria vascularis capillary filled with red blood cells. (Bottom) Section of stria adjacent to lesion of OHCs. Note the normal capillary and the avascular channel (arrow), the space in surrounding cells left by a previously existing capillary that has degenerated.

detached from the basilar membrane, and there is a longitudinal cleft between the second and third rows of OHCs. The detached segment of the organ of Corti will be absorbed in several days, leaving an undifferentiated layer of epithelial cells covering the basilar membrane (Theopold, 1978; Bohne & Rabbitt, 1983; Hamernik et al., 1984).

High levels of noise can also cause damage at the synapses of the IHCs with the 8th nerve fibers (Figure 15-1). During high-level noise exposure, the IHCs release large amounts of glutamate into the synapses with the afferent fibers of the 8th nerve. Excessive levels of glutamate in the synapses result in the condition of excitotoxicity, which can lead to swelling and rupturing of the dendritic terminals of the auditory nerve afferent fibers (Spoendlin, 1971). Application of a glutamate blocker limits the synaptic damage and reduces noise-induced threshold shift, suggesting that the damage is contributing to noise-induced threshold shift (Puel et al., 1996), possibly temporary threshold shift since recovery can be demonstrated.

The OHCs are most vulnerable to noise exposure. It is well known that prolonged exposure to 90+ dBA noise leads to a loss of OHCs, particularly in the basal third of the cochlea. Cochlear pathology limited to loss of OHCs can lead to hearing threshold shifts of 30 to 50 dB. For larger hearing losses, the IHCs and spiral ganglion cells are most likely destroyed as

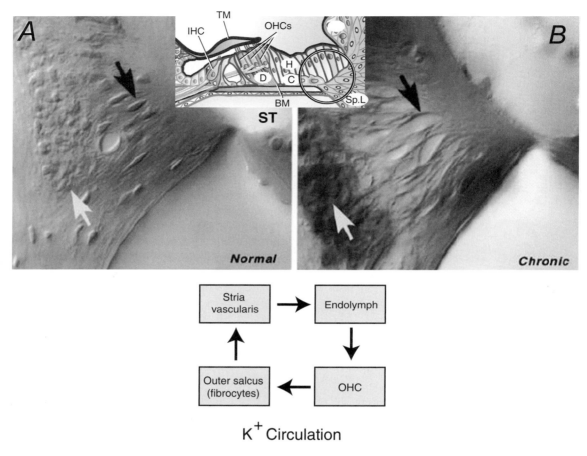

Figure 15-4. (A) Fibrocytes in outer sulcus region. (B) Missing fibrocytes after damaging noise. (Center) Schematic of potassium circuit.

well. Interestingly, the cochlea is more susceptible to higher-frequency sound (>3 kHz), and greater damage to the apical or low-frequency end of the cochlea requires exposures 10–20 dB higher than comparable high-frequency exposures. There have been a number of theories about the greater vulnerability of the basal end of the cochlea. One involves the physical impact of the stapes on the cochlea. The stapes force vector hits directly in the basal region, creating constant hydromechanical action (Hilding, 1953; Schuknecht & Tonndorf, 1960). Also, it has been hypothesized that the cochlear blood supply and the

supporting structures of the organ of Corti may be more vulnerable in the basal region (Bohne, 1976). A recent clue about the difference in susceptibility between the base and the apex may come from a publication by Sha and Schacht (2001), who reported that the OHCs' supply of the antioxidant glutathione is significantly lower in the basal end than in the apical end. The cuticular plate of the OHCs may be damaged, and endolymph can leak into the organ of Corti (Bohne & Rabbitt, 1983; Ahmad et al., 2003). Figure 15-7 shows examples of OHC pathology as well as a low-power view of the organ of Corti.

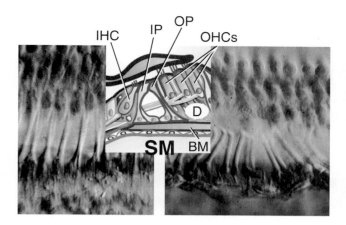

Figure 15-5. Example of structural damage to the cochlea. (Left) The inner pillar cells anchored at the basilar membrane and the top of the organ of Corti. (Right) Pillar anchorage disrupted at the top and bottom.

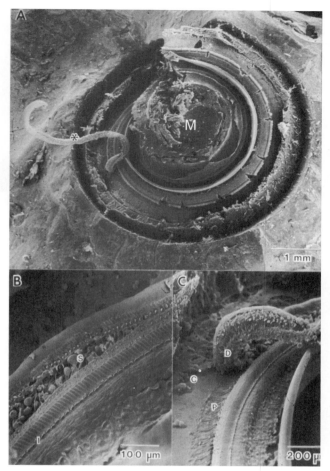

Figure 15-6. (A) Scanning electron microscopic view of the cochlea 15 minutes after exposure to simulated cannon fire. Note (asterisk) OHCs of lifted-off basilar membrane. (B) Adjacent to the detached organ of Corti is a longitudinal cleft between the first and second rows of OHCs. (C) Note that the top of pillar cells and IHCs are present and intact in spite of the OHC damage. M: modiolus; I: inner hair cells; D: Deiters' cells; P: pillar cells; S: split of the reticular lamina

Noise as a Stressor to the Cochlea

The cochlea normally operates at a high level of metabolism (Thalmann et al., 1975). The OHCs require high levels of energy because they elongate and contract in synchrony with the up and down movement of the basilar membrane. Their contractile activity enhances the basilar membrane sensitivity and tuning (Brownell et al., 1985). The other major demand for energy is at the stria vascularis, which constantly extrudes K^+ ions as it maintains the ionic balance and polarity of the endolymph (see review by Wangemann, 2002). The high energy demands are maintained by a large population of mitochondria in the OHCs and in the marginal, intermediate, and basal cells of stria vascularis.

The mitochondrial electron transport chain has long been recognized as a major source of reactive oxygen species (ROS) inside cells. Under normal physiological conditions, 98% of molecular oxygen (O_2) consumed by the mitochondria is used to promote phosphorylation of adenosine diphosphate (ADP) to generate adenosine triphosphate (ATP). The 1%–2% of O_2 that is not consumed is converted to superoxide ($O_2^{\cdot-}$) or to hydrogen peroxide (H_2O_2) at mitochondrial or extramitochondrial locations

(Chance et al., 1979). In a number of pathological processes or in the presence of drugs, toxins, electron chain inhibitors, and uncouplers, the mitochondrial generation of ROS can increase severalfold (Turrens et al., 1982). With high-level noise exposure, there is a large increase in cochlear ROS generation because of two factors. First, high-level noise drives the cochlea

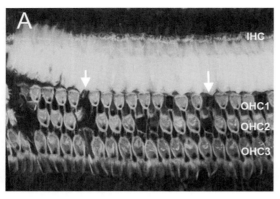
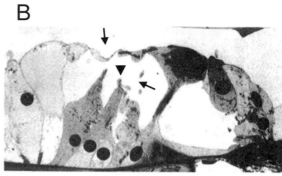

Figure 15-7. (A) Surface preparation showing missing OHCs. (B) Radial section showing missing OHCs and 8th nerve terminals. Arrows indicate the areas of missing OHCs. The arrowhead points to a stretched Deiters' cell.

at a much faster and demanding rate. Therefore, the absolute number of free radicals generated increases. Second, to exacerbate the situation, noise also influences cochlear blood flow (Miller & Dengerink, 1988). When the blood flow is reduced, ischemia develops in the organ of Corti and there is a shortage of O_2 for mitochondrial operation, leading to an even greater rate of superoxide generation. Conversely, with reperfusion (the return of blood flow to its preischemic level) there is an increased blood flow, which also increases availability of O_2 to the mitochondria, resulting in another burst of superoxide generation (Halliwell & Gutteridge, 1999). Finally, if the cells of the cochlea are damaged, cellular contents can be spilled into the extracellular matrix. Trace amounts of iron from the cell create the condition for the Fenton reaction (hydrogen peroxide [H_2O_2] and iron [FE]) (Figure 15-8), which can produce the highly reactive and toxic hydroxyl radical (OH•) (Beauchamp & Fridovich, 1970).

Several studies have reported increased free radical activity in the cochlea following traumatic noise exposure (Yamane et al., 1995; Ohlemiller et al., 1999). Those studies used biochemical techniques that provided a quantitative estimate of free radical activity on the cochlea after a noise exposure, but did not localize the ROS activity. Nicotera et al. (1999) exposed chinchillas to a 2-hour, 4 kHz octave band of noise. Fifteen minutes after the exposure, Nicotera et al.

labeled the cochleae with dichlorofluorescein and found increased ROS activity around the basal pole of the OHCs and along the neural plexus under the IHCs (Figure 15-9). Hu et al. (2002) also reported increased ROS activity for 4 days after exposure to traumatic noise (Figure 15-10). The persistent ROS activity is interesting because, in previous studies, it was reported by

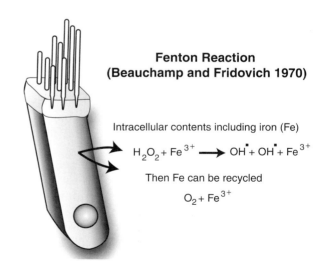

**Fenton Reaction
(Beauchamp and Fridovich 1970)**

Intracellular contents including iron (Fe)

$$H_2O_2 + Fe^{3+} \longrightarrow OH^• + OH^• + Fe^{3+}$$

Then Fe can be recycled

$$O_2 + Fe^{3+}$$

Figure 15-8. Fenton reaction. Trace amounts of iron (Fe) from damaged cells can react with hydrogen peroxide (H_2O_2) to create the highly reactive hydroxyl radical (•OH).

Bohne (1976) and Hamernik et al. (1986) that hair cells continue to die for days after an exposure.

The significance of the free radical activity in the cochlea raises a fundamental question: Is the free radical activity the consequence of dying cells, or are the dying cells initiated by increased free radical activity? The approach to that question was to expose the cochlea to paraquat, an herbicide that reacts with molecular O_2 to create O_2^- radicals (Nicotera et al., 2004; Bielefeld et al., 2005). Figure 15-11 shows the comparison of cell death patterns induced by paraquat and exposure to noise. The cochlea in the left panel was exposed to high-level noise and sacrificed 30 minutes after the exposure. The cochlea in the right panel had a 10 µl drop of 10 mM paraquat placed on the round window for 30 minutes. The cochlea was examined 18 hours after the drug application. There are similarities in the pattern of the two pathologies. Both have damaged OHCs while the IHCs are relatively intact. Additional experiments by Bielefeld et al. (2005) show that paraquat creates a high-frequency-based hearing loss. The significance of the paraquat experiments is that the superoxide activity alone is a sufficient cause to create a pattern of cochlear pathology very similar to the pathology found with noise exposure, but without the mechanical stress associated with noise.

Pathways of Sensory Cell Death

In the last few years, Hu et al. (2002) and Nicotera et al. (2003) have reported that noise exposures can produce both necrotic and apoptotic cell death. Both types of cell death are illustrated in Figure 15-12. The OHCs with swollen nuclei are dying by necrosis. The cell membrane has been compromised. Ca^{++} and water have leaked into the cell and expanded the cell volume; it will eventually rupture and spill its contents into the local area. The trace elements of the cell content will be available to react with H_2O_2 and create the very reactive and toxic $OH^\bullet$ (Ohlemiller et al., 1999). The OHCs with condensed nuclei are dying by apoptosis, where the proteins of the cell are being disassembled. Apoptosis is an active process, and both the cell membrane and mitochondria continue to function. In a normal functioning body, apoptosis is a very useful mechanism for ridding the body of unwanted cells. For example, in the developing brain, apoptosis is used to drastically reduce the number of neurons to maximize the efficiency of the pathways that remain. For that streamlining to be effective, the cells must be eliminated in an organized and controlled way. The cell death pathway of apoptosis allows for controlled cell death that prevents damage to the neighboring cells that survive. In the case of noise-induced OHC

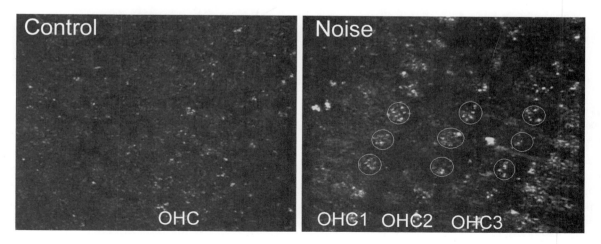

Figure 15-9. Organ of Corti labeled with dichlorofluorescein (DCF), a marker of free radical activity. (Left) In the nonexposed ear, notice a random low level of activity. (Right) A noise-exposed ear shows systematic labeling in the OHC region.

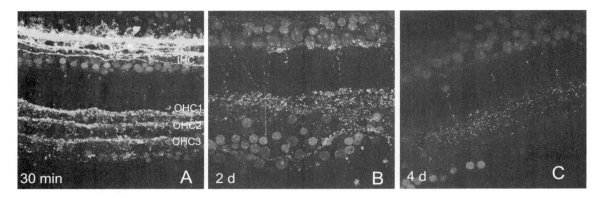

Figure 15-10. (A) DCF-labeled cochleae at 30 minutes, (B) 2 days, and (C) 4 days. Note that even at 4 days, there is still an orderly pattern of free radical labeling.

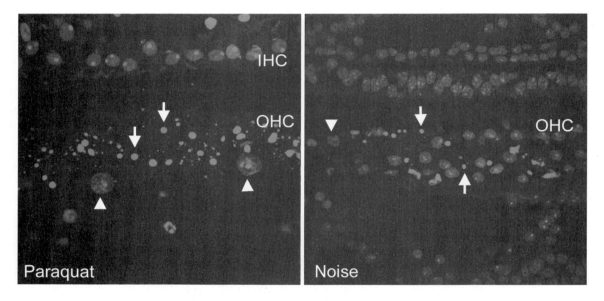

Figure 15-11. Cochleae labeled with propidium iodide, a nucleus dye. (Left) A paraquat-treated ear. (Right) A noise-exposed ear. Note that both treatments primarily affect the OHC region. Arrows show apoptotic OHCs. Arrowheads show necrotic OHCs.

death, apoptotic cell death is problematic because the population of OHCs is so small and the cells do not regenerate. Therefore, the loss of OHCs, even through the controlled death of apoptosis, leaves the cochlea in an impaired state because OHCs are essential for maximal sensitivity and tuning.

Apoptosis is regulated by a family of enzymes called caspases. Apoptosis can be initiated by cell death signals from the mitochondria, nucleus, or cell membrane. Caspase-8 is an initiator related to cell death signals from the cell mechanisms; caspase-9 is generated by cell death signals at the mitochondria;

caspase-3 is an effector caspase associated with the final stages of apoptosis (see Cohen, 1997, for a review of caspase activity in cell death). Figure 15-13 shows a cell labeled with propidium iodide (PI), a stain that is taken up by the nucleus of a dying or fixed cell. Notice that all of the darker red shrunken nuclei are also colabeled for caspase-3 (green staining) and that the swollen nuclei of necrotic cells do not express caspase-3. In a study to learn the pathways of cell death by noise exposure, Nicotera et al. (2003) reported that after a noise exposure, caspase-8 and caspase-9 were expressed, which implies that apoptosis in hair cells can be triggered into cell death through multiple pathways (Figure 15-13).

The course of apoptosis has a short latency. Hu et al. (2002) exposed chinchillas to continuous noise for 1 hour. Fifteen minutes after the exposure, hair cells were already missing and other cells showed both apoptosis and necrotic-like changes. Given the 1-hour period of the exposure, it is difficult to say when apoptosis began. To better define the latency of the cell death, the experiment was repeated; but the noise exposure was a 1-minute series of impulses at 155 dB peak SPL. Cochleae were evaluated at 5 minutes and

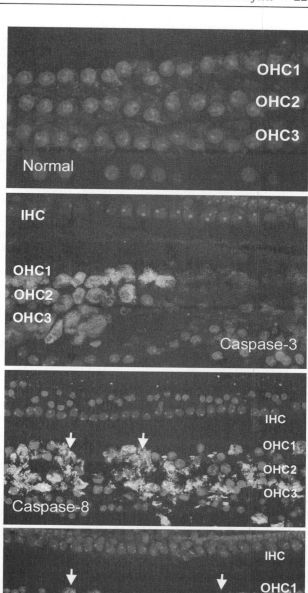

Figure 15-13. Noise-exposed cochlea colabeled with propidium iodide to mark cells in apoptosis and dyes that label either the effector caspases (caspases-3) or the initiator caspases (caspases-8 or caspases-9).

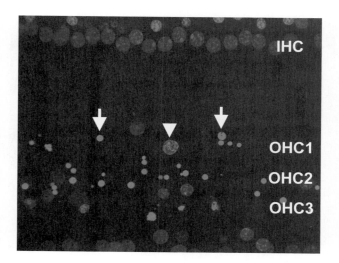

Figure 15-12. Section of organ of Corti 1 hour after exposure to damaging noise. Note the two classes of dying OHCs—apoptotic with a condensed nucleus (arrows) and necrotic with a swollen nucleus (arrowhead).

30 minutes after the exposure. Interestingly, at 5 minutes after the exposure, there was a small lesion consisting of only apoptotic cells; but at 30 minutes, the size of the lesion expanded and both apoptotic and necrotic cells were found (Figure 15-14). The necrotic cells may have been cells that began to die by apoptosis, but converted to necrosis because of a lack of energy to finish the active apoptosis process.

Experiments by Yang et al. (2004) and Hu et al. (2002) clearly show that the extent of the OHC lesion continues to expand for days after the exposure. The direction of expansion is primarily from the center of the lesion toward the basal end of the cochlea; and the mechanism driving the expansion is apoptosis, likely to be driven by lipid peroxidation because lipid peroxidation is self-perpetuating (Halliwell & Gutteridge, 1999).

Cell Death and Impulse Noise

Impulse noise from gunfire, explosions, etc., generate peak levels of 150 dB SPL or greater. Figure 15-6 illustrates an extreme reaction to such an exposure—a dramatic example of mechanical damage. Exposure to impulse noise produces a proliferation of ROS similar to exposure to continuous noise (i.e., concentration at the base of OHCs and neural plexus under IHCs (Figure 15-10). There are pathological changes that are characteristic of impulse noise, such as disassociation of the OHCs from their supporting Deiters' cup (Figure 15-15). Notice several changes. The OHC has shortened in length, and its diameter is larger; the nucleus has migrated from the basal pole to the middle of the cell; and, most importantly, the nucleus has shrunk. That may be an example of anoikis, a form of apoptosis where the triggering signal is a loss of attachment to the extracellular matrix. Using the same exposure, the chinchilla's cochlea expresses p53, a tumor suppressor gene that regulates the cellular response to DNA damage by mediating cell cycle arrest, DNA repair, and cell death (Ko & Prives, 1996). The mechanisms involved in p53-mediated cell death remain controversial, and regulation of p53 function is complicated. However, DNA damage and cell stress events, including oxidative stress (from ROS), are known to activate p53 (Finkel & Holbrook, 2000).

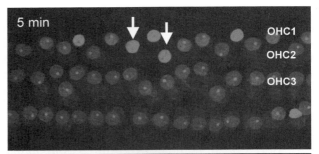

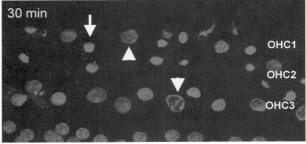

Figure 15-14. Progression of cell death after noise exposure. (Top) Propidium iodide-stained OHCs are shown 5 minutes after exposure to 150 dB peak SPL impulse noise. Notice that a few cells are beginning apoptosis as evidenced by slightly shrunken nucleus and brighter stain (arrows). (Bottom) Thirty minutes later the lesion is larger, apoptosis is further advanced and in more cells, and cells are dying by necrosis (arrowheads).

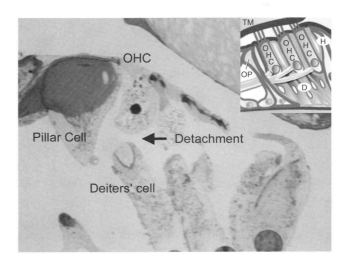

Figure 15-15. A radial section of the organ of Corti 15 minutes after an impulse noise exposure. Notice the separation of Deiters' cell cup and OHCs.

SUMMARY

Noise causes damage throughout the cochlea; but for hearing losses up to about 50 dB, the sensory targets are primarily the OHCs, especially in the basal third of the cochlea. Noise causes that damage by creating a large increase in toxic ROS, which, in turn, initiates cell death by necrosis and apoptosis.

A better understanding of the parameters of cell death (i.e., triggers for the initiation of apoptosis, the driving force behind prolonged cell death after an exposure, and factors that influence apoptosis versus necrosis) are interesting issues from a scientific perspective and may provide direction for the eventual development of drugs for prevention and treatment of acquired hearing loss.

REFERENCES

Ahmad, M., Bohne, B. A., & Harding, G. W. (2003). An in vivo tracer study of noise-induced damage to the reticular lamina. *Hear Res, 175*(1–2), 82–100.

Axelsson, A. (1988). Comparative anatomy of cochlear blood vessels. *Am J Otolaryngol, 9*(6), 278–290.

Beauchamp, C., & Fridovich, I. (1970). A mechanism for the production of ethylene from methional. The generation of the hydroxyl radical by xanthine oxidase. *J Biol Chem, 245*(18), 4641–4646.

Bielefeld, E. C., Hu, B. H., Harris, K. C., & Henderson, D. (2005). Damage and threshold shift resulting from cochlear exposure to Paraquat-generated superoxide. *Hear Res, 207*(1–2), 35–42.

Bohne, B. A. (1976). Mechanisms of noise damage in the inner ear. In D. Henderson, R. P. Hamernik, D. Dosanjh, & J. Mills (Eds.), *Effects of Noise on Hearing* (pp. 41–68). New York: Raven Press.

Bohne, B. A., & Rabbitt, K. D. (1983). Holes in the reticular lamina after noise exposure: Implication for continuing damage in the organ of Corti. *Hear Res, 11*(1), 41–53.

Brownell, W. E., Bader, C. R., Bertrand, D., & de Ribaupierre, Y. (1985). Evoked mechanical responses of isolated cochlear outer hair cells. *Science, 227*(4683), 194–196.

Chance, B., Sies, H., & Boveris, A. (1979). Hydroperoxide metabolism in mammalian organs. *Physiol Rev, 59*(3), 527–605.

Cohen, G. M. (1997). Caspases: The executioners of apoptosis. *Biochem J, 326* (Pt. 1), 1–16.

Cooper, J. C., & Owen, J. H. (1976). Audiologic profile of noise-induced hearing loss. *Arch Otolaryngol, 102*(3), 148–150.

Finkel, T., & Holbrook, N. J. (2000). Oxidants, oxidative stress and the biology of ageing. *Nature, 408*(6809), 239–247.

Halliwell, B., & Gutteridge, J. (1999). *Free Radicals in Biology and Disease*. Oxford: Oxford University Press.

Hamernik, R. P., Turrentine, G., & Roberto, M. (1986). Mechanically induced morphological changes in organ of Corti. In D. Henderson, R. P. Hamernik, & V. Colletti (Eds.), *Basic and Applied Mechanisms of Noise Induced Hearing Loss.* New York: Raven Press.

Hamernik, R. P., Turrentine, G., & Wright, C. G. (1984). Surface morphology of the inner sulcus and related epithelial cells of the cochlea following acoustic trauma. *Hear Res, 16*(2), 143–160.

Henderson, D., & Hamernik, R. P. (1986). Impulse noise: Critical review. *J Acoust Soc Am, 80*(2), 569–584.

Hilding, A. C. (1953). Studies on the otic labyrinth. VI. Anatomic explanation for the hearing dip at 4096 characteristic of acoustic trauma and presbycusis. *Ann Otol Rhinol Laryngol, 62*(4), 950–956.

Hu, B. H., Henderson, D., & Nicotera, T. M. (2002). Involvement of apoptosis in progression of cochlear lesion following exposure to intense noise. *Hear Res, 166*(1–2), 62–71.

Hudspeth, A. J., & Jacobs, R. (1979). Stereocilia mediate transduction in vertebrate hair cells (auditory system/cilium/vestibular system). *Proc Natl Acad Sci U S A, 76*(3), 1506–1509.

Hultcrantz, E. (1979). The effect of noise on cochlear blood flow in the conscious rabbit. *Acta Physiol Scand, 106*(1), 29–37.

Ko, L. J., & Prives, C. (1996). p53: Puzzle and paradigm. *Genes Dev, 10*(9), 1054–1072.

Lamm, K., & Arnold, W. (2000). The effect of blood flow promoting drugs on cochlear blood flow, perilymphatic pO(2) and auditory function in the normal and noise-damaged hypoxic and ischemic guinea pig inner ear. *Hear Res, 141*(1–2), 199–219.

Liberman, M. C., & Beil, D. G. (1979). Hair cell condition and auditory nerve response in normal and noise-damaged cochleas. *Acta Otolaryngol, 88*(3–4), 161–176.

Liberman, M. C., & Kiang, N. Y. (1984). Single-neuron labeling and chronic cochlear pathology. IV. Stereocilia damage and alterations in rate- and phase-level functions. *Hear Res, 16*(1), 75–90.

McGill, T. J., & Schuknecht, H. F. (1976). Human cochlear changes in noise induced hearing loss. *Laryngoscope, 86*(9), 1293–1302.

Miller, J. M., & Dengerink, H. (1988). Control of inner ear blood flow. *Am J Otolaryngol, 9*(6), 302–316.

Mulroy, M. J., & Curley, F. J. (1982). Stereociliary pathology and noise-induced threshold shift: A scanning electron microscopic study. *Scan Electron Microsc*(Pt. 4), 1753–1762.

Nicotera, T., Henderson, D., Zheng, X. Y., Ding, D. L., & McFadden, S. L. (1999). Reactive oxygen species, apoptosis and necrosis in noise-exposed cochleas of chinchillas. Paper presented at the 22nd Annual Midwinter Meeting of the Association for Research in Otolaryngology, St. Petersburg, FL.

Nicotera, T. M., Ding, D., McFadden, S. L., Salvemini, D., & Salvi, R. (2004). Paraquat-induced hair cell damage and protection with the superoxide dismutase mimetic m40403. *Audiol Neurootol, 9*(6), 353–362.

Nicotera, T. M., Hu, B. H., & Henderson, D. (2003). The caspase pathway in noise-induced apoptosis of the chinchilla cochlea. *J Assoc Res Otolaryngol, 4*(4), 466–477.

Nordmann, A. S., Bohne, B. A., & Harding, G. W. (2000). Histopathological differences between temporary and permanent threshold shift. *Hear Res, 139*(1–2), 13–30.

Ohlemiller, K. K., Wright, J. S., & Dugan, L. L. (1999). Early elevation of cochlear reactive oxygen species following noise exposure. *Audiol Neurootol, 4*(5), 229–236.

Perlman, H., & Kimura, R. (1962). Cochlear blood flow in acoustic trauma. *Acta Otolaryngolica, 54*, 99–110.

Prazma, J., Vance, S. G., Bolster, D. E., Pillsbury, H. C., & Postma, D. S. (1987). Cochlear blood flow. The effect of noise at 60 minutes' exposure. *Arch Otolaryngol Head Neck Surg, 113*(1), 36–39.

Puel, J.-L., d'Aldin, C. G., Saffiende, S., Eybalin, M., & Pujol, R. (1996). Excitotoxity and plasticity of IHC-auditory nerve contributes to both temporary and permanent threshold shift. In A. Axelsson, H. M. Borchgrevink, R. P. Hamernik, P.-A. Hellström, D. Henderson, & R. J. Salvi (Eds.), *Scientific Basis of Noise-induced Hearing Loss* (pp. 36–42). New York: Thieme.

Schuknecht, H. F., & Tonndorf, J. (1960). Acoustic trauma of the cochlea from ear surgery. *Laryngoscope, 70*, 479–505.

Sha, S. H., Taylor, R., Forge, A., & Schacht, J. (2001). Differential vulnerability of basal and apical hair cells is based on intrinsic susceptibility to free radicals. *Hear Res, 155*(1–2), 1–8.

Slepecky, N., Hamernik, R., Henderson, D., & Coling, D. (1981). Ultrastructural changes to the cochlea resulting from impulse noise. *Arch Otorhinolaryngol, 230*(3), 273–278.

Soudijn, E. R., Bleeker, J. D., Hoeksema, P. E., Molenaar, I., van Rooyen, J. P., & Ritsma, R. J. (1976). Scanning electron microscopic study of the organ of Corti in normal and sound-damaged guinea pigs. *Ann Otol Rhinol Laryngol, 85*(4 Pt. 2 Suppl. 29), 1–58.

Spicer, S. S., & Schulte, B. A. (1998). Evidence for a medial K+ recycling pathway from inner hair cells. *Hear Res, 118*(1–2), 1–12.

Spoendlin, H. (1971). Primary structural changes in the organ of Corti after acoustic overstimulation. *Acta Otolaryngol, 71*(2), 166–176.

Thalmann, R., Miyoshi, T., Kusakari, J., & Ise, I. (1975). Normal and abnormal energy metabolism of the inner ear. *Otolaryngol Clin North Am, 8*(2), 313–333.

Theopold, H. M. (1978). [The acoustic trauma in animal experiment: I. Morphological reaction in the guinea pig cochlea after traumatisation by shots (a scanning microscopical study)]. *Laryngol Rhinol Otol, 57*(8), 706–716.

Thorne, P. R., & Nuttall, A. L. (1987). Laser Doppler measurements of cochlear blood flow during loud sound exposure in the guinea pig. *Hear Res, 27*(1), 1–10.

Turrens, J. F., Freeman, B. A., Levitt, J. G., & Crapo, J. D. (1982). The effect of hyperoxia on superoxide production by lung submitochondrial particles. *Arch Biochem Biophys, 217*(2), 401–410.

Wang, Y., Hirose, K., & Liberman, M. C. (2002). Dynamics of noise-induced cellular injury and repair in the mouse cochlea. *J Assoc Res Otolaryngol, 3*(3), 248–268.

Wangemann, P. (2002). K+ cycling and the endo-cochlear potential. *Hear Res, 165*(1–2), 1–9.

Ward, W. D. (1979). General auditory effects of noise. *Otolaryngol Clin North Am, 12*(3), 473–492.

Yamane, H., Nakai, Y., Takayama, M., Konishi, K., Iguchi, H., Nakagawa, T., et al. (1995). The emergence of free radicals after acoustic trauma and strial blood flow. *Acta Otolaryngol Suppl, 519,* 87–92.

Yang, W. P., Henderson, D., Hu, B. H., & Nicotera, T. M. (2004). Quantitative analysis of apoptotic and necrotic outer hair cells after exposure to different levels of continuous noise. *Hear Res, 196*(1–2), 69–76.

Zwislocki, J. J. (1974). Cochlear waves: Interaction between theory and experiments. *J Acoust Soc Am, 55*(3), 578–583.

CHAPTER
16

Audiologic Monitoring for Ototoxicity and Patient Management

Stephen A. Fausti, PhD
VA RR&D National Center for Rehabilitative Auditory
Research (NCRAR)
Portland VA Medical Center, Portland, Oregon and
Department of Otolaryngology
Oregon Health & Science University, Portland, Oregon

Wendy J. Helt, MA, CCC-A
VA RR&D National Center for Rehabilitative Auditory
Research (NCRAR)
Portland VA Medical Center, Portland, Oregon

Jane S. Gordon, MS, CCC-A
VA RR&D National Center for Rehabilitative Auditory
Research (NCRAR)
Portland VA Medical Center, Portland, Oregon

Kelly M. Reavis, MS, CCC-A
VA RR&D National Center for Rehabilitative Auditory
Research (NCRAR)
Portland VA Medical Center, Portland, Oregon

David S. Phillips, PhD
VA RR&D National Center for Rehabilitative Auditory
Research (NCRAR)
Portland VA Medical Center, Portland, Oregon and
Department of Public Health and Preventive Medicine
Oregon Health and Science University, Portland, Oregon

Dawn L. Konrad-Martin, PhD
VA RR&D National Center for Rehabilitative Auditory
Research (NCRAR)
Portland VA Medical Center, Portland, Oregon and
Department of Otolaryngology
Oregon Health & Science University, Portland, Oregon

Acknowledgment: Work supported by the Office of Rehabilitation Research and Development Service, Department of Veterans Affairs (Grants C99-1794RA, C97-1256RA, E3239V, C3213R and C02-2637R).

INTRODUCTION

Therapeutic drug regimens including some medications used to treat cancer and infectious diseases can be toxic to inner ear tissues, or **ototoxic**. Nearly 200 prescription and over-the-counter drugs are recognized as having ototoxic potential, and changes in hearing or balance from those medications can be temporary or permanent. Two classes of medications that possess the greatest amount of ototoxic potential, often resulting in permanent hearing and balance changes, are aminoglycoside antibiotics and antineoplastic (chemotherapeutic) medications. The frequent use of ototoxic agents in health care settings directly impacts the occurrence of hearing loss. Approximately 4 million patients in the United States are at risk for hearing loss from aminoglycoside antibiotics (such as gentamicin) each year, with many more potentially affected by platinum-based chemotherapy agents (such as cisplatin). The incidence at which ototoxicity occurs is dependent on drug dosage, patient factors, and concomitant ototoxic medication administration. A list of commonly used medications with **cochleotoxic** (i.e., toxic to the cochlea) and **vestibulotoxic** (i.e., toxic to the vestibular end organs) potential is given in Table 16-1.

Clinical complaints related to cochleotoxicity are those commonly associated with hearing loss, such as **tinnitus** and difficulty understanding speech in noise. Vestibulotoxicity can result in conditions associated with peripheral vestibular disorder, including disequilibrium, instability of the visual field, and vertigo (Black et al., 2004; Halmagyi et al., 1994). Symptoms of ototoxicity can present after a single course of treatment or be delayed for days or months; symptoms are often progressive and permanent. The risk of hearing loss is often associated with high cumulative doses of ototoxic agents. However, the severity of hearing loss is poorly correlated with drug dosage (Blakley & Myers, 1993), peak serum levels (Black & Pesznecker, 1993), and other toxicities (e.g., renal toxicity) (Rougier et al., 2003). The only way to detect ototoxicity is by assessing auditory and vestibular function directly. Unfortunately, ototoxic hearing loss may go unnoticed by patients until a communication problem becomes apparent, signifying that hearing loss has

Table 16-1. Commonly Used Medications with Ototoxic Potential

Aminoglycoside Antibiotics	Antineoplastic Drugs
Amikacin	Cisplatin
Gentamicin*	Carboplatin
Neomycin*	Nitrogen mustard
Kanamycin	Methotrexate*
Netilmicin	Vincristine
Streptomycin*	Dactinomycin
Tobramycin*	Bleomycin

Other Antibiotics	Antimalarial Drugs
Erythromycin*	Quinine*
Vancomycin	Chloroquine
Chloramphenicol	Hydroxychloroquine*
Furazolidone*	Primaquine*
Polymyxin B and E	Quinidine*
Trimethoprim-sulfamethoxazole	Pyrimethamine

Loop Diuretics	Salicylates
Ethacrynic acid*	Aspirin
Furosemide*	Nonsteroidal anti-inflammatory agents
Bumetanide*	
	*also potentially vestibulotoxic

occurred within the frequency range important for speech understanding. Similarly, by the time a patient complains of dizziness, vestibular system damage probably has already occurred. Damage to the inner ear combined with any preexisting peripheral hearing loss or vestibular dysfunction can be debilitating, resulting in impaired speech communication, impaired balance, and reduced posttreatment quality of life. Thus, prospective audiometric testing, early identification of cochleotoxic changes in hearing and tinnitus, and awareness of clinical features of vestibulotoxicity are critical to minimize or prevent permanent impairment.

HEARING LOSS: EARLY IDENTIFICATION AND PREVENTION

Initial detection of ototoxicity typically corresponds with damage to the basal region of the cochlea, where higher-frequency sounds are processed. Damage progresses toward the cochlear apex, where lower frequency sounds are coded. As damage spreads along the length of the cochlea, outer hair cells are affected first, followed by inner hair cells and supporting cells (Barron & Daigneault, 1987; Kohn et al., 1988). Results of clinical studies have shown that ototoxic hearing loss typically presents first at the high frequencies and subsequently progresses to the lower frequencies (e.g., Fausti et al., 1992b; 1993; 1994a; MacDonald et al., 1994). Therefore, hearing assessment at the highest audible frequencies for each patient allows early detection of ototoxicity and is critical for detection of hearing changes before lower frequencies necessary for understanding speech are affected.

Noise exposure prior to treatment with an ototoxic drug does not appear to affect the potential for ototoxicity (Campbell & Durrant, 1993); however, excessive noise concomitant with treatment can enhance ototoxic effects (Brummett et al., 2001). Evidence suggests that noise exposure following treatment can act synergistically with aminoglycosides and platinum-based drugs that have not fully cleared from the inner ear (Federspil, 1981; Safirstein et al., 1983.) Counseling and training patients regarding proper use of ear protection even after cessation of treatment is important to prevent the adverse effects of noise.

Numerous studies mention tinnitus as a side effect of ototoxic medications (e.g., Schweitzer, 1993; Bokemeyer et al., 1998). Tinnitus has been linked to increased complaints of stress, pain, and neuro-psychiatric disorders (Shulman, 1999). The incidence of ototoxic drug-induced tinnitus is unknown, and the relationship between drug-related changes in tinnitus and hearing status has not been fully explored. Tinnitus can occur with or without other documented symptoms of ototoxicity. The onset of tinnitus or a change in preexisting tinnitus can be an indication of early auditory system damage, and the effect can be temporary or permanent. It is important to document tinnitus prior to drug administration.

Hearing loss and tinnitus adversely impact speech communication, coping skills, overall health, and quality of life (Mulrow et al., 1990). Communication ability is a central quality-of-life issue for patients with life-threatening illnesses that warrant treatment with ototoxic drugs. In addition, hearing impairment may impede a patient's ability to communicate with health care providers, which is critical for successful treatment. Equipment and testing methodology currently exist that can reliably identify ototoxic hearing changes up to the frequency limits of human hearing. Early identification of ototoxic-induced changes in hearing provides physicians the opportunity to adjust the therapeutic treatment to minimize or prevent hearing loss requiring rehabilitation, depending on a patient's overall treatment protocol. If hearing changes are identified, physicians may terminate or alter dosages of current medication, change to a less toxic drug, or prepare the patient and family to cope with hearing loss if continuation of the current medication regimen is necessary. If no hearing changes are noted, physicians may elect to treat the disease aggressively with increased confidence. Early identification and monitoring of ototoxic hearing loss provides audiologists an opportunity to counsel patients and their families regarding communication strategies and the synergistic effects of noise and ototoxic damage. Monitoring for ototoxic hearing loss also provides audiologists the opportunity to perform any rehabilitation required during and after treatment.

CRITERIA FOR HEARING CHANGE

Ototoxicity is determined clinically by comparing baseline data—ideally, obtained prior to ototoxic drug administration—to the results of subsequent monitoring tests. In that way, each subject serves as his or her own control. Detecting changes in pure-tone thresholds using serial audiograms is considered the most effective indicator of ototoxic hearing loss, particularly when **ultra-high frequency** (> 8 kHz) thresholds are included (Fausti et al., 1992b; 1993; 1994a; 1999). Serial monitoring tests for detection of ototoxic hearing loss typically categorize patients into two groups: those who exhibit hearing change and those who do not (based on a cutoff or hearing change criterion value). For serial audiograms, criteria for a clinically significant hearing change have been based on normal test-retest variability in subjects not receiving ototoxic drugs and results of large clinical studies in patients receiving ototoxic drugs.

Comparatively few studies have examined test performance, as the criterion (cutoff) is systematically varied. Test performance for ototoxicity monitoring can be determined by examining the sensitivity and specificity obtained using a particular criterion threshold shift to identify ototoxic hearing loss. The percentage of time patients exhibiting hearing change are identified as showing change using a criterion threshold shift is a measure of that test's **sensitivity** (i.e., hit rate). **Specificity** (i.e., correct rejection rate) refers to the percentage of times patients with stable hearing are correctly labeled using the criterion threshold shift. Sensitivity and specificity have related diagnostic errors. Failure to correctly identify hearing change results in a miss; diagnosing a hearing change when hearing sensitivity is unaltered results in a false positive. The likelihood of making diagnostic errors in ototoxicity monitoring depends on how a criterion threshold shift relates to normal test-retest variability intrinsic to serial testing. A statistical method for evaluating test performance borrows from clinical decision theory involving the construction of **receiver-operator characteristic (ROC) curves,** in which sensitivity or hit rates for a range of criterion threshold shifts can be plotted as a function of the corresponding **false positive rate**.

In 1994, the American Speech-Language-Hearing Association (ASHA) published "Guidelines for the Audiologic Management of Individuals Treated with Cochleotoxic Drug Therapy," which includes criteria for ototoxic pure-tone threshold changes. The following criteria for "clinically significant" changes in pure-tone thresholds following ototoxic drug exposure were noted: (1) ≥ 20 dB pure-tone threshold change at one test frequency; (2) ≥ 10 dB pure-tone threshold change at two adjacent test frequencies; (3) loss of responses at three consecutive test frequencies where responses were previously obtained; and (4) threshold change must be confirmed by retest.

Test-retest differences for behavioral pure-tone threshold testing are generally reported to be within ± 10 dB for frequencies above and below 8 kHz (Fausti et al., 1998; Frank, 2001; Matthews et al., 1997; Schmuziger et al., 2004). However, single frequency shifts of 10 dB have resulted in unacceptable false positive rates in patients receiving ototoxic drugs (Simpson et al., 1992). Threshold shifts at two or more adjacent test frequencies are thought to be comparatively strong indicators of a true hearing change because normal variability in pure-tone thresholds occurs at random frequencies (Pasic & Dobie, 1991; Simpson et al., 1992). Threshold shifts obtained on repeated tests are also more likely to indicate a true threshold change and reduce false positive rates (Royster & Royster, 1982). Although ASHA guidelines and variations of the guidelines have been implemented in many clinical and research settings (Campbell et al., 2003; Fausti et al., 1994a; 1999; 2003; Vasquez & Mattucci, 2003), use of well-accepted statistical methods for determining test performance in large groups of patients receiving ototoxic drugs and hospitalized (control) patients receiving nonototoxic drugs will likely be required for standard criteria to be fully acknowledged.

ULTRA-HIGH FREQUENCY TESTING

Numerous studies have demonstrated the increased sensitivity of ultra-high frequency (> 8 kHz) monitoring for the detection of ototoxicity compared to conventional audiometry (≤ 8 kHz) alone (Dreschler et al., 1989; Fausti et al., 1993, 1994b, 1999; Ress et al., 1999). Previous clinical use of ultra-high frequency audiometry was limited due to lack of instrumentation and headphone capabilities. Further, a lack of standardization in calibration, instrumentation, and methodological procedures (Fausti et al., 1985) has hindered the establishment of normative high-frequency sensitivity standards. There is also a high degree of **intersubject** threshold variability in high-frequency sensitivity, which appears to increase with age (Matthews et al., 1997; Schechter et al., 1986). Conversion to hearing level (HL), therefore, is not possible for frequencies above 8 kHz, although, ANSI S3.6 -1996 does provide standards for calibrating high frequencies in sound pressure level (SPL). While intersubject ultra-high frequency pure-tone sensitivity varies greatly across patients, the **intrasubject** threshold variability is within a clinically acceptable range.

Results from studies in subjects not receiving oto-toxic drugs have demonstrated greater than 94% of test-retest variability within ± 10 dB for frequencies between 9 and 14 kHz using many models of trans-ducers, such as KOSS HV/1A earphones (Matthews et al., 1997), modified KOSS Pro/4X Plus earphones (Fausti et al., 1998), Sennheiser HD 250 earphones (Frank, 1990; Frank & Dreisbach, 1991), Sennheiser HDA 200 earphones (Frank, 2001), Sennheiser HDA 200 and ER-2 insert earphones (Schmuziger et al., 2004), and modified KOSS Pro/4X Plus and ER-4B insert earphones (Gordon et al., 2005). Those results suggest that ultra-high frequency test-retest reliabil-ity is good when testing is performed in a sound booth. Table 16-2 compares false positive rates for three earphone types (modified KOSS Pro/4X Plus, ER-4B, and Sennheiser HDA 200) and two test condi-tions (soundproof booth and hospital ward) in which test-retest threshold shifts meeting the ASHA criteria for ototoxic hearing change were obtained in normal hearing subjects who did not receive ototoxic drugs. Results showed that intrasubject variability and false positive rates were low for each transducer exam-ined, even when thresholds were tested on the hospi-tal ward (Gordon et al., 2005).

Children six years of age and older can be evalu-ated using ultra-high frequency pure-tone audio-metry. (Schechter et al., 1986). However, to obtain accurate results in younger children (< 6 years of age), age-appropriate alteration of the audiological test procedures must be considered. **Objective measures** of hearing are particularly useful to include in a test battery for young children.

CONSIDERATIONS PRIOR TO PROGRAM IMPLEMENTATION

The following section outlines considerations that must be made prior to program implementation.

Determining Program Goals

Communication with potential members of a patient's health care team, such as the audiology, oncology, infectious disease, and nursing staff, are critical for determining perceived program needs and for implementing appropriate program goals. For example, if the purpose is to prevent or minimize spread of ototoxic hearing loss into frequencies important for understanding speech, including ultra-high frequency audiometry in the test protocol may be warranted. Ototoxic hearing loss, particularly in the pediatric population, may be tolerated in favor of survival. In such cases, family counseling and reha-bilitation planning is a major goal. If the program is to include patient counseling regarding realistic expectations, communication strategies, and aural rehabilitation, mechanisms must be in place to com-municate test results not only to a patient's medical provider, but also to the patient and family directly.

Determining Target Population

Prior to implementing an ototoxicity early detection and monitoring program, the population to be tested must be determined. A program should target patients scheduled to receive drugs showing a high

Table 16-2. Comparison of False Positive Rates for Three Types of Earphones in Two Test Environments

Earphone Type	Booth		Ward		
	≥ 20 dB at 1 Frequency	≥ 10 dB at 2 Consecutive Frequencies	≥ 20 dB at 1 Frequency	≥ 10 dB at 2 Consecutive Frequencies	Frequency Range
*KOSS Pro/4X Plus (modified)	0%	0%	0%	7%	2, 5–16 kHz
*ER-4B	0%	0%	0%	0%	2, 5–16 kHz
**Sennheiser HDA 200	0%	2%	n/a	n/a	8–16 kHz

Data were obtained from *Gordon et al., 2005 and **Frank, 2001.

incidence of ototoxicity, as well as those ototoxic medications prescribed most often at the hospital serviced by the program. Patients who are likely to be particularly susceptible to ototoxic damage include patients in poor general medical condition with low levels of red blood cells or serum proteins (Blakley et al., 1994) and poor renal function (Forge & Schacht, 2000). Factors such as advanced age, extreme youth (neonates), familial tendency for susceptibility to ototoxicity (hereditary factors), and size and physical condition of the patient also may increase an individual's susceptibility to ototoxicity (Black & Pesznecker, 1993). A target population including compromised adults confined to the hospital ward or young children will exhibit reduced ability to provide reliable behavioral data, which will impact the choice of tests to be used for ototoxicity monitoring.

Individualized Serial Monitoring Protocol

The effectiveness of particular tests for detecting and monitoring ototoxicity depends, in part, on the ability of target patients to provide reliable behavioral responses. Full-frequency pure-tone threshold testing is impractical for many patients receiving ototoxic medications because those individuals often are very ill, easily fatigued, and sometimes confined to hospital beds during treatment. Extensive behavioral testing also is inappropriate for children with limited attention spans. In such cases, responses to pure-tone threshold testing can be unreliable, as indicated by increased test-retest variability, which, in turn, increases the likelihood of undetected hearing loss and false positives. Abbreviated threshold monitoring procedures that are reliable, sensitive, and time-efficient have been developed for such patients; thus, they are clinically practical for most patients receiving ototoxic drugs (Fausti et al., 1993; 1999).

Ototoxic hearing changes tend to present first within a limited range of frequencies near the highest frequencies detected by each individual patient. That result is illustrated in Figure 16-1, which shows data obtained from large groups of hospitalized adult patients receiving ototoxic drugs (Fausti et al., 1999). Figure 16-1 is a histogram showing the number of times each test frequency corresponded to initial ototoxic change in ears

of hospitalized patients who were receiving aminoglycoside antibiotics (light gray bars) or cisplatin (dark gray bars) and incurred clinically significant threshold changes as determined using ASHA criteria described previously. Data shown for pure-tone thresholds were obtained in 1/6-octave steps. Test frequencies were normalized to each subject's highest audible frequency (R), which was defined during the baseline test as the highest frequency with a threshold nearest to and including, but not exceeding, 100 dB SPL. Thus, R-1 is 1/6 octave below R (the highest audible frequency), R-2 is 1/6 octave below R-1, etc.

Most changes occurred within one octave of the highest audible frequency in each patient. That range was found to be unique for each individual and was specific to the individual's hearing configuration. For patients receiving aminoglycoside antibiotics, the test frequency at which the greatest number of ears showed significant hearing change was at R-1, while cisplatin treatment most often resulted in changes at R-2. Thresholds above 100 dB SPL generally remained unchanged following drug exposure.

Those data led to the development of a shortened serial monitoring protocol individualized to each patient's hearing configuration. A limited frequency range sensitive to ototoxic insult is defined as "the highest frequency with a threshold at or below 100 dB SPL followed by the next six lower adjacent frequencies in 1/6-octave steps, or the one octave range near the highest audible frequency." This **sensitive range for ototoxicity (SRO)** is determined during the baseline evaluation prior to ototoxic drug administration and depends on an individual patient's hearing threshold configuration. Targeting the SRO for serial monitoring improves clinical efficiency by decreasing test time. A more complete monitor evaluation is necessary when hearing change is observed using the shortened protocol. Data obtained in the follow-up monitor evaluation allow hearing changes to be verified and any threshold shifts due to middle ear dysfunction to be identified.

Test sensitivity for pure-tone thresholds within the restricted SRO frequency range compared to full-frequency testing is shown in Table 16-3 for patients who had received ototoxic medications and demonstrated ototoxic hearing changes meeting the ASHA 1994 criteria. Thresholds were tested in 1/6-octave

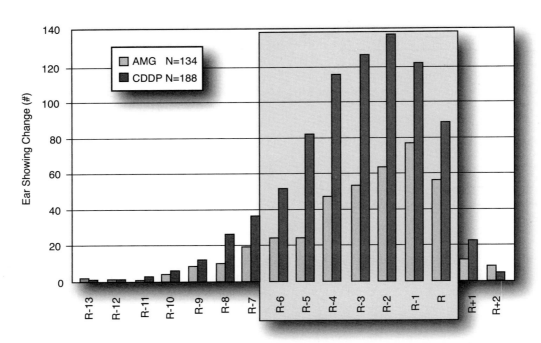

Figure 16-1. Comparison of test frequencies showing clinically significant pure-tone threshold changes in subjects receiving aminoglycoside antibiotics (AMG, n = 134 ears) or cisplatin (CDDP, n = 188 ears). *R* refers to the highest frequency with a threshold nearest to and including, but not exceeding, 100 dB SPL. Data surrounded by a rectangle refer to the sensitive region for ototoxicity (SRO). (Data are replotted from Fausti et al., 1999).

steps within the SRO, whether the SRO was located above or below 8 kHz. Of those ears demonstrating ototoxic change, 89% of all initial ototoxic hearing changes were detected within the seven-frequency SRO (Fausti et al., 2003). Thus, the shortened test protocol demonstrated a high degree of sensitivity to early decrements in hearing as a consequence of drug therapy, whether the SRO occurred within conventional audiometric frequencies or within the ultra-high frequency range (> 8 kHz).

Objective Measures of Ototoxicity

Currently, behavioral measures of hearing sensitivity are recommended for ototoxicity monitoring. However, even shortened behavioral protocols cannot be used for all patients. Objective techniques such as auditory brainstem response (ABR) and otoacoustic emissions (OAEs) have potential for ototoxicity monitoring in subjects unable to provide accurate behavioral data.

Auditory Brainstem Response (ABR)

Auditory brainstem responses (ABRs) consist of an electrophysiological potential from the ear (eighth cranial nerve or auditory centers located in the brain) evoked by an auditory stimulus and measured by electrodes placed on the scalp/forehead and proximal to the outer ears. ABRs can detect changes in waveform morphology and/or latency in subjects, which may indicate the occurrence of ototoxicity.

Table 16-3. SRO Initial Detection Rate. Of the ears with demonstrated ototoxic hearing changes, the percentage of time the initial change was detected within the individualized SRO using 1/6-octave steps is displayed here and grouped by drug. The sensitivity of the SRO using 1/6-octave steps to detect initial change is high, with an average of 89% for the aminoglycosides and platinum-based drugs.

	TOTAL (# ears)	Miss (# ears)	Hit (# ears)	Percent Hit
Aminoglycoside	54	8	46	85%
Cisplatin	226	19	207	92%
Carboplatin	59	9	50	85%
TOTAL	339	36	303	89%

Adapted from Fausti et al., 2003.

Advantages of ABR include the following: they show good test-retest reliability, they may be performed at bedside, they are noninvasive, and they are more likely to be present in ears with more severe preexisting hearing loss compared to OAE. The most common stimulus for eliciting the ABR is a 100 μs rectangular electrical signal, which produces an acoustic click when transduced by an earphone. The spectral properties of such clicks are broadband, usually with greatest acoustic energy between 2 and 4 kHz (Gorga et al., 1985; Mitchell et al., 1989), resulting in a strong correlation of ABR recordings and pure-tone thresholds within this frequency region.

Significant elongation of latency and/or disappearance of wave V is concomitant with diminishing hearing in early studies by Bernard et al. (1980) with aminoglycoside-treated neonates and by Piek et al. (1985) with comatose adult patients receiving aminoglycosides. Those studies demonstrated the potential that the click-evoked ABR has for monitoring auditory changes in nonresponsive individuals. However, a disadvantage of the traditional click-evoked ABR response is that sensitivity information is limited to 4 kHz and below. Therefore, hearing loss can progress to the point of communication impairment before being detected with ABR using conventional click stimuli.

The use of tone bursts to obtain frequency-specific responses has substantially increased the amount of information to be obtained from the ABR (Fausti et al., 1991, 1994b). Just as ultra-high frequency pure-tone stimuli are used in behavioral evaluation, ultra-high frequency tone burst stimuli can be used in ABR testing to identify ototoxic changes before the speech frequency range is affected, thus preserving communication ability. Ultra-high frequency (8–14 kHz) tone burst stimuli ABR testing has been shown to have good intersession test-retest reliability, a requirement for serial monitoring of ototoxicity (Fausti et al., 1991). Studies comparing ABR response data from conventional acoustic clicks to response data from ultra-high frequency tone bursts have demonstrated that ultra-high frequency tone bursts are more sensitive than conventional clicks in the detection of ototoxicity for those patients with measurable hearing above 8 kHz (Fausti et al., 1992a). Although ABR elicited with ultra-high frequency tone bursts has proven effective for reliably estimating behavioral thresholds and detecting ototoxicity (84% in Fausti et al., 1992b), the test is lengthy, could lack frequency specificity depending on how it is measured, and has limited high-frequency output. In addition, response interpretation at ultra-high frequencies is variable and subjective. To reduce ABR test time, tone bursts in multiple sequences have been developed to allow more stimuli to be presented in a shorter time period and has shown to be as reliable and useful as single stimuli (Fausti et al., 1994b; Mitchell et al., 1999; Henry et al., 2000).

Otoacoustic Emissions (OAEs)

OAE testing has also been proposed as an objective measure of ototoxic hearing change as OAEs are acoustic responses that are thought to originate from the vibratory motion of the outer hair cells (Brownell, 1990), which are the sensory cells in the cochlear end organ that are most vulnerable to damage by ototoxic agents (Hodges & Lonsbury-Martin, 1998). Consequently, OAEs may be more sensitive to ototoxic damage compared to behavioral testing or ABR.

OAEs recorded in response to clicks or tones are referred to as evoked OAE. Responses to clicks or tone bursts are referred to as **transient evoked OAE (TEOAE)**. Responses elicited by single tones or two tones presented simultaneously are called **stimulus frequency OAE (SFOAE)** and **distortion product OAE (DPOAE),** respectively. TEOAE are most often elicited by clicks that activate the entire basilar membrane simultaneously and are arguably the most complex in terms of their response generation and interpretation. The DPOAE stimuli also result in a complex basilar membrane activity pattern with two mechanisms or sources combining to produce the DPOAE measured in the ear canal (Shera & Guinan, 1999). SFOAE at low and moderate stimulus levels are thought to be generated by a single mechanism (Shera & Guinan, 1999; Zweig & Shera, 1995). The emissions most analogous to pure-tone behavioral testing are SFOAE because of their relatively simple stimulus and response generation. Considerable literature exists with respect to TEOAE and DPOAE, and there are reports concerning their use in detecting ototoxicity in small numbers of subjects. Use of SFOAE for ototoxicity monitoring is an active area of investigation.

DPOAE have particular value because the testing stimuli can be directed to elicit frequency-specific responses across most of the speech frequency range (Hodges & Lonsbury-Martin, 1998). In addition, DPOAE are more effective at eliciting responses in patients with hearing loss compared to TEOAE (Harris & Probst, 1997). The potential of DPOAE testing for objective detection of incipient ototoxicity has been recognized by a number of researchers (Arnold et al., 1997; Lonsbury-Martin & Martin, 2001; Ress et al., 1999; Stavroulaki et al., 2001; Kimberley, 1999).

Advantages of OAE include good test-retest reliability, time-efficiency, and the ability to be performed at a patient's bedside. DPOAE also have frequency specificity and the ability to be measured over a wide frequency range. Furthermore, OAE may indicate "preclinical" damage and can be influenced by damage at frequencies higher than the OAE test frequency (Arnold et al., 1999). Thus, OAE have the potential to identify ototoxic damage prior to behavioral detection, particularly when pure-tone thresholds are limited to the conventional frequency range.

The use of DPOAE for ototoxicity detection is limited by the frequency range of most OAE systems, which have been developed for use up to 8 kHz. DPOAE systems tend to have insufficient output for stimuli above 8 kHz and increased system distortion at the higher frequencies. In addition, standard calibration procedures produce errors at high frequencies. Those errors depend on probe insertion depth, which adds variability for repeated DPOAE measures at the high

frequencies. Another potential disadvantage of using DPOAEs is that they are not analogous to behavioral threshold measurements. Unlike pure-tone thresholds and ABR thresholds, DPOAEs are preneural and specifically test outer hair cell system function. There is marked variability in the relationship between audiometric thresholds and OAE amplitude, signal-to-noise ratios, and OAE threshold (Gorga et al., 2003; Janssen et al., 1998; Kummer et al., 1998). In spite of this variability, changes in the measures are observed as hearing thresholds become poorer. The stimulus eliciting the OAE and the OAE response coming out of the ear must pass through the middle ear; therefore, the responses are reduced or absent in ears with middle ear dysfunction. OAEs cannot be used for serial monitoring in ears with fluctuating middle ear disorder. Another limitation of OAE use involves monitoring changes in hearing sensitivity where thresholds are already poor at baseline. Those changes may not be detectable using DPOAE measures because DPOAE levels are correlated with hearing sensitivity only for behavioral thresholds less than about 60 dB SPL, and hearing loss may preclude obtaining measurable DP responses prior to drug administration.

Determining effective ototoxicity detection and monitoring strategies using objective measures of auditory function such as ABR and OAE is an active area of research. In contrast to behavioral methods, however, there are no accepted protocols for ototoxicity monitoring using objective measures. Moreover, the sensitivity and specificity of objective tests for detecting ototoxicity has not been determined in large groups of patients receiving ototoxic drugs and in hospitalized controls. Most reports in patients receiving ototoxic drugs have focused on ABR or OAE test sensitivity, in which sensitivity was defined as "a clinically significant change in the value of the objective measure."

Test-retest variability in subjects not receiving ototoxic drugs has been used to provide criteria for a clinically significant response change and to estimate false positive rates. Such studies have been useful for developing potential objective protocols for ototoxicity, which need to be validated. Further research is needed comparing test performance for each objective test (i.e., its sensitivity and specificity) to a behavioral standard.

IMPLEMENTING A HOSPITAL OTOTOXICITY MONITORING PROGRAM

Fundamental components exist when one is considering the implementation of an effective and efficient ototoxicity monitoring program. These elements include test location and equipment, patient identification, testing, counseling, report to physician, and patient tracking.

Test Location and Equipment

Ototoxicity monitoring can occur in either a sound attenuation booth or on a hospital ward at bedside. However, use of a sound booth is always preferable. It is essential that ambient room noise be kept to a minimum if testing is to be conducted on a hospital ward (e.g., turn off the television and put a sign on the door that reads "Quiet please. Hearing test in progress."). Sound level meter recordings of ambient room noise should be documented to ensure reliable results. Additionally, if hearing changes are noted, thresholds must be retested as soon as possible to confirm test results. If all testing is conducted on the hospital ward and a hearing change is noted, it is essential to compare sound level meter recordings between the baseline and current test to ensure that excessive ambient room noise did not affect the hearing test results. Maintaining consistent methods, test location, and environment is critical for reducing diagnostic errors during serial monitoring.

Once the test location is chosen, the appropriate testing equipment must be identified. To obtain behavioral thresholds for ototoxicity monitoring purposes, the audiometer must have the following features: (1) conventional (0.5–8 kHz) and ultra-high frequency capabilities (9–20 kHz), (2) portability for hospital ward testing, and (3) high output levels ($\geq$ 100 dB SPL) with low distortion across all test frequencies. Capability of testing in 1/6-octave intervals is useful for increasing hit rates and results in acceptable false positive rates. Most major audiometer manufacturers produce audiometers with ultra-high frequency options, and some will allow testing in 1/6-octave intervals.

In addition to audiometer selection, it is critical to consider the frequency response of the headphones that will be used. Earphones typically used for conventional audiometry (e.g., ER-3A insert earphones and TDH 39/49/50 circumaural headphones) have a reduced frequency response above 8 kHz and, therefore, are not useful for ultra-high frequency testing. It is also essential to consider the output limitations of the headphones. Some headphones may be capable of producing higher frequencies but may have insufficient output. The headphone should be capable of producing frequencies at or near 100 dB SPL to determine the upper-frequency limit of the SRO. Headphones that have demonstrated effectiveness for high-frequency audiometry are the Sennheiser HDA 200 and modified KOSS Pro/4X Plus circumaural headphones and the ER-4B insert earphones (see Table 16-2) (Frank, 2001; Gordon et al., 2005).

All audiometric testing instrumentation should be calibrated in a sound-attenuated booth. It is important to use an artificial ear that simulates the impedance of the human ear canal. However, most artificial ears are not simulated beyond 8 kHz. Continued calibration with the same equipment should yield consistent SPL output and would be sufficient for repeated measures in the ultra-high frequencies. Headphones used for conventional frequency evaluation should be calibrated according to ANSI standards S3.6-1996. Headphones with ultra-high frequency capabilities should be calibrated in SPL, utilizing the same equipment as for the conventional frequencies, using a flat-plate adapter. Consistent headphone placement during calibration measures is imperative to obtain reliable pure-tone thresholds. Frequencies greater than 8 kHz must be calibrated in SPL due to the lack of standards for conversion to HL. Consistent calibration is imperative to ensure that any threshold changes are due to hearing loss and not the equipment. See ANSI S3.6-1996 for further suggestions on ultra-high frequency calibration.

Patient Identification

Identifying patients who should receive ototoxicity monitoring as part of their therapeutic management should be a coordinated effort of the audiologist, oncologist, physician, nurse, and other health care professionals. Two primary resources for patient identification include key medical personnel and hospital pharmacy medication lists, which are often computer-generated. It is essential for the audiologist to establish a rapport with key medical personnel such as nurse practitioners, physicians, and hospital pharmacists. Nurse practitioners can provide valuable assistance to the audiologist by identifying patients requiring ototoxicity monitoring, coordinating hearing test times, and tracking patients. Nurses are a direct link to the patients. Ideally, before the audiologist makes initial contact, nurses will discuss with patients the purpose and benefit of hearing monitoring. Therefore, it is important that nurses be informed regarding the purpose and benefits of ototoxicity early detection and monitoring. It cannot be overemphasized that nurses are an indispensable resource for audiologists. They are a wealth of information in terms of knowing what the patient's treatment schedule is, when the patient is available for a hearing test, and how a patient may be feeling the day of the test.

Another means of identifying patients who should receive ototoxicity monitoring is by accessing a hospital pharmacy list. Careful coordination with the pharmacy staff or the hospital's computer support team can assist in creating this resource. It is a valuable tool for identifying patients receiving aminoglycoside antibiotics and other potentially ototoxic medications. The pharmacy list can be queried to identify patients' names, treatment medications, and patients' locations on hospital wards. Additionally, an e-mail notification from the pharmacy can be generated once a potentially ototoxic medication has been prescribed.

Once a patient has been scheduled to receive ototoxic drug therapy, the next step is to make initial contact with the patient. The audiologist should introduce himself or herself to the patient and explain the purpose, benefits, and procedures involved with ototoxicity monitoring. It is important to explain to the patient why he or she might be at risk for ototoxic hearing loss, without causing undo anxiety or alarm. The audiologist, along with the nurse, should then coordinate test scheduling with the patient's appointments and treatment regimens and with other aspects of the patient's schedule.

Patient Testing

The particular test protocol used may vary depending upon the target population being tested. The following ototoxicity monitoring guidelines can be modified for use in children, sedated adults, or patients confined to

hospital wards. For any population, it is important to consider: 1) the patient's level of alertness or ability to respond reliably; 2) the most appropriate times during the treatment protocol for test administration, and; 3) the tests that should comprise the baseline, monitoring and posttreatment evaluations.

Determining Patient Status

Before ototoxicity monitoring can be conducted, it is important to determine the status of the patient. Patients with life-threatening illnesses that warrant treatment with ototoxic drugs often fatigue easily. Therefore, patient status in this context refers to the ability of a patient to provide reliable behavioral responses. Patient status can be determined, in part, by physician or nurse reports in the patient's medical chart. If a patient is responsive, he or she is capable of completing a full audiometric evaluation. If a patient tires easily or shows limited responsiveness, impaired orientation, or acuity, a long test battery will not be feasible. The limited responsiveness category may also include small children with reduced attention. The nonresponsive adult patient, as well as infants, are likely to be in intensive care and may be sedated. Therefore, it is useful to include objective measures of auditory status, even in fully responsive patients, so that hearing status can be screened despite a reduction in responsiveness over the course of treatments. It is also important to consider that patients may become confined to the hospital ward, thus requiring bedside testing.

When to Test

Three types of audiometric evaluations are necessary to conduct effective and efficient ototoxicity early detection and monitoring. They are baseline, monitor, and posttreatment follow-up evaluations. Ototoxicity is determined by comparing baseline data (ideally obtained prior to ototoxic drug administration) to the results of subsequent monitoring tests. The timing of the baseline evaluation is dependent on the medication the patient is receiving. Animal studies have demonstrated that ototoxicity does not occur with aminoglycoside antibiotics until after doses are administered for 72 hours (Brummett & Fox, 1982). Cisplatin, however, can cause ototoxicity following a single treatment (Durrant et al., 1990). Based on these studies and according to "Guidelines for the Audiologic Management of Patients Treated with Ototoxic Medications" (ASHA, 1994), the baseline evaluation should occur no later than 24 hours after the administration of chemotherapeutic drugs and no more than 72 hours following administration of aminoglycoside antibiotics. A recheck of thresholds within 24 hours of the baseline test can be helpful for determining patient reliability for pure-tone threshold testing.

The frequency of monitor evaluations depends on a patient's particular drug regimen, which can be determined by reviewing the patient's medical chart. Monitoring and appropriate referrals for further auditory and vestibular testing also are warranted any time a patient reports increased hearing difficulties, tinnitus, aural fullness, or dizziness. Monitor evaluations, which may be a streamlined version of the baseline evaluation, are performed periodically throughout treatment, usually prior to each dose for chemotherapy patients and one or two times per week for patients receiving ototoxic antibiotics. Confirming significant changes by retest will reduce false positive rates and is recommended by ASHA (1994). Posttreatment evaluations are necessary to confirm that hearing is stable as ototoxic hearing loss can continue for several months following drug exposure (Safirstein et al., 1983).

The timing of initial detection of ototoxic effects is variable in that a significant hearing loss may occur following a single-dose administration or may present as a late onset and not be detected for months following treatment (Aran, 1995; Blakley & Myers, 1993). Thus, posttreatment evaluations should be conducted as soon as possible after the medication is discontinued and repeated at one, three, and six months following treatment. If ASHA significant hearing change is noted, repeat testing should be performed to verify the change. The determination of how long to follow up may be guided by the stability of hearing. It may be necessary to continue monitoring longer than six months if hearing has not stabilized. Follow-up evaluations are important in that they are useful for documenting ASHA significant hearing change, identifying latent hearing changes, and/or documenting any hearing recovery.

Test Protocol

Test protocols for the baseline, monitor evaluations, and posttreatment evaluations will be examined separately, below.

Baseline Evaluation. Obtaining accurate baseline hearing results is essential since all future tests will be compared to those results. The baseline evaluation is a full audiometric test battery that begins with a brief medical case history. Additional history information includes previous noise exposure and radiation treatment, current symptoms related to vestibular dysfunction (disequilibrium, ability to maintain a steady visual field, or vertigo), and current levels of tinnitus. The Tinnitus Ototoxicity Monitoring Interview (TOMI) included with this chapter (Table 16-6), was developed as a clinical tool to detect tinnitus onset or changes in the tinnitus percept during treatment with potentially ototoxic drugs. Portions of the TOMI were adapted from the Tinnitus Retraining Therapy Initial Interview (Henry et al., 2003). The TOMI is a one-page instrument that usually can be completed in about five minutes. Ideally, an audiologist or otolaryngologist familiar with clinical tinnitus issues should administer the TOMI. A nurse or another health care professional can also administer the TOMI because it is fully scripted; however, an audiologist or otolaryngologist should review the patient's responses.

Baseline audiometric tests include otoscopy, tympanometry, and acoustic reflexes to assess the integrity of the outer and middle ear. Bilateral pure-tone air conduction thresholds should be obtained for pulsed tones at 0.5, 1, 2, 3, 4, 6, 8, 9, 10, 11.2, 12.5, 14, 16, 18, and 20 kHz using the modified Hughson-Westlake technique (Carhart & Jerger, 1959). Patients with tinnitus and/or sensorineural hearing loss prefer pulsed tones over continuous tones for difficult listening situations such as listening for high frequencies and low intensities (Burk & Wiley, 2004), and use of pulsed tones results in comparatively fewer false positive responses (Burk & Wiley, 2004; Mineau & Schlauch, 1997).

The authors advocate the use of a shortened pure-tone threshold protocol for subsequent monitoring tests. The shortened protocol serves as a screening test for ototoxic hearing change and targets those frequencies most likely to be affected using small frequency steps. Thus, the next procedure in the baseline test involves determining the individualized SRO by locating the uppermost frequency (R) with a threshold of ≤ 100 dB SPL followed by the adjacent six lower frequencies in 1/6-octave steps, R-1 through R-6 (all ≤ 100 dB SPL). The baseline SRO will provide the reference from which all further tests are compared (see Table 16-4 for an example).

Ideally, the entire SRO is tested in 1/6-octave steps. Many audiometers on the market have the ability to test up to 20 kHz, and most will allow testing in 1/6-octave intervals in the ultra-high frequencies. Fewer clinical audiometers, however, allow testing in 1/6-octave steps below 8 kHz. If 1/6-octave testing is not possible within the targeted SRO frequencies, it is recommended that testing be conducted in as discrete resolution as the audiometer allows. For example, if the patient's SRO top frequency is 11.2 kHz (i.e., 11.2 kHz is the highest frequency with a pure-tone threshold not exceeding 100 dB SPL), then the SRO in 1/6-octave steps should include test frequencies of 5.66, 6.35, 7.13, 8, 9, 10, and 11.2 kHz. However, if the audiometer does not allow for 1/6-octave steps below 8kHz, then the SRO test frequencies would include 6, 8, 9, 10, and 11.2 kHz. The SRO is reduced from seven to five frequencies. Test sensitivity may be decreased if the ultra-high test frequencies and smaller step size are not utilized.

Baseline evaluation should also include bilateral pure-tone bone conduction thresholds obtained at 0.5, 1, 2, 3, and 4 kHz to identify conductive pathologies. If a patient presents with a nonfluctuating conductive pathology (i.e., stable tympanograms, acoustic reflexes, and bone conduction thresholds), serial ototoxicity monitoring could still be effective. If the conductive pathology is fluctuating, ototoxicity monitoring results are rendered invalid because changes in hearing sensitivity cannot be attributed solely to damage by ototoxic medications.

Next, an objective measure should be chosen should the patient become too ill to respond during serial monitoring, as is commonly seen with patients receiving chemotherapeutic medications. Consider the pure-tone audiometry results and status of the middle ear when selecting the objective measure.

Finally, speech reception thresholds and speech discrimination should be collected. Speech audiometry typically is not an early indicator of ototoxic hearing loss. However, if ototoxic hearing changes are identified and confirmed, a comparison of speech results to those taken at the baseline test can provide essential information for counseling and aural rehabilitation.

Comorbidities (e.g., pain, coughing, and fatigue) associated with the target patient population may result in increased test-retest errors. Therefore, a baseline recheck is necessary and appropriate to verify baseline results. It is recommended that procedures likely to be used in subsequent monitoring tests (e.g., SRO and DPOAE testing) be repeated. Recheck of behavioral thresholds should initially be obtained at

Table 16-4. Identification of Individualized SRO, Using 1/6-Octave Intervals. Example values represent behavioral thresholds in SPL and 1/6-octave intervals. The SRO is shaded. The individualized sensitivity range for this patient starts at 12.5 kHz. This is the uppermost frequency with a threshold ≤ 100 dB SPL.

Test Frequency (Hz)	Baseline Hearing Thresholds	Monitor Hearing Thresholds
500	25	
1000	25	
2000	35	
2240		
2520		
2830		
3170		
3560		
4000	55	
4490		
5040		
5660		
6350	55	R-6
7130	60	R-5
8000	70	R-4
9000	75	R-3
10000	85	R-2
11200	90	R-1
12500	100	R
14000	110	
16000	> 115	
18000	> 115	
20000	> 115	

Adapted with permission from Fausti et al., 2003.

the patient's SRO frequencies, followed by the remaining audiometric frequencies. While the SRO is the behavioral frequency region where initial ototoxic change is to be expected, further progression to the lower frequencies is not uncommon. Repeating full-frequency pure-tone thresholds will ensure accurate measures for comparison in the event ototoxicity progresses beyond the SRO to include lower frequencies.

Monitor Evaluations.   Monitor evaluations can be modified by condensing tests to target particular information or stimuli and should include follow-up questionnaires that query for recent excessive noise exposure, tinnitus, dizziness, and radiation treatment. It has been documented that radiation treatment prior to or concurrent with cisplatin may increase the degree of ototoxic hearing impairment (McHaney et al., 1992) (see example baseline/follow-up and tinnitus questionnaires in Tables 16-5 and 16-6). When utilizing questionnaires for ototoxicity monitoring purposes, the interviewer must ask the questions in a consistent manner so that changes in patient responses can be attributed to a true alteration and are not a result of variation in question presentation by the interviewer. In addition, otoscopy, tympanometry, and acoustic reflexes should be included to ensure that potential ototoxic-induced hearing threshold changes are not otherwise being confounded by middle ear dysfunction and/or blockage of the ear canal. Pure-tone air conduction thresholds should be obtained within the patient's defined SRO. ASHA 1994 guidelines should be used to identify ototoxic change. If an ASHA significant hearing change is noted within the SRO, full-frequency testing should be conducted within the same session to document hearing change. Full-frequency testing should then be repeated as soon as possible on another day to confirm hearing change. If it is not possible to use behavioral measures to monitor the patient, the objective measure selected during baseline for monitoring (OAE or ABR) should be conducted. The objective measure should be repeated on another day if changes are detected. If further changes are identified, frequent testing should continue until hearing has stabilized.

Posttreatment Evaluations.   Testing should be conducted one month and three months after final treatment

with the potentially ototoxic agent, using the same procedures outlined for monitor evaluations. Six months following cessation of treatment, a repeat of the full baseline audiometric test battery should be completed to assess the patient's overall hearing health. Figure 16-2 summarizes the steps necessary to obtain early identification of ototoxicity.

Patient Counseling

Patient counseling is an additional element necessary to achieve effective ototoxicity prevention, identification, and monitoring. There are three different phases of patient counseling for the audiologist: (1) initiating contact with and educating the patient about potentially ototoxic medications, (2) counseling the patient about possible hearing changes and posttreatment rehabilitation, and (3) emphasizing the importance of hearing protection during and following therapeutic treatment.

The audiologist's responsibility is to initiate contact with the patient and educate him or her about potentially ototoxic drugs and the importance of ototoxicity early identification and monitoring. Additionally, patients must be counseled regarding the risks of hearing loss associated with their treatment. Counseling will help the patient prepare for realistic expectations regarding symptoms, including hearing loss and tinnitus (Huang & Schacht, 1989; Seligmann et al., 1996). It is also important to counsel patients to avoid excessive noise exposure during and up to approximately six months after treatment due to the increased risk or susceptibility to noise-induced hearing damage. Therefore, the audiologist should strongly advise the patient to wear appropriate hearing protection when he or she is exposed to excessive noise (e.g., use of earplugs when using power tools).

Report to Physician

Communication between the audiologist and health care team regarding the identification of ototoxic hearing change is essential to a successful ototoxicity monitoring program. Once the patient has been tested and a hearing change has been confirmed, the

Table 16-5. Example Baseline/Follow-up Questionnaire

1. Test date:	
2. Type of test performed today:	❏ Baseline ❏ Baseline Recheck ❏ Monitor
	❏ Immediate Postdrug ❏ 1 Month follow-up
	❏ 3 Month follow-up
	❏ 6 Month follow-up
	❏ Retest (*check with one of the above*)
3. How well is the patient feeling today?	❏ 1 ❏ 2 ❏ 3 ❏ 4 ❏ 5 ❏ 6 ❏ 7 ❏ 8 ❏ 9 ❏ 10
1 = very poor 10 = very well	
4. Has the patient had tinnitus since the last test?	❏ No ❏ Yes
5. Does the patient report excessive noise exposure since the last test?	❏ No ❏ Yes
5a. If yes, indicate type and extent:	
6. Does the subject report dizziness?	❏ No ❏ Yes
7. Was otoscopy unremarkable?	❏ No ❏ Yes
7a. If no, why:	
8. Was tympanometry within normal limits?	❏ No ❏ Yes
8a. If no, why:	
9. Was any ototoxic change noted in behavioral hearing thresholds?	❏ No ❏ Yes
9a. If yes, which ear(s) showed change?	❏ Right ❏ Left ❏ Both
9b. If yes, which frequencies showed a change?	
10. Has radiation been added to the treatment regimen?	❏ No ❏ Yes
10a. If yes, note duration and location:	
11. Date and type of next test:	

physician must be notified so appropriate decisions regarding potential alternative medications or dosing regimens can be considered. The physician report should include the following: (1) test type (e.g., monitor evaluation) and results, (2) any ASHA significant hearing change noted compared to baseline and most recent test date, and (3) any other symptoms (e.g., tinnitus). If objective measures are used and a change is noted, the change should be reported if it is greater than normal test-retest variability, is repeatable, and/or is spreading to surrounding frequencies.

Two examples of chart notes are as follows:

Monitor evaluation completed. Otoscopy, tympanometry, and acoustic reflex measures were within normal limits. Behavioral thresholds indicated no change compared to baseline evaluation.

Patient denies tinnitus, dizziness, and recent noise exposure. Will obtain next monitor evaluation prior to next treatment.

Monitor re-test completed. Otoscopy, tympanometry, and acoustic reflex measures were within normal limits. Behavioral thresholds confirmed an ASHA significant hearing change compared to baseline evaluation. Change noted between 8–12.5 kHz in the right ear. No hearing changes were noted in the left ear. Patient denies dizziness and recent noise exposure, but reports recent onset of tinnitus in the right ear. Will continue to follow.

A successful ototoxicity monitoring program must emphasize early identification, thus enabling physicians, medical personnel, and patients to make informed decisions related to ototoxic medications

Table 16-6. Example Tinnitus Questionnaire: Tinnitus Ototoxicity Monitoring Interview (TOMI)

You are being treated with a medication that has the potential to affect the auditory system. One possible effect is tinnitus, which is ringing, humming, buzzing, or other noises in your ears or head.

1. [Clinician: ask only at first visit] Did you have persistent tinnitus before the start of treatment?
   ❏ No   ❏ Yes

   1a. If yes, how long have you had tinnitus?
   ❏ Less than 1 year   ❏ 1–2 years   ❏ 3–5 years
   ❏ 6–10 years   ❏ 11–20 years   ❏ More than 20 years
   ❏ Not sure

2. Have you noticed any persistent tinnitus since you started the treatment?
   ❏ No   ❏ Yes

   If no, the interview is complete. No further questions are required.

   If yes, continue to question 3.

3. What does your tinnitus sound like? (Mark all that apply.)
   ❏ Ringing   ❏ Hissing   ❏ Buzzing   ❏ Sizzling
   ❏ Crickets   ❏ Whistle   ❏ Hum
   ❏ Other: _____

4. Does your tinnitus have a pulsing quality to it?
   ❏ No   ❏ Yes

5. Where is your tinnitus located?
   ❏ Left ear only   ❏ Right ear only
   ❏ Both ears   ❏ Inside head
   ❏ Other: _____

6. Is your tinnitus louder on one side of your head than the other?
   ❏ Right is louder than left.
   ❏ Left is louder than right.   ❏ Equal

7. How loud is your tinnitus on average?
   ❏ Not loud at all   ❏ Slightly loud   ❏ Moderately loud
   ❏ Very loud   ❏ Extremely loud

8. How much of the time do you think your tinnitus is present?
   ❏ Occasionally   ❏ Some of the time
   ❏ Most of the time   ❏ Always

9. On average, how much of a problem is your tinnitus?
   ❏ Not a problem   ❏ Slight problem   ❏ Moderate problem
   ❏ Big problem   ❏ Very big problem

[Clinician: Ask the following questions only if the patient (1) had tinnitus before the start of treatment or (2) reported tinnitus previously with this TOMI. The objective is to determine if the patient's tinnitus is being affected by the drug treatment. If the patient has previously responded to this interview, each response should reflect the period of time since the last interview. Otherwise, each response reflects the period of time since before the start of treatment.]

10. Has the sound of your tinnitus changed?
    ❏ No   ❏ Yes   ❏ Not sure
    If yes, how is it different? _____

11. Has the location of your tinnitus changed?
    ❏ No   ❏ Yes   ❏ Not sure
    If yes, how is it different? _____

12. Has the loudness of your tinnitus changed?
    ❏ No   ❏ Yes, louder now
    ❏ Yes, quieter now   ❏ Not sure

13. Has the amount of time your tinnitus is present changed?
    ❏ No   ❏ Yes, more often
    ❏ Yes, less often   ❏ Not sure

and their effects. Audiologists are integral in this process. Potential treatment options the physician may consider include (1) changing the drug to one that has a reduced risk for ototoxicity; (2) terminating treatment; (3) altering the drug dosage; and (4) if no change in hearing is detected, possibly treating the patient more aggressively. Therefore, ototoxicity monitoring may prevent or preserve hearing damage

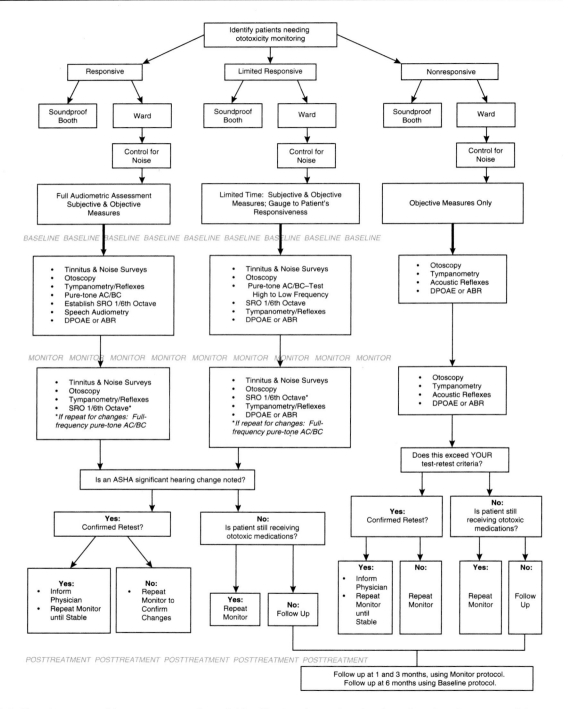

Figure 16-2. Flow chart summarizing test sequences for early identification of ototoxicity. Top-down flow chart depicting guidelines to determine an optimal test battery based on subject responsiveness. The sequence that should be followed is shown diagrammatically on the chart.

that can have a devastating effect on communication and posttreatment quality of life.

Patient Tracking

To ensure early detection of ototoxicity, patients should be evaluated according to the recommended schedule; and the audiologist must know when the patient is to receive his or her next treatment. It is recommended that the audiologist's patient tracking database be computer-generated so that weekly and/or monthly lists of patients receiving ototoxic drugs can be created and patients scheduled accordingly. The audiologist can coordinate his or her monitor evaluations with patients' next medication treatments. Patient tracking can be the most difficult and time-consuming aspect of ototoxicity monitoring. Participation by medical staff is critical to assist with the process. Staff can inform the audiologist regarding dates of patients' treatments, dosages, etc. There is, however, potential for communicative breakdowns; and, ultimately, the responsibility for tracking patients lies with the audiologist.

SUMMARY

Ototoxic agents are commonly prescribed to aggressively treat various infections and cancers with the desired outcome of extending patients' lives. Treatment with therapeutic medications such as the aminoglycoside antibiotics and the platinum-based chemotherapeutic agents can cause hearing loss with potentially severe vocational and social consequences. Millions of patients are placed at risk for ototoxic hearing loss as a consequence of treatment with ototoxic drugs. Because ototoxic hearing loss can severely affect quality of life, early identification of hearing loss due to ototoxicity is important to health care providers and patients alike.

Implementation of clinically efficient, evidence-based ototoxicity early identification and monitoring programs is essential. Requirements to an efficacious ototoxicity early identification and monitoring program using behavioral and objective techniques have been outlined in this chapter. Results of clinical studies in individuals receiving ototoxic drugs have demonstrated

that ototoxic damage progresses from high to low frequencies. For that reason, hearing assessment at the highest audible frequencies for each patient not only allows early detection of ototoxic changes, but also is critical for detection of hearing changes before lower frequencies necessary for understanding speech are affected. Numerous studies have demonstrated that monitoring of behavioral thresholds at frequencies from 250–8,000 Hz and 9,000–20,000 Hz is a sensitive indicator of ototoxicity but is lengthy and labor-intensive.

A time-efficient behavioral technique that provides reliable early detection and monitoring of ototoxicity while maintaining a high degree of sensitivity has been developed. Research results have demonstrated approximately 90% of initial ototoxic threshold changes occur within a small range of frequencies at or near the highest frequencies heard by each individual. A test protocol targeting this SRO in 1/6-octave increments has proven to be a sensitive, reliable, and time-efficient behavioral ototoxicity early detection and monitoring strategy. Thus, a time-efficient, evidence-based behavioral technique is now available for audiologists to use with patients who are receiving potentially ototoxic medications and who are too ill to participate in the lengthier full-frequency monitoring tests. Unfortunately, some patients who are treated with pharmacological agents having ototoxic potential are too ill or are unable to provide reliable responses, even when using a shortened behavioral protocol. Nonbehavioral objective tests can be used in this compromised patient population. Most reports of objective tests used for monitoring ototoxic hearing loss have focused on the use of auditory evoked potentials and OAEs.

Determining effective ototoxicity detection and monitoring strategies using objective measures of auditory function is an active area of research. However, there currently are no accepted protocols or criteria for ototoxic change using objective measures. Test-retest variability in subjects not receiving ototoxic drugs has been used to provide criteria for a clinically significant response change and to estimate false positive rates. Such studies, which need to be validated, have been useful for developing potential objective protocols for ototoxicity. Further research is needed comparing test performance for each objective test (i.e., its sensitivity and specificity) to a behavioral standard.

REFERENCES

American National Standards Institute. (1996). *Specifications for Audiometers*. (ANSI S3.6-1996). New York: ANSI.

American Speech-Language-Hearing Association. (1994). Guidelines for the audiologic management of individuals receiving cochleotoxic drug therapy. *ASHA, 36*, 11–19.

Aran, J. M. (1995). Current perspectives on inner ear toxicity. *Otolaryngology Head & Neck Surgery, 112*(1), 133–144.

Arnold, D. J., Lonsbury-Martin, B. L., & Martin, G. K. (1999). High-frequency hearing influences lower-frequency distortion–product otoacoustic emissions. *Arch Otolaryngol Head Neck Surg, 125*, 215–222.

Barron, S. E., & Daigneault, E. A. (1987). Effect of cisplatin on hair cell morphology and lateral wall Na,K-ATPase activity. *Hear Res, 26*(2), 131–137.

Bernard, P. A., Pechere, J. C., & Hebert, R. (1980). Altered objective audiometry in aminoglycosides-treated human neonates. *Arch Otorhinolaryngol, 228*(3), 205–210.

Black, F. O., & Pesznecker, S. C. (1993). Vestibular ototoxicity. Clinical considerations. *Otolaryngologic Clinics of North America, 26*, 713–736.

Black, F. O., Pesznecker, S., & Stallings, V. (2004). Permanent gentamicin vestibulotoxicity. *Otol Neurotol, 25*(4), 559–569.

Blakley, B. W., & Myers, S. F. (1993). Patterns of hearing loss resulting from cis-platinum therapy. *Otolaryngol Head Neck Surg, 109*, 385–391.

Blakley, B. W., Gupta, A. K., Myers, S. F., & Schwan, S. (1994). Risk factors for ototoxicity due to cisplatin. *Arch Otolaryngol Head Neck Surg, 120*(5), 541–546.

Bokemeyer, C., Berger, C. C., Hartmann, J. T., Kollmannsberger, C., Schmoll, H. J., Kuczyk, M. A., & Kanz, L. (1998). Analysis of risk factors for cisplatin-induced ototoxicity in patients with testicular cancer. *Br J Canc, 77*, 1355–1362.

Brownell, W. E. (1990). Outer hair cell electromotility and otoacoustic emission. *Ear Hear, 11*(2), 82–92.

Brummett, R. E., & Fox, K. E. (1982). Studies of aminoglycoside ototoxicity in animal models. In A. Whelton & H. C. Neu (Eds.), *The Aminoglycosides* (pp. 419–451). New York: Marcel Dekker, Inc.

Brummett, R. E., Fox, K. E., & Kempton, J. B. (1992). Quantitative relationships of the interaction between sound and kanamycin. *Arch Otolaryngol Head Neck Surg, 118*, 498–500.

Burk, M. H., & Wiley, T. L. (2004). Continuous versus pulsed tones in audiometry. *American Journal of Audiology, 13*, 54–61.

Campbell, K. C. M., & Durrant, J. (1993). Audiologic monitoring for ototoxicity. *Otolaryngologic Clinics of North America, 26*, 903–914.

Campbell, K. C. M., Kelly, E., Targovnik, N., Hughes, L., Van Saders, C., Gottlieb, A. B., Dorr, M. B., & Leighton, A. (2003). Audiologic monitoring for potential ototoxicity in a phase I clinical trial of a new glycopeptide antibiotic. *Journal of the American Academy of Audiology, 14*, 157–168.

Carhart, R., & Jerger, J. (1959). Preferred method for clinical determination of pure-tone thresholds. *Journal of Speech and Hearing Disorders, 24*, 330–345.

Dreschler, W. A., van der Hulst, R. J., Tange, R. A., & Urbanus, N. A. (1989). Role of high-frequency audiometry in the early detection of ototoxicity. II. *Clinical Aspects, 28*(4), 211–220.

Durrant, J. D., Rodgers, G., Meyers, E. N., & Johnson, J. T. (1990). Hearing loss-risk factor for cisplatin ototoxicity? Observations. *American Journal of Otology, 11*, 375–377.

Fausti, S. A., Frey, R. H., Henry, J. A., Olson, D. J., & Schaffer, H. I. (1992a). Early detection of ototoxicity using high-frequency, tone burst-evoked auditory brainstem responses. *J Am Acad Audiol, 3*, 397–404.

Fausti, S. A., Frey, R. H., Rappaport, B. Z., & Schechter, M. A. (1985). High-frequency audiometry with an earphone transducer. *Sem Hear, 6*, 347–357.

Fausti, S. A., Helt, W. J., Phillips, D. S., Gordon, J. S., Bratt, G. W., Sugiura, K. M., & Noffsinger, D. (2003). Early detection of ototoxicity using 1/6th octave steps. *Journal of the American Academy of Audiology, 14*, 444–450.

Fausti, S. A., Henry, J. A., Hayden, D., Phillips, D. S., & Frey, R. H. (1998). Intrasubject reliability of high-frequency (9-14 kHz) thresholds: Tested separately vs. following conventional-frequency testing. *J Amer Acad Audiol, 9,* 147–152.

Fausti, S. A., Henry, J. A., Helt, W. J., Phillips, D. S, Noffsinger, D., Larson, V. D., & Fowler, C. G. (1999). An individualized, sensitive frequency range for early detection of ototoxicity. *Ear & Hearing, 20,* 497–505.

Fausti, S. A., Henry, J. A., Schaffer, H. I., Olson, D. J., Frey, R. H., & Bagby, G. C. (1993). High-frequency monitoring for early detection of cisplatin ototoxicity. *Archives of Otolaryngology Head & Neck Surgery, 119,* 661–665.

Fausti, S. A., Henry, J. A., Schaffer, H. I., Olson, D. J., Frey, R. H., & McDonald, W. J. (1992b). High-frequency audiometric monitoring for early detection of aminoglycoside ototoxicity. *Journal of Infectious Disease, 165,* 1026–1032.

Fausti, S. A., Larson, V. D., Noffsinger, D., Wilson, R. H., Phillips, D. S. & Fowler, C. G. (1994a). High-frequency audiometric monitoring strategies for early detection of ototoxicity. *Ear & Hearing, 15,* 232–239.

Fausti, S. A., Olson, D. J., Frey, R. H., Henry, J. A., Schaffer, H. I., & Phillips, D. S. (1994b). High-frequency toneburst-evoked ABR latency-intensity functions in sensorineural hearing-impaired humans. *Scand Audiol, 24,* 19–25.

Fausti, S. A., Rappaport, B. Z., Frey, R. H., Henry, J. A., Phillips, D. S., Mitchell, C. R, & Olson, D. J. (1991). Reliability of evoked responses to high-frequency (8-14 kHz) tone bursts. *J Am Acad Audiol, 2,* 105–114.

Federspil, P. (1981). Pharmacokinetics of aminoglycoside antibiotics in the perilymph. In S. A. Lerner, G. J. Matz, & J. E. Hawkins (Eds.), *Amingolycoside Ototoxicity.* Boston: Little, Brown and Company.

Forge, A., & Schacht, J. (2000). Aminoglycoside antibiotics. *Audiol Neurootol, 5*(1), 3–22.

Frank, T. (1990). High-frequency hearing thresholds in young adults using a commercially available audiometer. *Ear Hear, 11,* 450–454.

Frank, T. (2001). High-frequency (8-16 kHz) reference thresholds and intrasubject threshold variability relative to ototoxicity criteria using a Sennheiser HDA 200 earphone. *Ear Hear, 22,* 161–168.

Frank, T., & Dreisbach, L. E. (1991). Repeatability of high-frequency thresholds. *Ear Hear, 12,* 294–295.

Gordon, J. S., Phillips, D., Helt, W. J., Konrad-Martin, D., & Fausti, S. A. (2005). The evaluation of insert earphones for high-frequency bedside ototoxicity monitoring. *Journal of Rehab Rsch & Dev, 42*(3), 353–361.

Gorga, M. P., Neely, S. T., Dorn, P. A., & Hoover, B. M. (2003). Further efforts to predict pure-tone thresholds from distortion product otoacoustic emission input/output functions. *J Acoust Soc Am, 113*(6), 3275–3284.

Gorga, M. P., Worthington, D. W., Reiland, J. K., Beauchaine, K. A., & Goldgar, D. E. (1985). Some comparisons between auditory brainstem response thresholds, latencies, and the pure-tone audiogram. *Ear & Hearing, 6,* 105–112.

Halmagyi, G. M., Fattore, C. M., Curthoy, I. S., & Wade, S. (1994). Gentamicin vestibulotoxicity. *Otolaryngol Head Neck Surg, 111*(5), 571–574.

Harris, F. P., & Probst, R. (1997). Otoacoustic emissions. *Adv Otorhinolaryngol, 53,* 182–204.

Henry, J. A., Fausti, S. A., Kempton, J. B., Trune, D. R., & Mitchell, C. R. (2000). Twenty-stimulus train for rapid acquisition of auditory brainstem responses in humans. *J Am Acad Audiol, 11*(2), 103–113.

Henry, J. A., Jastreboff, M. M., Jastreboff, P. J, Schechter, M. A., & Fausti, S. A. (2003). Guide to conducting tinnitus retraining therapy initial and follow-up interviews. *Journal of Rehabilitation Research & Development, 40*(2), 157–178.

Hodges, A. V., & Lonsbury-Martin, B. L. (1998). Hearing management. In P. A. Sullivan, & A. M. Guilford (Eds.), *Best Practices in Oncology Management: Focus on Swallowing and Communication Disorders* (pp. 269–290). San Diego: Singular Press.

Huang, M. Y., & Schacht, J. (1989). Drug-induced ototoxicity. Pathogenisis and prevention. *Medical Toxicology & Adverse Drug Experience, 4,* 452–467.

Janssen, T., Kummer, P., & Arnold, W. (1998). Growth behavior of the $2f_1$-f_2 distortion product otoacoustic emission in tinnitus. *J Acoust Soc Am, 103,* 3418–3430.

Kimberley, B. P. (1999). Applications of distortion-product emissions to an otological practice. *Laryngoscope, 109*(12), 1908–1918.

Kohn, S., Fradis, M., Pratt, H., Zidan, J., Podoshin, L., Robinson, E., & Nir, I. (1988). Cisplatin ototoxicity in guinea pigs with special reference to toxic effects in the stria vascularis. *Laryngoscope, 98*(8), 865–871.

Kummer, P., Janssen, T., & Arnold, W. (1998). The level and growth behavior of the 2 f$_1$-f$_2$ distortion product otoacoustic emission and its relationship to auditory sensitivity in normal hearing and cochlear hearing loss. *J Acoust Soc Am, 103,* 3431–3444.

Littman, T., & Emery, C. (1997). Distortion product otoacoustic emissions in children at risk for progressive sensorineural loss. *Abstr Assoc Res Otolaryngol, 20,* 21.

Lonsbury-Martin, B. L., & Martin, G. K. (2001). Evoked otoacoustic emissions as objective screeners for ototoxicity. *Seminars in Hearing, 22*(4), 377–391.

MacDonald, M. R., Harrison, R. V., Wake, M., Bliss, B., & Macdonald, R. E. (1994). Ototoxicity of carboplatin: Comparing animal and clinical models at the Hospital for Sick Children. *Journal of Otolaryngology, 23,* 151–159.

Matthews, L. J., Lee, F. S., Mills, J. H., & Dubno, J. R. (1997). Extended high-frequency thresholds in older adults. *J Speech Lang Hear Res, 40,* 208–214.

McHaney, V., Kovnar, E., Meyer, W., Furman, W., Schell, M., & Kun, L. (1992). Effects of radiation therapy and chemotherapy on hearing. *Late Effects of Treatment for Childhood Cancer* (pp. 7–10). Wilmington, DE: Wiley-Liss, Inc.

Mineau, S. M., & Schlauch, R. S. (1997). Threshold measurement for patients with tinnitus: Pulsed or continuous tones. *American Journal of Audiology, 6,* 52–56.

Mitchell, C. R., Kempton, J. B., Creedon, T. A., & Trune, D. R. (1999). The use of a 56-stimulus train for the rapid acquisition of auditory brainstem responses. *Audiol Neurootol, 4*(2), 80–87.

Mitchell, C. R., Phillips, D. S., & Trune, D. R. (1989). Variables affecting the auditory brainstem response: Audiogram, age, gender, and head size. *Hearing Research, 40,* 75–86.

Moore, R. D., Smith, C. R., & Leitman, P. S. (1984). Risk factors for the development of auditory toxicity in patients receiving aminoglycosides. *J Infect Dis, 149,* 23–30.

Mulrow, C. D., Aguilar, C., Endicott, J. E., Tuley, M. R., Velez, R., Charlip, W. S., Rhodes, M. C., Hill, J. A., & DeNino, L. A. (1990). Quality of life changes and hearing impairment: A randomized trial. *Annals of Internal Med, 113,* 188–194.

Pasic, T. R., & Dobie, R. A. (1991). Cis-platinum ototoxicity in children. *Laryngoscope, 101,* 985–91.

Piek, J., Lumenta, C. B., & Bock, W. J. (1985). Monitoring of auditory function in comatose patients in therapy with potentially ototoxic substances using acoustically evoked brain stem potentials. *Anasth Intensivther Notfallmed, 20*(1), 1–5.

Ress, B. D., Sridhar, K. S., Balkany, T. J., Waxman, G. M., Stagner, B. B., & Lonsbury-Martin, B. L. (1999). Effects of cis-platinum chemotherapy on otoacoustic emissions: The development of an objective screening protocol. *Otolaryngol Head Neck Surg, 121,* 693–701.

Rougier, F., Claude, D., Maurin, M., Sedoglavic, A., Ducher, M., Corvaisier, S., Jelliffe, R., & Maire, P. (2003). Aminoglycoside nephrotoxicity: Modeling, simulation, and control. *Antimicrobial Agents & Chemother, 47*(3), 1010–1016.

Royster, J. D., & Royster, L. H. (1982). Comparing the effectiveness of significant threshold shift criteria for industrial hearing conservation programs. Unpublished report commissioned by Occupational Safety and Health Administration, U.S. Department of Labor.

Safirstein, R., Daye, M., & Guttenplan, J. (1983). Mutagenic activity and identification of excreted platinum in human and rat urine and rat plasma after administration of cisplatin. *Cancer Lett, 18,* 329.

Schechter, M. A., Fausti, S. A., Rappaport, B. Z., & Frey, R. H. (1986). Age categorization of high-frequency auditory threshold data. *J Acoust Soc Am, 79,* 767–771.

Schmuziger, N., Probst, R., & Smurzynski, J. (2004). Test-retest reliability of pure-tone thresholds from 0.5 to 16 kHz using Sennheiser HDA 200 and Etymotic Research ER-2 earphones. *Ear Hear, 25,* 127–132.

Schweitzer, V. G. (1993). Cisplatin-induced ototoxicity: The effect of pigmentation and inhibitory agents. *Laryngoscope, 103,* 1–52.

Seligmann, H., Podoshin, L., Ben-David, J., Fradis, M., & Goldsher, M. (1996). Drug-induced tinnitus and other hearing disorders. *Drug Safety, 13*(3), 198–212.

Shera, C. A., & Guinan, J. J. (1999). Evoked otoacoustic emissions arise by two fundamentally different mechanisms: A taxonomy for mammalian OAEs. *J Acoust Soc Am, 105,* 782–798.

Shulman, A. (1999). The cochleovestibular system/ ototoxicity/clinical issues. *Ann NY Acad Sci, 884,* 433–436.

Simpson, T. H., Schwan, S. A., & Rintelmann, W. F. (1992). Audiometric test criteria in the detection of cisplatin ototoxicity. *J Am Acad Audiol, 3*(3), 1976–1985.

Stavroulaki, P., Apostolopoulos, N., Segas, J., Tsakanikos, M., & Adamopoulos, G. (2001). Evoked otoacoustic emissions—an approach for monitoring cisplatin induced ototoxicity in children. *Int J Pediatr Otorhinolaryngol, 59*(1), 47–57.

Tan, C. T., Hsu, C. J., Lee, S. Y., Liu, S. H., & Lin-Shiau, S. Y. (2001). Potentiation of noise-induced hearing loss by amikacin in guinea pigs. *Hearing Research, 161*(1–2), 72–80.

Vasquez, R., & Mattucci, K. F. (2003). A proposed protocol for monitoring ototoxicity in patients who take cochleo- or vestibulotoxic drugs. *Ear, Nose & Throat Journal, 82*(3), 181–184.

Zweig, G., & Shera, C. (1995). The origin of periodicity in the spectrum of evoked otoacoustic emissions. *J Acoust Soc Am, 98,* 2018–2047.

CHAPTER
17

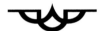

Vestibular Ototoxicity

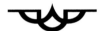

F. Owen Black, MD
Susan Pesznecker, RN, BA
Legacy Clinical Research and Technology Center
Department of Neurotology Research
Portland, Oregon

Sponsored in part by NIH/NIDCD 00205, NIH 19221, NASA NAG5-6329 and the Legacy Research Advisory Committee (RAC).

INTRODUCTION

Ototoxicity—toxic damage to (and potential destruction of) the hearing and balance end organ sensory cells and/or their neural connections—can be a devastating consequence of exposure to certain medications, particularly the **aminoglycoside** antibiotics. Although specific conditions predispose or increase risk for ototoxicity, anyone exposed to or receiving potentially ototoxic drugs or agents are at risk for ototoxicity. Damage to hearing and balance may be difficult to detect clinically, especially during the acute phases of ototoxicity. Most health care systems (including hospitals) do not have the facilities necessary to detect early ototoxicity. While there is no such thing as a "safe dose" of some ototoxic medications, patients may sustain less permanent damage and recover some residual function if ototoxic agents are stopped immediately upon suspicion or detection of ototoxicity. Because drugs that cause conscious-level hearing loss are more readily identified, most have been removed from clinical use or have been appropriately labeled for risk. Recent studies confirm conclusions from earlier studies that vestibular organ damage—**vestibular ototoxicity**—may occur more often than cochleotoxicity from some commonly prescribed drugs and may be more disabling depending on occupation. By developing familiarity with the mechanisms and causality of vestibular ototoxicity, health care providers will be in a better position to recognize and prevent vestibular ototoxicity.

Almost all of the severe to profound vestibular-deficient patients due to ototoxicity studied in this laboratory, prospectively and retrospectively, are supported by public assistance. Consequently, the socioeconomic consequences of vestibular ototoxicity are, potentially, enormous.

INTRODUCTION TO VESTIBULAR OTOTOXICITY

Ototoxicity may be defined as "the destructive or damaging effects of an exogenous chemical substance on the structure and function of labyrinthine (vestibular and cochlear) **hair cells,** their supporting structures, and/or the 8th cranial nerve. Some ototoxic drugs—such as dihydrostreptomycin—preferentially affect the pars inferior (cochlea and saccular macula). Other ototoxic drugs—such as gentamicin—preferentially affect the pars superior (semicircular canal cristae and utricular maculae) hair cells. At high cumulative doses, most ototoxic drugs affect both vestibular and cochlear hair cells. Drugs, such as neomycin, that produce both auditory and vestibular ototoxicity have, for the most part, been removed from hospital formularies for parenteral administration. This chapter focuses on vestibular ototoxicity.

Vestibular ototoxicity may be therapeutic or unintentional (iatrogenic). In therapeutic ototoxicity, vestibulotoxic drugs are administered selectively and incrementally to reduce vestibular hair cell responses to vestibular pathologies that produce vestibular hair cell stimulation unrelated to head and body motion (e.g., **endolymphatic hydrops**—disordered control of inner ear fluid homeostasis). Ototoxic drugs may be administered systemically (e.g., for bilateral endolymphatic hydrops) or topically to the round window (e.g., for unilateral endolymphatic hydrops) (de Waele et al., 2002; Diamond, O'Connell, Hornig, & Liu, 2003; Lange, Maurer, & Mann, 2004; Longridge & Mallinson, 2000; Minor, 1999; Perez, Martin, & Garcia-Tapia, 2003; Wu & Minor, 2003).

Unintentional ototoxicity—the focus of this chapter—is an unwanted, unplanned, and highly damaging consequence of exposure to vestibular ototoxic medications used to treat systemic—often life-threatening—infections or to treat potential infections prophylactically. For example, the patients in the authors' NIH-funded prospective and retrospective studies have received vestibular ototoxic medications for treatment of bacterial endocarditis, osteomyelitis, septic arthritis, cellulitis, wound infections, septicemia, bowel infarcts, and certain kinds of cancer.

If potentially ototoxic drugs are the only option for treatment of life-threatening infections, early detection and intervention is particularly important in the prevention of vestibular ototoxicity. While damage caused by ototoxins may be primarily auditory, primarily vestibular, or mixed (Table 17-1), recent prospective and retrospective studies of gentamicin ototoxicity in humans show that susceptible patients experience vestibular damage much earlier than auditory damage. Evidence from those studies also suggests that discontinuing ototoxic medication upon earliest evidence of vestibular ototoxicity greatly improves the likelihood of recovery (Black, Gianna-Poulin, & Pesznecker, 2001; Black, Pesznecker, & Stallings, 2004).

CAUSES AND MECHANISMS OF VESTIBULAR OTOTOXICITY

Almost every major group of medications contains compounds known to be ototoxic, some with temporary and others with permanent effects (Table 17-2). Tobacco, alcohol, heavy metals, and many chemical and organic solvents are potentially ototoxic, as are certain antibiotics, diuretics, and chemotherapeutic agents (Black & Pesznecker, 1993). Ototoxic mechanisms vary depending on the biochemistry of specific ototoxic agents (Schacht, 1993).

The most problematic vestibulotoxic agents are the aminoglycoside antibiotics, especially gentamicin. Aminoglycoside antibiotics are inexpensive, readily available, and widely used to treat serious, life-threatening gram-negative infections. Aminoglycosides are

typically given parenterally (intravenously) but may be administered via peritoneal lavage, intrathecal, or intra-articular injection. They may also be inspired via respiratory therapy treatments. All of those administration routes have resulted in vestibular ototoxicity. Neomycin is particularly dangerous in this regard, resulting in both cochlear and vestibular ototoxicity (Chong, Piraino, & Bernardini, 1991; DeBeukelaer, Travis, & Dodge, 1971; Gerharz et al., 1995; Gibson, 1967; Johnsson, Hawkins, Kingsley, Black, & Matz, 1981; Kalbian, 1972; Kavanaugh & McCabe, 1983; Kunin, Chalmers, & Leevy, 1960; Langman, 1994; Last & Sherlock, 1960; Wersäll, 1995).

The means by which systemically administered ototoxic antibiotics enter the inner ear is under intensive investigation. The agents may diffuse into the inner ear fluid spaces passively or may be actively secreted into the endolymph (by the stria vascularis) or the perilymph (via the spiral ligament). An in-depth discussion of the cellular and subcellular actions of vestibular ototoxicity exceeds the scope of this chapter, and the reader is referred to recent reviews (Black & Pesznecker, 1993; Miller, 1985; Rybak & Matz, 1986; Schacht, 1993, 1998, 1999; Taylor & Forge, 2005; Ali & Goetz, 1997; Aran, 1995; Aust,

Table 17-1. Auditory, Vestibular, and Mixed Ototoxicity of the More Common Ototoxins

Ototoxins that Primarily Cause Auditory (Cochlear) Toxicity	Ototoxins that Primarily Cause Vestibular Toxicity	Ototoxins that Cause Mixed (Auditory and Vestibular) Toxicity
Carbon monoxide	Alcohol	6-Amino nictonamide (6-AN)
Carboplatin	Barbiturates	Aminoglycoside antibiotics (amikacin,
Chloramphenical	Carbon disulfide	dihydrostreptomycin, gentamicin, kanamycin,
Cisplatin (cis-platinum)	Hexane	neomycin, netilmycin, streptomycin, and
Erythromycin	Lipid solvents	tobramycin)
Loop diuretics (bumetanide,	Manganese	Lead
ethacrynic acid, furosemide,	Marijuana	Nitrogen mustard
and torsemide)	Mercury	Nonsteroidal anti-inflammatory agents (NSAIDs)
Salicylates	Minocycline	Polymixin
Vincristine and vinblastine	Styrene	Quinine and cinchona bark preparations
	Tin	Quinine and its derivatives (chloroquine,
	Toluene	quinidine, quinine, and tonic water)
	Trichloroethylene	Tobacco
	Xylene	Vancomycin

Source: Black & Pesznecker, 1993; Brummett, 1993; Gagnaire & Langlais, 2005; Jung, Rhee, Lee, Park, & Choi, 1993; Matz, 1993; Schweitzer, 1993; Sulkowski et al., 2002

Table 17-2. Agents Known to Produce Temporary Versus Permanent Ototoxicity in Humans

Agents that May Cause Temporary Toxicity	Agents that May Cause Permanent Toxicity
Alcohol	6-Amino nictonamide (6-AN)
Barbiturates	Aminoglycoside antibiotics (amikacin, dihydrostreptomycin,
Chloramphenical	gentamicin, kanamycin, neomycin, netilmycin, streptomycin,
Erythromycin	and tobramycin)
Loop diuretics (bumetanide, ethacrynic acid, furosemide, and torsemide)	Carboplatin and cisplatin (cis-platinum)
Marijuana	Hazardous chemicals (butyl nitrite and carbon disulfide)
Minocycline	Heavy metals (lead, manganese, mercury, and tin)
Nonsteroidal anti-inflammatory agents (ibuprofen, naproxen, etc.)	Lipid solvents
Polymixin	Nitrogen mustard
Quinine and its derivatives (chloroquine, quinidine, quinine, and tonic water)	Organic solvents (styrene, toluene, trichloroethylene, and xylene)
Salicylates	Quinine and cinchona bark preparations
Tobacco	Toxic inhalants (carbon monoxide and hexane)
	Vancomycin
	Vincristine and vinblastine

Comment: Some of the above agents may also produce neural toxicity, especially when a person is exposed to high doses or experiences prolonged exposure.

Source: Black & Pesznecker, 1993; Brummett, 1993; Gagnaire & Langlais, 2005; Jung et al., 1993; Matz, 1993; Schweitzer, 1993; Sulkowski et al., 2002

2001; Blakley et al., 1991; Brummett, 1993; Calder & Jacobson, 2000; Carey & Wichter, 1977; de Vries, Verkooyen, Leguit, & Verbrugh, 1990; Doretto, Marseillan, Pinto-Gonçalves, Oliveira, & Corrado, 1994; English & Williams, 2000; Forge & Schacht, 2000; Halmagyi, Fattore, Curthoys, & Wade, 1994). However, the abnormal (pathophysiological) effect of vestibular ototoxicity is destruction of vestibular hair cells (Figure 17-1). The elucidation of vestibular ototoxic drug pharmacodynamics, including partition dynamics (i.e., circulating versus intracellular drug concentrations), is particularly important in light of ongoing advances in hair cell regeneration studies (Taylor & Forge, 2005).

THE NATURAL HISTORY OF VESTIBULAR OTOTOXICITY

The clinical presentation of vestibulotoxicity may vary from asymptomatic partial (incomplete) damage— detectable only by objective testing—to complete or profound bilateral loss of vestibular (balance) function. The rapidity of bilateral ototoxicity onset and preexisting asymmetric vestibular disorders determine patient symptoms, depending on rapidity of vestibular receptor (hair cell) damage.

Complete or profound bilateral loss of vestibular function is always accompanied by permanent, disabling symptoms, especially upon attempts to reengage in normal activities (Black, Wade, & Nashner, 1996). The severely vestibulotoxic patient experiences constant postural instability (dysequilibrium) upon attempts to walk. Those patients are in constant danger of falling and are at constant risk of injury. Most severely vestibulotoxic patients complain of **oscillopsia.** When they move, everything in their field of view "bounces" or appears to move. Attempts to use a computer, read, or recognize faces while walking are impaired by the lack of ocular globe stability. While many severely ototoxic patients drive a car, none can do so safely. In addition, vestibular ototoxic patients also may suffer from hearing loss, tinnitus, and various neurocognitive difficulties, including short-term memory loss and problems with concentration (Black et al., 2004).

Because of those symptoms, patients with severe ototoxicity typically spend their postvestibulotoxic lives not being able to work, subsisting on public

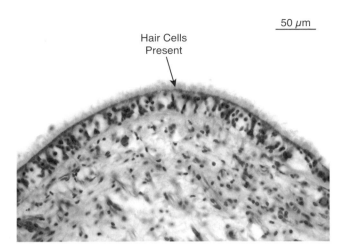

Figure 17-1a. Cross section of the horizontal semicircular canal crista from a patient with no known inner ear disease. Postmortem time was 19 hours.

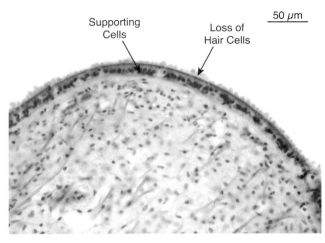

17-1b. Comparable cross section of a horizontal semicircular canal crista from a fifty-three-year old male who received 1 gm of Streptomycin by systemic administration every day for 10 days at the age of forty-seven. Following this medication, he became ataxic and developed oscillopsia. There was no response to ice water caloric testing in either ear. Histologic studies show a severe loss of hair cells in all cristae of both ears. Postmortem time was 11 hours. (Images courtesy of Saumil N. Merchant, M.D., Otopathology Laboratory, Massachusetts Eye and Ear Infirmary and Harvard Medical School, Boston, MA.).

disability, and experiencing a very poor quality of life. In recent years, severe vestibular ototoxicity has generated a large number of personal injury lawsuits, many of which have resulted in multimillion-dollar settlements. Fortunately, vestibular ototoxicity is preventable in most cases.

FACTORS PREDISPOSING TO VESTIBULAR OTOTOXICITY

Aminoglycosides are primarily excreted via glomerular filtration in the kidney. Patients with renal disease or insufficiency clear the drug more slowly, and the slow clearance extends the drug's effective half-life (increased concentration of the drug in body fluids); therefore, patients with impaired renal clearance are at higher risk for developing aminoglycoside vestibular ototoxicity (Walsh, 2000). Many aminoglycoside antibiotics are also nephrotoxic, further increasing potential for vestibular ototoxic damage.

Dehydration impairs drug clearance by the kidneys, produces relative increases in serum concentration with respect to standard dose regimens, and consequently increases the risk of toxicity. Loop diuretics commonly used in treating seriously ill patients—e.g., furosemide and ethacrynic acid—are potentially ototoxic themselves. Anemia may increase ototoxic risk by altering the oxygen-carrying capability of the blood and creating hypoxia that, when combined with direct effects of ototoxic drugs, produces the potential for cumulative damage to vestibular hair cells.

Although studies have failed to clearly correlate serum drug levels and ototoxicity, higher serum levels lead to higher tissue concentrations and longer clearance times, which lengthen the period of exposure to the medications and increase the potential for ototoxicity. Very young and very old patients are at greater risk of ototoxicity, with high serum concentrations occurring unpredictably even with recommended reductions in drug doses.

Infants may develop congenital ototoxicity due to prenatal maternal exposure to ototoxins. Some studies suggest genetic predisposition to ototoxicity (Bacino, Prezant, Bu, Fournier, & Fischel-Ghodsian, 1995; Casano et al., 1999; el-Schahawi et al., 1997; Estivill et al., 1998; Hamasaki & Rando, 1997; Prezant et al., 1993; Tessa et al., 2001; Usami et al., 2000; Yoshida et al., 2002; Zhao et al., 2004).

Ototoxic damage is thought to be cumulative, and a history of prior treatment with or exposure to known ototoxic substances may predispose to the future development of ototoxicity (Lerner, Schmitt, Seligsoh, & Matz, 1986). Patients who are to receive ototoxic medications should be questioned carefully about having received ototoxic agents in the past, and medical records should be reviewed before potentially ototoxic agents are administered. Some patients are unaware that they have received ototoxic drugs, verifying the need to obtain and review hospital and outpatient intravenous drug records. In addition, the concomitant administration of some potentially ototoxic medications may augment the risk of ototoxicity (Riggs, Brummett, Guitjens, & Matz, 1996; Riggs et al., 1999).

In the past, it was believed that by keeping the weight-based dose, per treatment dose, cumulative dose, and treatment duration within tightly proscribed boundaries, the patient would be protected from ototoxicity (Peloquin et al., 2004). We now know that this isn't the case (Bakri, Pallett, Smith, & Duncombe, 1998; Barza, Ioannidis, Cappelleri, & Lau, 1996; Black et al., 2004; Fee, 1980; Galløe, Graudal, Christensen, & Kampmann, 1995; Halmagyi et al., 1994; Munckhof, Grayson, & Turnidge, 1996). It was also once believed that maintaining peak and serum trough levels of drug within "safe ranges" would protect against ototoxicity. We now know that concept to be incorrect with respect to vestibular ototoxicity (Barza et al., 1996; Black et al., 2004).

It is important to detect subclinical vestibular abnormalities during pretreatment baseline testing, as patients with preexisting vestibular abnormalities may be at additional risk of ototoxicity. Subjects with preexisting unilateral loss of vestibular function are also more likely to develop symptoms at onset of ototoxicity; the ototoxic change in vestibular function creates an additional asymmetry between the two ears and may induce nystagmus, **vertigo,** nausea, and/or vomiting. In patients with normal baseline function, bilateral ototoxic loss typically does not result in those symptoms—particularly if the change occurs slowly—as the loss is symmetrical (unpublished observations from lead author's NIH prospective study).

SUBJECTIVE COMPLAINTS (SYMPTOMS) OF VESTIBULAR OTOTOXICITY

Symptoms may be separated into two groups: (1) those associated with acute or developing ototoxicity and (2) those accompanying permanent ototoxicity. Symptoms resulting from the sudden changes in vestibular function (e.g., the acute development of ototoxicity) may include nausea, vomiting, dizziness, vertigo, tinnitus, and hearing loss. If the patient is able to ambulate, he or she may also note the sudden onset of ataxia (unsteadiness, dysequilibrium, sensation of falling, etc.). Patients who are ambulatory throughout treatment may present with disequilibrium as the first manifestation of ototoxicity (Black & Pesznecker, 1993). The functional change may not progress symmetrically in both ears, particularly if superimposed on preexisting vestibular abnormalities.

The idea that symptoms can be used to detect the onset or gauge the severity of vestibular ototoxicity is common but erroneous, as is the equally unsupported notion that potentially ototoxic symptoms are due to "something else" and that they will "get better over time" (Black et al., 2004; Halmagyi et al., 1994). To further compound the problem of relying solely on symptoms for detection of vestibular ototoxicity, most patients receiving ototoxic medications are seriously ill—often with life-threatening illness. They may be receiving other medications that cause nausea and vomiting (N&V) or may be receiving sedatives or narcotics that alter their mentation and make them unreliable reporters of potentially significant symptoms. For patients unable to ambulate, vestibular symptoms may go unnoticed until activity is resumed. That point is important because many critically ill patients will not resume activities for weeks or months, long after the ototoxic medications have done their damage.

N&V are rarely associated with bilateral vestibular ototoxicity unless onset is rapid. When present, N&V usually occur in the acute phase of ototoxicity and most often occur because of a sudden change in subjects with preexisting asymmetric loss of vestibular function. N&V are mediated by the autonomic nervous system (ANS), which is subdivided into the sympathetic and parasympathetic nervous systems (Figure 17-2) (see review by Yates, 1998). The vestibular and cerebellar nuclei both have extensive connections with the ANS. The sympathetic nervous system prepares the body for a perceived emergency by increasing heart rate and blood pressure, opening the bronchi, inhibiting digestion, increasing blood flow to the skeletal muscles, dilating the pupils, inhibiting urination, and stimulating the release of glycogen. The parasympathetic nervous system works in "opposition" to return the body to a normal physiologic state (i.e., slowing the heart rate, decreasing blood pressure, returning the airways to normal, increasing digestive activity, constricting pupils, etc.). Either or both autonomic systems can be activated by sudden changes in vestibular function (Yates & Miller, 1996). For the clinician, interpretation of the varying stages and presentations of autonomic responses to sudden changes in vestibular function can be confusing. Some patients who have chronic or preexisting vestibular disorders may present a different autonomic response compared to subjects who have not previously experienced a vestibular disorder.

Vestibular receptors respond to linear and angular accelerations acting on the head. Through a subconscious, automatic process, information about the head in inertial space provided by vestibular receptors is distributed to muscles controlling the ocular globes and other body segments (Figure 17-3). Vestibular and more ambiguous spatial orientation reference information from visual and somatosensory systems is modified (modulated), depending on the task at hand, by the midline cerebellar nuclei. The vestibular and cerebellar nuclei both have extensive connections with the ANS. A schematic of vestibular connections to ocular and body muscles and interactions with central nervous control systems is summarized in Figure 17-3 (Correia & Guedry, 1978).

In patients with permanent (chronic) ototoxicity who are one year or more from their last dose of medication, the most common symptoms are dysequilibrium and oscillopsia (Black et al., 2004). Both dysequilibrium and oscillopsia result from failure of the vestibulospinal and **vestibulo-ocular reflexes** (VORs) to stabilize body segments (head, ocular globes, trunk—body center of mass). For example, the inability to stabilize the ocular globe (eyeball) relative to inertial space—normally accomplished by the VOR—results in the inability to stabilize retinal images for clear vision during active and passive head movements.

Most ototoxic patients also complain of fatigue, visual "sensitivity" (i.e., exacerbation or provocation of symptoms when exposed to movement in the visual periphery), and neurocognitive difficulties, symptoms seen in all types of vestibular disorders (Black et al., 2004). Some patients with vestibular ototoxicity also develop signs of **auditory toxicity** (e.g., tinnitus and hearing loss).

Because many of the above symptoms have multiple causes, ototoxic symptoms may be incorrectly attributed to other sources, delaying diagnosis and potentially increasing severity of ototoxic damage. A severely ill patient may not be able to relate accurate, subjective complaints to the staff caring for him or her. Even when a patient is alert and coherent, the symptoms may or may not be a reliable indicator of onset, severity, progression, or permanence of vestibulotoxicity. Severely ototoxic patients sometimes report few symptoms, while patients with only a minimal change in VOR are sometimes severely symptomatic (Black et al., 2004). For those reasons, objective testing—beginning with establishing baseline vestibular function—is critical for adequate monitoring (evidence-based medicine) of patients receiving ototoxic medications.

DETECTION AND MONITORING OF OTOTOXICITY

The clinical diagnosis of vestibular ototoxicity relies on the documentation of reduced (relative to baseline—pretreatment vestibular function) or absent

A. Vestibulo-spinal and vestibulo-ocular reflexes

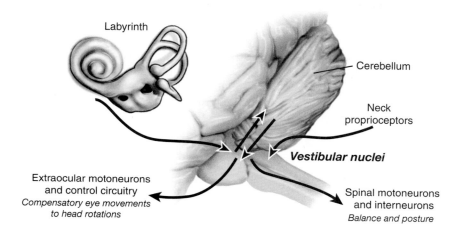

B. Vestibulo-autonomic regulation

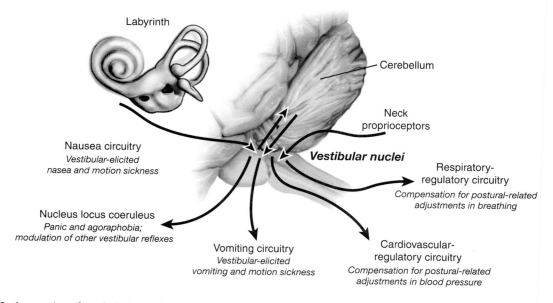

Figure 17-2. An overview of vestibular inputs for motor and autonomic control. (A) Schematic of vestibular inputs to the brainstem and cerebellum for maintenance of balance and eye position, respectively. (B) Vestibular inputs to brainstem and cerebellum for autonomic control. With permission from Yates BJ and Miller AD, Overview of vestibular autonomic regulation, in Yates BJ and Miller AD, *Vestibular Autonomic Regulation*; CRC Press: Boca Raton; 1996, p. 109. (Yates & Miller, 1996).

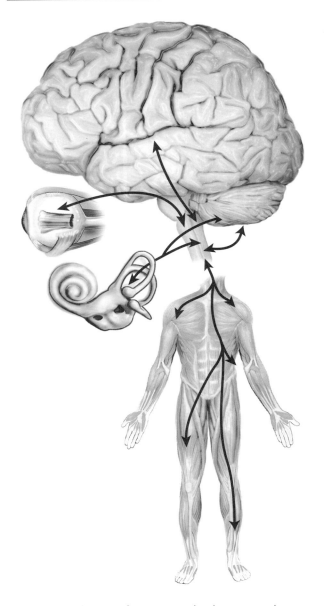

Figure 17-3. Schematic of primary neural and neuromuscular connections of the peripheral vestibular receptors. With permission from Correia, M. J. and Guedry, F. E. Jr. The vestibular system: Basic biophysical and physiological mechanisms. In *Handbook of Behavioral Neurobiology. Volume 1. Sensory Integration.* Masterson, RB (Ed.) New York: Plenum, 1978. p. 312.

vestibular function. In most facilities, VOR responses are used to establish baseline vestibular function and to monitor patients receiving ototoxic agents. Caloric tests have long been used for VOR testing (Fee, 1980). Unfortunately, the caloric test has many drawbacks, including but not limited to the following: (1) they have the ability to provide only low-frequency stimulation—well below ranges of most normal head movements; (2) test-retest variability is too high to detect changes in vestibular function reliably (caloric responses do correlate with changes in rotational VOR **time constants** (TCs) (Wade, Halmagyi, Black, & McGarvie, 1999)); (3) absent caloric responses do not correlate with higher-frequency VOR responses from rotary stimuli; and (4) caloric tests stimulate only one of the five spatially separate vestibular end organs (Kaplan et al., 2001; Saadat, O'Leary, Pulec, & Kitano, 1995).

Today the most accurate and reliable methods for detecting reduced angular (rotational) VOR are either rotary chair testing (Black et al., 2004) or vestibular autorotation (VAT) (O'Leary, Davis-O'Leary, & Li, 1995). The most dependable and informative test of VOR function is full-frequency rotary chair testing, which tests the passive VOR over a broad frequency range (Figure 17-4). Rotary chair testing can be used in patients who are unable to stand unassisted (Black et al., 2001; Black et al., 2004).

If a rotary chair is not available or the patient's condition makes rotary chair testing impossible, VAT is another reliable means of assessing VOR (Figure 17-4). VAT differs from passive rotary chair testing in that it assesses the VOR in response to active head movements. An advantage of the VAT is that it tests the vertical or horizontal plane in pace with a sweep frequency auditory stimulus. VAT thus requires an alert subject with normal ranges of neck motion. An important advantage of VAT is that it may be used at the bedside of patients too ill for passive rotary chair tests. VAT testing obviously cannot be used in deaf or extremely hard-of-hearing patients (O'Leary et al., 1995).

Symptoms of severe or profound vestibular ototoxicity occur when the magnitude of vestibular loss prevents ocular globe stabilization during active and passive head movements. When the VOR **gain constant** (GC) drops below about 0.3 (Black et al., 1996), most patients cannot achieve a visual-vestibulocular gain of

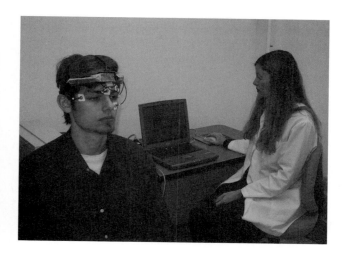

Figure 17-4. Subject seated during VAT test. Note the recording electrodes (around eyes) and head-mounted accelerometer. The subject is focusing on a spot on the wall several feet away. An adjacent laptop computer generates an auditory sweep tone from 2–6 Hz; the subject moves his or her head in synchrony with auditory stimuli. The computer records and analyzes eye movement responses in both the horizontal and pitch planes.

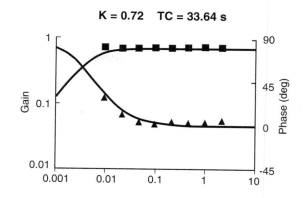

Figure 17-5a. Baseline VOR gain and phase responses.

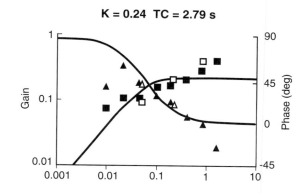

Figure 17-5b. VOR gain and phases 90 days after receiving streptomycin. Both gain and time constants are severely reduced (abnormal), and there is a phase lead throughout. Note: Because of poor response amplitudes, fits are not accurate; however, results were confirmed by single frequency (sinusoidal stimuli) responses.

unity (i.e., 1.0). In other words, the subject cannot stabilize the ocular globe with respect to a visual target and, thus, cannot achieve clear vision during active or passive head movements, resulting in oscillopsia "jumping" of the visual target or visual environment. Also note that if a patient's baseline VOR is already abnormal (before receiving any ototoxic medication), the patient is at additional risk for ototoxicity; any changes in GC and TC must be considered in terms of the abnormal baseline. The first indication of ototoxicity in the VOR rotational response is a decline in VOR TC followed by decrement in VOR GC (Black et al., 2001; Black et al., 2004). In the authors' published studies, criteria for VOR decline were VOR GC or TC below the fifth percentile range of their published normal database (Black et al., 2004; Peterka, Black, & Schoenhoff, 1990a, 1990b). Figure 17-5 shows one patient's VOR responses to rotation before and after receiving 42 grams of intramuscular streptomycin.

Electronystagmography (ENG) and, more recently, infrared videonystagmography (VNG) are widely used as tests of VOR function (Figure 17-6).

Complete ENG or VNG always includes caloric testing. While long considered a "gold standard" for assessing human VOR function, the caloric test is inadequate for either diagnosing or monitoring vestibular ototoxicity for the reasons noted above. In addition, most patients with severe or profound bilateral loss of vestibular function due to ototoxicity retain some high-frequency (>0.8 Hz) VOR functions, which are missed by caloric tests but easily detected with rotary chair testing or VAT. Those are critical distinctions, as patients with even a small

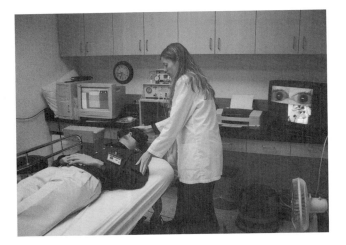

Figure 17-6. Subject reclining on stretcher during videonystagmography testing. Note that the subject is wearing infrared camera-goggles. Video images of the subject's eyes are visible on the monitor to the right of the picture. Eye movements can be recorded in response to visual targets, using dichroic mirrors or goggles occluded (complete darkness). Images are recorded for later analysis.

amount of residual VOR may recover over time and/or may be more amenable to VRT than those whose vestibular function is completely ablated (Black et al., 2001; Black & Pesznecker, 2003; Black et al., 1996).

Computerized dynamic posturography (CDP) (Figure 17-7) is useful for monitoring ambulatory patients receiving potentially vestibulotoxic drugs. CDP tests the interactions of a patient's visual, proprioceptive, and vestibular inputs through a series of sensory organization tests (SOTs) (Figure 17-8). Patients experiencing either acute or chronic vestibular ototoxicity will typically show a classic "vestibular deficient" pattern of SOTs, with falls on SOTs 5 and 6 (the test conditions requiring intact vestibular function) and a decreased composite score (Black, 1985; Nashner, 1993; Nashner, Black, & Wall, 1982). Normal and abnormal responses to CDP are shown in Figure 17-9a and 17-9b, respectively. Prospective studies suggest that shift of SOTs 5 and 6 from normal to abnormal during drug administration often occurs before objective changes in the VOR (Black & Pesznecker, 1993).

CDP is likewise useful in monitoring progress and/or recovery after the drug is stopped and is an important outcome measure for vestibular rehabilitation therapy (VRT) (Black & Pesznecker, 2003).

New dynamic visual acuity (DVA) tests—performed while sitting (Goebel, Sangasilp, & Lindberg, 2005) and during treadmill walking (Peters & Bloomberg, 2004)—are currently being evaluated as potential methods for assessing VOR integrity as a function of vestibular function. Testing of vestibular evoked myogenic potentials (VEMPs) has also been

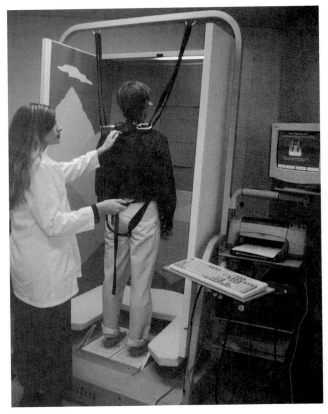

Figure 17-7. Subject standing within computerized dynamic posturography platform (NeuroCom EquiTest). Note the safety harness securing the patient to a bolt in the ceiling. Computer equipment at the right controls and administers test stimulus, analyzes data, and prints a hard copy of results.

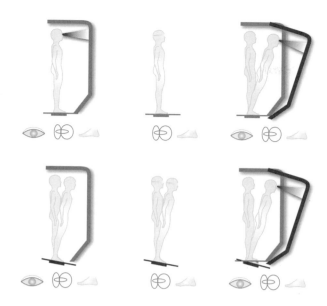

Figure 17-8. The six sensory organization trials. SOTs 5 and 6 require intact vestibular function for the patient to maintain a normal stance. Reprinted with permission from EquiTest System Version 4.0, Data Interpretation Manual. NeuroCom International, Inc. Clackamas, OR. 1994. (EquiTest System. Version 4.0. Data Interpretation Manual, 1994).

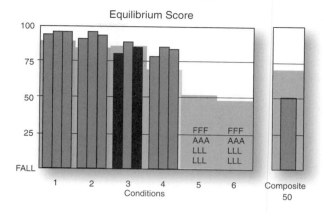

Sensory Organization Test
(Sway Referenced Gain: 1.0)

Equilibrium Score

17-9b. CDP results from the same ototoxic patient shown in Figure 17-5b. The patient is normal on SOTs 1, 2, and 4. Two of three trials are mildly abnormal on SOT 3. On SOTs 5 and 6, the patient is clearly abnormal, falling on all trials and showing a classical vestibular-deficient pattern of postural dyscontrol. The composite score is well below normal.

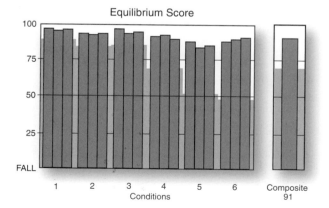

Sensory Organization Test
(Sway Referenced Gain: 1.0)

Equilibrium Score

Figure 17-9a. Normal computerized dynamic posturography (CDP) responses from the same patient shown in Figure 17-5a. Solid bars show responses for three trials at each of six sensory organization tests (SOTs, or conditions), with 100 being a perfect score (no sway). Gray background boxes show 95 %tile responses from a large-n study of normal subjects (see Peterka, Balck, & Schoenhoff: Age-related changes in human posture control: Sensory organization tests). The composite score—a weighted averaging of performance on all SOTs—is normal.

suggested as an objective method of evaluating vestibulotoxic changes (de Waele et al., 2002).

An oft-encountered practical problem is the testing and monitoring of the seriously or critically ill patient who receives potentially ototoxic agents. The seriously ill patient who is alert but bedridden may be monitored using the test for "dynamic illegible E" (Longridge & Mallinson, 1987) until he or she has recovered sufficiently to undergo rotary chair or other objective tests of vestibular function. VAT testing may also be used to document onset, progression, and recovery of ototoxicity at the bedside of patients who are alert enough to participate and who have no limitation of neck motion or loss of hearing (Kitsigianis, O'Leary, & Davis-O'Leary, 1988).

After establishing a pretreatment baseline, periodic monitoring is essential for following each patient's vestibular function response to the ototoxic medication and for the objective detection of vestibular ototoxicity. The authors recommend that the baseline tests (or, at a minimum, rotary chair testing or VAT) be repeated weekly (patient's condition permitting) while the patient is receiving the potentially ototoxic drug. Testing should also be performed if symptoms emerge during treatment that could herald ototoxicity.

Once the course of drug has been completed in patients demonstrating loss of vestibular function, (some patients may undergo multiple courses), follow-up testing should be repeated periodically (ideally at monthly intervals) for one year. In prospective studies, ototoxic-induced reduction in VOR GC and TC often continued for several months after the drug was discontinued and full recovery of VOR function required up to one year for some vestibulotoxic patients (Black, Elardo, Mirka, Peterka, & Shupert, 1988; Black et al., 2001; Black, Peterka, & Elardo, 1987). Based on those findings, the authors recommend that ototoxic patients be monitored for at least one year after the ototoxic drugs have been discontinued (Black et al., 2004).

Administration of Ototoxic Medications

Studies have repeatedly shown that there is no such thing as a "safe dose" of ototoxic medication, especially as concerns gentamicin, the most widely used aminoglycoside antibiotic (Halmagyi et al., 1994). Prospective studies of patients receiving aminoglycosides have shown that patients became ototoxic even when recommended weight-based, daily maximum, and cumulative maximum limit guidelines were observed. In some cases, a cumulative dose far below the recommended safe limits caused catastrophic vestibular ototoxicity, while in others, doses that appeared excessive sometimes failed to cause ototoxic (including vestibular) damage (Black et al., 2001; Black et al., 2004).

Although several researchers have investigated the safety versus efficacy of once- versus multiple daily dose administrations of gentamicin, there appears to be no significant relationship between gentamicin administration schedule and onset or severity of ototoxicity (Barclay & Begg, 1994; Barclay, Begg, & Hickling, 1994; Bates & Nahata, 1994; Elhanan, Siplovich, & Raz, 1992; Galløe et al., 1995; Munckhof et al., 1996; Raz, Adawi, & Romano, 1995). Serum drug levels (e.g., baselines, peaks, and troughs) likewise appear to be of no value for prediction onset, occurrence, or severity of either vestibular ototoxicity or cochleotoxicity (Barclay & Begg, 1994; Barclay et al., 1994; Black et al., 2004; Matz, 1993).

Recovery from Vestibular Ototoxicity

Prospective studies have demonstrated that partial recovery of vestibular function may occur following severe vestibular ototoxicity (Figure 17-10) (Black et al., 2004). While studies suggest that adaptive mechanisms may play a role in recovery from vestibular

Legend: VOR recovery dynamics in the same patient shown in Figure 17-5. The subject received 42 gm of intramuscular streptomycin. K = gain constant; TC = time constant.

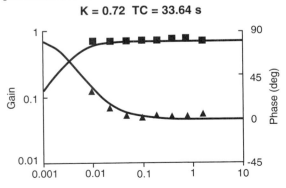

Figure 17-10a. Baseline VOR gain and phase responses. Gain and time constants are normal.

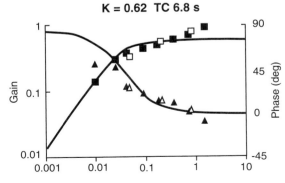

17-10b. VOR gain and phase responses 397 days after receiving streptomycin. Gain constant has recovered to normal range; time constant remains severely reduced (abnormal phase lead). The patient continues to experience dysequilibrium and oscillopsia.

ototoxicity, adaptation or compensatory mechanisms probably cannot explain the observed differential GC and TC recovery dynamics characteristic of some types of ototoxicity. (Kramer et al. have demonstrated differential gain and phase adaptation in the human (Kramer, Shelhamer, & Zee, 1995).) VOR adaptive changes in gain occur rapidly in the human, usually within hours to days (Gonshor & Melvill-Jones, 1976a, 1976b; Kramer et al., 1995). Therefore, it is unlikely that those mechanisms can account for the late (usually after six months) recovery of vestibular function following ototoxicity. Hair cells may be sublethally damaged, allowing subsequent recovery. Hair cell recovery may also involve metabolic and intracellular repair mechanisms requiring long periods (possibly weeks to months) for completion (Schacht, 1993). Given the often-prolonged time course of recovery observed in this study, it is likely that intracellular and neural connectivity mechanisms play key roles in recovery from vestibular ototoxicity (Taylor & Forge, 2005).

Recovery of VOR function associated with hair cell regeneration following aminoglycoside-induced ototoxicity has been demonstrated in avians (Carey, Fuchs, & Rubel, 1996) and mammals. Forge et al. (1993) and Warchol et al. (1993) reported regeneration of guinea pig and human vestibular hair cells *in vivo* and *in vitro*, respectively, after ototoxic destruction. The rates of regeneration observed suggested that the process occurred more slowly in mammals than in other species. Warchol et al. (1995) and Wersäll et al. (1993) also suggested that support cell transformation to functioning hair cells following aminoglycoside destruction might explain the recovery sometimes observed following aminoglycoside ototoxicity. Rubel et al. (1995) proposed nonproliferative mechanisms such as repair of damaged stereocilia bundles and cellular recovery as alternative explanations. Rubel et al. (1995) also presented evidence supporting vestibular hair cell regeneration *in vivo* (guinea pigs) following gentamicin toxicity, but questioned cellular transformation as the mechanism.

Prevention of Vestibular Ototoxicity

It is clear from the above review and results that clinicians and investigators cannot rely solely or reliably on symptoms for detecting or monitoring human vestibular ototoxicity. Nor can one adhere to published dosage schedules or rely on serum drug levels to avoid ototoxicity. Consequently, prevention takes on heightened importance. The best way to prevent ototoxicity is to avoid use of potentially ototoxic medications when clinically feasible. Managed care often plays an unwanted role here, for even though culture and sensitivities may point to safer alternative medications, many of the most dangerous medications (in terms of potential ototoxicity) are among the least expensive and, thus, are often found at the top of formulary lists as "preferred medications" (Black et al., 2004). In such cases, the treating physician and patient may opt for a different—albeit more expensive—choice of medication (English & Williams, 2000). If that is not possible, potentially ototoxic drugs should be given in the smallest possible dose for the shortest possible time period.

Obtaining a proper informed consent is essential when using ototoxic medications and plays a key role in preventing ototoxicity. In a recent retrospective study, none of the patients received a complete informed consent before the ototoxic drug was administered (Black et al., 2004). Most were warned of kidney damage and a few of hearing loss, but none were warned of the possibility of life-altering vestibular function loss.

Even though the signs and symptoms are unreliable for early detection and documentation of vestibular ototoxicity, it is very important that the entire medical team be aware of them. Two recent reports indicated that virtually all vestibulotoxic subjects went undiagnosed while hospitalized despite the fact that some of them reported symptoms compatible with ototoxicity onset before discharge (Black et al., 2004; Halmagyi et al., 1994).

Management of Vestibular Ototoxicity

Once severe to profound bilateral, permanent vestibular ototoxicity has occurred, it cannot be treated. While some ototoxic patients may recover some vestibular function, residual damage if severe or profound may cause life-changing disability.

Patients with mild to moderate ototoxicity may benefit from VRT, which is aimed at improving the patient's reliance on accurate visual and somatosensory cues, as well as at overall conditioning (Black & Pesznecker, 2003).

All types of vestibulotoxic patients will benefit from rehabilitative measures designed to modify their home and other environments, including reduction of fall risk. Patients experiencing severe and profound bilateral vestibular loss are at heightened risk for falls, especially when walking in the dark and on unstable surfaces and when negotiating stairs (especially going down the stairs). Severe to profound bilateral vestibular loss patients should be taught to leave nightlights on and to remove obstacles—such as throw rugs and electric cords—from walking paths because they have difficulty recovering from perturbations of gait (tripping or stumbling). Severe to profound BVL subjects may benefit from using a walking staff, which provides additional proprioception information that will aid balance. (The authors do not recommend using canes, as they cause patients to lean forward, which shifts their center of gravity forward and further increases their risk of falling.) Vestibulotoxic patients should use care on slick or graveled surfaces and should stay off step stools and ladders. Patients with severe and profound bilateral vestibular loss should not drive an automobile. Until generally accepted criteria can be developed, the response for patients with severe to profound bilateral loss who want to drive is characterized by the following questions: (1) Can you drive? Yes. (2) Should you drive? No.

SUMMARY

This chapter introduces the subject of vestibular ototoxicity that sometimes does not occur with cochleotoxicity, depending on the ototoxic agent. If the ototoxic agent affects both auditory and vestibular function, it is much easier clinically to monitor auditory system function especially in bed-ridden or obtunded patients. Use of otoacoustic emissions has recently been introduced as a sensitive method of monitoring for early ototoxicity, providing the patient has sufficient baseline auditory function. Extended high-frequency audiometry may also be used for monitoring for ototoxic effects.

Although potentially ototoxic medications are sometimes essential for treatment of life-threatening medical and surgical crises, vestibular ototoxicity can result in life-altering debilitation. While certain medical conditions are known to predispose to ototoxicity, it is impossible to predict with certainty who will develop ototoxicity and how severe it will be if it does occur. Studies have shown that there are no safe doses of some ototoxic medications, nor is there a safe schedule of administration. Serum drug levels are likewise of no value in predicting the onset, occurrence, or severity of vestibular ototoxicity. Because of those factors, the decision to use potentially ototoxic medications must be weighed against the potential outcome, and the patient must be properly and completely informed of all risks. Establishing a baseline of objective vestibular function is of critical importance in monitoring patients receiving medications known to be ototoxic, particularly since symptom reporting may not be consistent with objective vestibular changes. Patient condition permitting, objective monitoring should continue throughout the period of administration and for one year after the drug has been discontinued. Termination of gentamicin upon appearance of suspicious signs or symptoms may reduce the likelihood or severity of permanent vestibular ototoxicity and may enhance some recovery of vestibular function. In most cases, equally effective and less toxic but more expensive drugs are available.

Ototoxic medications are sometimes used for therapeutic purposes. The reader is encouraged to become familiar with known mechanisms of ototoxicity to fully understand what the clinical course is and how best to monitor for intended ototoxic effects of the agent employed.

Patients with vestibular toxicity, both temporary and permanent, should undergo VRT. Achievement of rehabilitation goals of (1) more rapid recovery for the more fortunate recovering patients, (2) reduction of risk, including falls and injuries; and (3) improved quality of life have been demonstrated for patients with vestibular ototoxicity (Black, Angel, Pesznecker, & Gianna, 2000; Herdman & Clendaniel, 2000; Herdman & Whitney, 2000).

Development of criteria for risky activities by vestibular loss patients is under development. At present, there are no quantitative guidelines for determining when it is safe for a patient with bilateral vestibular loss to drive an automobile. However, some states are requiring physicians to report patients who have conditions that may impair their ability to drive safely. Some states include as part of their criteria (1) functional impairments (including motor planning and coordination) and (2) cognitive impairments (including attention; judgment and problem solving; reaction time; planning; and sequencing, visuospatial, and memory). All of those processes can be impaired by vestibular disorders (Grimm, Hemenway, LeBray, & Black, 1989; Jacob, Furman, Durrant, & Turner, 1996; Jacob, Lilienfeld, Furman, Durrant, & Turner, 1989; Jacob, Lillinfield, Furman, & Turner, 1989; Jacob et al., 1993).

REFERENCES

Ali, M. Z., & Goetz, M. B. (1997). A meta-analysis of the relative efficacy and toxicity of single daily dosing versus multiple daily dosing of aminoglycosides. *Clinical Infectious Disease, 24*(5), 796–809.

Aran, J. M. (1995). Current perspectives on inner ear toxicity. *Otolaryngology—Head and Neck Surgery, 112,* 133–144.

Aust, G. (2001). Vestibulotoxicity and ototoxicity of gentamicin in newborn at risk. *International Tinnitus Journal, 7*(1), 27–29.

Bacino, C., Prezant, T. R., Bu, X., Fournier, P., & Fischel-Ghodsian, N. (1995). Susceptibility mutations in the mitochondrial small ribosomal RNA gene in aminoglycoside induced deafness. *Pharmacogenetics, 5*(3), 165–172.

Bakri, F. E., Pallett, A., Smith, A. G., & Duncombe, A. S. (1998). Ototoxicity induced by once-daily gentamicin. *Lancet, 351,* 1407–1408.

Barclay, M. L., & Begg, E. J. (1994). Aminoglycoside toxicity and relation to dose regimen. *Adverse Drug React Toxicol Rev, 13* (4), 207–234.

Barclay, M. L., Begg, E. J., & Hickling, K. G. (1994). What is the evidence for once-daily aminoglycoside therapy? *Clinical Pharmacokinetics, 27,* 32–48.

Barza, M., Ioannidis, J. P., Cappelleri, J. C., & Lau, J. (1996). Single or multiple daily doses of aminoglycosides: A meta-analysis. *British Medical Journal, 312*(7027), 338–345.

Bates, R. D., & Nahata, M. C. (1994). Once-daily administration of aminoglycosides. *Annals of Pharmacotherapy, 28,* 757–766.

Black, F. O. (1985). Vestibulospinal function assessment by moving platform posturography. *American Journal of Otology, 6,* 39–45.

Black, F. O., Angel, C. R., Pesznecker, S. C., & Gianna, C. C. (2000). Outcome analysis of individualized vestibular rehabilitation protocols. *American Journal of Otology, 21,* 543–551.

Black, F. O., Elardo, S. E., Mirka, A., Peterka, R. J., & Shupert, C. L. (1988). Vestibulo-ocular and vestibulospinal function changes during titrated streptomycin treatment for Meniere's disease. In J. B. Nadol (Ed.), *Second International Symposium on Meniere's Disease* (pp. 433-441). Amsterdam: Kugler & Ghedini Publications.

Black, F. O., Gianna-Poulin, C., & Pesznecker, S. C. (2001). Recovery from vestibular ototoxicity. *Otology & Neurotology, 22,* 662–671.

Black, F. O., & Pesznecker, S. C. (1993). Vestibular ototoxicity. Clinical considerations. *Otolaryngologic Clinics of North America, 26*(5), 713–736.

Black, F. O., & Pesznecker, S. C. (2003). Vestibular adaptation and rehabilitation. *Current Opinion in Otolaryngology, 11*(5), 355–360.

Black, F. O., Pesznecker, S. C., & Stallings, V. (2004). Permanent gentamicin vestibulotoxicity. *Otology & Neurotology, 25,* 559–569.

Black, F. O., Peterka, R. J., & Elardo, S. E. (1987). Vestibular reflex changes following aminoglycoside induced ototoxicity. *Laryngoscope, 97*(5), 582–586.

Black, F. O., Wade, S. W., & Nashner, L. M. (1996). What is the minimal vestibular function required for compensation? *American Journal of Otology, 17*(3), 401–409.

Blakley, B. W., Black, F. O., Myers, S. F., Rintelmann, W. F., Schweitzer, V., & Schwan, S. A. (1991, January–February). Ototoxicity. *Head & Neck,* 2–3.

Brummett, R. E. (1993). Ototoxicity of vancomycin and analogues. *Otolaryngologic Clinics of North America, 26,* 821–828.

Calder, J. H., & Jacobson, G. P. (2000). Acquired bilateral peripheral vestibular system impairment: Rehabilitative options and potential outcomes. *Journal of the American Academy of Audiology, 11*(9), 514–521.

Carey, J. P., Fuchs, A. F., & Rubel, E. W. (1996). Hair cell regeneration and recovery of the vestibuloocular reflex in the avian vestibular system. *Journal of Neurophysiology, 76*(5), 3301–3312.

Carey, J. T., & Wichter, M. D. (1977, May 12). Testing for ototoxicity: Amikacin and gentamicin. *New England Journal of Medicine.*

Casano, R. A., Johnson, D. F., Bykhovskaya, Y., Torricelli, F., Bigozzi, M., & Fischel-Ghodsian, N. (1999). Inherited susceptibility to aminoglycoside ototoxicity: Genetic heterogeneity and clinical implications. *American Journal of Otolaryngology, 20*(3), 151–156.

Chong, T. K., Piraino, B., & Bernardini, J. (1991). Vestibular toxicity due to gentamicin in peritoneal dialysis patients. *Peritoneal Dialysis International, 11,* 152–155.

Correia, M. J., & Guedry, F. E., Jr. (1978). The vestibular system: Basic biophysical and physiological mechanisms. In R. B. Masteron (Ed.), *Handbook of Behavioral Neurobiology. Volume 1. Sensory Integration* (pp. 311–351). New York: Plenum.

DeBeukelaer, M. M., Travis, L. B., & Dodge, W. F. (1971). Deafness and acute tubular necrosis following parenteral administration of neomycin. *American Journal of Diseases of Children, 121,* 250.

de Vries, P. J., Verkooyen, R. P., Leguit, P., & Verbrugh, H. A. (1990). Prospective randomized study of once-daily versus thrice-daily netilmicin regimens in patients with intraabdominal infections. *European Journal of Clinical Microbiology and Infectious Disease, 9*(3), 161–168.

de Waele, C., Meguenni, R., Freyss, G., Zamith, F., Bellalimat, N., Vidal, P. P., et al. (2002). Intratympanic gentamicin injections for Meniere disease: Vestibular hair cell impairment and regeneration. *Neurology, 59*(9), 1442–1444.

Diamond, C., O'Connell, D. A., Hornig, J. D., & Liu, R. (2003). Systematic review of intratympanic gentamicin in Meniere's disease. *Journal of Otolaryngology, 32*(6), 351–361.

Doretto, M. C., Marseillan, R. F., Pinto-Gonçalves, R., Oliveira, J. A. A., & Corrado, A. P. (1994). Reduction of streptomycin-induced acute and chronic toxicities. *Laryngoscope, 104,* 631–637.

el-Schahawi, M., Lopez de Munain, A., Sarrazin, A. M., Shanske, A., Basirico, M., Shanske, S., et al. (1997). Two large Spanish pedigrees with nonsyndromic sensorineural deafness and the mtDNA mutation at nt 1555 in the 12s rRNA gene: Evidence of heteroplasmy. *Neurology, 48*(2), 453–456.

Elhanan, K., Siplovich, L., & Raz, R. (1992). Gentamicin once-daily versus thrice-daily in children. *Journal of Antimicrobial Chemotherapy, 35,* 327–332.

English, W. P., & Williams, M. D. (2000). Should aminoglycoside antibiotics be abandoned? *American Journal of Surgery, 180*(6), 512–516.

EquiTest System. Version 4.0. Data Interpretation Manual. (1994). Clackamas, OR: NeuroCom International, Inc.

Estivill, X., Govea, N., Barcelo, E., Badenas, C., Romero, E., Moral, L., et al. (1998). Familial progressive sensorineural deafness is mainly due to the mtDNA A1555G mutation and is enhanced by treatment of aminoglycosides. *American Journal of Human Genetics, 62*(1), 27–35.

Fee, W. E., Jr. (1980). Aminoglycoside ototoxicity in the human. *Laryngoscope, 1*(Suppl. 24), 1–19.

Forge, A., Li, L., Corwin, J. T., & Nevill, G. (1993). Ultrastructural evidence for hair cell regeneration in the mammalian inner ear. *Science, 259*(5101), 1616–1619.

Forge, A., & Schacht, J. (2000). Aminoglycoside antibiotics. *Audiology and Neurootology, 5*(1), 3–22.

Gagnaire, F., & Langlais, C. (2005, January 20). Relative ototoxicity of 21 aromatic solvents. *Archives of Toxicology.*

Galløe, A. M., Graudal, N., Christensen, H. R., & Kampmann, J. P. (1995). Aminoglycosides: Single or multiple daily dosing? *European Journal of Clinical Pharmacology, 49,* 39–43.

Gerharz, E. W., Weingärtner, K., Melekos, M. D., Varga, S., Feiber, H., & Riedmiller, H. (1995). Neomycin-induced perception deafness following bladder irrigation in patients with end-stage renal disease. *British Journal of Urology, 76,* 479–481.

Gibson, W. S., Jr. (1967). Deafness due to orally administered neomycin. *Archives of Otolaryngology, 86*(2), 163–165.

Goebel, J. A., Sangasilp, N., & Lindberg, B. (2005, February 19–24). *Comparison of Dynamic Subjective Visual Vertical (DSVV) Test and Computerized Dynamic Posturography (CDP) for Evaluation of Patients with Postural Instability.* Paper presented at the 28th MidWinter Meeting, Association for Research in Otolaryngology, New Orleans, LA.

Gonshor, A., & Melvill-Jones, G. (1976a). Extreme vestibulo-ocular adaptation induced by prolonged optical reversal of vision. *Journal of Physiology, 256,* 381–414.

Gonshor, A., & Melvill-Jones, G. (1976b). Short-term adaptive changes in the human vestibulo-ocular reflex arc. *Journal of Physiology, 256,* 361–379.

Grimm, R. J., Hemenway, W. G., LeBray, P. R., & Black, F. O. (1989). The perilymph fistula syndrome defined in mild head trauma. *Acta Otolaryngologica Suppl, 464,* 5–40.

Halmagyi, G. M., Fattore, C. M., Curthoys, I. S., & Wade, S. W. (1994). Gentamicin vestibulotoxicity. *Otolaryngology—Head and Neck Surgery, 111,* 571–574.

Hamasaki, K., & Rando, R. R. (1997). Specific binding of aminoglycosides to a human rRNA construct based on a DNA polymorphism which causes aminoglycoside-induced deafness. *Biochemistry, 36*(40), 12323–12328.

Herdman, S. J., & Clendaniel, R. A. (2000). Assessment and treatment of complete vestibular loss. In S. J. Herdman (Ed.), *Vestibular Rehabilitation* (pp. 424–450). Philadelphia: FA Davis.

Herdman, S. J., & Whitney, S. L. (2000). Treatment of vestibular hypofunction. In S. J. Herdman (Ed.), *Vestibular Rehabilitation* (pp. 387–423). Philadelphia: FA Davis.

Jacob, R. G., Furman, J. M. R., Durrant, J. D., & Turner, S. M. (1996). Panic, agoraphobia, and vestibular dysfunction. *American Journal of Psychiatry, 153,* 503–512.

Jacob, R. G., Lilienfeld, S. O., Furman, J. M. R., Durrant, J. D., & Turner, S. M. (1989). Panic disorder with vestibular dysfunction: Further clinical observations and description of space and motion phobic stimuli. *Journal of Anxiety Disorders, 3,* 117–130.

Jacob, R. G., Lillinfield, S. O., Furman, J. M. R., & Turner, S. M. (1989). Space and motion phobia in panic disorder with vestibular dysfunction. *Journal of Anxiety Disorders, 3,* 117–130.

Jacob, R. G., Woody, S. R., Clark, D. B., Lilienfeld, S. O., Hirsch, B. E., Kucera, G. D., et al. (1993). Discomfort with space and motion: A possible marker of vestibular dysfunction assessed by the situational characteristics questionnaire. *Journal of Psychopathology and Behavioral Assessment, 15*(4), 299–324.

Johnsson, L. G., Hawkins, J. E., Jr, Kingsley, T. C., Black, F. O., & Matz, G. J. (1981). Aminoglycoside-induced cochlear pathology in man. *Acta Otolaryngologica Suppl, 383,* 3–19.

Jung, T. T., Rhee, C. K., Lee, C. S., Park, Y. S., & Choi, D. C. (1993). Ototoxicity of salicylate, nonsteroidal anti-inflammatory drugs, and quinine. *Otolaryngologic Clinics of North America, 26*(5), 791–810.

Kalbian, V. (1972). Deafness following oral use of neomycin. *Southern Medical Journal, 65*(4), 499–501.

Kaplan, D. M., Marais, J., Ogawa, T., Kraus, M., Rutka, J. A., & Bance, M. L. (2001). Does high-frequency pseudo-random rotational chair testing increase the diagnostic yield of the ENG caloric test in detecting bilateral vestibular loss in the dizzy patient? *Laryngoscope, 111*(6), 959–963.

Kavanaugh, K. T., & McCabe, B. F. (1983). Ototoxicity of oral neomycin and vancomycin. *Laryngoscope, 93*(5), 649–653.

Kitsigianis, G. A., O'Leary, D. P., & Davis-O'Leary, L. L. (1988). Vestibular autorotation testing of cisplatin chemotherapy patients. In C. R. Pfaltz (Ed.), *Advances in Oto-Rhino-Laryngology* (pp. 250–253). Basel, Switzerland: Karger.

Kramer, P. D., Shelhamer, M., & Zee, D. S. (1995). Short-term adaptation of the phase of the vestibulo-ocular reflex (VOR) in normal human subjects. *Experimental Brain Research, 106*(2), 318–326.

Kunin, C. M., Chalmers, T. C., & Leevy, C. M. (1960). Absorption of orally administered neomycin and kanamycin with special reference to patients with severe hepatic and renal disease. *New England Journal of Medicine, 262,* 393.

Lange, G., Maurer, J., & Mann, W. (2004). Long-term results after interval therapy with intratympanic gentamicin for Meniere's disease. *Laryngoscope, 114*(1), 102–105.

Langman, A. W. (1994). Neomycin ototoxicity. *Otolaryngology—Head and Neck Surgery, 110,* 441–444.

Last, P. M., & Sherlock, S. (1960). Systemic absorption of orally administered neomycin in liver disease. *New England Journal of Medicine, 262,* 385.

Lerner, S. A., Schmitt, B. A., Seligsoh, R., & Matz, G. J. (1986). Comparative study of ototoxicity and nephrotoxicity in patients randomly assigned to treatment with amikacin or gentamicin. *American Journal of Otology, 80,* 98–104.

Longridge, N. S., & Mallinson, A. I. (1987). The dynamic illegible E (DIE) test: A simple technique for assessing the ability of the vestibulo-ocular reflex to overcome vestibular pathology. *Journal of Otolaryngology, 16,* 97–103.

Longridge, N. S., & Mallinson, A. I. (2000). Low-dose gentamicin treatment for dizziness in Meniere's disease. *Journal of Otolaryngology, 29*(1), 35–39.

Matz, G. J. (1993). Aminoglycoside cochlear ototoxicity. *Otolaryngologic Clinics of North America, 26,* 705–712.

Miller, J. J. (1985). *CRC Handbook of Ototoxicity.* Boca Raton, Florida: CRC Press, Inc.

Minor, L. B. (1999). Intratympanic gentamicin for control of vertigo in Meniere's disease: Vestibular signs that specify completion of therapy. *American Journal of Otology, 20,* 209–219.

Munckhof, W. J., Grayson, M. L., & Turnidge, J. D. (1996). A meta-analysis of studies on the safety and efficacy of aminoglycosides given either once daily or as divided doses. *Journal of Antimicrobial Chemotherapy, 37,* 645–663.

Nashner, L. M. (1993). Computerized dynamic posturography: Clinical applications. Part IV: Posturographic testing. In G. P. Jacobson, C. W. Newman, & J. M. Kartush (Eds.), *Handbook of Balance Function Testing* (pp. 308–334). St. Louis: Mosby Year Book.

Nashner, L. M., Black, F. O., & Wall, C., III. (1982). Adaptation to altered support and visual conditions during stance: Patients with vestibular deficits. *Journal of Neuroscience, 2*(5), 536–544.

O'Leary, D. P., Davis-O'Leary, L. L., & Li, S. (1995). Predictive monitoring of high-frequency vestibulo-ocular reflex rehabilitation following gentamicin ototoxicity. *Acta Otolaryngologica Suppl, 520,* 202–204.

Peloquin, C. A., Berning, S. E., Nitta, A. T., Simone, P. M., Goble, M., Huitt, G. A., et al. (2004). Aminoglycoside toxicity: Daily versus thrice-weekly dosing for treatment of mycobacterial diseases. *Clinical Infectious Disease, 38*(11), 1538–1544.

Perez, N., Martin, E., & Garcia-Tapia, R. (2003). Results of vestibular autorotation testing at the end of intratympanic gentamicin treatment for Meniere's disease. *Acta Otolaryngologica, 123*(4), 506–514.

Peterka, R. J., Black, F. O., & Schoenhoff, M. B. (1990a). Age-related changes in human vestibulo-ocular and optokinetic reflexes: Pseudorandom rotation tests. *Journal of Vestibular Research, 1*(1), 61–71.

Peterka, R. J., Black, F. O., & Schoenhoff, M. B. (1990b). Age-related changes in human vestibulo-ocular reflexes: Sinusoidal rotation and caloric tests. *Journal of Vestibular Research, 1*(1), 49–59.

Peters, B. T., & Bloomberg, J. J. (2004). Dynamic visual acuity using "far" and "near" targets. *Acta Otolaryngologica, 125,* 353–357.

Prezant, T. R., Agapian, J. V., Bohlman, M. C., Bu, X., Oztas, S., Qiu, W. Q., et al. (1993). Mitochondrial ribosomal RNA mutation associated with both antibiotic-induced and non-syndromic deafness. *Nat Genet, 4*(3), 289–294.

Raz, R., Adawi, M., & Romano, S. (1995). Intravenous administration of gentamicin once daily versus thrice daily in adults. *European Journal of Clinical Microbiology and Infectious Disease, 14,* 88–91.

Riggs, L. C., Brummett, R. E., Guitjens, S. K., & Matz, G. J. (1996). Ototoxicity resulting from combined administration of cisplatin and gentamicin. *Laryngoscope, 106,* 401–406.

Riggs, L. C., Shofner, W. P., Shah, A. R., Young, M. R., Hain, T. C., & Matz, G. J. (1999). Ototoxicity resulting from combined administration of metronidazole and gentamicin. *American Journal of Otology, 20*, 430–434.

Rubel, E. W., Dew, L. A., & Roberson, D. W. (1995). Mammalian hair cell regeneration (Technical Comments). *Science, 267*, 701–707.

Rybak, L. P., & Matz, G. J. (1986). Auditory and vestibular effects of toxins. In C. W. Cummings, J. M. Fredrickson, L. A. Harker, C. J. Krause, & D. E. Schuller (Eds.), *Otolaryngology—Head and Neck Surgery* (pp. 3161–3172). St. Louis: C.V. Mosby.

Saadat, D., O'Leary, D. P., Pulec, J. L., & Kitano, H. (1995). Comparison of vestibular autorotation and caloric testing. *Otolaryngology—Head and Neck Surgery, 113*(3), 215–222.

Schacht, J. (1993). Biochemical basis of aminoglycoside ototoxicity. *Otolaryngologic Clinics of North America, 26*, 845–856.

Schacht, J. (1998). Aminoglycoside ototoxicity: Prevention in sight? *Otolaryngology—Head and Neck Surgery, 118*(5), 674–677.

Schacht, J. (1999). Antioxidant therapy attenuates aminoglycoside-induced hearing loss. *Annals of the New York Academy of Sciences, 884*, 125–130.

Schweitzer, V. G. (1993). Ototoxicity of chemotherapeutic agents. *Otolaryngologic Clinics of North America, 26*, 759–789.

Sulkowski, W. J., Kowalska, S., Matyja, W., Guzek, W., Wesolowski, W., Szymczak, W., et al. (2002). Effects of occupational exposure to a mixture of solvents on the inner ear: A field study. *International Journal of Occupational Medicine and Environmental Health, 15*(3), 247–256.

Taylor, R., & Forge, A. (2005). Developmental biology. Life after deaf for hair cells? *Science, 307*(5712), 1056–1058.

Tessa, A., Giannotti, A., Tieri, L., Vilarinho, L., Marotta, G., & Santorelli, F. M. (2001). Maternally inherited deafness associated with a T1095C mutation in the mDNA. *European Journal of Human Genetics, 9*(2), 147–149.

Usami, S., Abe, S., Akita, J., Namba, A., Shinkawa, H., Ishii, M., et al. (2000). Prevalence of mitochondrial gene mutations among hearing impaired patients. *Journal of Medical Genetics, 37*(1), 38–40.

Wade, S. W., Halmagyi, G. M., Black, F. O., & McGarvie, L. M. (1999). Time constant of nystagmus slow phase velocity to yaw-axis rotation as a function of the severity of unilateral caloric paresis. *American Journal of Otology, 20*(4), 471–478.

Walsh, P. (2000). *Physician's Desk Reference* (54th ed.). Montvale, NJ: Medical Economics Company, Inc.

Warchol, M. E., Lambert, P. R. R., Goldstein, B. J., Forge, A., & Corwin, J. T. (1993). Regenerative proliferation in inner ear sensory epithelia from adult guinea pigs and humans. *Science, 259*(5101), 1619–1622.

Wersäll, J. (1995). Ototoxic antibiotics: A review. *Acta Otolaryngologica, Suppl, 519*, 26–29.

Wu, I. C., & Minor, L. B. (2003). Long-term hearing outcome in patients receiving intratympanic gentamicin for Meniere's disease. *Laryngoscope, 113*(5), 815–820.

Yates, B. J. (1998). Autonomic reaction to vestibular damage. *Otolaryngology—Head and Neck Surgery, 119*(1), 106–112.

Yates, B. J., & Miller, A. D. (1996). Overview of vestibular autonomic regulation. In B. J. Yates & A. D. Miller (Eds.), *Vestibular Autonomic Regulation* (pp. 1–3). Boca Raton: CRC Press.

Yoshida, M., Shintani, T., Hirao, M., Himi, T., Yamaguchi, A., & Kikuchi, K. (2002). Aminoglycoside-induced hearing loss in a patient with the 961 mutation in mitochondrial DNA. *ORL Journal of Otorhinolaryngology and Related Specialties, 64*(3), 219–222.

Zhao, H., Li, R., Wang, Q., Yan, Q., Deng, J. H., Han, D., et al. (2004). Maternally inherited aminoglycoside-induced and nonsyndromic deafness is associated with the novel C1494T mutation in the mitochondrial 12S rRNA gene in a large Chinese family. *American Journal of Human Genetics, 74*(1), 139–152.

CHAPTER
18

Audiologic Findings in Vestibular Toxicity

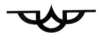

Jaynee A. Handelsman, PhD
University of Michigan

INTRODUCTION

Ototoxicity is a problem that is encountered by audiologists and other health care professionals. It is a negative consequence of the availability and use of medications that prolong life through the treatment of serious illness, including infection and cancer. As has been discussed in preceding chapters in this text, numerous agents are known to be toxic to the delicate structures of the inner ear and in many cases, the toxic effect of the agent is affected by the patient's overall health as well as prior or concomitant exposure to other agents. While the literature is replete with evidence of ototoxicity and protocols exist for monitoring the effects of toxic agents on hearing, less is known about the impact of medications and other agents on the vestibular system. Specifically, a relative paucity of information exists about the prevalence of vestibular toxicity among patients who are exposed to toxic agents, and there are no commonly accepted protocols for monitoring the vestibular system function during exposure.

The purpose of this chapter is to discuss the audiological management of vestibular toxicity. The discussion will include a description of the clinical features of vestibular toxicity, the tools that can be employed in monitoring vestibular system function, and experimental evidence of the impact of various toxic agents on the vestibular system. Case examples will be described in an effort to illustrate the variable presentation of vestibular toxicity, as well as its relationship to auditory changes. Finally, suggestions will be made for monitoring vestibular system function in patients who are exposed to potentially toxic agents.

CLINICAL FEATURES OF VESTIBULAR TOXICITY

One of the earliest accounts of vestibular toxicity resulting from aminoglycoside use was written by a physician who described his own symptoms resulting from a 76-day course of streptomycin to treat sepsis of the knee (J. C., 1952). He described a sudden onset of symptoms that are typically associated with bilateral vestibular loss, including oscillopsia and **ataxic gait**. His symptoms reportedly progressed over a 2–3 day period to the point that his own pulse caused enough head motion that he had difficulty reading without head stabilization. Over time, he learned to minimize head movements, particularly when trying to read. He also learned how to use visual and somatosensory information to compensate for the loss of vestibular function, which resulted in improved gait and balance.

While the symptoms that J. C. (1952) described are consistent with a sudden loss of bilateral vestibular system function, vestibular toxicity occurs with a variable presentation. Specifically, the onset can be sudden, as was the case with J. C., or it can be gradual. For example, in a case report presented by Minor (1998), the patient gradually noticed unsteadiness and oscillopsia over a two-month period following treatment with a two-week course of gentamicin. The final gentamicin course occurred after 30 days of induction chemotherapy as well as pre-chemotherapy treatment with vancomycin and ciprofloxin and a three-week course of gentamicin. Minor's patient illustrates a more delayed and gradual onset of symptoms relative to the timing of the administration of toxic agents. As is often the case because of the severity of the illnesses that are being treated with toxic agents, patients may not notice symptoms until weeks or months after the administration of the medication. It is difficult to know in those instances when the actual toxic effect occurred. As was true with Minor's patient, although peak levels of the medications are typically maintained within the appropriate therapeutic ranges, damage to the inner ear occurred. What is not clear is whether the damage progressed gradually over time in the posttreatment period or whether the damage was present immediately but was not realized by the patient until his activity level was sufficient to require vestibular input for gaze stabilization and postural control.

Vestibular toxicity resulting from the systemic use of potentially ototoxic agents is typically bilateral, but that is not always the case. As illustrated in the cases presented later in this chapter, intravenous (IV) aminoglycoside use can result in unilateral vestibular loss. Furthermore, in patients with bilateral vestibular loss, one ear is often relatively more affected than the other, resulting in symptoms that are consistent both with unilateral and bilateral vestibular paresis. For example, affected patients might report oscillopsia and unsteadiness that are characteristic of bilateral loss of function, as well as positional vertigo that is typically associated with an imbalance between the peripheral vestibular systems. In addition, according to Black, Gianna-Poulin, and Pesznecker (2001), there is some evidence that patients can recover vestibular function following loss due to aminoglycoside toxicity. In their longitudinal investigation of twenty-eight subjects who received ototoxic medications, of the eleven subjects who had evidence of vestibular ototoxicity following medication use, five displayed some recovery of function at one year. Interestingly, they reported that the onset of vestibular ototoxicity was not dose-related and that the presence and severity of the symptoms were unrelated to the development of objective evidence of ototoxicity and to the type or cumulative dose of medications administered. It is clear that vestibular ototoxicity is variable in presentation as well as in terms of its functional impact on the individuals affected.

EVALUATION TOOLS

The tools that are available for evaluating vestibular system function fall into two broad categories: bedside tests and laboratory tests. Because ototoxic medications are often administered to patients who are critically ill, their ability to cooperate with testing might be limited. In addition, it is not always practical to transport patients to a clinical laboratory for evaluation. Consequently, tests that can be performed at the patient's bedside are useful. Unfortunately, the bedside tests that are typically performed to assess vestibular function are relatively gross and can only provide evidence that damage has already occurred. Because there is no objective information about the relationship between performance on those measures and the extent of vestibular damage present, it is not clear whether they are useful in monitoring subtle changes in function over time. Therefore, laboratory tests, which have results that are more easily quantified and are relatively stable over time, are important. Bedside and laboratory vestibular tests are summarized in the following sections.

Bedside Tests

Limitations in the availability of laboratory evaluations of vestibular function for all patients being exposed to potentially ototoxic medications increase the practical role of bedside tests for monitoring changes in vestibular function over time. Perhaps the most important part of the bedside evaluation is inquiry about and consideration of patients' subjective complaints. Unfortunately, too often health care workers ignore patients' reports of vague changes in status or symptoms, resulting in delayed evaluation and prolonged exposure to the toxic agents. Questioning patients about symptoms such as changes in vision associated with head movement and unsteadiness is an essential component of any monitoring program.

Head-Shaking Nystagmus

The presence of **nystagmus** following head shaking is suggestive of an asymmetry in the peripheral vestibular system. During back-and-forth rotation of the head on the horizontal plane, the vestibular system on both sides is being stimulated. In the case of a relative weakness on one side, the stronger response on the intact side builds up and is stored in a central velocity storage mechanism. When the head shaking stops, stored energy is released in the form of slow eye movement away from the stronger ear, resulting in nystagmus beating away from the weaker ear (Desmond, 2004). In the context of a bedside evaluation, head-shaking testing is performed using Frenzel lenses or infrared video goggles. The patient is instructed to shake his or her head back and forth rapidly for 20–30 seconds and then stop. The eyes are observed for the presence of nystagmus within the first 10 seconds following the cessation of head shaking. When nystagmus of more than a couple of beats is present, it is suggestive of a relative weakness in the vestibular system of one ear.

Head Thrust Testing

Head thrust testing as originally described by Halmagyi and Curthoys (1988) is useful in detecting both unilateral and bilateral vestibular system loss.

Because the vestibulo-ocular reflex (VOR) is required for maintenance of gaze stability during rapid head movements, individuals with vestibular loss will display catch-up saccades during this procedure. To perform the test, the examiner holds the patient's head and slowly oscillates it in a side-to-side manner. The patient is instructed to maintain his or her gaze on the examiner's nose or on some other stationary object. The examiner then gently applies brief, high-acceleration head thrusts, with the eyes beginning slightly off center and ending in the primary position of center gaze. The hallmark of a positive head thrust test, which is suggestive of low VOR gain, is the presence of a **corrective saccade** in the same direction as the head thrust. The corrective saccade is required to compensate for the inappropriate slow phase of the VOR in an impaired vestibular system (Zee & Fletcher, 1996). For example, a corrective saccade with a right head thrust is suggestive of a right peripheral vestibular system paresis, and corrective saccades in both directions suggest a bilateral vestibular paresis. Testing can also be performed on the vertical plane.

Dynamic Visual Acuity

Dynamic visual acuity testing involves comparing the patient's visual acuity with the head still against visual acuity with the head in motion. It can be assessed in a number of ways, one of the most simple of which is to have the patient read from a Snellen chart without and with head turning or tilting. A decrease in visual acuity that represents more than a two-line shift on the chart as a result of head turning at 1–2 Hz is considered to be indicative of oscillopsia. Inasmuch as oscillopsia can affect both the horizontal and vertical planes and since there is no evidence that improved performance from therapy on one plane affects changes in the other, it is important to evaluate both. Provided the patient is reasonably alert and able to cooperate by performing repeated head turns, dynamic visual acuity testing may be one of the most valuable tools for monitoring changes in vestibular system function over time.

Postural Control

Bedside tests of postural control are designed to assess the vestibulo-spinal reflexes that are mediated by the lateral and vertical semicircular canals as well

as the otolith-spinal reflexes. Specifically, tandem walking with eyes open and eyes closed and the Fukuda stepping test (marching for 30 seconds with eyes closed) are sensitive measures of a static imbalance in the lateral canal reflexes, whereas the various Romberg tests are sensitive to an imbalance affecting the vertical canal reflexes. A static imbalance that affects the otolith-spinal reflexes can result in excessive postural sway in the form of lateral head and body tilt. Observation of postural stability during rapid body turns as well as in response to external perturbations that are imposed by the examiner can be used to assess dynamic vestibulo-spinal function (Zee & Fletcher, 1996).

Laboratory Tests

The purpose of the laboratory tests of vestibular function is to determine whether the peripheral and central components of the system are functioning normally. Advantages of laboratory tests are that the stimulus is precise and known and the results are more easily quantified than those from bedside tests. As a result, these tools provide a more accurate means of monitoring changes in vestibular system function. A brief overview of each of the components of the battery is provided in the following sections.

Electronystagmography (ENG)/ Videonystagmography (VNG)

Horizontal and vertical eye movements are recorded using electrodes (by way of the corneoretinal potential) during electronystagmography (ENG) or infrared video cameras during videonystagmography (VNG) and are digitally stored. Although both techniques provide evidence of nystagmus, VNG has distinct advantages over ENG, including cleaner traces that enable the examiner to record more subtle eye movements and the ability to view and record torsion. The ENG/VNG battery typically consists of oculomotor tests, recording and measurement of spontaneous eye movements, positional and positioning tests, and caloric tests. While assessing vestibular end organ function is most important in monitoring potential ototoxic effects, normal responses require normal central vestibulo-ocular pathway function. For that reason, at least during baseline testing, completion of the entire battery is essential.

Bithermal caloric testing is the only portion of the test battery that allows the examiner to evaluate individual ear function; and for that reason, it is valuable in assessing the relative strength of the vestibular end organs. In caloric testing, a nonphysiologic stimulus (air or water) is utilized to induce endolymph flow in the semicircular canals by creating a temperature gradient from one side of the canal to the other. Four irrigations are typically completed (warm and cool into each ear individually), the nystagmus that results is recorded and analyzed to determine peak slow component eye velocity (SCEV) for each irrigation, and the responses from each ear and for each nystagmus direction are compared. Establishment of normal criteria for each laboratory is important because test technique, including stimulus type, temperature, and duration, directly impacts the strength of the responses obtained. For example, responses to air irrigations are typically weaker than those obtained in response to open loop water. Similarly, reducing the caloric flow time can result in weaker responses. When calorics are used to assess the impact of potentially toxic medications over time, it is important that testing be conducted in the same manner each time. Even when that is the case, however, because various patient factors (e.g., anxiety, degree of alertness, body temperature, and medications) can impact the absolute slow component velocity of the caloric responses, caution should be used when interpreting changes in total eye speed from one test session to another.

Rotational Testing

Rotational testing involves stimulating the vestibular system by turning the patient along an earth-vertical axis in a sinusoidal, pseudorandom, or constant velocity fashion. It provides some distinct advantages over VNG testing for assessing overall vestibular system function in that both labyrinths are stimulated simultaneously using a quantifiable physiologic stimulus (rotation) and testing is conducted over a range of frequencies from 0.01–0.64 or 1.28 Hz. Unlike caloric stimulation, which is equivalent to a very low

frequency rotation of 0.002–0.004 Hz (Furman, Wall, & Kamerer, 1988) that falls substantially below the range of typical head movements, the frequencies evaluated during rotational testing more closely approximate those that occur normally. Testing is conducted in darkness, and eye movement responses to acceleration are recorded using electrodes or infrared cameras. The dependent measures of gain, phase, and symmetry are calculated by comparing the amplitude and velocity of the nystagmus with the movement of the chair. Specifically, gain is the ratio of eye velocity to chair velocity, phase describes the timing relationship between chair (head) movement and eye movement, and symmetry describes the relationship between responses for clockwise rotations and for counterclockwise rotations. Significant gain reductions are indicative of bilateral vestibular loss. Because testing is conducted over a range of frequencies, rotational testing is useful in quantifying the extent of bilateral involvement, which, in turn, provides information that can be used to estimate prognosis for functional recovery. For example, a patient with absent caloric responses would be expected to do well following vestibular rehabilitation if higher frequency responses were preserved. On the other hand, gain reductions present throughout the frequency range tested would suggest a more guarded prognosis for functional recovery.

Dynamic Posturography

Computerized dynamic posturography (CDP) provides a battery of tests that is designed to assess a person's ability to use vision, vestibular, and somatosensory cues in the maintenance of postural control. During the sensory organization subtest, anterior and posterior sway and sheer are measured during upright stance while the patient's access to vision and somatosensory cues is systematically altered. For example, the patient has access to accurate somatosensory cues in the first three conditions since the support surface remains fixed, while access to vision is systematically altered in Conditions 1–3 from normal vision (eyes open) to absent vision (eyes closed) followed by inaccurate vision (sway-referenced surround). In Conditions 4–6, the same progression in vision changes occurs with the additional component of loss of accurate somatosensory cues as the support surface is sway-referenced. The results are interpreted based on patterns of performance across the six testing conditions. Patients with uncompensated peripheral vestibular system involvement typically have difficulty in the conditions in which they do not have access to accurate vision or somatosensory cues. Specifically, with uncompensated unilateral or bilateral vestibular loss, patients will exhibit increased postural sway or falls in Conditions 5 (sway-referenced support and absent vision) and Condition 6 (sway-referenced support and vision). The motor control subtest provides information about a patient's ability to respond to forward and backward support surface perturbations, as well as adaptation to repeated changes in the ankle angle. Although CDP is useful in the assessment of postural control function, in and of itself it does not delineate the site of lesion within the vestibular system (Kisilevsky, Tomlinson, Ranalli, & Prepageran, 2004).

Tests of Auditory Function

Clearly, ototoxicity can affect both auditory and vestibular system function, and it is impossible to predict for a given individual whether hearing or balance system function will be affected first. For that reason, all patients receiving potentially ototoxic medications should be monitored for changes in both. Refer to Chapter 16 for a discussion of protocols that are appropriate for monitoring hearing status.

Assessment of Handicap/Disability

The Dizziness Handicap Inventory (DHI) is a validated 25-item, self-perceived disability/handicap scale that is designed to assess the impact of dizziness and unsteadiness on quality of life (Jacobson & Newman, 1990; Newman & Jacobson, 1993a; Newman & Jacobson, 1993b). The items included in the DHI are divided into three groups, each of which is designed to evaluate the impact of the symptoms on one aspect (emotional, functional, or physical) of daily living. Each of the items is answered by the patient with a "yes" (scored as 4 points), "sometimes" (scored as

2 points), or "no" (scored as 0 points) response. A minimum score of 0 relates to no self-perceived disability/handicap, and a maximum score of 100 represents profound self-perceived handicap. The DHI has been broadly used as a tool for assessing patients' perceptions regarding the functional impact of their disorders. For example, in an effort to characterize the self-perceived balance disability of patients with bilateral vestibular loss, Jacobson and Calder (2000) compared the DHI total and subscale scores of subjects with normal vestibular system function to the scores of subjects demonstrating unilateral peripheral vestibular loss, partial bilateral vestibular loss, and complete bilateral vestibular loss. Jacobson and Calder found significant group differences for DHI total and physical subscale scores. Specifically, they found that as a group, patients with bilateral vestibular loss experience greater degrees of self-perceived handicap than do those with unilateral vestibular loss. Similarly, in a case report discussing vestibular rehabilitation for treatment of acquired bilateral vestibular impairment secondary to ototoxicity, the DHI provided evidence of perceived functional change over time (Calder & Jacobson, 2000).

RECENT DATA REGARDING VESTIBULAR OTOTOXICITY

In a recent study of 33 patients demonstrating evidence of vestibular toxicity secondary to exposure to gentamicin alone or in combination with other aminoglycosides, Black, Pesznecker, and Stallings (2004) examined the objective findings and subjective symptoms at least one year following cessation of antibiotic treatment. At the time of the initial evaluation, all subjects reported disequilibrium and ataxia; all but one reported oscillopsia; and approximately two-thirds reported tinnitus, cognitive dysfunction, nausea, or **visual sensitivity**. In addition, all subjects demonstrated abnormal horizontal canal vestibulo-ocular reflex (HCVOR) responses to single-frequency and pseudorandom rotational stimuli in terms of gain and/or time constant measures. Of the 25 subjects who underwent caloric testing, 12 had bilaterally absent responses and 12 had asymmetrically reduced responses; the other subject had borderline normal results. Twenty-eight subjects also completed CDP; all but one of them demonstrated abnormal performance on Conditions 5 and 6, and 13 of 28 performed abnormally on three or more sensory organization conditions. Of the 28 subjects for whom audiological testing was completed, 11 demonstrated normal hearing sensitivity while 17 subjects without pretreatment hearing loss subjectively had sensorineural hearing loss after gentamicin treatment that the authors believed was not attributable to other causes.

In an attempt to investigate the relationship between the development of ototoxicity and factors related to gentamicin dose and serum levels, the authors examined records of ten of thirty-three subjects. Interestingly, the authors were not able to correlate development of ototoxicity to either dose regimens (single versus multiple dose) or peak and trough serum levels. They concluded, as a result, that there is no "safe" dose of gentamicin. The authors also reported that although twenty-nine of thirty-three subjects complained of symptoms consistent with the development of ototoxicity prior to discharge from the hospital, only one was diagnosed at that time. The authors reported further that subjects were often told that their symptoms would cease as soon as the gentamicin was stopped. Unfortunately, all 33 subjects in the study were disabled as the result of vestibular toxicity (Black et al., 2004).

A recent report by Dhanireddy, Liles, and Gates (2005) included a discussion of three cases in which vestibular toxicity resulted from once-daily doses of gentamicin. Each subject received a three-, four-, or six-week course of gentamicin—two for postsurgical infections and one for preoperative treatment of a sinus infection. In all three cases, subjects began to develop symptoms of dizziness within two weeks of initiation of treatment. One individual also noticed the onset of tinnitus without subjective hearing loss at the end of his treatment course. In no case was auditory or vestibular function evaluated at the time of symptom onset, nor was the treatment course modified. At the time vestibular testing was completed, two subjects had completely absent caloric responses while the other had minimal responses, rotational testing demonstrated low gains and absent responses in the two subjects evaluated, and CDP results were abnormal in all three. Dynamic visual acuity was also severely impaired in all three subjects, confirming the presence of oscillopsia. None of the subjects is able to work. Of note, despite the severity of the vestibular toxicity that was evident in all three subjects, hearing was apparently unaffected.

CASE REPORTS

As mentioned, vestibular toxicity presents in various ways in terms of timing, symptoms, and degree of loss. Some individuals have auditory complaints in addition to vestibular symptoms, but many do not. And while most patients are bilaterally affected, that is not always the case. The following cases are intended to illustrate the clinical presentation of patients with vestibular system involvement that is presumed to be secondary to aminoglycoside exposure. Unfortunately, since none of them were evaluated prior to treatment, the premorbid status is unknown.

Case 1

A 55-year-old gentleman underwent surgery to repair a ruptured colon related to diverticulitis. His recovery was complicated by the development of peritonitis, for which he was treated with a 10-day course of IV tobramycin. One day prior to his final treatment, he noticed significant disequilibrium; and by the final day of treatment, he had difficulty walking and said his head felt "dazed." At the time of testing a month later, the patient continued to experience occasional nausea, unsteadiness, disturbed vision, and a funny sensation in his head associated with movement. He also reported having trouble concentrating. Audiological testing was completed and revealed a mild to moderate sensorineural hearing loss beginning at 3K Hz with excellent word recognition ability bilaterally. VNG testing revealed a 91%

left caloric weakness, as well as significant positional and post head-shaking nystagmus (see Figure 18-1). Oculomotor testing yielded normal results. Rotational testing revealed significant phase leads at 0.01–0.16 Hz with normal gain and symmetry at all frequencies tested. Rotational step testing revealed the presence of short time constants for both clockwise and counterclockwise steps. Overall the findings suggest a left peripheral vestibular system paresis in a partially uncompensated state physiologically (for eye movements). Although formal postural control testing was not completed, an assessment of gait and balance was completed by a physical therapist and revealed slight increases in postural sway during tests of static balance without vision, and mildly disturbed gait with head movement, suggesting lack of complete functional compensation.

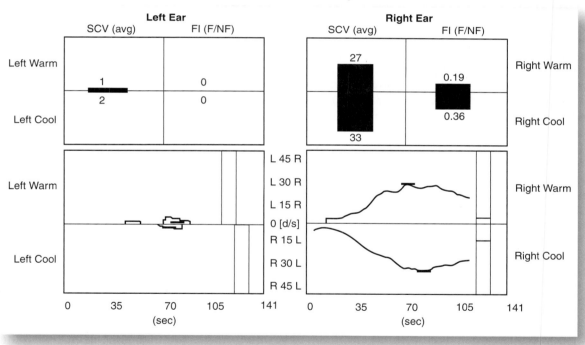

Caloric Summary

RVR (UW): Left Ear Response 91% weaker
DP: Left beating response 9% stronger
Total Eye Speed: 63 (deg/sec)
Spontaneous Nystagmus: None

Figure 18-1. Caloric Summary for Case 1. Summary plot for bithermal caloric results demonstrating a 91% left caloric weakness. The left-hand column shows the SCEV for the left ear to warm and cool irrigations, respectively, while the right-hand column displays the same data for the right ear. Data are supplied in numeric and graphic form. Finally, the summary at the bottom of the figure specifies the caloric asymmetry and directional preponderance as a percentage as well as the total eye speed for all four calorics. No spontaneous nystagmus was present.

Case 2

A thirty-seven-year old woman with cystic fibrosis was seen for evaluation of dizziness following a recent three-week course of IV tobramycin and ceftazidime. She has had a long, complicated history of cystic fibrosis that included multiple prior courses of IV tobramycin in conjunction with other antibiotics, as well as frequent use of nebulized tobramycin. At some point during the most recent course of tobramycin, which the patient reported was given at a higher dose than usual, she began to experience the sensation of rocking and general instability coupled with vague visual disturbances. She reported that the symptoms waxed and waned since their onset, but she had not felt normal at any time. The patient reported a long-standing history of bilateral tinnitus and aural fullness, but did not notice any change in either symptom. Audiological testing was completed and revealed normal hearing sensitivity and excellent word recognition ability bilaterally. Tympanograms and acoustic reflexes were also normal. VNG testing revealed persistent left-beating spontaneous nystagmus, significant post head-shaking nystagmus, and a 55% right caloric weakness (see Figure 18-2). Oculomotor tests yielded normal results. Rotational testing revealed normal phase, gain, and symmetry at all sinusoidal frequencies tested, as well as normal time constants for rotational step testing. Dynamic visual acuity was borderline normal, with the patient dropping two lines on the Snellen chart with head rotation. **Clinical Test of Sensory Integration and Balance (CTSIB)** revealed normal postural control.

Overall, then, the results suggest right peripheral vestibular system paresis in a partially uncompensated state physiologically and a compensated state functionally (for maintenance of stance). Given the timing of the onset of symptoms, the vestibular system paresis is presumed to be secondary to aminoglycoside toxicity. Despite the high level of suspicion regarding the cause, an MRI was completed to rule out the presence of an acoustic neuroma, which yielded normal results. Unfortunately, at no time prior to the symptom onset was the patient involved in an audiologic monitoring program. Rather, she reported that she had been advised to listen to her tinnitus and to alert her physicians in the event that she noticed a change. It is noteworthy that the patient said that the busyness of taking care of her three children prevented her from focusing attention on any of her symptoms.

Case 3

A 33-year-old woman was seen for evaluation during her most recent hospital stay. She reported that she had felt dizzy and unsteady for over a month. She described the dizziness as the perception that things in her environment seem to be off kilter. With additional questioning, the symptoms she described are consistent with oscillopsia. She also reported that she was unable to walk without touching something. Her previous medical history is complicated and significant for multiple pulmonary issues, primary hyperparathyroidism, hemoptysis, right knee avascular necrosis secondary to steroid use, arthritis, anxiety disorder, hypertension, and allergic rhinitis. At the time of testing, she was being treated with IV gentamicin, zosyn, and vancomycin for treatment of recurrent pneumonia. She reported multiple prior courses of IV gentamicin. Rotational testing revealed significant gain reductions at 0.01–0.32 Hz (see Figure 18-3). Phase and symmetry data were not calculated due to the severity of the gain reductions that were noted. In addition, no response was present during rotational step testing for either clockwise or counterclockwise steps (see Figure 18-4). Oculomotor testing revealed normal findings for lateral and vertical stationary gaze. Formal saccade testing using individual eye recordings revealed hypometric and slow saccades. Phase lags were also noted during pursuit tracking of sinusoidal velocity tracking presentations. Formal dynamic visual acuity testing was not completed because the patient was unable to read

Caloric Summary

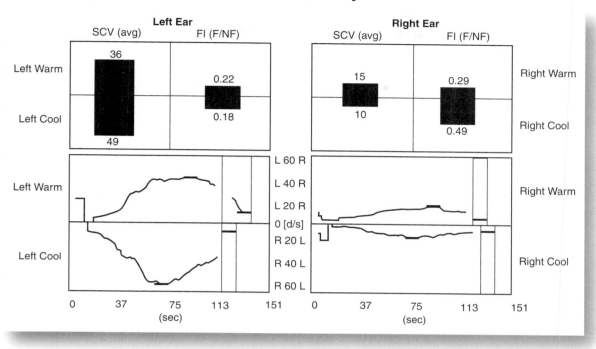

Figure 18-2. Caloric Summary for Case 2: Summary plot for bithermal caloric results demonstrating a 55% right caloric weakness. The left-hand column shows the SCEV for the left ear to warm and cool irrigations, respectively, while the right-hand column displays the same data for the right ear. Data are supplied in numeric and graphic form. Finally, the summary at the bottom of the figure specifies the caloric asymmetry and directional preponderance as a percentage as well as the total eye speed for all four calorics. The spontaneous nystagmus that is noted represents the 1 deg/sec left-beating precaloric nystagmus that was present. As indicated, the summary data are corrected for the presence of precaloric nystagmus.

even the largest line on the Snellen chart with head rotation.

Overall the findings suggest profound bilateral vestibular system paresis. It is noteworthy that in addition to the IV antibiotics mentioned above, the patient was on multiple CNS suppressant medications including methadone, which could have been contributing factors to her profound bilateral weakness in addition to her abnormal performance on oculomotor testing. Even if the findings are partially due to those medications, however, it is important to consider the fact that abnormal oculomotor control, regardless of the cause, can have a negative impact on the patient's ability to compensate from the loss of vestibular system function. Furthermore, bilateral vestibular system paresis—whether a permanent result of ototoxicity, a temporary condition that is caused by medications that suppress function, or a combination of the two—results in symptoms, including

VOR Summary

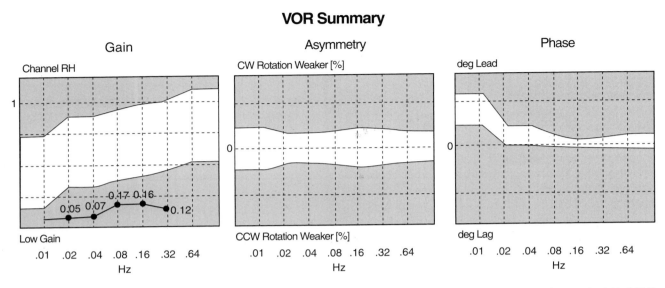

Figure 18-3. Rotational Chair VOR Summary for Case 3. Summary plot of gain, asymmetry, and phase data for sinusoidal frequencies 0.01–0.32 Hz. The gain values that are noted in the left-hand plot are all well below the normal range. No responses are indicated in the asymmetry and phase plots because those data are not calculated for gains less than 0.2. The highest gain value that was noted is 0.17 at 0.08 Hz.

oscillopsia and unsteadiness, that have a profound negative impact on the patient's quality of life.

As suggested by Calder and Jacobson (2000), vestibular rehabilitation is an essential component in the management of patients with bilateral vestibular loss and rapid initiation of a therapy program has a positive impact on outcome. This patient immediately began gaze stabilization exercises at home; and at the time of her follow-up at two weeks, there was a noticeable improvement in her oscillopsia. She was also able to shift from the use of a walker to a cane. While it is unlikely that she will ever be able to resume all of her previous activities, without additional exposure to ototoxic medications, with therapy, she will be able to improve the quality of her life substantially and to resume many normal activities. Unfortunately, as is often the case with patients being given ototoxic medications, despite the fact that she repeatedly mentioned her symptoms to the physicians involved in her care, they discounted them. In fact, one note mentioned the possibility that they were entirely psychologically based. At no point over the course of more than a month was the patient referred for evaluation of vestibular system function.

Case 4

A nineteen-year-old woman with cystic fibrosis was seen for evaluation of a two-month history of unsteadiness and dizziness. The patient began to feel a constant sense of unsteadiness while receiving IV gentamicin for treatment of an infection secondary to her cystic fibrosis. She also reported a recent onset of episodic motion-provoked vertigo, the onset of which followed the cessation of treatment. Previous additional medical history is significant for a "lazy" left eye and prior exposure to potentially ototoxic medications. The patient denied tinnitus, aural fullness, hearing loss, previous middle ear pathology, and otologic surgery. Audiological testing was completed and revealed normal hearing sensitivity and excellent

RVS Summary

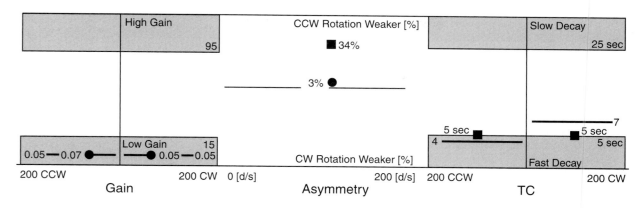

Figure 18-4. Rotational Step Summary for Case 3. Summary plots of the gain and time constant data for clockwise and counterclockwise rotational steps. The left-hand plot represents the gain values, which approximate zero for all four steps. The right-hand plot represents the time constant for each of the four steps. Numbers less than 10 seconds are considered to be abnormal. However, in the presence of minimal responses to chair acceleration, time constant values are not meaningful.

word recognition ability bilaterally. Acoustic immittance testing also yielded normal results. VNG testing revealed significant oblique right and up-beating positional and post head-shaking nystagmus, as well a mild bilateral caloric weakness with a significant (36%) relative left weakness (see Figure 18-5).

Oculomotor test results revealed the presence of disconjugate eye movements consistent with the "lazy eye" as reported by the patient, but were otherwise normal. Rotational testing revealed increased phase leads at 0.01–0.08 Hz and significant left greater than right slow component velocity asymmetries at 0.01–0.04 Hz. Response gain was normal at all test frequencies, as were the time constants in rotational step testing (see Figure 18-6).

The overall findings, then, suggest a mild bilateral peripheral vestibular system paresis with a relative left

weakness that is in a partially uncompensated status physiologically. An assessment of balance and gait was performed by a physical therapist, which revealed moderately increased postural sway with eyes closed and mild unsteadiness when walking with reciprocal head movement. The therapist noted that from a functional perspective, the subject's presentation was more like that seen with a unilateral peripheral vestibular loss rather than a bilateral loss, which is most likely due to the fact that the loss in the stronger (right ear) was mild. Her response gains in rotational testing were normal, suggesting preserved function in the frequencies that are most relevant to head movements associated with the activities of daily life. The patient was given a home therapy program consisting of habituation and gaze stabilization/VOR exercises, and her potential for functional recovery was reported to be excellent.

SUMMARY

Vestibular ototoxicity is a complex problem for health care professionals. Because the clinical presentation of vestibular toxicity is highly variable, the symptoms of toxicity are frequently ignored or are attributed to

other factors. Furthermore, there is no generally accepted protocol for monitoring vestibular function during exposure to potentially ototoxic agents. Ideally, adequate monitoring would include determination of baseline vestibular function prior to the initiation of treatment, as well as sequential testing

Caloric Summary

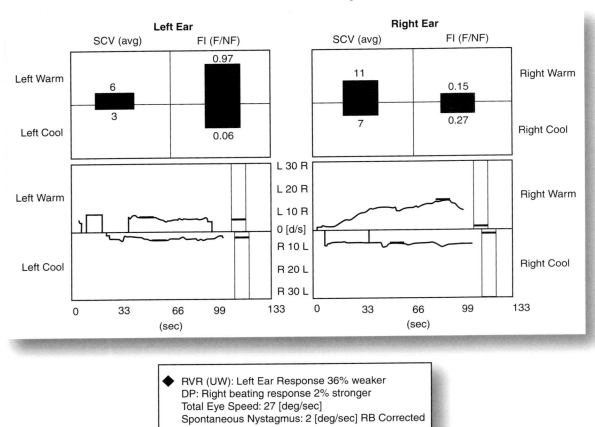

Figure 18-5. Caloric Summary for Case 4. Summary plot for bithermal caloric results demonstrating a 36% relative left caloric weakness with slightly weak responses noted in the better ear as well. The left-hand column shows the SCEV for the left ear to warm and cool irrigations, respectively, while the right-hand column displays the same data for the right ear. Data are supplied in numeric and graphic form. Finally, the summary at the bottom of the figure specifies the caloric asymmetry and directional preponderance as a percentage, as well as the total eye speed for all four calorics. The spontaneous nystagmus that is noted represents the 2 deg/sec right-beating precaloric nystagmus that was present. As indicated, the summary data are corrected for the presence of precaloric nystagmus.

throughout and following termination of therapy. Because it is not yet clear which tests are most sensitive to the early identification of vestibular toxicity, the monitoring program should utilize a test battery approach and tests should be conducted frequently. Clearly, monitoring changes in dynamic visual acuity is essential. While is it also important to evaluate changes in auditory function as a part of a monitoring protocol, it is clear from the evidence presented to date that vestibular toxicity often occurs in the absence of any clinical evidence of change in auditory status. For that reason, merely monitoring hearing during treatment with potentially ototoxic medications is inappropriate.

Table 18-1 provides a summary of the bedside and laboratory test findings that are most typically

VOR Summary

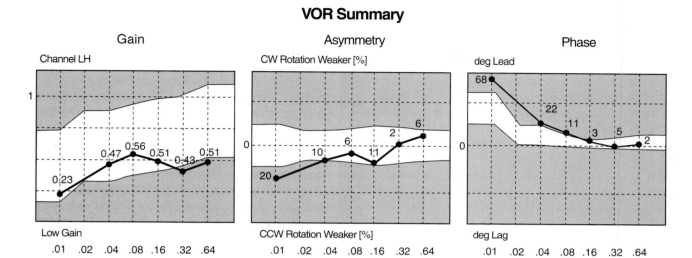

Figure 18-6.   Rotational Chair VOR Summary for Case 4. Summary plot of gain, asymmetry, and phase data for sinusoidal frequencies 0.01–0.64 Hz. The gain values that are noted in the left-hand plot are all normal or borderline normal, suggesting preserved vestibular function in the sinusoidal frequency range tested. The presence of significant left greater than right asymmetries is consistent with the relative left weakness that was noted in caloric testing. Increased phase leads at 0.01–0.08 Hz that are noted in the right-hand plot support the presence of peripheral vestibular system involvement.

Table 18-1.   Comparative Test Results

This table summarizes the typical findings for bilateral and unilateral vestibular loss. The left-hand column lists the bedside and laboratory test results that are most consistent with an uncompensated bilateral peripheral vestibular system paresis, while the right-hand column represents the findings that are most consistent with an uncompensated unilateral vestibular system loss. In the event of a bilateral paresis with a significant asymmetry as noted in Case 4, the results obtained would most likely represent some combination of findings from each column. With compensation secondary to formal therapy or informal recovery, improved outcomes would be expected across many of the tests.

Bilateral Vestibular Paresis	Unilateral Vestibular Paresis
No post head-shaking nystagmus	Significant post head-shaking nystagmus
Bilaterally positive head thrust	Positive head thrust toward impaired ear
Abnormal dynamic visual acuity	Normal/abnormal dynamic visual acuity
Abnormal gait and standing balance	Abnormal gait with reciprocal head movement
Bilaterally weak/absent caloric responses	Significant caloric asymmetry
Low response gains to rotational tests	Normal response gains to rotational tests
Increased phase leads (if calculated)/ no significant asymmetries (if calculated)	Increased phase leads/significant asymmetries possible
Falls in Conditions 5, 6 in CDP	Increased sway in Conditions 5, 6 in CDP
Normal/abnormal hearing sensitivity	Normal/abnormal hearing sensitivity
High self-perceived handicap/disability	Moderate self-perceived handicap/disability

associated with bilateral and unilateral vestibular system paresis. As was evident from the cases presented and from the data that were discussed from the recent literature, systemic use of ototoxic agents can result in varying degrees of loss affecting one or both ears. It appears as though there is no safe level of aminoglycoside dose and that maintaining serum levels within recommended ranges does not prevent damage to the vestibular system. The symptoms associated with vestibular loss are devastating; and although therapy results in improved functional status, the lives of affected individuals are permanently altered. Audiologists and other health care professionals must be vigilant in facilitating the ongoing assessment of vestibular and auditory system status in all patients for whom potentially ototoxic agents are prescribed.

REFERENCES

Black, F. O., Gianna-Poulin, C., & Pesznecker, S. C. (2001). Recovery from vestibular ototoxicity. *Otology and Neurotology, 22,* 662–671.

Black, F. O., Pesznecker, S., & Stallings, V. (2004). Permanent gentamicin vestibulotoxicity. *Otology and Neurotology, 25,* 559–569.

Calder, J. H., & Jacobson, G. P. (2000). Acquired bilateral peripheral vestibular system impairment: Rehabilitative options and potential outcomes. *Journal of the American Academy of Audiology, 11,* 514–521.

Desmond, A. L. (2004). *Vestibular Function: Evaluation and Treatment* (pp. 45–62). New York: Thieme.

Dhanireddy, S., Liles, W. C., & Gates, G. A. (2005). Vestibular toxic effects induced by once-daily aminoglycoside therapy. *Archives of Otolaryngology Head and Neck Surgery, 131,* 46–48.

Furman, J. M., Wall, C. III, & Kamerer, D. B. (1988). Alternate and simultaneous bithermal caloric testing: A comparison. *Annals of Otology, Rhinology, and Laryngology, 97,* 359.

Halmagyi, G. M., & Curthoys, I. S. (1988). A clinical sign of canal paresis. *Archives of Neurology, 45,* 737–739.

Jacobson, G. P., & Calder, J. H. (2000). Self-perceived balance disability/handicap in the presence of bilateral peripheral vestibular system impairment. *Journal of the American Academy of Audiology, 11,* 76–82.

Jacobson, G. P., & Newman, C. W. (1990). The development of the Dizziness Handicap Inventory (DHI). *Archives of Otolaryngology Head and Neck Surgery, 116,* 424–427.

J. C. (1952). Living without a balance mechanism. *New England Journal of Medicine, 246,* 458–460.

Kisilevsky, V. E., Tomlinson, R. D., Ranalli, P. J., & Prepageran, N. (2004). Monitoring vestibular ototoxicity. In P. S. Roland & J. A. Rutka (Eds.), *Ototoxicity* (pp. 161–169). London: BC Decker Inc.

Minor, L. B. (1998). Gentamicin-induced bilateral vestibular hypofunction. *Journal of the American Medical Association, 279,* 541–544.

Newman, C. W., & Jacobson, G. P. (1993). Application of self-report scales in balance function testing, handicap assessment and management. *Seminars in Hearing, 14,* 363–376.

Newman, C. W., & Jacobson, G. P. (1993). Assessing balance handicap. In G. P. Jacobson, C. W. Newman, & J. Kartush (Eds.), *Handbook of Balance Function Testing* (pp. 380–391). Chicago: Mosby-Yearbook.

Zee, D. S., & Fletcher, W. A. (1996). Bedside examination. In R. W. Baloh & G. M. Halmagyi (Eds.), *Disorders of the Vestibular System* (pp. 178–190). New York: Oxford University Press.

CHAPTER

19

Otoprotective Agents

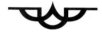

Kathleen C. M. Campbell, PhD
Professor & Director of Audiology Research

Leonard P. Rybak, MD, PhD
Professor of Otolaryngology
Southern Illinois University School of Medicine
Springfield, IL

INTRODUCTION

Currently, no otoprotective agents are FDA approved, but several agents are in or approaching clinical trials. In the future, the audiologist may have the opportunity not only to monitor ototoxic- or noise-induced hearing loss as it occurs, but also to work with the patient's physician in deciding when an otoprotective agent may be advisable. It is also possible that otoprotective agents for platinum-based chemotherapeutic- and aminoglycoside-induced hearing loss will be so safe and effective that they will be routinely administered and that ototoxic hearing loss from those two drugs will no longer be an audiologic clinical concern. Perhaps more likely is the possibility that those agents will not fully protect all patients, depending on dosing and agent, so audiologic monitoring will still be required. It is also possible that due to cost or other factors, otoprotective agents, at least in some patients, will only be employed once an initial ototoxic threshold shift has been discovered. Only clinical trials and ongoing clinical studies will elucidate the best approach.

For noise-induced hearing loss, it is unlikely that the otoprotective agents under current study will fully protect against all types of noise exposures in all situations. Pharmacologic otoprotective and rescue agents are being designed to augment, not supplant, measures to reduce noise exposure at the source and through use of physical hearing protectors such as muffs or earplugs. Even so, at high noise exposure levels, mechanical as well as oxidative damage to the cochlea can occur. Further, in some situations, individuals may be exposed to a combination of solvents and noise exposure in the work environment. Some workers may not want to take a protective agent on an ongoing basis for chronic or repeated noise exposure. Instead, they may use a protective or rescue agent only when a shift in hearing threshold is noted.

Some audiologists may choose to focus their research on otoprotective agents. For that purpose, they will generally need to expand their course work to emphasize chemistry and pharmacology. Multidisciplinary research is needed to improve patient care. Other audiologists may be involved in translational research, running clinical trials of new otoprotective agents.

In the not-to-distant future, clinical audiologists may also be involved with otoprotective agents by monitoring the hearing of patients exposed to ototoxic drugs and/or noise and determining whether a protective agent is needed and, if so, whether it is adequately protecting hearing. If a protective agent is being used and is not fully protecting hearing, the audiologist may then work with the physician in altering the dose or changing the otoprotective agent. Eventually, combinations of otoprotective agents may also be used, just as combinations of chemotherapeutic agents are used today. Consequently, all audiologists should have some knowledge of otoprotective agents to facilitate their communication with the pharmacist, physician, and patient in preserving hearing. Preventing hearing loss is always preferable to treating it.

However, the audiologist must be cautious in recommending any therapy that is not approved by the Food and Drug Administration (FDA) and, therefore, does not have the FDA-required extensive safety and efficacy testing through clinical trials. Some agents that initially looked promising were later found to have side effects of their own or were found to interfere with the therapeutic efficacy of the treatment drug (e.g., cisplatin). Other pharmacologic agents may be relatively safe as nutritional supplements, but have marginal or questionable clinical efficacy as otoprotective agents. Because nutritional supplements are not regulated by the FDA, claims should be considered with caution. Before recommending them to patients, the audiologist should carefully read published peer-reviewed efficacy data in humans. If those studies are not available, it is difficult to justify recommending the agent. Although some purported protective agents may be relatively safe, patients' sometimes limited financial resources may be wasted or patients may have an unwarranted sense of safety when using supplements with limited efficacy. The risk/benefit ratio must always be considered, as should spending money for treatments with little efficacy.

MECHANISMS OF OTOPROTECTIVE AGENTS

Throughout this text, various mechanisms of toxicity and cell death have been discussed. A variety of otoprotective agents have been used to counteract those mechanisms. Sometimes the protective agents are investigated to elucidate mechanisms, rather than to develop a clinical agent. Some protective agents may never be safe enough for general clinical use, but provide valuable insights into how drugs or noise damage the auditory system. Other therapies, such as gene therapy, provide insights into the mechanisms underlying ototoxic damage and may also underlie useful genetic therapies in the future. However gene therapies will probably not be in clinical trials or in use in the next few years. Other agents are being used in or are approaching clinical trials. While those agents can also elucidate mechanisms, they show promise for clinical use, perhaps within the next decade.

Many agents being studied as potential otoprotective agents fall under the general category of antioxidants. Generally, antioxidants work by detoxifying free radicals. However antioxidants may work in a number of ways. Some antioxidants may act by reducing the formation of free radicals. The goal is not to eliminate all free radicals because some free radical formation is essential for normal physiologic function. Rather, the goal is to keep the body's oxidative system in balance because excessive free radical formation can be damaging.

Agents may act as direct or indirect antioxidants or, in some cases, both. Direct antioxidants, such as free radical scavengers, may detoxify free radicals by donating an electron to stabilize the outer shell of an atom or group of atoms with an unpaired electron in its outer shell. Indirect antioxidants may act by increasing levels of the body's endogenous antioxidant systems, such as the enzymes superoxide dismutase (SOD) and catalase (CAT). Glutathione (GSH) prodrugs are another form of indirect antioxidant. Rather than directly donating an electron to detoxify a free radical, they act by increasing the level of GSH, one of the body's most important endogenous antioxidant systems. The GSH prodrug may provide the substrate for the body to form more GSH in response to oxidative stress. However, other drugs may work by keeping the GSH in a reduced rather than oxidized state so the reduced GSH can then donate electrons and detoxify free radicals. Some agents may mimic or enhance the levels of the enzymes glutathione peroxidase (GSHpx), which is necessary for reduced GSH to donate its electron to detoxify a free radical and be converted to oxidized glutathione (GSSG). Other agents may work by enhancing the enzyme glutathione reductase (GR), which converts GSSG back to GSH so it can once again donate an electron, or by enhancing glutathione-S-transferase (GST), which acts by binding the GSH to the atoms to be detoxified. Iron chelators may also reduce oxidative stress in some cases. Iron chelators bind to iron. Because iron has been found to facilitate aminoglycosides' ability to generate free radicals, iron chelators may reduce that reaction.

Other agents may act by blocking cell death pathways. For example, some ototoxins may activate the c-Jun-terminal protein kinase (JNK) pathway, which converts precursors to gene transcription factors via phosphorylation. JNK activation is one of several often interconnecting pathways that can lead to cell death. JNK inhibitors can sometimes reduce cell death induced by certain ototoxins. Similarly, a number of caspases are involved in apoptotic cell death. Caspases can cleave other proteins, which can lead to apoptotic cell death. Some protective agents may act by inhibiting caspases, thus preventing cell death. However, it would not be desirable to inhibit all apoptotic cell death in the body. Failure of apoptosis could lead to cancer or autoimmune disease. As in controlling free radicals, the idea is not to eliminate all free radicals or to eliminate all apoptosis, but rather to keep the physiologic system in balance to prevent damage to normal tissues.

N-methyl-D-aspartate (NMDA) receptor antagonists limit the binding of glutamate, the primary excitatory neurotransmitter in the auditory system. The NMDA receptor is a specific type of glutamate receptor. While glutamate excitation is essential for the function of the auditory system, excessive glutamate levels may cause excitotoxicity and be damaging to cells.

Neurotrophins, molecules that encourage nervous tissue survival, have also been tested as otoprotectants.

Neurotrophic factors prohibit or inhibit neurons from entering apoptosis. The neurotrophins include nerve growth factor (NGF), brain-derived neurotrophic factor (BDNF), neurotrophin 3 (NT-3), and neurotrophin 4 (NT-4).

However, many times a single agent has multiple effects. For example, some of the neurotrophins also have antioxidant properties that augment or account for their protective action. Some antioxidants are both direct and indirect antioxidants. Even for drugs that have been on the market for a long time, such as aspirin, scientists are discovering new information about their mechanisms of action. Thus, scientists frequently discuss "putative mechanisms of action."

Genetic studies including gene therapies are an interesting area of ototoxicity research. For example, the mitochondrial A1555G mutation renders some humans highly susceptible to aminoglycoside ototoxicity. In the future, doctors may test for certain genetic profiles before administering certain medications. At some point, doctors may also be able to correct certain genetic defects; but otoprotective agents are closer on the horizon. Pharmacogenomics, the study of drug and genetic interactions, is also a growing area of research. At some point, each patient may have a genetic profile in each medical chart and drug therapies will be chosen accordingly to maximize efficacy and minimize side effects, such as ototoxicity.

Some genetic studies explore animal models that over- or underproduce certain enzymes or alter other factors that can elucidate mechanisms of ototoxicity but may not lead directly to new therapies. However, new information is being obtained all the time although scientists don't always know exactly where it will lead. Albert Einstein was once asked the value of new basic science research; in reply, he asked, "What is the value of an infant?"

PROTECTIVE AGENTS FOR AMINOGLYCOSIDE OTOTOXICITY

Aminoglycoside ototoxicity has been recognized for decades, but it is only in the last decade that otoprotective agents have appeared truly promising. The authors have been working with D-methionine

(D-met) for over a decade. To their knowledge, no otoprotective agent other than D-met is patented, is licensed, and is approaching FDA-approved clinical trials for protection against aminoglycoside-induced ototoxicity in the next few years. However, in the world of drug development, agents are sometimes developed with little or no public disclosure until they are close to being market-ready. Thus, other agents may be in the development or clinical trials stages.

However, thus far, D-met, which can be given by injection or by mouth, is one of the most promising agents to protect against aminoglycoside-induced ototoxicity. For example, Sha and Schacht (2000) administered twice daily injections of 200 mg/kg D-met 7 hours apart in guinea pigs administered 120 mg/kg/day gentamicin. Gentamicin-induced threshold shifts were reduced from approximately 60 dB SPL to 20 dB SPL at 18 kHz and from 50 dB SPL to 30 dB SPL at 9 kHz. In that same study, histidine, another antioxidant, provided substantially less otoprotection. Sha and Schacht also tested D-met, using once daily instead of twice daily 200 mg/kg D-met dosing prior to the gentamicin; they found less, although significant, protection. Dr. Campbell's lab had earlier tested 300 mg/kg D-met prior to 200 mg/kg/day for 28 days and also found partial, but not complete, otoprotection. Thus, it appears that D-met is effective against the ototoxicity of at least two of the aminoglycosides, but multiple daily dosing of D-met may further enhance protection. More research is needed to test D-met dosing strategies and otoprotection for other aminoglycosides such as kanamycin and tobramycin. In the authors' studies thus far, D-met does not appear to interfere with the antimicrobial action of aminoglycosides (Herr et al., 2001) and does not alter serum levels of gentamicin (Sha & Schacht, 2000); but the authors plan to expand their studies further.

D-met has been found to be protective against cisplatin (CDDP)-induced and noise- induced hearing loss, as well as aminoglycoside-induced ototoxicity. An oxidative mechanism could explain why D-met protects against those ototoxins because free radical formation appears to be a common mechanism underlying all three toxicities (Yamane et al., 1995; Kopke et al., 1997; Ohlemiller & Dugan, 1999; Sha & Schacht, 2000). Methionine is reversibly oxidized and serves as a free radical scavenger (Vogt, 1995). Methionine's free radical scavenging ability could explain why it is protective against multiple types of cochlear toxins.

Methionine may also act as an indirect antioxidant by increasing intracellular reduced GSH (Lu, 1998) and particularly mitochondrial GSH (Fernandez-Checa et al., 1998). Although aminoglycosides do not alter cochlear GSH levels (Lauterman et al., 1997), if D-met administration increases GSH or the GSH/GSSG ratio in the presence of aminoglycosides, that action could be protective. For aminoglycosides, D-met appears to protect against ototoxicity primarily as a direct free radical scavenger, but further research is needed to fully understand the mechanisms of protection.

However, many other agents have been tested as aminoglycoside otoprotectants. Systemic lipoic acid administration, another antioxidant, reduced amikacin-induced ototoxicity, as measured by action potential threshold shifts in pigmented guinea pigs (Conlon et al., 1999). However, Sinswat et al. (2000) reported that lipoic acid enhanced weight loss and animal mortality in a gentamicin guinea pig model. Round window administration of lipoic acid slowed the rate of deterioration of neomycin-induced ototoxicity, but significant cochlear damage still occurred (Conlon & Smith, 2000). Additionally, an otoprotective agent that can be delivered by mouth or by injection will probably receive faster clinical acceptance than an agent that requires direct round window delivery.

Several investigators have found that iron chelators such as deferoxamine and 2,3-dihydroxybenzoate can reduce aminoglycoside-induced ototoxicity and free radical formation (Song et al., 1998; Conlon et al., 1998; Sha & Schacht, 2000; Sinswat et al., 2000; Dehne et al., 2002). While the studies are valuable in elucidating mechanisms, those iron chelators can also be ototoxic (Kanno et al., 1995; Ryals et al., 1997). Additionally, iron chelators may not be advisable for chronic administration, particularly in certain patient populations, such as women of child-bearing age. Further, the agents have not yet been tested to determine if they interfere with the antimicrobial activity of aminoglycoside antibiotics.

Salicylate, which may act as an antioxidant and as an iron chelator in tissues undergoing oxidative stress, can reduce gentamicin-induced outer hair cell (OHC) loss and auditory brainstem response (ABR) threshold shift without interfering with antimicrobial efficacy (Sha & Schacht, 1999). Clinical trials have been conducted in China and showed that 3 grams of aspirin per day reduced the incidence of ototoxicity (as defined as threshold shifts of 15 dB or more at 6 and 8 kHz) from 13% in the control group to 3% in the aspirin treated group (Schacht et al 2006). It is unclear whether salicylate will ever obtain widespread clinical acceptance as an otoprotective agent considering its possible gastrointestinal and hematologic effects, its role as an ototoxin at high dosing levels, and the fact that it cannot be used in children because of the possibility of Reye's syndrome. Nonetheless, it is an intriguing, well-known, and inexpensive compound.

CEP-1347 and D-JNKI-1, which block JNK pathway activation (and thus may block caspase activation), protected against neomycin-induced ototoxicity in *in vitro* and *in vivo* experiments (Pirvola et al., 2000; Wang et al., 2003). However, it has not been determined whether those compounds interfere with the antimicrobial action of aminoglycoside antibiotics or what their efficacy is in an *in vivo* model.

Caspase inhibitors such as z- VAD-fmk can reduce gentamicin-induced hair cell loss from avian basilar papillae *in vitro* (Cheng et al., 2002); however, the long-term safety of systemic administration of general caspase inhibitors has not been established, nor has it been determined whether they interfere with the antimicrobial action of aminoglycosides. Although the studies provide valuable information in establishing the mechanisms of aminoglycoside-induced ototoxicity, they may not directly lead to clinical therapies.

Other investigators have explored the use of neurotrophins as protective agents against aminoglycoside-induced ototoxicity with varying degrees of success. Zheng and Gao (1996) reported that neither neurotrophin 4/5, BDNF, nor NT-3 prevented gentamicin-induced hair cell loss in rat cochlear explants. Duan et al. (2000) reported that NT-3, when administered to guinea pigs pretreated with MK-801, an NMDA antagonist, prevented amikacin-induced

OHC loss and reduced hearing loss, but that MK-801 pretreatment alone provided only a partial protection of hearing. Ernfors et al. (1996) reported that NT-3 significantly reduced spiral ganglion cell loss in amikacin-exposed animals, but that hair cells could be identified in only one of the five animals. Spiral ganglion cell protection with NT-3 could not be explored in the Zheng and Gao 1996 study because their gentamicin model did not induce spiral ganglion cell loss even in the absence of a protective agent.

Gene therapies that were delivered directly into the cochlea (Kawamoto et al., 2004) or that utilized transgenic mice (Sha et al., 2001) have shown some promise in reducing aminoglycoside ototoxicity by increasing expression of CAT or SOD. Similarly, transgenic GDNF expression can reduce aminoglycoside-induced (Suzuki et al., 2000) or combined aminoglycoside- and loop diuretic-induced (Yagi et al., 1999) ototoxicity. Those studies hold promise for the future and support the oxidative stress theory for aminoglycoside-induced ototoxicity, but will probably not undergo clinical trials in the near future.

The hope is that in the future, many otoprotective agents for aminoglycoside ototoxicity will be FDA approved and available for clinical use. Certainly physicians and audiologists would welcome the option to have more than one otoprotective agent at their disposal when selecting patient therapies.

PROTECTIVE AGENTS FOR CDDP OTOTOXICITY

A variety of antioxidant compounds have been tested against CDDP ototoxicity. Several of them contain thiol (SH) groups and are effective protective agents against CDDP ototoxicity. The sulfur in these compounds has a high affinity for platinum. For example, D-met may react directly with the hydrated form of CDDP; D-met's sulfur groups may bind to the CDDP, thus protecting sulfur-containing enzymes and proteins (Melvik & Pettersen, 1987; Jones & Basinger, 1989; Miller & House, 1990; Jones et al., 1991a, 1991b). Thiol-containing compounds can scavenge free radicals. Those compounds include sodium thiosulfate, diethyldithiocarbamate, D- or L-methionine, methylthiobenzoic acid, lipoic acid, N-acetylcysteine (NAC),

tiopronin, GSH ester, and amifostine (Rybak & Whitworth, 2005).

To date, the only protective agent that has been successful in animal experiments and has been used in human trials is amifostine. This drug is also used as a protectant against radiation injury. Although amifostine was effective in preventing CDDP toxicity to the hamster cochlea, the central auditory conduction times were prolonged on ABR testing, suggesting neurotoxicity (Church et al., 2004). Clinical trials have shown that it was not effective in preventing hearing loss in patients with metastatic melanoma treated with CDDP. Ototoxicity in those patients was unacceptable (Ekborn et al., 2004). No protection against CDDP ototoxicity was found in children with germ cell tumors who were treated with amifostine in combination with CDDP, etoposide, and bleomycin (Marina et al., 2005; Sastry & Kellie, 2005). Although sodium thiosulfate administered to guinea pigs by perfusion of the cochlea was effective in preventing CDDP ototoxicity (Wang et al., 2003), it is not likely that this highly invasive method would be used on patients. On the other hand, when sodium thiosulfate was applied to the round window membrane by a minipump, it did not protect against CDDP ototoxicity in guinea pigs (Wimmer et al., 2004).

NAC was found to be effective in protecting against CDDP ototoxicity when administered intravenously to rats (Dickey et al., 2004) or when injected into the middle ear cavity of guinea pigs (Choe et al., 2004). Both sodium thiosulfate and NAC may covalently bind to CDDP, thereby inactivating the drug (Dickey et al., 2005). They may also displace CDDP after it is bound to target molecules (Schweitzer, 1993). Similarly, coadministration of NAC and CDDP reduces the tumor-killing effects in two cancer cell lines (Wu et al., 2005).

D-met provides excellent protection against CDDP ototoxicity whether applied by injecting it intraperitoneally in rats (Campbell et al., 1996) or by placing a D-met solution on the round window membrane of chinchillas (Korver et al., 2002). D-met not only protected the cochlear hair cells, but also prevented damage to the stria vascularis of rats (Meech et al., 1998). D-met also prevented the depletion of antioxidant enzymes and the elevation of malondialdehyde that otherwise occurs in the cochlea of rats treated with CDDP (Campbell et al., 2003). It is interesting to note that radioactively labeled D-met was found to readily pass through the round window membrane into the cochlea of the rat. Not only did D-met enter the organ of Corti, it also intensely labeled the stria vascularis (Laurell et al., 2002). Other antioxidant agents shown to protect the cochlea against CDDP ototoxicity in animal experiments include vitamin E (alpha-tocopherol), either alone or in combination with tiopronin; aminoguanidine; sodium salicylate; and ebselen combined with allopurinol (Lynch et al., 2005; Rybak & Whitworth, 2005).

Drugs that interact with adenosine receptors, such as R-PIA, applied to the chinchilla round window membrane provide very good protection against CDDP ototoxicity. Hair cells were preserved and ABR threshold shifts were minimized in these animal studies (Whitworth et al., 2004). Previous studies had shown that those agents increase the activity of the antioxidant enzymes in the cochlea (Ford et al., 1997).

Neurotrophins such as NT-3 provide protection against CDDP-induced ototoxicity in aged mice. Animals treated with a herpes simplex virus vector expressing NT-3 had a reduced incidence of cell death in the spiral ganglion from CDDP compared with mice treated with a control virus (Bowers et al., 2002).

Several *in vitro* experiments with organ of Corti cultures have shown some interesting findings. Flunarizine cotreatment with CDDP provided complete protection against cell death in the cultured cells (So et al., 2005). Protection against CDDP ototoxicity was obtained using inhibitors of caspases in cochlear cultures (Liu et al., 1998) and in guinea pigs (Wang et al., 2004). The p53 inhibitor pifithrin-alpha applied to cultures of the organ of Corti exposed to CDDP prevented p53 expression and caspase activation and protected hair cells from damage (Zhang et al., 2003). However, it is not known whether caspase inhibitors and pifithrin-alpha are safe to use in patients.

The possible interference with the antitumor effects of CDDP by protective agents needs to be considered (Blakley et al., 2002). For example, sodium thiosulfate inhibits the antitumor effects of CDDP in a human squamous cell carcinoma line *in vitro* (Viallet et al., 2006). There appears to be no difference in protective effects for sodium thiosulfate against CDDP toxicity in normal cells compared to tumor cells (Dickey et al., 2005). However, when the administration of sodium thiosulfate after CDDP treatment is delayed in guinea pigs, ototoxicity is reduced and antitumor activity preserved (Muldoon et al., 2000).

Sodium butyrate is a histone deacetylase inhibitor that possesses anticancer activity. It is also classified as a neuroprotective agent. Treatment of guinea pigs with this drug before and after CDDP provided nearly complete protection against ototoxicity (Drottar et al., 2006). Since sodium butyrate has antitumor effects, perhaps it will not interfere with the therapeutic effect of CPPD. That possibility would need to be tested before using it in clinical trials.

The potential for interference with the antitumor effects of CDDP may also be avoided by administering the agent into the tympanic cavity or directly on the round window membrane. L-met applied to the round window membrane prevented CDDP ototoxicity but did not compromise the antitumor effectiveness in tumor-bearing rats (Li et al., 2001).

PROTECTIVE AGENTS FOR NOISE-INDUCED HEARING LOSS

Although no pharmacologic agent is FDA approved for the purpose of preventing noise-induced hearing loss, a wide variety of agents have been tested in animals to determine whether they can prevent temporary or permanent noise-induced hearing loss. As for aminoglycoside-induced and CDDP-induced hearing loss, most of those agents have been tested as protective agents and administered prior to noise exposure. Some agents also prevent permanent noise-induced hearing loss when they are first administered within hours or a few days after the noise exposure. Those agents are frequently referred to as rescue agents. They are not designed to provide hair cell regeneration in the presence of long-standing noise-induced hearing loss, however. They are designed to act before the cochlear damage is permanent.

The classes of putative otoprotective agents for noise-induced hearing loss overlap the putative otoprotective agents for aminoglycoside-induced and

CDDP-induced hearing loss, including direct and indirect antioxidants that include GSH prodrugs and antioxidant enzymes, cell death inhibitors, NMDA antagonists, and iron chelators. Additionally, glucocorticoids, growth factors, and magnesium have been studied. As discussed for otoprotection from aminoglycoside-induced and CDDP-induced ototoxicity, some of these agents, such as iron chelators, are interesting in elucidating mechanisms but may have toxicities of their own, thus limiting promise for clinical utility (Yamasoba et al., 1999). Other agents such as carbamathione, an NMDA antagonist, show some efficacy but less than other tested agents (Kopke et al., 2002.) Agents showing less protection in preclinical animal studies will probably not progress to clinical trials.

Currently, the pharmacologic agents closest to approaching or in clinical trials to provide protection or rescue from permanent noise-induced hearing loss are D-met, ebselen, and NAC. Because acetyl-L-carnitine (ALCAR) has also shown good efficacy in animal studies, it may also proceed to clinical trials in the future. All of those agents act as direct and/or indirect antioxidants. Further, all of them can be effectively delivered orally, which is particularly important for an otoprotective agent for noise exposure. While hospitalized patients receiving aminoglycoside antibiotics or CDDP chemotherapy may prefer an orally administered otoprotective agent, they also may be able to accept an agent delivered by injection. However, for protection or rescue from noise-induced hearing loss, acceptance of an agent that can be administered only parenterally seems unlikely.

Magnesium, a metal present in many foodstuffs, has already been tested in clinical trials with some significant protection noted against temporary and permanent noise-induced hearing loss (Attias et al., 1994, 2004). In animal studies, magnesium deficiency exacerbated noise-induced hearing loss (Gunther et al., 1989). But in soldiers, no significant correlation between noise-induced hearing loss and endogenous magnesium levels was found (Walden et al., 2000).

For protection from permanent noise-induced hearing loss in chinchillas, both D-met and ALCAR provided virtually complete protection from permanent threshold shift (< 10 dB ABR threshold shift in treated animals) and OHC loss (< 10% in treated animals) secondary to a 6-hour 105 dB HL 4 kHz octave band of noise. In that same study, carbamathione, an NMDA antagonist, provided poorer protection than D-met or ALCAR with OHC preservation, measuring only 30%–40% versus 60% in nonprotected controls (Kopke et al., 2002). NAC, in combination with salicylate, showed substantially less OHC preservation (50%–60%) (Kopke et al., 2000) for the same noise-exposure protocol when compared to D-met and ALCAR, which provided over 90% OHC preservation (Kopke et al., 2002). However in a study of impulse noise exposure (155 dB SPL for 150 repetitions), both NAC (without additional salicylate in this study) and ALCAR provided significant protection from permanent noise-induced hearing loss and OHC loss (Kopke et al., 2005).

Similarly, ebselen has been demonstrated to provide excellent protection from permanent noise-induced ABR threshold shift and OHC loss in both rats and guinea pigs (Pourbakht & Yamasoba, 2003; Lynch et al., 2004; Lynch & Kil, 2005), although direct comparisons with D-met, ALCAR, and NAC have not been performed within the same study. Further studies will be needed to compare the relative efficacy and of those various otoprotective agents.

In the future, the health care field may have not only single agents delivered to protect against noise induced hearing loss, but also combination or "cocktail" agents. Coleman et al. (2002) reported that preadministration of a combination of low-dose D-met and NAC markedly reduced permanent noise-induced ABR threshold shift in chinchillas and that the protection afforded by the D-met component alone was similar to the combined administration of D-met and NAC. However, when the NAC component was delivered alone, no protection was provided. Thus, for that particular combination of agents, D-met alone provided as much protection as the combination of D-met and NAC. However, further studies will be needed to determine if protection from noise-induced hearing loss can be optimized by combining a variety of otoprotective agents.

In some situations, noise-exposure may not always be anticipated in advance. For example, a person may attend an unexpectedly loud concert and notice tinnitus or temporary threshold shift afterward. A car airbag may deploy in a motor vehicle accident, causing noise-induced hearing loss. In some professions, such as the military or emergency services, sudden noise exposure from weapons or sirens may exceed safe noise exposure limits. In those instances, a protective agent may not always be given in advance, as the noise was not anticipated and many people do not want to ingest agents chronically just in case they are exposed to noise. In those cases, a rescue agent administered immediately after the noise exposure could be very helpful. In rats, D-met can be administered an hour after noise exposure cessation and still provide excellent protection from permanent noise-induced hearing loss (Campbell 2005). Similarly, a combination of salicylate and trolox, an analogue of vitamin E, delivered rescue from permanent noise-induced hearing loss in guinea pigs even when started 3 days after the noise exposure. Many other compounds need to be tested to determine whether they can provide rescue from noise-induced hearing loss. It is also unknown at this time how many of those compounds will proceed to clinical trials for that purpose.

However, there is hope of being able to prevent noise-induced hearing loss in many thousands of patients every year through protective or rescue agents. Although reduction of noise exposure and use of physical hearing protectors will always be advisable, the potential of augmenting those precautions with pharmacologic agents to reduce permanent hearing loss is an exciting one. Only clinical trials will resolve the safety and efficacy of those agents.

SUMMARY

Over the last few decades, a number of potential otoprotective agents have been investigated. Some agents protect against aminoglycoside-induced ototoxicity, others protect against the ototoxicity of CDDP and carboplatin, and still others protect against noise-induced hearing loss. Some agents can even protect against noise-induced hearing loss when first given after the noise exposure. Those agents are sometimes called rescue agents. The hope is that within the next decade, several otoprotective agents will be FDA approved for clinical use. Some otoprotective agents are near or already in clinical trials.

However, the study of otoprotective agents may have several purposes. In some cases, the agent being studied will probably not be suited for clinical use. It may have safety concerns for systemic use in humans, or it may require such high dosages to achieve efficacy that clinical use would be unrealistic. Nonetheless, the study of some of the agents can often elucidate the mechanisms of ototoxicity. By understanding the underlying mechanisms, the health care field increases its chances of successfully preventing or treating ototoxic hearing loss.

Otoprotective agents may work through a variety of mechanisms. Those mechanisms include working as direct or indirect antioxidants, working as iron chelators, blocking cell death pathways through caspase inhibitors or JNK inhibitors, limiting glutamate binding, encouraging nervous tissue survival with neurotrophins, and working to induce a variety of genetic manipulations. While not all of the mechanisms will lead directly to clinical otoprotective agents, they may help in the development of nonototoxic therapies or other related otoprotective agents.

For aminoglycoside-induced hearing loss a number of otoprotective agents have been investigated, including caspase inhibitors, JNK inhibitors, NMDA receptor antagonists, neurotrophins, and direct and indirect antioxidants. To the authors' knowledge, the only otoprotective agent currently approaching clinical trials for that purpose is D-met, which does not appear to inhibit the antimicrobial action of the aminoglycosides and may enhance it. Only clinical trials will fully determine its safety and efficacy.

A variety of genetic manipulations have also been investigated for their relationship to aminoglycoside-induced ototoxicity. In the more distant future, that information may lead to new therapies. It is also interesting that the A1555G genetic mutation, which has been discovered to predispose individuals to severe aminoglycoside-induced hearing loss, may eventually decrease the incidence of aminoglycoside-induced hearing loss by allowing patients to be genetically screened before receiving aminoglycosides. Currently, however, most patients need to start their antimicrobial therapy before genetic testing can be completed.

For CDDP-induced hearing loss, otoprotective agents also include cell death inhibitors, neuroprotective agents including neurotrophins, and direct and indirect antioxidants. Some otoprotective agents may also bind to the CDDP. Some of those agents are in or are approaching clinical trials for CDDP otoprotection, including delayed sodium thiosulfate and D-met. Again, the clinical trials process will determine whether those and other agents are suitable for widespread clinical use.

For prevention of permanent noise-induced hearing loss, several pharmacologic agents are in or approaching clinical trials. Protective agents are given prior to noise exposure and generally are continued after the noise exposure. Some agents, often called rescue agents, can be first initiated within hours or days after the noise exposure and still provide significant protection from permanent noise-induced hearing loss. The agents approaching or already being used in clinical trials include D-met, NAC, ebselen, and potentially ALCAR. Magnesium has already been tested in some clinical trials and demonstrated some significant otoprotection.

Currently, the FDA has not approved any agents for use as otoprotective agents. In the future, it appears probable that one or more otoprotective agents will be FDA approved for clinical use. When that happens, the role of the audiologist may change from simply monitoring for ototoxic change to working with the physician and patient to determine when an otoprotective agent may be appropriate and what its efficacy is. At that time, hearing loss may be preventable in many thousands of patients every year.

REFERENCES

Attias, J., Sapir, S., Bresloff, I., Reshef-Haran, I., & Ising, H. 2004. Reduction in noise-induced temporary threshold shift in humans following oral magnesium intake. *Clinical Otolaryngology 29*, 635–641.

Attias, J., Weisz, G., Almog, S., Shahar, A., Wiener, M., Joachims, Z., Netzer, A., Ising, H., Rebentisch, E., & Guenther, T. 1994. Oral magnesium intake reduces permanent hearing loss induced by noise exposure. *Am J Otolaryng, 15*(1), 26–32.

Blakley, B. W., Cohen, J. I., Doolittle, N. D., Muldoon, L. L., Campbell, K. C., Dickey, D. T., & Neuwelt, E. A. (2002). Strategies for prevention of toxicity caused by platinum-based chemotherapy: Review and summary of the annual meeting of the Blood-Brain Barrier Disruption Program, Gleneden Beach, Oregon, March 10, 2001. *Laryngoscope, 112*, 1997–2001.

Bobbin, R. P., Fallon, M., LeBlanc, C., & Baber, A. (1995). Evidence that glutathione is the unidentified amine (Unk 2.5) released by high potassium into cochlear fluids. *Hearing Research, 87*, 49–54.

Bowers, W. J., Chen, X., Guo, H., Frisina, D. R., Federoff, H. J., & Frisina, R. D. (2002). Neurotrophin-3 transduction attenuates cisplatin spiral ganglion neuron ototoxicity in the cochlea. *Mol Ther, 6*, 12–18.

Campbell, K. C. M., Larsen, D. L., Meech, R. P., Rybak, L. P., & Hughes, L. F. (2003a). Glutathione ester but not glutathione protects against cisplatin-induced ototoxicity in a rat model. *Journal of the American Academy of Audiology, 14*(3), 124–133.

Campbell, K. C. M., Meech, R. P., Jackson, R. L., Hughes, L. F., Rybak, L. P., Coleman, J. K. M., & Kopke, R. D. (2003b). Noise exposure alters cochlear oxidized and reduced glutathione levels as a function of noise exposure duration in the chinchilla [Abstract]. *Association for Research in Otolaryngology, 1296*.

Campbell, K. C. M. "Prevention of Noise- and Drug-Induced Hearing Loss with D-methionine" Presentation at International Symposium-Pharmacologic Strategies for Prevention and Treatment of Hearing Loss and Tinnitus" Niagara Falls, Canada October 12, 2005.

Campbell, K. C. M., Meech, R. P., Rybak, L. P., & Hughes, L. F. (1999). D-methionine protects against CDDP damage to the stria vascularis. *Hear Res, 138*, 13–28.

Campbell, K. C., Meech, R. P., Rybak, L. P, & Hughes L. F. (2003c). The Effect of D-methionine on cochlear oxidative state with and without CDDP administration: Mechanisms of otoprotection. *JAAA, 14*(3), 144–156.

Campbell, K. C. M., Rybak, L. P., Meech, R. P., & Hughes, L. (1996). D-methionine provides excellent protection from CDDP ototoxicity in the rat. *Hear Res, 102*, 90–98.

Cheng, A. G., Cunningham, L. L., & Ruble, E. W. (2002). Hair cell death in the avian basilar papilla: Characterization of the in vitro model and caspace activation. *JARO, 04,* 91–105.

Choe, W. T., Chinosornvatana, N., & Chang, K. W. (2004). Prevention of cisplatin ototoxicity using transtympanic N-acetylcysteine and lactate. *Otol Neurotol, 25,* 910–915.

Church, M. W., Blakley, B. W., Burgio, D. L., & Gupta, A. K. (2004). WR-2721 (amifostine) ameliorates cisplatin-induced hearing loss but causes neurotoxicity in hamsters. *J Assoc Res Otolaryngol, 5,* 227–237.

Coleman, J. K. M., Liu, J., Wood, K., & Kopke, R. D. (2002). Low dose methionine with N-Acetyl-Cysteine reduces noise-induced threshold shift in the chinchilla [Abstract]. *Association for Research in Otolaryngology,* 861.

Conlon, B., Perry, B., & Smith, D. (1998). Attenuation of neomycin ototoxicity by iron chelation. *Laryngoscope, 108,* 284–287.

Conlon, B. J., Aran, J. M., Erre, J. P., & Smith, D. W. (1999). Attenuation of aminoglycoside-induced cochlear damage by the metabolic antioxidant alpha-lipoic acid. *Hear Res, 128*(1–2), 40–44.

Conlon, B. J., & Smith, D. W. (2000). Topical aminoglycoside ototoxicity: Attempting to protect the cochlea. *Acta Otolaryngol, 120*(5), 596–599.

Dehne, N., Rauen, U., deGroot, H., & Lautermann, J. (2002). Involvement of the mitochondrial permeability transition in gentamicin ototoxicity. *Hear Res, 169,* 47–55.

Dickey, D. T., Muldoon, L. L., Kraemer, D. F., & Neuwelt, E. A. (2004). Protection against cisplatin ototoxicity by N-acetylcysteine in a rat model. *Hear Res, 193,* 25–30.

Dickey, D. T., Wu, Y. J., Muldoon, L. L., & Neuwelt, E. A. (2005). Protection against cisplatin-induced toxicities by N-acetylcysteine and sodium thiosulfate as assessed at the molecular, cellular and in vivo levels. *J Pharmacol Exp Ther, 314,* 1052–1058.

Drottar, M., Liberman, M. C., Ratan, R. R., & Roberson, D. W. (2006). The histone deacetylase inhibitor sodium butyrate protects against cisplatin-induced hearing loss in guinea pigs. *Laryngoscope, 116,* 292–296.

Duan, M., Agerman, K., Ernfors, P., & Canlon, B. (2000). Complementary roles of neurotrophin 3 and a N-methyl-D-aspartate antagonist in the protection of noise and aminoglycoside induced ototoxicity. *PNAS, 97*(13), 7597–7602.

Ekborn, A., Hansson, J., Ehrsson, H., Eksborg, S., Wallin, I., Wagenius, G., & Laurell, G. (2004). High dose cisplatin with amifostine: Ototoxicity and pharmacokinetics. *Laryngoscope, 114,* 1660–1667.

Ernfors, P., Duan, M. L., ElShamy, W., & Canlon, B. (1996). Protection of auditory neurons from aminoglycoside toxicity by neurotrophin-3. *Nature Medicine, 2*(4), 263–267.

Fernandez-Checa, J. C., Kaplowitz, N., Garcia-Ruiz, C., & Colell, A. (1998). Mitochondrial glutathione: Importance and transport. *Seminars in Liver Disease, 18*(4), 389–401.

Ford, M. S., Nie, Z., Whitworth, C., Rybak, L. P., & Ramkumar, V. (1997). Up-regulation of adenosine receptors in the chinchilla cochlea by cisplatin. *Hear Res, 111,* 143–152.

Ghibelli, L., Fanelli, C., Rotilio, G., Lafavia, E., Coppola, S., Colussi, C., Civitareale, P., & Ciriolo, M. R. (1998). Rescue of cells from apoptosis by inhibition of active GSH extrusion. *FASEB Journal, 12*(6), 479–486.

Gunther, T., Ising, H., & Joachims, Z. (1989). Biochemical mechanisms affecting susceptibility to noise-induced hearing loss. *American Journal of Otology, 10*(1), 36–41.

Herr, L., Koirala, J., Campbell, K., Starks, S. & Khardori, N. (2001). D-methionine does not interfere with antimicrobial effectiveness. Abstract of the Infectious Disease Society of America Conference in San Francisco, California, 457.

Hyde, G. E., & Rubel, E. W. (1995). Mitochondrial role in hair cell survival after injury. *Otolaryngology— Head & Neck Surgery, 113*(5), 530–540.

Jones, M. M., & Basinger, M. A. (1989). Thiol and thioester suppression of cis-platinum-induced nephrotoxicity in rats bearing the Walker 256 carcinosarcoma. *Anticancer Res, 9,* 1937–1942.

Jones, M. M., Basinger, M. A., & Holscher, M. A. (1991a). Relative effectiveness of some compounds for the control of CDDP-induced nephrotoxicity. *Toxicology, 68,* 227–247.

Jones, M. M., Basinger, M. A., & Holscher, M. A. (1991b). Thioether suppression of CDDP nephrotoxicity in the rat. *Anticancer Research, 11*, 449–454.

Kanno, H., Yamanobe, S., & Rybak, L. P. (1995). The ototoxicity of deferoxamine mesylate. *American Journal Otolaryngology, 16*, 148–152.

Kawamoto, K., Sha, S., Minoda, R., Izumikawa, M., Kuriyama, H., Schacht, J., & Rafael, Y. (2004). Antioxidant gene therapy can protect hearing in hair cells from ototoxicity. *Molecular Therapy, 9*(2), 173–181.

Kopke, R., Bielefeld, E., Liu, J., Zheng, J., Jackson, R., Henderson, D., & Coleman, J. (2005). Prevention of impulse noise-induced hearing loss with antioxidants. *Acta Oto-Laryngologica, 125*, 235–243.

Kopke, R. D., Coleman, J. K. M., Liu, J., Campbell, K. C. M., & Riffenburgh, R. H. (2002). Enhancing intrinsic cochlear stress defenses to reduce noise-induced hearing loss. *Laryngoscope, 112*, 1515–1532.

Kopke, R. D., Liu, W., Gabaizeadeh, R., Jacono, A., Feghali, J., Spray, D., Garcia, P., Steinman, H., Malgrange, B., Ruben, R., Rybak, L. P., & Van De Water, T. (1997). Use of organotypic cultures of Corti's organ to study the protective effects of antioxidant molecules on CDDP-induced damage of auditory hair cells. *Am J Otol, 18*, 559–571.

Kopke, R. D., Weisskopf, P. A., Boon, J. L., Jackson, R. L., Wester, D. C., Hoffer, M. E., Lambert, D. C., Charon, C. C., Ding, D. L., & McBride, D. (2000). Reduction of noise-induced hearing loss using L-NAC and salicylate in the chinchilla. *Hear Res, 149*, 138–146.

Korver, K. D., Rybak, L. P., Whitworth, C. A., & Campbell, K. C. M. (2002). Round window application of D-methionine provides complete CDDP otoprotection. *Otolaryngol Head Neck Surg, 126*(6), 683–689.

Laurell, G., Teixeira, M., Sterkers, O., Bagger-Sjoback, D., Eksborg, S., Lidman, O., & Ferrary E. (2002). Local administration of antioxidants to the inner ear: Kinetics and distribution. *Hear Res, 173*, 198–209.

Lautermann, J., Crann, S. A., McLaren, J., & Schacht, J. (1997). Glutathione dependent antioxidant systems in the mammalian inner ear: Effects of aging, ototoxic drugs and noise. *Hear Res, 114*, 75–82.

Li, G., Frenz, D. A., Brahmblatt, S., Feghali, J. G., Ruben, R. J., Berggren, D., Arezzo, J., & Van De Water, T. R. (2001). Round window membrane delivery of L-methionine provides protection from cisplatin ototoxicity without compromising chemotherapeutic efficacy. *NeuroToxicol, 22*, 163–176.

Liu, W., Staecker, H., Stupak, H., et al. (1998). Caspase inhibitors prevent cisplatin-induced apoptosis of auditory sensory cells. *Neuroreport, 9*, 2609–2614.

Lu, S. (1998). Regulation of hepatic glutathione synthesis. *Sem in Liver Dis, 18*, 331–334.

Lynch, E., Gu, R., Pierce, C., & Kil, J. (2004). Ebselen-mediated protection from single and repeated noise exposure in rat. *Laryngoscope, 114*(2), 333–337.

Lynch, E., & Kil, J. (2005). Compounds for prevention and treatment of noise-induced hearing loss. *Drug Discovery Today, 10*(19), 1291–1298.

Lynch, E. D., Gu, R., Pierce, C., & Kil, J. (2005). Reduction of acute cisplatin ototoxicity in rats by oral administration of allopurinol and ebselen. *Hear Res, 201*, 81–89.

Marina, N., Chang, K. W., Malogolowkin, M., London, W. B., Frazier, A. L., Womer, R. B., Rescoria, F., Billmire, D. F., Davis, M. M., Perlman, E. J., Giller, R., Lauer, S. J., & Olson, T. A. (2005). Amifostine does not protect against the ototoxicity of high-dose cisplatin combined with etoposide and bleomycin in pediatric germ-cell tumors: A children's oncology group study. *Cancer, 104*, 841–847.

Meech, R. P., Campbell, K. C. M., Hughes, L. P., & Rybak, L. P. (1998). A semiquantitative analysis of the effects of cisplatin on the rat stria vascularis. *Hear Res, 124*, 44–59.

Melvik, J., & Pettersen, E. (1987). Reduction of cis-dichloro diammine platinum-induced cell inactivation by methionine. *Inorganica Chimica Acta, 137*, 115–118.

Miller, S. E., & House, D. A. (1990). The hydrolysis products of cis-dichlorodiammineplatinum (II). 3. Hydrolysis kinetics at physiological pH. *Inorgan Chem Acta, 173*, 53–60.

Muldoon, L. L., Pagel, M. A., Kroll, R. A., Brummett, R. E., Doolittle, N. D., Zuhowski, E. G., Egorin, M. J., & Neuwelt, E. A. (2000). Delayed administration of sodium thiosulfate in animal models reduces platinum ototoxicity without reduction of anti-tumor activity. *Clin Cancer Res, 6,* 309–315.

Ohlemiller, K. K., & Dugan, L. L. (1999). Elevation of reactive oxygen species following ischemia-reperfusion in mouse cochlea observed in vivo. *Audiol Neurootol, 4*(5), 219–228.

Pirvola, U., Xing-Qun, L.,Virkkala, J., Saarma, M., Murakata, C., Camoratto, A. M., Walton, K. M., & Ylikoski, J. (2000). Rescue of hearing, auditory hair cells, and neurons by CEP-1347/KT 7515, an inhibitor of c-Jun N-Terminal kinase activation. *J Neurosci, 20*(1), 43–50.

Pourbakht, A., & Yamasoba, T. (2003). Ebselen attenuates cochlear damage caused by acoustic trauma. *Hearing Research, 181,* 100–108.

Reser, D., Rho, M., Dewan, D., Herbst, L., Li, G., Stupa, H., Zur, K., Romaine, J., Frenz, D., Goldblum, L., Kopke, R., Arezzo, J., & Van De Water, T. (1999). L- and D-methionine provide equivalent long term protection against CDDP-induced ototoxicity in vivo, with partial in vitro and in vivo retention of antineoplastic activity. *Neurotoxicology, 20*(5), 731–748.

Ryals, B., Westbrook, A., & Schacht, J. (1997). Morphological evidence of ototoxicity of the iron chelator deferoxamine. *Hear Res, 112,* 44–48.

Rybak, L. P., & Whitworth, C. A. (2005). Ototoxicity: Therapeutic opportunities. *Drug Discovery Today, 10,* 1313–1321.

Sastry, J., & Kellie, S. J. (2005). Severe neurotoxicity, ototoxicity and nephrotoxicity following high-dose cisplatin and amifostine. *Pediatr Hematol Oncol, 22,* 441–445.

Scha, S.H., Qiu J.H., & Schacht J. (2006) Aspirin to prevent gentamicin-induced hearing loss. *N Engl J Med.* 354(170), 1856–1857.

Schweitzer, V. G. (1993). Ototoxicity of chemotherapeutic agents. *Otolaryngol Clin North Am, 26,* 759–785.

Sha, S., & Schacht, J. (1999). Stimulation of free radical formation by aminoglycoside antibiotics. *Hear Res, 128,* 112–118.

Sha, S. H., & Schacht, J. (2000). Antioxidants attenuate gentamicin-induced free radical formation in vitro and ototoxicity in vivo: D-methionine is a potential protectant. *Hear Res, 142,* 34–40.

Sha, S. H., Taylor, R., Forge, A., & Schacht, J. (2001). Differential vulnerability of basal and apical hair cells is based on intrinsic susceptibility to free radicals. *Hear Res, 155,* 18.

Sinswat, P., Wu, W., Sha, S., & Schacht, J. (2000). Protection from ototoxicity of intraperitoneal gentamicin in guinea pig. *Kidney Int, 58*(6), 2525–2532.

So, H. S., Park, C., Kim, H. J., Lee, J. H., Park, S. Y., Lee, J. H., Lee, Z. W., Kim, H. M., Kalinec, F., Lim, D., & Park, R. (2005). Protective effect of T-type calcium channel blocker flunarizine on cisplatin-induced death of auditory cells. *Hear Res, 204,* 127–139.

Song, B., Sha, S., & Schacht, J. (1998). Iron chelators protect from aminoglycoside-induced cochleo- and vestibulo-toxicity. *Free Radic Biol Med,* 25(2), 189–195.

Suzuki, M., Yagi, M., Brown, J. N., Miller, A.L., & Rafael., Y. (2000). Effect of transgenic GDNF expression and gentamicin-induced cochlear and vestibular toxicity. *Gene Therapy, 7,* 1046–1054.

Viallet, N. R., Blakley, B. B., Begleiter, A., & Leith, M. K. (2006). Sodium thiosulphate impairs the cytotoxic effects of cisplatin on FADU cells in culture. *J Otolaryngol, 35,* 19–21.

Vogt, W. (1995). Oxidation of methionyl residues in protein: Tools, targets and reversal. *Free Radic Biol Med, 18,* 93–105.

Walden, B. E., Henselman, L. W., & Morris, E. R. (2000). The role of magnesium in the susceptibility of soldiers to noise-induced hearing loss. *Journal of the Acoustical Society of America, 108*(1), 453–456.

Wang, J., Faulconbridge, R. V. L., Fetoni, A., Guitton, M. J., Pujol, R., & Puel, J. L. (2003). Local application of sodium thiosulfate prevents cisplatin-induced hearing loss in the guinea pig. *Neuropharmacol, 45,* 380–393.

Wang, J., Ladrech, S., Pujol, R., Brabet, P., Van De Water, T. R., & Puel, J. L. (2004). Caspase inhibitors, but not c-Jun NH2-terminal kinase inhibitor treatment, prevent cisplatin-induced hearing loss. *Cancer Res, 64,* 9217–9224.

Whitworth, C. A., Ramkumar, V., Jones, B., Tsukasaki, N., & Rybak, L. P. (2004). Protection against cisplatin ototoxicity by adenosine antagonists. *Biochem Pharmacol, 67,* 1801–1807.

Wimmer, C., Mees, K., Stumpf, P., Welsch, U., Reichel, O., & Suckfull, M. (2004). Round window application of D-methionine, sodium thiosulfate, brain-derived neurotrophic factor, and fibroblast growth factor-2 in CDDP induced ototoxicity. *Otol. Neurotol, 25*(1), 33–40.

Wu, Y. J., Muldoon, L. L., & Neuwelt, E. A. (2005). The chemoprotective agent N-acetylcysteine blocks cisplatin-induced apoptosis through caspase signaling pathway. *J Pharmacol Exp Ther, 312*, 424–431.

Yagi, M., Magal, E., Sheng, Z., Ang, K., & Raphael, Y. (1999). Hair cell protection for aminoglycoside ototoxicity by adenovirus-mediated overexpression of glial cell line-derived neurotrophic factor. *Hum Gene Ther, 10*, 813–823.

Yamane, H., Yoshiaki, N., Takayama, M., Konishi, K., Iguchi, H., Nakagawa, T., Shibata, S., Kato, A., Sunami, K., & Kawakatsu, C. (1995). The emergence of free radicals after acoustic trauma and strial blood flow. *Acta Otolaryngol Suppl, 519*, 87–92.

Yamasoba, T., Harris, C., Shoji, F., Lee, R. J., Nuttall, A. L., & Miller, J. M. (1998a). Influence of intense sound exposure on glutathione synthesis in the cochlea. *Brain Research, 804*(1), 72–78.

Yamasoba, T., Nuttall, A. L., Harris, C., Raphael, Y., & Miller, J. M. (1998b). Role of glutathione in protection against noise-induced hearing loss. *Brain Res, 784*, 82–90.

Yamasoba, T., Schacht, J., Shoji, F., & Miller, J. M. (1999). Attenuation of cochlear damage from noise trauma by an iron chelator, a free radical scavenger and glial cell line-derived neurotrophic factor in vivo. *Brain Research, 815*, 317–325.

Zhang, M., Liu, W., Ding, D., & Salvi, R. (2003). Pifithrin-alpha suppresses p53 and protects cochlear and vestibular hair cells from cisplatin-induced apoptosis. *Neuroscience 120*, 191–205.

Zheng, J. L., & Gao, W. (1996). Differential damage to auditory neurons in hair cells by ototoxins and protection by specific neurotrophins and cochlear organotypic cultures. *Eur J Neurosci, 8*, 1897–1905.

CHAPTER 20

Regeneration of Hair Cells

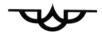

Brenda M. Ryals, PhD
Department of Communication Sciences and Disorders
James Madison University
Harrisonburg, VA

Jonathan I. Matsui, PhD
Department of Molecular and Cellular Biology
Harvard University
Cambridge, MA
Department of Otolaryngology and
Communication Disorders
Children's Hospital Boston
Boston, MA

Douglas A. Cotanche, PhD
Department of Otolaryngology
Children's Hospital
Boston, MA
Department of Otology and Laryngology
Harvard Medical School
Cambridge, MA

Acknowledgments: Dr. Ryals' research on hair cell regeneration is supported in collaboration with Dr. Robert Dooling by research grant DC001372 from the National Institute on Deafness and Other Communication Disorders, National Institutes of Health. Dr. Cotanche's research is supported by NIH Grant DC01689, Deafness Research Foundation, Samuel P. Rosenthal and Dossberg Foundation, and the Sarah Fuller Fund. Dr. Matsui's research is supported by a grant from the National Organization for Hearing Research Foundation, the American Hearing Research Foundation, and the National Eye Institute EY14790.

INTRODUCTION

In the late 1980s, several researchers discovered that birds could regenerate their sensory hair cells following deafening (Corwin & Cotanche, 1988; Ryals & Rubel, 1988). That discovery contradicted everything audiologists, physicians, and auditory neuroscientists knew about hair cell loss and permanent sensorineural hearing loss. After over fifty years of studying the mammalian inner ear, scientists did not suspect that the inner ear of any warm-blooded vertebrates could restore damaged or lost sensory hair cells. Did that simply mean the scientists hadn't looked hard enough? Or did it mean that birds were somehow special, perhaps retaining a capacity lost in higher-order vertebrates? It was quickly determined that the birds' capacity to spontaneously regenerate hair cells within the auditory portion of the inner ear was unique among warm-blooded vertebrates. Experiments similar to those performed in birds were performed in small mammals (e.g., rats and guinea pigs), but no evidence of spontaneous regeneration or restoration of auditory hair cells was found. Scientists interpreted this lack of spontaneous hair cell regeneration in mammals to mean that some factor or combination of factors may be needed to stimulate a dormant capacity for self-repair or to stimulate mechanisms similar to those in birds to act in the mammalian inner ear. Thus, an entirely new field of investigation in hearing and deafness was begun. A literature search using the phrase *hair cell regeneration* the first year following the discovery of hair cell regeneration revealed seven peer-reviewed publications; a similar search conducted in 2005 yielded more than forty such publications.

Auditory scientists in laboratories around the world are actively studying ways in which medicine may someday restore lost or damaged sensory cells of the inner ear in mammals, including humans. New discoveries in molecular genetics, cell cycle, cell signaling, stem cell research, and **gene therapy** happen on a daily basis. The goal of this chapter is to provide an overview of the current understanding of the cellular and molecular mechanisms underlying hair cell regeneration and to highlight the potential application of those mechanisms to prevent and/or treat sensorineural hearing loss. Providing an overview of current information in a rapidly advancing field of research is risky since new advances will occur prior to publication of the textbook. Therefore, the intention of this chapter is to provide the reader with an appreciation of the current understanding of the underlying mechanisms of hair cell regeneration so they will have a strong basis for interpreting the exciting scientific and clinical advances to come.

REGENERATING HAIR CELLS IN BIRDS

In mammals, the complete complement of auditory hair cells is present at birth and no new hair cells are spontaneously added to replace hair cells lost after injury or aging (Ruben, 1967; Roberson & Rubel, 1994; Roberson et al., 2004) although some evidence shows that there may be limited replacement of vestibular hair cells (Forge et al., 1993; Warchol et al., 1993; Kirkegaard & Jorgensen, 2000). That is why mammalian hair cells are said to have reached terminal mitosis and are postmitotic. Those cells are fully differentiated and do not reenter the cell cycle spontaneously, even when neighboring cells are destroyed.

That is not the case for birds, where new hair cells are produced continuously in the vestibular epithelium (Jorgensen & Mathiesen, 1988; Roberson et al., 1992) and after hair cell loss (Cotanche, 1987; Cruz et al., 1987; Corwin & Cotanche, 1988; Ryals & Rubel, 1988; Oesterle & Rubel, 1993; Warchol & Corwin, 1996). The principal mechanism of hair cell regeneration in birds is mitosis of supporting cells (Girod et al., 1989; Stone & Cotanche, 1994; Stone & Rubel, 2000). That is, when hair cells are lost or destroyed, the cells lying just beneath and surrounding them (supporting cells) reenter the cell cycle to become two new cells—a supporting cell and a hair cell. The evidence for this cell division comes from studies using markers that label DNA synthesis that confirms DNA replication and cell division to produce the new cells. Since these avian supporting cells, which are usually quiet and do not divide, can be stimulated to reenter the cell cycle, divide, and differentiate to become hair

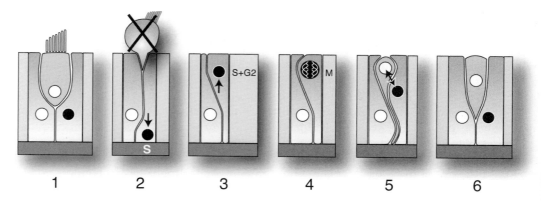

Figure 20-1.   Graphic representation of the time course for supporting cell reentry into the cell cycle after hair cell loss (1 and 2) to DNA synthesis and growth (3), mitosis (4 and 5), and regenerated hair cell and supporting cell (6). The time from hair cell loss to the appearance of immature stereocilia bundles on a regenerated hair cell is about forty-eight hours. (Adapted from Stone and Cotanche, 1992.)

cells, they have been termed precursor cells. Figure 20-1 is a graphic representation of the time course after hair cell loss for supporting cells to leave their quiescent state, reenter *cell cycle*, divide, and differentiate into a new supporting cell and hair cell. The time course from initiation of hair cell loss to appearance of immature hair cell stereocilia bundles is approximately forty-eight hours (Stone & Cotanche, 1992).

Recent studies suggest there may be a subset of supporting cells in birds and other nonmammals that have the ability to directly differentiate into hair cells without undergoing cell division (Roberson et al., 1996; Stone et al., 1998; Roberson et al., 2004). Figure 20-2 shows representative photomicrographs of regenerated hair cells labeled for postmitotic cell division and hair cells without labels that were formed via direct differentiation from supporting cell to hair cell.

This direct differentiation from supporting cell to hair cell has been variously termed direct **trans-differentiation**, cell conversion, and nonmitotic hair cell regeneration. The first evidence for nonmitotic hair cell regeneration was seen in amphibian lateral line organs (Balak et al., 1990) and later confirmed in the bullfrog sacculus (Baird et al., 1996; Steyger et al., 1997) and chick basilar papilla (Adler & Raphael, 1996; Adler et al., 1997). Roberson et al. (2004) demonstrated that the earliest hair cells produced after hair cell loss

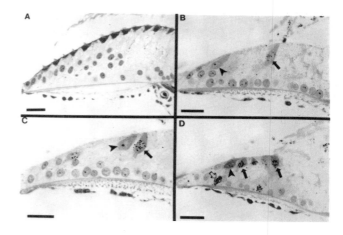

Figure 20-2.   (A) Photomicrograph of section through normal chick cochlea. (B) Section through a chick cochlea five days after gentamicin injection. Two regenerating hair cells are seen, one labeled for postmitotic division (long arrow) and one unlabeled (arrowhead). (C) Section through a chick cochlea five days after gentamicin injection. As in (B), two characteristic regenerating hair cells are seen, one labeled (long arrow) and one unlabeled (arrowhead). (D) Section through a chick cochlea twelve days after gentamicin injection. Two supporting cells are labeled (open arrow). Three cells are present with the characteristic morphology of regenerating hair cells, two labeled (long arrows) and one unlabeled (arrowhead). (Adapted from Roberson et al. (1996), with permission.)

in the avian inner ear are produced via direct transdifferentiation. Their findings suggest that direct transdifferentiation is a simpler, faster process that produces the first new hair cells and that mitotic regeneration is somewhat slower but ultimately produces the majority of new hair cells. Although the transdifferentiation of supporting cells through nonmitotic means may seem to be a simpler way of replacing dead hair cells than stimulating local cells to reenter the cell cycle, such nonmitotic sensory cell replacement could significantly alter the structural integrity of the sensory organ. For example, if local resident supporting cells transdifferentiated into hair cells without replacing themselves, the mechanical structure of the organ of Corti could be compromised. On the other hand, if nonresident cells within the sensory organ could transdifferentiate into hair cells and migrate to the appropriate position to replace lost hair cells, the nonmitotic mechanism could be quite effective.

Thus, avian hair cells are regenerated after chemical or traumatic injury either through precursor cell division or through precursor cell transdifferentiation. To apply that information to the critical issue of mammals' inability to spontaneously regenerate hair cells, scientists must address the following fundamental questions. Each question will be addressed in detail in this chapter.

1. Are precursor cells available in the mammalian cochlea?

2. What are the triggers that stimulate normally quiescent cells to enter the cell cycle and divide?

3. What are the triggers that terminate cell cycle so the optimal numbers of cells are produced?

4. What are the factors that provide the signals that make an undifferentiated cell become a hair cell?

Finally, it is important to note that the ultimate goal of regenerating hair cells is to restore hearing. Regenerated hair cells without neural connections to the brain are useless. Therefore, the final sections of this chapter will address the current understanding of the interaction of neural connections and avian regenerated hair cells on the return of hearing, as well as the potential for neural connections on mammalian regenerated hair cells.

PRECURSOR CELLS IN THE MAMMALIAN COCHLEA

In order to discuss the development of specific cell types, such as hair cells, it is important to define the different types of cells that play a roll in the formation of that cell. As was previously stated, supporting cells in mature avian inner ears are precursor cells; they are committed to develop as a specific cell type but are quiescent (postmitotic) within the epithelium. Thus, avian supporting cells can be induced either through cell division or transdifferentiation to become a hair cell but not, for example, a red blood cell; they have limited cell fate capability. Another term for *precursor cell* is *progenitor cell*; the terms are synonymous. Other cell types that have less limited cell fate are called **stem cells.** Embryonic stem cells are pluripotent, so they have the capacity to become any of the many cell types that exist in the body. Nonembryonic stem cells (e.g., neural stem cells) are multipotent. They are limited in the types of cells they can become. For example, neural stem cells can become neurons or glial cells, but they cannot be induced to become other cell types, such as blood cells. Either precursor cells or stem cells need to be present for regeneration of hair cells to occur in the mammalian cochlea.

Figure 20-3 shows the organ of Corti viewed by scanning electron microscopy. The elegant pattern of sensory hair cells and adjacent supporting structures are apparent. Could any of those supporting structures retain the capacity to reenter the cell cycle or to change their fate and become a hair cell? Are stem cells or precursor cells present within the mature mammalian cochlea, just waiting to be stimulated?

In the past, investigators looking into hair cell regeneration in mammals had to consider the possibility that nonsensory cells in the mammalian cochlea had reached such a state of final differentiation that they could no longer be induced to reenter the cell cycle or to transform into another cell type. Investigators turned to studies conducted by developmental biologists to determine which cells were originally responsible for hair cell production. Cells that eventually become hair cells are derived from specific regions of the embryonic **otocyst** and receive genetic and local signals that determine whether they will

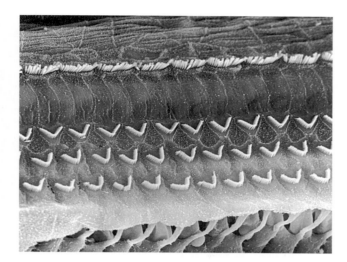

Figure 20-3. Scanning electron photomicrograph of hair cells and supporting cells in the mammalian organ of Corti. (Photomicrograph provided by Dr. Marc Lenoir.)

become sensory hair cells or nonsensory supporting cells (e.g., pillar cells). The factors that control the exact positioning of these cells to form the organ of Corti are not well understood, but probably involve signals from the adjacent neural tube and underlying mesenchyme (Rubel, 1978; Ladher et al., 2000). So all of the cells within the cochlea derive from the same cell type; they have a different final cell fate depending on local and genetic factors. An excellent review of the issues surrounding determination and commitment of inner ear cell fate can be found in Kelley (2002).

Several lines of investigation have led to the conclusion that postmitotic, nonsensory cells naturally exist within the mammalian inner ear and can be induced to become hair cells. The mammalian vestibular system houses some stem cells that have the capacity to become hair cells in the developing chick otocyst (Li et al., 2003). Furthermore, evidence that some nonsensory cells in mammalian cochlea retain their capacity to become hair cells was recently found using markers for precursor cells in the cochlea (Lopez et al., 2004). Finally, one study found that by removing local cues (separating each cell type into a separate "dish") and applying known genetic

cues that direct hair cell fate, nonsensory cells within the mammalian cochlea were able to become sensory hair cells (Doetzlhofer et al., 2004; Doetzlhofer et al., 2005). Thus, it is *not* the lack of precursor or stem cells within the mature mammalian cochlea that is the limiting factor for regenerating hair cells.

CELL CYCLE

Since cells within the mature mammalian cochlea can form hair cells, why don't they? During normal development of the inner ear, cells in the otocyst divide to eventually form the optimal number of cells in the cochlear duct. The cells then stop dividing and begin to differentiate into the various cell types that make up the inner ear. The signals that are critical for starting and stopping cell division to form the inner ear will be critical in starting and stopping the cell division that may be necessary to regenerate hair cells in humans. Thus, it is important to have a fundamental grasp of the nature of the cell cycle. Much of the following discussion regarding the cell cycle and hair cell regeneration has been presented previously (Ryals, 2000b; Ryals & Cunningham, 2003). For those interested in a more thorough discussion, the following references are informative: Stone et al. (1998) and Ryan (2003). For a comprehensive review of the basic biology of the cell cycle, the reader is referred to Nasmyth (1996) and the Nobel Foundation Web page at http://www.nobel.org (click "Medicine," then "Educational." Scroll down and click "Are you able to work as a Cell Division Supervisor?")

Figure 20-4 is a diagram of the cell cycle. Each phase in the cycle represents a point at which the cell may remain until stimulated to enter the next stage.

Cells that have completed a cell cycle may initiate a new cycle, "rest" between cycles, or be terminally differentiated (do not cycle again). This phase of "rest," or terminal differentiation, is termed G0. The *G* stands for gap in the cell cycle and indicates a point at which the cell may remain indefinitely or where the cell may be stimulated to initiate growth (G1). In the G1 phase, the cell grows until it has reached its appropriate size and can enter the phase of DNA synthesis, or S phase. The S phase is the point at which

DNA replication occurs. This is the phase where the chromosomes reproduce themselves so that each

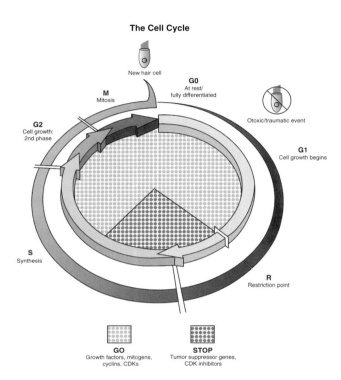

Figure 20-4. The cell cycle is an orderly set of events that culminate in cell division into two daughter cells. *G* stands for "gap" in the cell cycle. The stages of the cell cycle pictured here are G0-G1-S-G2-M. When cells are quiet, not getting ready to divide or grow, they are said to be in G0 phase. This is the usual stage for sensory and nonsensory cells in the mammalian cochlea. The next gap in time, G1, represents the time when the cell is just beginning to get ready to divide. This stage is initiated in birds when hair cells are lost after trauma or ototoxicity. Some "go" signal is initiated by this loss (growth factors, mitogens, cyclins, etc.), which stimulates the cell to reenter the cell cycle. After cells enter G1, they may proceed to the synthesis stage (S) when the DNA replicates within the nucleus of the cell. Or they may receive a signal that restricts or stops the cell from dividing (tumor suppressor genes, CDK inhibitors, etc.). Those restriction points are critical for controlling overproduction of cells and tumor formation. If the cell is not inhibited from division, there is another gap, G2, which represents the period just before the cell finally divides into two separate cells; nutrients are important at this point in the cell cycle for appropriate cell growth. The M stages (*M* stands for "mitosis") is when the nuclear chromosomes separate and two new cells are formed. Mitosis is the creation of two new cells with identical DNA from a single cell. In the case of hair cell regeneration, mitotic division of supporting cells gives rise to a supporting cell and a hair cell.

new cell will have a complete set of identical chromosomes. Most cells that are stimulated to enter the S phase are said to be "committed" to proceed to G2 and M (mitosis). Gap 2 (G2) is the gap or pause between DNA synthesis and the onset of actual cell division (called mitosis, or M phase). During G2, more cell growth and maturation occurs as the cell prepares to enter M phase. The time it takes to reach mitosis can vary depending on the signals and the cell type. During mitosis, the nuclear chromosomes separate and the cell divides to form two new cells.

Regulation of the Cell Cycle

One reason hair cells don't spontaneously regenerate in mammals may be that the precursor cells aren't stimulated to divide when hair cells are lost or damaged. Another reason might be that the supporting or precursor cells are inhibited or prevented from dividing. Both of these situations may represent fundamental differences between bird and mammal inner ears. Therefore, studying the molecular and genetic regulation of the cell cycle may provide clues for future efforts aimed at inducing hair cell regeneration in mammals.

Agents that stimulate a cell to move from G0 to G1 are called mitogens. Several molecular controls are in place for signaling the cell to proceed through the cell cycle. Strict control must be maintained when progressing through the cell cycle so the right numbers of cells are produced. When these regulatory controls go awry, mitogens can become oncogenes (factors that stimulate the uncontrolled proliferation of cells) and may result in the formation of tumors. The following discussion reviews the factors that are critical to regulating the cell cycle during normal development and relates some of those factors to current knowledge about their potential roles during hair cell regeneration.

Cyclins and Cyclin-Dependent Kinases (CDKs)

Proteins called cyclins and enzymes called kinases are found within the cell's cytoplasm and control the passage of the cell through the cell cycle. One specific kinase has been designated as cyclin-dependent kinase (CDK); interactions between this CDK and cyclins play a critical role in regulating the cell cycle. CDK and cyclin form an enzyme that activates other proteins by chemical modification (phosphorylation). The level of CDK is constant during the cell cycle, but its enzymatic activity varies because of the regulatory function of the cyclins (their level rises and falls during the cell cycle). One might compare the function of CDKs on the movement of cells through the cell cycle to a car engine (cell) that is driven by CDKs to accelerate, brake, or idle, depending on the amount of cyclin present. So cyclins and CDKs are critical in stimulating cells to leave G0 and begin the cell cycle. They are also critical to stopping the cell cycle, so that too many cells (tumor) are not formed. One particular kinase, mitogen-activated protein kinase (MAPK), plays a significant role in regulating cells entering S phase in the avian inner ear (Witte et al., 2001), while phosphatidylinositol 3-kinase is a key element in the signaling cascades that lead to the proliferation of cells in mammalian vestibular epithelia *in vitro* (Montcouquiol & Corwin, 2001).

Growth Factors and the Immune Response

A growth factor is a biological substance (protein, hormone, vitamin, etc.) that stimulates cellular growth and is critical for the cell to move from G1 to S phase and from G2 to mitosis. A multitude of different **growth factors** promote cell division and growth throughout the body; however, only a few have been shown to be particularly effective in the inner ear. Oesterle and Hume (1999) provide a detailed review of growth factor regulation of the cell cycle in the developing and mature inner ear. Table 20-1 summarizes some growth factors that have been found to stimulate cell proliferation in the mammalian inner ear.

While growth factors have only been found to stimulate cell proliferation in the mammalian inner ear, growth factors may also inhibit cell proliferation in the avian inner ear (Warchol, 1999; Oesterle et al., 2000).

One way that growth factors might enter the inner ear after damage or hair cell loss is through macrophage activity. **Macrophages** are specialized white blood cells that are part of the immune system's response to injury. They are actively involved in "cleaning up" dead cells and have been known to secrete growth hormones to stimulate wound repair. Macrophages are found within the inner ear soon after hair cell damage. Investigators have suggested that macrophages may provide the growth factors that initiate progenitor cell division or transdifferentiation (Warchol, 1997; Bhave et al., 1998; Warchol & Matsui, 2001; Warchol et al., 2001).

Table 20-1.   Growth Factors That Have Been Shown to Stimulate Cell Proliferation in Mammalian Inner Ear

Growth Factor	Cochlear	Vestibular	Reference
EGF+I*		+	Oesterle & Hume, 1999**
TGFα*	+	+	Oesterle & Hume, 1999**
			Daudet et al., 2002
TGFα+I*			Oesterle & Hume, 1999**
FGF-4, FGF-6, FGF-7		+	Oesterle & Hume, 1999**
GGF2		+	Oesterle & Hume, 1999**
Heregulin		+	Zheng et al., 1999; Hume et al., 2003
IGF-1		+	Oesterle & Hume, 1999**
IGF-II		+	Oesterle & Hume, 1999**
TGFß-1, TGFß-2, TGFß-3, TGFß-5		+	Oesterle & Hume, 1999**

*effect in both developing and mature mammalian inner ear
**review article contains original citations

(Adapted from Oesterle & Hume, 1999.)

The potential therapeutic benefit (if any) of using growth factors to stimulate hair cell regeneration *in vivo* may be limited by their potent mitogenic effects. It seems likely that growth factors will have to be used in combination with other inhibitory factors that can act to decrease the action of growth factors so the optimal numbers of cells are produced.

CDK Inhibitors—Tumor Suppressor Proteins

There are several "checkpoints" in the cell cycle where the cell can either proceed to the next phase of the cycle, stop (arrest) the cell cycle, or initiate cell death. Those checkpoints are necessary to regulate the cell cycle so that overproduction of cells doesn't occur and damaged cells don't proliferate. Because failure of the "checkpoint" regulators can result in tumor formation, the genetically controlled proteins are called tumor suppressors. Cells in the organ of Corti appear to be maintained in a postmitotic state through the action of CDK inhibitor signaling pathways. The first evidence for the role of a specific CDK inhibitor, or genetically controlled tumor suppressor protein, in the organ of Corti was provided in 1999 (Chen & Segil, 1999; Lowenheim et al., 1999). p27(Kip1) inhibits the progression of the cell cycle and is required to keep supporting cells in the organ of Corti in a "quiescent" state. When the p27(Kip1) gene is "knocked out" in mice, the result is ongoing supporting cell proliferation in the embryonic and mature organ of Corti well after the developmental period when mitosis in the sensory epithelia ceases. In fact, these p27(Kip1) knock out mice have an over-abundance of hair cells and supporting cells, never hear normally, and do not live to maturity (Chen & Segil, 1999). Thus, the presence of p27(Kip1) is critical to limiting the number of hair cells that are produced; when the gene is not present, the number of hair cells increases (Figure 20-5). Unfortunately, too many hair cells are just as bad as too few in terms of the ability to hear normally.

Two other tumor suppressor proteins, p19/ink4d (Chen et al., 2003) and Rb1 (Sage et al., 2005), are also involved in regulating the cell cycle in the inner ear. For example, targeted deletion of p19/ink4d, another inhibitor of cell cycle progression, causes the initiation of DNA synthesis in hair cells, but then leads to the precocious death of those cells and a subsequent hearing loss (Chen et al., 2003). Thus, it appears that these cell cycle inhibitors are used by the cochlear tissues to suppress mitosis in the sensory epithelium and promote the establishment of a mature, nonproliferating sensory epithelium. The elimination of these suppressors initially leads to continued proliferation and overproduction of hair cells. However, these cell cycle suppressors must also have some other critical function in the cells since eliminating either gene results in premature death of the hair cells and sometimes the entire animal. So while these studies are a proof of principal that regeneration in the mammalian cochlea can be activated by elimination of specific mitotic suppressors, additional consequences to the loss of these inhibitors need to be understood before they can be used as a therapeutic approach to hearing loss. So if scientists are to stimulate endogenous cells in the mammalian cochlea to leave G0 and enter the cell cycle, they need to understand how to manipulate the inhibitory genetic controls that regulate the number of hair cells produced in order to maintain the delicate balance necessary for normal hearing function.

CELL FATE DETERMINATION

This chapter has discussed the elements necessary to move cells within the mature organ of Corti out of their quiescent state and into mitotic division. Research has shown that precursor cells are available in the mammalian cochlea, as are at least some of the stimulatory (growth factors) and inhibitory factors (tumor suppressor genes) that are critical for these precursor cells to reenter the cell cycle. The next questions must then be, what are the factors that provide the signals that make an undifferentiated cell become a hair cell, and what are the factors involved in determining the correct number and organization of cells within the sensory epithelium? Certainly the answers to those questions will be fundamental to regenerating the appropriate number and organization of both sensory and nonsensory cells to reestablish the organ of Corti.

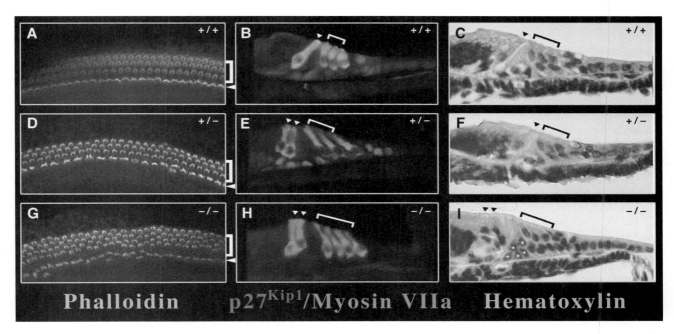

Phalloidin   p27^{Kip1}/Myosin VIIa   Hematoxylin

Figure 20-5. A comparison of the structure of organ of Corti from p27$^{+/+}$ wild-type (A–C), p27$^{+/-}$ heterozygous (D–F), and p27$^{-/-}$ homozygous mutant (G–I) mice, age P6. Loss of p27^{Kip1} expression due to a targeted gene deletion causes the development of supernumerary hair cells and supporting cells in the organ of Corti. (A, D, and G) Confocal images of surface preparations used to compare the overall arrangement of sensory cells in the organ of Corti. They were stained with rhodamine-conjugated phalloidin to visualize the actin-rich stereocilia of the sensory hair cells. (B, E, and H) Cross sections through the organ of Corti in the mid-cochlear region stained with antibody to the hair cell-specific antigen myosin VIIa. (C, F, and I) Alternate sections stained with hematoxylin to reveal the cellular architecture of the organ of Corti. Brackets mark multiple rows of outer hair cells, three in the p27$^{+/+}$ and p27$^{+/-}$ animals and four in the p27$^{-/-}$ animals. Arrowheads point to the single row of inner hair cells present in the wild-type organ of Corti, as well as to the rows of inner hair cells containing supernumerary hair cells in the p27$^{+/-}$ and p27$^{-/-}$ mutant animals. Sections from wild-type animals contain the normal number of inner and outer hair cells (B and C). The occasional presence of supernumerary inner hair cells in heterozygotes is illustrated in (E) but not in (F). Note the supernumerary cells present in the pillar cell region of the organ of Corti from p27$^{-/-}$ animals, where normally one inner pillar cell and one outer pillar cell are present (compare (C) with (I), asterisks). (From Chen and Segil, 1999 with permission The Company of Biologists, Ltd. Publisher.)

Two excellent review articles are available that discuss the cellular, molecular, and genetic mechanisms that guide hair cell fate and organization of the sensory epithelium (Bryant et al., 2002; Kelley, 2002). The following is a summary of the controls that appear to be critical during development and regeneration in the inner ear.

Genetic Controls

In developing mammals, hair cells express a specific **transcription factor,** *Math1* (the mammalian homologue of the Drosophila basic helix-loop-helix (bHLH)

gene *atonal* (Akazawa et al., 1995), while nonsensory cells do not. bHLH transcription factors are an evolutionarily conserved classification of transcription factors that either initiate or regulate transcription and include a specific DNA-binding structural motif. In animals, they are important regulators of embryonic development, particularly in the development of the nervous system and muscles. Some bHLH family members (e.g., *Math1*) are involved in cell-fate determination in different cell lineages including the initial determination of specific types of neurons, whereas other factors (e.g., *Nero-D*) facilitate differentiation of the cell. Genetically altered mice deficient in *Math1* fail to develop sensory hair cells, so the *Math1* gene is both necessary and sufficient to determine hair cell fate (Bermingham et al., 1999; Chen et al., 2002; Woods et al., 2004). Moreover, when *Math1* is over-expressed in cultured mouse ears, the result is an overabundance of hair cells (Zheng & Gao, 2000). Thus, when *Math1* is present in the cochlea, some cells become hair cells and have the morphologic and genetic attributes of mechanosensory hair cells; when *Math1* is absent, cells do not become hair cells. Recently the gene *Sox2* was identified as acting upstream of *Math1* and providing essential signals for hair cell fate in the developing mouse ear (Kiernan et al., 2005). Mice lacking *Sox2* and/or *Math1* failed to establish differentiated supporting cells and hair cells and, thus, had a severe to profound hearing impairment. Other genes have been identified as playing a negative role in hair cell fate. *Hes1* and *Hes5*, two members of the bHLH transcription gene family, act as negative regulators of hair cell fate (Zheng et al., 2000; Zine et al., 2001). Mice with targeted deletions for those genes showed a significant increase in the number of inner and outer hair cells. The authors conclude that *Hes1* and *Hes5* likely participated together, through a negative regulation of *Math1*, to control hair cell fate. As development of the inner ear proceeds, the level of *Math1* is reduced so that some cells become nonsensory supporting cells (Bermingham et al., 1999; Lanford et al., 2000). Thus, the regulation and expression of these genes are critical to final cell fate. It seems likely that upregulation or increased availability of such a hair cell gene is involved in the observed transdifferentiation of supporting cells to hair cells during regeneration in the avian ear. As will be discussed later, introduction of the *Math1* gene has successfully induced hair cell regeneration in the mammalian cochlea (Kawamoto et al., 2003; Izumikawa et al., 2005).

As has been discussed, several genes have been found to be critical for inducing cells to become hair cells during normal development of the mammalian inner ear. The *Sox2* gene is required for sensory organ development and acts upstream of *Math1* during inner ear development. Its discovery is relatively recent (Kiernan et al., 2005), and it will be interesting to see whether *Sox2* is important for the establishment and/or maintenance of sensory cell progenitors in the inner ear. Thus far, however, experiments have centered on the positive effect of the *Math1* gene on hair cell differentiation. Recent *in vivo* experiments from Raphael and colleagues (Kawamoto et al., 2003; Izumikawa et al., 2005) have demonstrated that *Math1* transfected into the cochleas of guinea pigs deafened by the aminoglycoside antibiotic kanamycin led to an extensive structural and functional recovery of the organ of Corti. In all cases, the new hair cells appear to arise from direct transdifferentiation of existing non-sensory cells rather than through the mitotic production of new cells. Even though those studies are in their beginning stages, it appears that **transfection** of *Math1* into the deafened cochlea may prove to be a promising option for gene therapy. However, as is the case in some gene therapy paradigms, target specificity can be problematic (Parker & Cotanche, 2004). For instance, when Raphael and colleagues successfully introduced *Math1*-encoding viral particles into the cochlea, there was an ectopic production of hair cells in addition to those seen in the organ of Corti (Kawamoto et al., 2003). Therefore, to reestablish the proper connections after damage, there is a need to establish a model where *Math1* may be more effectively delivered directly to the site of hair cell loss.

Cell-Cell Interaction and Notch Signaling

Whether a cell becomes a hair cell or a supporting cell is also influenced by local cell-cell contact signals or by lateral inhibition (Bryant et al., 2002) where neighboring cells generate a signal that prevents the overproduction of a particular cell type. This lateral inhibition is mediated through the Notch signaling pathway (Zine et al., 2000; Bryant et al., 2002; Kelley, 2002). Notch is a membrane-bound receptor that is activated when a membrane-bound ligand (Delta, Serrate, or Jagged) binds to the receptor. A detailed description of the interactions of the Notch signaling pathway and hair cell fate can be found in Kelley (2002). Briefly, soon after the onset of the expression of *Math1*, cells within the *Math1* domain begin to express other ligands such as Delta1 and/or Jagged2 that interact with the Notch receptor; as development continues, cells expressing those ligands go on to differentiate as hair cells. Cells located adjacent to the ligand-expressing cells upregulate Notch target genes such as *Hes5* and *Hes1*, resulting in the correct number of sensory and nonsensory cells (Kelley, 2002; Zine & de Ribaupierre, 2002). Since birds do not regenerate hair cells unless a hair cell is lost from the sensory epithelium, it is reasonable to assume that the Notch signaling pathway may be stimulated during regeneration. Stone and Rubel (1999) showed that Delta1 is expressed in cells arising from postmitotic divisions during hair cell regeneration, which suggests that the Notch-Delta signaling pathway may be involved in correct cell differentiation and patterning of the sensory epithelium during hair cell regeneration. Figure 20-6 is a summary diagram for the molecular signals that play a role in determination of hair cell fate.

In summary, cell fate determination during development involves the genetic signaling for hair cell fate (*Math1* and *Sox2*) and cell-cell contact inhibition signaling involving the Notch signaling pathway. Recent experiments have shown that it may be possible to induce nonsensory cells within the mammalian sensory epithelium to change their postmitotic state to become hair cells (Kawamoto et al., 2003) and that these new cells may be functional (Izumikawa et al., 2005).

STEM CELLS AND HAIR CELL REGENERATION

As has been shown from the above review, the issues that are likely to be most relevant to regenerating hair cells in mature mammalian cochleae involve controlling cell cycle and/or determining cell fate. Scientists have taken those fundamental issues and designed experiments along three lines of inquiry in an attempt to regenerate hair cells in the damaged mammalian cochlea. Those experiments include:

1. Controlling cell cycle—i.e., experimentally manipulating (knockouts or transgenics) genes that inhibit proliferation in the organ of Corti—tumor suppressor genes.

2. Controlling cell fate—i.e., intentionally transfecting (gene therapy) cochlear cells with viruses carrying genes for inducing hair cell differentiation (insertion of the "hair cell" gene *Math1*).

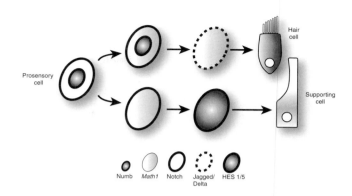

Figure 20-6. Graphic illustration of the molecular signals that play a role in the determination of hair cell fate. Initially, an epithelial, prosensory cell divides to form two daughter cells. During the final division, Numb becomes restricted to one of the cells, leading to a relative decrease in the level of Notch in that cell. Following mitosis, each of the daughter cells begins to express an *Math1* protein. Next, the cell that will develop as a hair cell upregulates the expression of one or more Notch ligands (e.g., Jagged2 or Delta1). Activated Notch induces a downstream signaling pathway that results in the expression of the inhibitory bHLH proteins *Hes5* and/or *Hes1*. Expression of *Hes* proteins leads to inhibition and downregulation of *Math1*. As a result, these cells are diverted from developing as hair cells and ultimately become supporting cells. (Adapted from Kelley, 2002.)

3. Activating or inserting stem cells—i.e., replacing lost cochlear cells with either intrinsic or extrinsic (transplanted) stem cells.

This chapter has reviewed experiments designed to control cell cycle through the use of knockout and transgenic mice (see "Regulation of the Cell Cycle"). Experiments designed to control cell fate through intentional transfection of genes that control cell fate have also been reviewed (see "Cell Fate Determination"). The following section reviews the third area of research in hair cell regeneration—activation or insertion of stem cells.

Stem cells have received considerable attention in the scientific field and in the popular press over the last several years because of their potential to repair or regenerate damaged cells and tissues in the human body. Li et al. (2004) have written an excellent review of their potential for therapy within the inner ear. Embryonic stem cells have the capacity to give rise to any cell type in the body; nonembryonic stem cells have the potential to give rise to a limited number of related cell types, and both types of stem cells may have therapeutic potential within the inner ear (Li et al., 2003; Li et al., 2003; Li et al., 2004). If intrinsic stem cells in the inner ear could be activated or extrinsic stem cells could be transplanted into the ear, they could produce new hair cells and/or neurons to replace those that have been lost.

Recently investigators (Li et al., 2003) have isolated a population of cells from the utricles of mice that they describe as end organ stem cells. These cells exhibit the capacity to self-renew and to produce cell types with the morphologies and biological markers of hair cells (myosin VIIa and Brn-3.1) and supporting cells (pancytokeratin and p27^{Kip1}). In other studies, researchers have manipulated identified stem cell populations to express characteristics of neural or hair cell precursors. Li et al. (2003) induced mouse embryonic stem cells down a pathway that resembles neural progenitor cells. When those "neural progenitor cells" were transplanted into an embryonic chick otocyst, the transplanted cells gave rise to new hair cells. Kanda et al. (2004) induced mouse embryonic stem cells to form neuronlike cells by overexpression of bHLH genes. Similarly, treatment of mouse bone marrow stem cells with the signaling molecules sonic hedgehog and retinoic acid enabled them to differentiate into neuronlike cells (Kondo et al., 2005). Strategies like these may enable readily available stem cells to be primed to become cells with a more cochlear fate that could be transplanted into damaged cochleas.

Some scientific groups have transplanted neural stem cells into the inner ears of mammals. Ito et al. (2001) injected rat hippocampal stem cells into the cochleas of newborn rat pups and observed that some of the transplanted hippocampal cells had integrated into the cochlear epithelium. Hu et al. (2005) transplanted adult neurospheres into the cochleas of normal and neomycin-treated guinea pigs. They saw a higher survival rate of the stem cells in the neomycin-treated cochleas and reported that some of the surviving cells were beginning to express neuronal markers. Preliminary experiments in the Cotanche laboratory (Parker et al., in preparation) have transplanted immortalized neural stem cells into the noise-damaged cochleas of mice and guinea pigs. Those stem cells have survived up to 6 weeks and have integrated into the spiral ganglion and organ of Corti in the damaged regions.

Studies using stem cells are still in rudimentary stages, but they do indicate that there may be a resident mammalian stem cell population, at least in the vestibular end organs. Moreover, the introduction of pluripotent stem cells into a damaged ear may result in those cells integrating into the remains of the sensory epithelium and deriving the necessary signals for differentiating into hair cells, supporting cells, and neurons that could repopulate and repair the damaged sensory epithelium. Before stem cells can be considered for therapeutic applications in humans, however, their capacity for integrating into the site of lesion; for forming neural/synaptic connections; and, ultimately, for restorating functional hearing, must be established in other animal models. It is conceivable that stem cell based therapy may work best, at least in the short term, in combination with gene therapy and drug treatment or used in conjunction with technical devices such as cochlear implants (Li et al., 2004).

CAN REGENERATED HAIR CELLS RESTORE FUNCTIONAL HEARING AND BALANCE?

Molecular and genetic cues for hair cell regeneration are critical if scientists are to discover a way to regenerate hair cells in humans. The final goal, though, is to restore hearing. For that to happen, the supporting cells need to differentiate into hair cells and the newly differentiated hair cells need to grow stereocilia bundles, form the appropriate ion channels for transduction, and be reinnervated by the eighth cranial nerve fibers to connect the sensory receptor to the central nervous system. The animals must also be able to access the new sensory information and use it to make behaviorally meaningful responses. At least two book chapters and two review articles have been published concerning neural innervation and functional recovery of hearing following sound- and drug-induced damage and hair cell regeneration

(Ryals & Dooling, 1996; Smolders, 1999; Ryals, 2000; Bermingham-McDonogh & Rubel, 2003).

Although numerous studies have examined the physiology of regenerated sensory hair cells, few studies have examined complex properties of perceptual processing and behavioral plasticity. Compensatory behaviors such as oculomotor, gaze, and postural responses that occur during movement largely depend on a functioning vestibular system. The vestibular ocular reflex (VOR) and the vestibular colic reflex (VCR) disappear after hair cells in the crista of the semicircular canals are killed with aminoglycoside antibiotics (Jones & Nelson, 1992; Carey et al., 1996; Goode et al., 1999; Goode et al., 2001; Matsui et al., 2003). Those reflexes, however, reappear as the hair cells regenerate (Carey et al., 1996; Jones et al., 1998; Goode et al., 1999; Goode et al., 2001). Dickman and Lim (2004) trained adult pigeons to run along a long chamber and peck an illuminated key to receive a fluid reward. Multiple behavioral measures assessing performance, posture, and head stability were quantified. Once normative values were obtained, the animals received aminoglycoside antibiotics, which killed the sensory hair cells in the vestibular system and resulted in severe postural and head instability. As the regeneration process progressed, the tremor and head shakes diminished and spatial orientation and navigation ability improved to pretreatment levels.

In the auditory system, recognition and production of vocal signals depend on hearing and are necessary for communication. Dooling and colleagues used budgerigars (Australian parrots) to examine the return of complex auditory perception and vocal production after hair cell regeneration (Dooling et al., 1997; Ryals & Dooling, 2000). Budgerigars mimic sounds and readily learn new vocalizations throughout life, which has been likened to language acquisition in humans. The birds were trained to precisely match their vocalizations to specific acoustic templates. Aminoglycoside antibiotic treatment induced a high-frequency hearing loss, which disrupted both auditory perception and vocal production. Behavioral tests of auditory sensitivity showed that audiometric thresholds returned to near normal levels (within 20 dB) within 4 weeks. Difference thresholds for frequency and intensity

returned to normal levels as well. More complex perceptual tasks, such as vocal call discrimination and/or recognition, took much longer (up to 5 months) but also returned to normal levels after hair cell regeneration. Precision in vocal production initially declined, but was restored to pretreatment levels well before the full recovery of auditory function. Those data suggested that relatively little acoustic feedback from a few regenerated hair cells was necessary to guide full recovery of vocal precision. These results may have particular relevance for understanding the relationship between hearing loss and human speech production especially when one is considering an auditory prosthetic device, such as a cochlear implant.

Woolley and colleagues conducted another series of studies that examined complex communication behavior in Bengalese finches (Woolley & Rubel, 1997; Woolley et al., 2001; Woolley & Rubel, 2002). Male Bengalese finches are songbirds that learn a single sequence of "syllables" early in life and reliably produce the same song throughout life. After each animal's song was recorded and its stability verified, the birds were treated with a combination of sound exposure and aminoglycoside antibiotics to cause hearing loss; the songs rapidly deteriorated (Woolley & Rubel, 1999). As hearing was restored by hair cell regeneration as assessed by auditory brainstem responses (ABRs) (Woolley et al., 2001), the song returned to its preexposure structure (Woolley & Rubel, 2002). Restoration of hearing allowed each bird to access a stored "template" of its own learned vocalization and gradually match its new vocalizations to the stored memory.

While scientists have no behavioral measurement for the return of hearing after hair cell regeneration in mammals, electrophysiological measurements of the ABR in guinea pigs that were first deafened by kanamycin and then were given gene therapy to deliver *Math1* to the cochlea showed evidence of hair cell regeneration and improved threshold sensitivity for all frequencies tested (Kawamoto et al., 2003; Izumikawa et al., 2005). Previous studies from that group had also shown preliminary evidence of neural reinnervation of regenerated hair cells (Kawamoto et al., 2003).

SUMMARY

The cellular, molecular, and genetic aspects of hair cell regeneration have been well documented in birds. Scientists are just beginning to see the fruits of their efforts in inducing hair cell regeneration in the mammalian cochlea. While inherent genetic inhibitory controls prohibit spontaneous hair cell regeneration in mammals, recent discoveries suggest that the use of externally introduced factors and/or stem cells may override this inhibition. Advances in genomics, adenovirus gene therapy, and stem cell technology have raised hopes that these techniques will eventually lead to a cure for sensorineural hearing loss. Safe and effective means of delivering genes and/or stem cells need to be developed for these therapies to be of any clinical relevance. Moreover, being able to direct stem cells and/or gene delivery systems (viral vectors) to the correct locations to promote supporting cell proliferation and then hair cell differentiation is paramount to the return of function. Future studies of the molecular and genetic mechanisms underlying hair cell regeneration in mammals are likely to focus on those important issues. Finally, scientists will need to understand the impact of induced hair cell regeneration on neural connections and the brain in order to predict the ultimate impact of mammalian hair cell regeneration on restoring the complex mechanisms involved in hearing and understanding human speech.

This chapter addressed the current state of basic science regarding the status of hair cell regeneration in mammals. While that information is vital to initiating some form of therapeutic advance, it is relatively far removed from everyday clinical practice. Forward-thinking clinicians have questions regarding the impact of potential therapies on their clinical practice. Significant among these questions are as follows: When will hair cell regeneration be a reality for patients? What will the measures of candidacy be? What will the impact of hair cell regeneration be in patients who are or have been candidates for hearing aids or other amplification devices? Will hearing aids or cochlear implants continue to be necessary in the face of hair cell regeneration? We have addressed these questions individually in a previous review

(Matsui & Ryals, 2006) but will summarize our thoughts here.

The time frame for human hair cell regeneration therapy is certainly much closer now than it was in 1988 when the first papers on hair cell regeneration were published. Scientists now know that it is possible to regenerate in mature mammals, at least to a limited extent, hair cells and many other cells within the inner ear. That is a huge step forward, but not big enough to begin regenerating hair cells in humans. Many questions remain to be answered in other mammalian animal models before physicians can begin human therapy. Certainly, the overarching issue is whether mammalian hair cell regeneration is sufficiently safe and robust to restore hearing and balance function. The fact that regenerating avian hair cells results in the restoration of hearing sensitivity, complex perception, and vestibular function is promising for the future potential of hair cell regeneration to restore hearing and balance function in mammals.

The question of candidacy for hair cell regeneration therapy must be considered in light of scientists' understanding of the mechanisms of hearing and hair cell regeneration. The unique and elegant architecture and electrochemical environment of the cochlea is critical to hearing function. For example, hair cell regeneration in the absence of a tectorial membrane or an endocochlear potential is not likely to be sufficient for hearing restoration. Candidacy therapeutic intervention involving hair cell regeneration must be evaluated in terms of the underlying genetic, anatomical, and biochemical mechanisms that contribute to the origin of the hearing loss. Therefore, it will be essential in the coming years to develop the most accurate and specific diagnostic assessments possible for the multiple etiologies underlying sensorineural hearing loss.

Hair cell regeneration occurs spontaneously in birds immediately after damage and cell loss. Therefore, research in birds has done little to increase scientists' understanding of hair cell regeneration or their ability to restore hearing in the face of long-term hair cell damage and hearing loss. The influence of duration of hearing loss/cochlear damage on candidacy for treatments through hair cell regeneration is as yet unknown. However, since experience with cochlear implantation in adults with long-standing hearing loss has been positive, it seems likely that duration of hair cell loss will not obviate potential treatment through hair cell regeneration.

Studies of hair cell regeneration in a bird with genetic, progressive deafness (Gleich et al., 1995c; Dooling et al., 1997; Wilkins et al., 2001) show that hair cell regeneration neither fully restores the number of hair cells nor restores hearing. In this bird (Belgian Waterslager canary), the genetic disorder appears to be localized to the hair cells themselves; the auditory nerve fibers are minimally affected (Gleich et al., 2001; Kubke et al., 2002c). Therefore, hair cell regeneration may not be a viable therapy in some humans with genetic abnormalities at the level of the hair cell. More research on the influence of existing genetic abnormalities on hair cell regeneration is needed in order to more fully answer questions of candidacy in patients with genetic inner ear abnormalities.

Once regeneration has been stimulated in birds, other structures within the ear also appear to repair (Cotanche, 1999). Recent evidence in mature mammals has shown that stem cells have the potential to regenerate several cell types within the cochlea (Matsui & Cotanche, 2004; Parker & Cotanche, 2004). It is certain that regenerating more than one cell type, such as restoring both hair cells and supporting cells, will be more complex than regenerating a single cell type. That is particularly true when cell differentiation is guided primarily by genetic cues as opposed to local environmental cues. Therefore, scientists will need to understand the structural integrity of the cochlea prior to treatment through regenerative therapy. The prognosis for restoring hearing through hair cell regeneration will certainly be influenced by the inherent structural integrity of the cochlea. However, again taking a cue from cochlear implant research, it seems likely that damage to cells other than hair cells will not necessarily preclude the possibility of help through regenerative therapy.

Finally, some clinicians have questioned the impact of future regenerative therapies on patients who have been treated with amplification devices or cochlear implants. Will hair cell regeneration eliminate the need for hearing aids and cochlear implants? The short answer to that question is that it is highly unlikely that hair cell regenerative therapies will restore a fully functioning cochlea. If the potential for safely initiating hair cell regeneration in humans does become a possibility, the first attempts will probably result in incomplete replacement of all structures necessary for normal hearing. Even incomplete replacement, however, could be very good news for patients with sensorineural hearing loss and for audiologists. Patients with difficult-to-fit hearing losses (very severe to profound, corner audiograms, or severe to profound sharply sloping high-frequency hearing loss) could benefit greatly from the restoration of just a few hair cells. Adding a few hair cells connected to the appropriate neural fibers might increase sensitivity to the point where amplification can be useful. Therefore, hair cell regeneration therapy might increase the number of patients benefiting from amplification. For those individuals with less severe hearing loss but with unsatisfactory hearing aid use, scientists could expect that restoring some outer hair cells might result in an ear with better tuning and less loudness distortion.

It seems hard to imagine that improved medical treatment of sensorineural hearing loss through therapies such as hair cell regeneration can be anything but positive for audiologists and the patients they treat. Further research into the basic cellular, molecular, and genetic mechanisms underlying hair cell regeneration, always done with an eye to translation into clinical practice, can hold only a positive potential for all patients with heretofore permanent sensorineural hearing loss.

REFERENCES

Adler, H., Komeda, M., et al. (1997). Further evidence for supporting cell conversion in the damaged avian basilar papilla. *Int J Dev Neurosci, 15*, 375–385.

Adler, H., & Raphael, Y. (1996). New hair cells arise from supporting cell conversion in the acoustically damaged chick inner ear. *Proc Natl Acad Sci USA, 97*, 11722–11729.

Akazawa, C., Ishibashi, M., et al. (1995). A mammalian helix-loop-helix factor structurally related to the product of Drosophila proneural gene atonal is a positive transcriptional regulator expressed in the developing nervous system. *J Biol Chem, 270,* 8730–8738.

Baird, R. A., Steyer, P. S., et al. (1996). Mitotic and nonmitotic hair cell regeneration in the bullfrog vestibular otolith organs. *J Neurosci, 781,* 59–70.

Balak, K., Corwin, J, et al. (1990). Regenerated hair cells can originate from supporting cell progeny: Evidence from phototoxicity and laser ablation experiments in the lateral line system. *J Neurosci, 10*(8), 2502–2512.

Bermingham, N., Gassan, B., et al. (1999). Math1: An essential gene for the generation of inner ear hair cells. *Science, 284,* 1837–1841.

Bermingham-McDonogh, O., & Rubel, E. W. (2003). Hair cell regeneration: Winging our way towards a sound future. *Curr Opin Neurobiol, 13*(1), 119–126.

Bhave, S., Oesterle, E. C., et al. (1998). Macrophage and microglia-like cells in the avian inner ear. *J Comp Neurol, 398*(2), 241–256.

Bryant, J., Goodyear, R., et al. (2002). Sensory organ development in the inner ear: Molecular and cellular mechanisms. *British Medical Bulletin, 63,* 39–57.

Carey, J. P., Fuchs, A. F., et al. (1996). Hair cell regeneration and recovery of the vestibulo-ocular reflex in the avian vestibular system. *J Neurophysiol, 76*(5), 3301–3312.

Carey, J. P., Fuchs, A. F., et al. (1996). Hair cell regeneration and vestibulo-ocular reflex recovery. *J Neurosci, 781*(47), 47–58.

Chen, L., & Segil, N. (1999). p27(Kip1) links cell proliferation to morphogenesis in the developing organ of Corti. *Development, 126,* 1581–1590.

Chen, P., Johnson, J., et al. (2002). The role of Math1 in inner ear development: Uncoupling the establishment of the sensory primordium from hair cell fate determination. *Development, 129*(10), 2495–24505.

Chen, P., Zindy, F., et al. (2003). Progressive hearing loss in mice lacking the cyclin-dependent kinase inhibitor Ink4d. *Nature Cell Biology, 5,* 422–426.

Corwin, J. T. & Cotanche, D. A. (1988). Regeneration of sensory hair cells after acoustic trauma. *Science, 240*(4860), 1772–1774.

Cotanche, D. A. (1987). Regeneration of hair cell stereociliary bundles in the chick cochlea following severe acoustic trauma. *Hearing Research, 30*(2–3), 181–195.

Cotanche, D. A. (1999). Structural recovery from sound and aminoglycoside damage in the avian cochlea. *Audiol Neurootol, 4*(6), 271–285.

Cruz, R. M., Lambert, P. R., et al. (1987). Light microscopic evidence of hair cell regeneration after gentamicin toxicity in chick cochlea. *Arch Otolaryngol Head Neck Surg, 113*(10), 1058–1062.

Doetzlhofer, A., White, P., et al. (2004). In vitro growth and differentiation of mammalian sensory hair cell progenitors: A requirement for EGF and periotic mesenchyme. *Dev Biol, 272*(2), 432–447.

Doetzihofer, A., White, P., et al. (2005). Mitotic hair cell generation by postnatal cochlear supporting cells. *ARO,* 819.

Dooling, R. J., Ryals, B. M., et al. (1997). The paradox of the Belgian Waterslager canary: Congenital hair cell abnormalities and hearing loss despite post mitotic hair cell replacement. In A. R. Palmer, A. Rees, A. Q. Summerfield, & R. Meddis (Eds.), Proceedings of the 11th International Symposium on Hearing: *Psychophysical and physiological advances in hearing* (pp. 145–152). London: Whurr Publishers.

Dooling, R. J., Ryals, B. M., et al. (1997). Recovery of hearing and vocal behavior after hair cell regeneration. *PNAS, 94,* 14206–14210.

Forge, A., Li, L., et al. (1993). Ultrastructural evidence for hair cell regeneration in the mammalian inner ear. *Science, 259,* 1616–1619.

Girod, D., Duckert, L., et al. (1989). Possible precursors of regenerated hair cells in the avian cochlea following acoustic trauma. *Hear Res, 42,* 175–194.

Gleich, O., Dooling, R. J., et al. (2001). A quantitative analysis of the nerve fibers in the VIIIth nerve of Belgian Waterslager canaries with a hereditary sensorineural hearing loss. *Hear Res, 151*(1–2), 141–148.

Gleich, O., Klump, G. M., et al. (1995c). Peripheral basis for the auditory deficit in Belgian Waterslager canaries (Serinus canarius). *Hear Res, 82*(1), 100–108.

Goode, C.T., C., Carey, J. P., et al. (1999). Recovery of the vestibulocolic reflex after aminoglycoside ototoxicity in domestic chickens. *J Neurophysiol, 81*(3), 1025–1035.

Goode, C.T., C., Maney, D., et al. (2001). Visual influences on the development and recovery of the vestibulo-ocular reflex in the chicken. *J Neurophysiol, 85*(3), 1119–1128.

Izumikawa, M., Minoda, R., et al. (2005). Auditory hair cell replacement and hearing improvement by Atoh1 gene therapy in deaf mammals. *Nature Medicine, 11,* 271–276.

Jones, S. M., Ryals, B., et al. (1998). Vestibular function in Belgian Waterslager canaries (Serinus canarius). *Hear Res, 121*(1–2), 161–169.

Jones, T. A., & Nelson, R. C. (1992). Recovery of vestibular function following hair cell destruction by streptomycin. *Hear Res, 62*(2), 181–186.

Jorgensen, J. M. & Mathiesen, C. (1988). The avian inner ear. Continuous production of hair cells in vestibular sensory organs, but not in the auditory papilla. *Naturwissenschaften, 75,* 319–320.

Kawamoto, K., Ishimoto, S., et al. (2003). Math1 gene transfer generates new cochlear hair cells in mature guinea pigs in vivo. *J Neurosci, 23*(11), 4395–4400.

Kelley, M. W. (2002). Determination and commitment of mechanosensory hair cells. *Scientific World Journal, 2,* 1079–1094.

Kiernan, A., Pelling, A., et al. (2005). Sox2 is required for sensory organ development in the mammalian inner ear. *Nature, 434*(7036), 1031–1035.

Kirkegaard, M., & Jorgensen, J. (2000). Continuous hair cell turnover in the inner ear vestibular organs of a mammal, the Daubenton's bat (Myotis daubentonii). *Naturwissenschaften, 87,* 83–86.

Kondo, T., Johnson, S., et al. (2005). Sonic hedgehog and retinoic acid synergistically promote sensory fate specification from bone marrow-derived pluripotent stem cells. *Proc Natl Acad Sci USA, 102*(13), 4789–4794.

Kubke, M. F., Dent, M. L., et al. (2002c). Nucleus magnocellularis and nucleus laminaris in Belgian Waterslager and normal strain canaries. *Hear Res, 164*(1–2), 19–28.

Ladher, R., Anakwe, K., et al. (2000). Identification of synergistic signals initiating inner ear development. *Science, 290,* 1965–1967.

Lanford, P., Shailam, R., et al. (2000). Expression of Math1 and HES5 in the cochleae of wildtype and Jag2 mutant mice. *JARO, 1,* 161–170.

Li, H., Corrales, C., et al. (2004). Stem cells as therapy for hearing loss. *Trends Mol Med, 10*(7), 309–315.

Li, H., Liu, H., et al. (2003). Pluripotent stem cells from the adult mouse inner ear. *Nat Med, 9*(10), 1293–1299.

Li, H., Roblin, G., et al. (2003). Generation of hair cells by stepwise differentiation of embryonic stem cells. *Proc Natl Acad Sci USA, 100*(23), 13495–13500.

Lopez, I., Zhao, P., et al. (2004). Stem/progenitor cells in the postnatal inner ear of the GFP-nestin transgenic mouse. *Int J Dev Neurosci, 22*(4), 205–213.

Lowenheim, H., Furness, D., et al. (1999). Gene disruption of p27(Kip1) allows cell proliferation in the postnatal and adult organ of Corti. *Proc Natl Acad Sci USA, 96*(7), 4084–4088.

Matsui, J. I., & Cotanche, D. A. (2004). Sensory hair cell death and regeneration: Two halves of the same equation. *Curr Opin Otolaryngol Head Neck Surg, 12*(5), 418–425.

Matsui, J. I., Haque, A., et al. (2003). Caspase inhibitors promote vestibular hair cell survival and function after aminoglycoside treatment in vivo. *J Neurosci, 23*(14), 6111–6122.

Matsui, J. I., & Ryals, B. (2006). Hair cell regeneration: An exciting phenomenon, but will it be possible to restore hearing and balance? *Journal of Rehabilitation Research and Development, 42*(4):187–198

Montcouquiol, M., & Corwin, J. T. (2001). Intracellular signals that control cell proliferation in mammalian balance epithelia: Key roles for phosphatidylinositol-3 kinase, mammalian target of rapamycin, and S6 kinases in preference to calcium, protein kinase C, and mitogen-activated protein kinase. *J Neurosci, 21*(2), 570–580.

Oesterle, E. C., Bhave, S., et al. (2000). Basic fibroblast growth factor inhibits cell proliferation in cultured avian inner ear sensory epithelia. *J Comp Neurol, 424*(2), 307–326.

Oesterle, E. C., & Rubel, E. W. (1993). Postnatal production of supporting cells in the chick cochlea. *Hear Res, 66*(2), 213–224.

Parker, M., & Cotanche, D. A. (2004). The potential use of stem cells for cochlear repair. *Audiol & Neuro-Otol, 9,* 72–80.

Roberson, D., & Rubel, E. W. (1994). Cell division in the gerbil cochlea after acoustic trauma. *Am J Otol, 15,* 28–34.

Roberson, D. W., Alosi, J., et al. (2004). Direct transdifferentiation gives rise to the earliest new hair cells in regenerating avian auditory epithelium. *J Neuroscience Res, 78,* 461–471.

Roberson, D. W., Kreig, C., et al. (1996). Light microscopic evidence that pre-mitotic transdifferentiation may give rise to new hair cells in the regenerating avian auditory epithelium. *Aud Neurosci, 2,* 195–205.

Roberson, D. W., Weisleder, P., et al. (1992). Ongoing production of sensory cells in the vestibular epithelium of the chick. *Hear Res, 57*(2), 166–174.

Rubel, E. W. (1978). Ontogeny of structure and function in the vertebrate auditory system. In M. Jacobson (Ed.), *Handbook of Sensory Physiology* (pp. 135–237). New York: Springer-Verlag.

Ruben, R. (1967). Development of the inner ear of the mouse: A radioautographic study of terminal mitoses. *Acta Otolaryngol Suppl, 220,* 221–244.

Ryals, B. (2000). Regeneration of the auditory pathway. Valente, M., Hosford-Dunn, H., & Roeser, R. In *Audiology Treatment* (pp. 755–771). New York: Thieme Medical Publishers.

Ryals, B., & Dooling, I. R. J. (1996). Changes in innervation and auditory sensitivity following acoustic trauma and hair cell regeneration in birds. Salvi R. J., Henderson, D., Fiorino, F., & Colletti, V. In *Auditory Plasticity and Regeneration* (pp. 84–100). New York: Thieme Medical Publishers.

Ryals, B. M. (2000b). Regeneration of the auditory pathway. Valente, M., Hosford-Dunn, H., & Roeser, R. In *Audiology Treatment* (pp. 755–771). New York: Thieme Medical Publishers.

Ryals, B. M., & Cunningham, L. (2003). A primer on biology of hair cell regeneration, rescue, and repair. *Seminars in Hearing, 24*(2), 99–110.

Ryals, B. M., & Dooling, R. J. (2000). Discussion: Changes in vocal production and auditory perception after hair cell regeneration. *J Communication Disorder, 33*(4), 313–319.

Ryals, B. M., & Rubel, E. W. (1988). Hair cell regeneration after acoustic trauma in adult Cotumix quail. *Science, 240,* 1774–1776.

Ryan, A. (2003). The cell cycle and the development and regeneration of hair cells. *Curr Top Dev Biol, 57,* 449–466.

Sage, C., Huang, M., et al. (2005). Proliferation of functional hair cells in vivo in the absence of the retinoblastoma protein. *Science, 307*(5712), 1114–1118.

Smolders, J. W. (1999). Functional recovery in the avian ear after hair cell regeneration. *Audiol Neurootol, 4*(6), 286–302.

Steyger, P. S., Burton, M., et al. (1997). Calbindin and parvalbumin are early markers of non-mitotically regenerating hair cells in the bullfrog vestibular otolith organs. *Int J Dev Neurosci, 15,* 417–432.

Stone, J., Oesterle, E., et al. (1998). Recent insights into regeneration of auditory and vestibular hair cells. *Curr Opin Neurol, 11*(1), 17–24.

Stone, J. S., & Cotanche, D. A. (1992). Synchronization of hair cell regeneration in the chick cochlea following noise damage. *J Cell Sci, 102*(Pt. 4), 671–680.

Stone, J. S., & Contache, D. A. (1994). Identification of the timing of S phase and the patterns of cell proliferation during hair cell regeneration in the chick cochlea. *J Comp Neurol, 341*(1), 50–67.

Stone, J. S., & Rubel, E. W. (2000). Cellular studies of auditory hair cell regeneration in birds. *Proc Natl Acad Sci USA 97,* 11714–11721.

Warchol, M. E. (1997). Macrophage activity in organ cultures of the avian cochlea: demonstration of a resident population and recruitment to sites of hair cell lesions. *J Neurobiol, 33*(6), 724–734.

Warchol, M. E. (1999). Immune cytokines and dexamethasone influence sensory regeneration in the avian vestibular periphery. *J Neurocytol, 28*(10–11), 889–900.

Warchol, M. E., & Corwin, J. T. (1996). Regenerative proliferation in organ cultures of the avian cochlea: Identification of the initial progenitors and determination of the latency of the proliferative response. *J Neurosci, 16,* 5466–5477.

Warchol, M. E., Lambert, P. R., et al. (1993). Regenerative proliferation in inner ear sensory epithelia from adult guinea pigs and humans. *Science, 259,* 1619–1622.

Warchol, M. E., & Matsui, J. I. (2001). Ongoing cell death and immune influences on regeneration in the vestibular sensory organs. *J Neurosci, 942,* 34–45.

Warchol, M. E., Matsui, J. I., et al. (2001). Ongoing cell death and immune influences on regeneration in the vestibular sensory organs. *J Neurosci, 942,* 34–45.

Wilkins, H. R., Presson, J. C., et al. (2001). Hair cell death in a hearing-deficient canary. *J Assoc Res Otolaryngol, 2*(1), 79–86.

Witte, M., Montcouquiol, M., et al. (2001). Regeneration in avian hair cell epithelia: Identification of intracellular signals required for S-phase entry. *Eur J Neurosci, 14*(5), 829–838.

Woods, C., Montcouquiol, M., et al. (2004). Math1 regulates development of the sensory epithelium in the mammalian cochlea. *Nature Neuroscience, 7*(12), 1310–1318.

Woolley, S. M., & Rubel, E. W. (1997). Bengalese finches Lonchura Striata domestica depend upon auditory feedback for the maintenance of adult song. *J Neurosci, 17*(16), 6380–6390.

Woolley, S. M., & Rubel, E. W. (1999). High-frequency auditory feedback is not required for adult song maintenance in Bengalese finches. *J Neurosci, 19*(1), 358–371.

Woolley, S. M., & Rubel, E. W. (2002). Vocal memory and learning in adult Bengalese finches with regenerated hair cells. *J Neurosci, 22*(17), 7774–7787.

Woolley, S. M., Wissman, A. M., et al. (2001). Hair cell regeneration and recovery of auditory thresholds following aminoglycoside ototoxicity in Bengalese finches. *Hear Res, 153*(1–2): 181–195.

Zheng, J., & Gao, W. (2000). Overexpression of Math1 induces robust production of extra hair cells in postnatal rat inner ears. *Nat Neurosci, 3*(6), 580–586.

Zheng, J. L., Shou, J., et al. (2000). Hes1 is a negative regulator of inner ear hair cell differentiation. *Development, 127*(21), 4551–4560.

Zine, A., Aubert, A., et al. (2001). Hes1 and Hes5 activities are required for the normal development of the hair cells in the mammalian inner ear. *J Neurosci, 21*(13), 4712–4720.

Zine, A., & de Ribaupierre, F. (2002). Notch/Notch ligands and Math1 expression patterns in the organ of Corti of wild-type and Hes1 and Hes5 mutant mice. *Hear Res, 170*(1–2), 22–31.

Zine, A., Van De Water, T., et al. (2000). Notch signaling regulates the pattern of auditory hair cell differentiation in mammals. *Development, 127,* 3373–3383.

CHAPTER

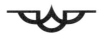

21

From Pharmacology to Function: Using Drugs as Tools to Dissect the Cochlea

Sharon G. Kujawa, PhD[1,2,3,4]
Department of Audiology
Massachusetts Eye and Ear Infirmary

William F. Sewell, PhD[1,3,4,5]
Eaton Peabody Laboratory
Massachusetts Eye and Ear Infirmary

[1]Department of Otology and Laryngology, Harvard Medical School; [2]Department of Audiology, Massachusetts Eye and Ear Infirmary; [3]Eaton-Peabody Laboratory, Massachusetts Eye and Ear Infirmary; [4]Harvard-MIT Speech and Hearing Bioscience and Technology Program; [5]Program in Neuroscience, Harvard Medical School.

INTRODUCTION

A drug, broadly defined, is a chemical with the ability to affect some process in a living system (organism or cell). Clinicians may want to use drugs as tools in the diagnosis, treatment, and prevention of human disease. They also may be concerned with drugs that have toxic side effects that compromise health by impairing function. Another use of drugs that has both basic science and clinical application is as tools to dissect physiological and biochemical processes supporting normal function. That application is the focus of this chapter.

The role of a cell or a system can be probed by perturbing its function. Perturbations introduced using pharmacologic tools have provided important insights on the functioning of complex and poorly accessible systems. In the ear, for example, drugs have helped identify the origins of certain cochlear versus neural responses, they have helped to characterize the unique roles of outer hair cells (OHCs) versus inner hair cells (IHCs) in hearing, they have been used to delineate the role of the endocochlear potential (EP) in cochlear function, and they have clarified the classes and properties of receptors mediating afferent and efferent neurotransmission.

This chapter reviews some traditional pharmacologic approaches and tools to study biologic function in general and cochlear function in particular. Effective use of drugs in this fashion requires understanding the biochemistry of their interactions with components of biological systems; thus, common cellular sites, mechanisms, and consequences of drug action will be considered. The inaccessibility of the cochlea poses specific challenges to pharmacologic study; methods developed to address those challenges also will be discussed. Finally, the chapter will consider some of the newer, combined pharmacologic-microbiologic/genetic approaches that could yield new drugs to provide powerful and sophisticated ways to dissect cochlear function and remediate dysfunction.

SITES, MECHANISMS, AND CONSEQUENCES OF DRUG ACTION

Receptors

Whether used as research probes or therapeutic agents, most drugs exert their biological actions by interacting with receptors. The term *receptor* is used in pharmacology to identify a biological molecule to which a drug (ligand) binds. Receptors are almost always membrane proteins; other targets, such as enzymes and DNA, exist as well. Most pharmacologically useful receptors are those to which some endogenous biological compound normally binds. Exogenously-applied drugs that bind to the receptor and mimic the endogenous compound are called agonists, and those that prevent the endogenous compound from acting are called antagonists.

The interaction between drugs and receptors is usually a reversible chemical reaction governed by the law of mass action. That is, the magnitude of the effect is directly related to the concentration of the drug and the number of available receptors. In practice, the effect also is limited by the range over which the system can respond. Some drugs have a high affinity for the receptor and, thus, are very potent (acting at very low concentrations). Drugs acting on the same receptor can differ in their ability to block or stimulate the receptor. Traditionally, a dose-response curve (Figure 21-1) is used to express the magnitude of the effect as a function of the concentration of the drug. From the dose response curve, one can determine the efficacy, or maximal effect (Emax), of the drug and the potency of the drug. A measure of potency is the EC50, which is the concentration at which the drug produces its half-maximal effect.

Most drugs begin to influence multiple processes as concentration increases. The selectivity of a drug is the separation in dose between the desired effect and unintended effects. Selectivity of a drug (and, consequently, its value as a probe of function) increases with decreasing concentration. The more potent a drug, the more likely the drug will act selectively.

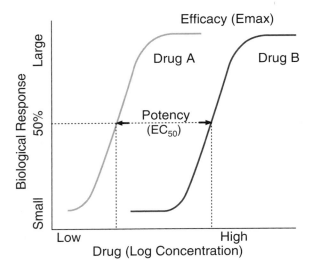

Figure 21-1. The dose-response relation for two drugs. Drugs A and B produce the same maximum biological effect, shown by Emax; however, Drug A achieves its effect at a much lower concentration than Drug B. Drugs are often compared in terms of the concentration required to produce a half-maximal effect (EC50). Drug A in this example is said to be more potent than Drug B, and Drug A's actions will likely be more selective in the system under study.

Receptors as Drug Targets

Many receptors span the cell membrane. Those receptors are often used in communicating between cells or in taking up compounds special to the function of that cell and, thus, are particularly useful as drug targets. Examples of membrane proteins that can be probed pharmacologically include neurotransmitter receptors, some hormone receptors, and metabolic transporters.

A second major class of receptors includes intracellular or extracellular proteins. Drugs most useful at these targets are those that affect proteins specific to a specific type of cell. Examples include intracellular and extracellular enzymes, and proteins used in cell motility, those involved in generation of cytoplasmic second messengers, and those regulating intracellular calcium. Some hormones bind intracellularly to DNA in the nucleus and through that binding can alter protein transcription.

Neurotransmitter Receptors

Neurons communicate with one another by releasing chemical messengers (neurotransmitters), which tend to be relatively small molecules. The neurotransmitter diffuses across a synaptic cleft to bind to its receptor on the receiving neuron. Neurotransmitter receptors fall into one of two categories. Ionotropic receptors are those that comprise an ion channel. The receptor spans the membrane, forming a pore. The pore is normally closed until binding of the neurotransmitter opens it, allowing certain ions to flow (Figure 21-2). The resulting change in membrane permeability and flow of charged ions results in an electrical change in the cell. Antagonism of such receptors can be chemical, wherein the agonist and antagonist agents physically combine, with inactivation of the agonist a possible result; physiological, in which the agonist and antagonist ligands bind to two different sites on the receptor, inducing effects that oppose one another; or pharmacological, resulting in agonist-antagonist competition for occupancy and/or activity at the same binding site.

Less directly, and with a correspondingly longer time course, transmitter binding to its receptor may be communicated to the interior of the cell through one or several intermediate steps, as shown in Figure 21-3 for metabotropic receptors. Metabotropic receptors are those that include a G protein binding site. Here the first messenger (neurotransmitter) or an exogenously applied agonist binds to the receptor, leading to activation of GTP-binding proteins (G proteins). Those proteins may interact directly with a membrane ion channel (left panel), changing its open probability and, thus, the likelihood that ions will flow through its pore. Alternatively, they may modulate second messenger-mediated processes in the cell that regulate the activity of specific cell-signal effector proteins (middle panel). Effector proteins can be enzymes, ion channels, or transport proteins.

Drugs affecting neurotransmitter receptors have been particularly useful in neurobiology since they can be used to selectively block communication between neurons. Substances that alter the ability of a neuron to assemble and package neurotransmitter substrates or release the neurotransmitter are said to act presynaptically, while those that act on the

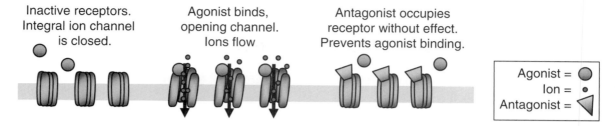

Figure 21-2. Ionotropic (ligand-gated) receptors. Signal transduction is initiated by the binding of an agonist to the receptor. A conformational change in the receptor opens the integral ion channel, allowing flow of ions and resulting in a change in electrical activity of the cell. In this simplified example, antagonist binding to the agonist binding site produces no postsynaptic effect of its own, but prevents the agonist binding and, hence, agonist-activated effects. Other arrangements are possible; for example, antagonists can bind to other sites on the receptor and act in a fashion competitive to the agonist. Agonist = ◯; Ion = •; Antagonist = ◁. (Adapted from Dale and Hylett)

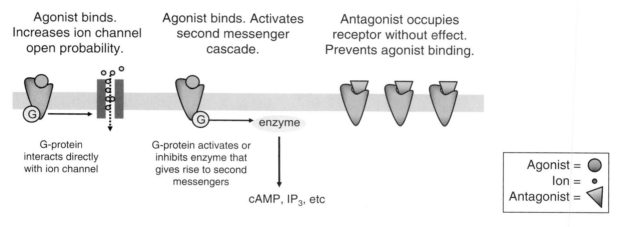

Figure 21-3. Metabotropic (G protein coupled) receptors. Neurotransmitter binding activates G proteins that, in turn, modulate ion channel opening/closing or enzyme activity and "second messenger"-mediated cascades within the cell that regulate various intracellular effector proteins. Antagonism can be achieved by several mechanisms (see Figure 21-2 legend). Agonist = ◯; Ion = •; Antagonist = ◁. (Adapted from Dale and Hylett)

neurotransmitter receptor as ligands or on the released transmitter substance to alter its time window of availability for binding are said to act postsynaptically. Indeed, in addition to drugs that activate or block the endogenous transmitter's actions at the postsynaptic receptor, the toolbox for modulating synaptic transmission also may include agents that act by any of the pre- or postsynaptic mechanisms depicted in Figure 21-4.

Ion Channels

Ion channels provide controlled access through the otherwise poorly penetrable lipid bilayer of the cell membrane. In addition to those that are ligand gated, some ion channels are gated by changes in the electrical activity of cells and some are gated by mechanical stimulation. Voltage-gated ion channels are sensitive to membrane potential. Thus, processes

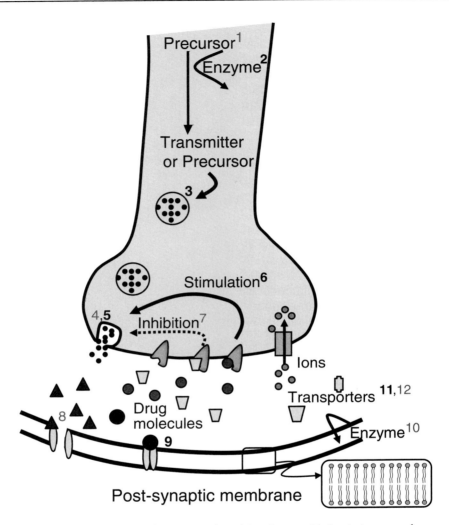

Figure 21-4. Drug modulation of synaptic transmission. This can occur through interference with chemical precursors[1] or enzymes[2] required for transmitter manufacture. interference with packaging and storing transmitter or precursors in vesicles[3], stimulating[4] or inhibiting[5] vesicle fusion and transmitter release, activating[6] or blocking[7] presynaptic autoreceptors, activating[8] or blocking[9] postsynaptic receptors for the transmitter, interfering with enzymes[10] required for breakdown of the released transmitter, or enhancing[11] or interfering[12] with transporters required for reuptake and recycling of the by-products. Drugs that interfere with transmission are coded in **gray** (red in color plates); those that facilitate transmission, in **black**. (Adapted from Jackson)

that alter the potential difference between the interior and exterior of the cell (e.g., the flow of ions through receptor-mediated ion channels) may gate such channels and allow ions to flow. Some ion channels, such as the hair cell transduction channel, are said to be mechanically gated. Deflection of the hair cell

stereocilia in the excitatory direction opens those channels. The hair cell transduction current and its modulation by drugs are discussed in greater detail later in this chapter.

Ion channels act as filters. Some are highly specific and allow only ions of a certain ionic species through the cell membrane; thus, there are calcium channels, potassium channels, sodium channels, and so on. Other ion channels are less specific and may allow families of ions that can be grouped on the basis of charge or size to pass through. Interference with ion channels by drugs can alter basic functions of cells and systems.

Voltage-dependent sodium channels, for example, are crucial to the excitation of excitable cells (e.g., neurons). Those channels play a central role in the generation and conduction of action potentials. The function of these channels is subject to modulation by various naturally occurring toxins (e.g., tetrodotoxin from puffer fish, spider, bee, and scorpion venoms). The small molecules act with a high degree of potency and selectivity and, thus, are valuable pharmacologic tools in the investigation of neurotransmission. Drugs are available that can block the sodium channels needed to generate action potentials (tetrodotoxin), various forms of calcium-activated potassium conductances (apamin, charybdotoxin, and iberiotoxin), and voltage-dependent calcium channels (dihydropyridines).

Other Membrane Receptors

Neurotransmitter receptors are important for relatively rapid cell-to-cell communication, but other intracellular signals also can act on membrane receptors. Examples include some hormones and other factors that control cell growth and development. These receptors generally have an extracellular binding domain for the communication signal and an intracellular domain that is usually either a protein kinase (enzyme), which acts by phosphorylating intracellular proteins to change their properties, or a guanylyl cyclase (enzyme), which synthesizes the second messenger cyclic GMP.

Transporter Proteins

Transporters are proteins used to move substances from one side of the lipid bilayer to the other. All cells contain transporters, but some cells contain high amounts of specific transporters related to their special function. Transporters are highly specific for their intended substrate. Transporters either facilitate movement of a compound down a concentration gradient (often called facilitated diffusion) or use metabolic energy (ATP) to transport a compound against a concentration gradient. Many cells rely on ATP-dependent pumps to maintain an ionic balance in the cell. An enzyme, Na,K-ATPase, for example, is used extensively in the cochlea to maintain high-potassium/low-sodium concentrations in the cells. Because many hair cell processes are regulated by intracellular calcium, several forms of Ca-ATPase are present in hair cells.

DNA-binding hormones

Many hormones, including steroid hormones, thyroid hormones, and vitamin D, diffuse into the cell to interact with receptor sites specific to nuclear DNA. The hormones and drugs that interact with those sites can control transcription of proteins in the cell.

Enzymes

Enzymes serve as catalysts in the transformation of one compound into another. Enzymes are needed for virtually every function in the cell. Some enzymes perform roles special to certain cell types. For example, neurons that communicate via the neurotransmitter acetylcholine often secrete acetylcholinesterase (AChE) into the synaptic cleft. That enzyme is used to break down acetylcholine after it is released as a neurotransmitter. Drugs that target enzymes provide powerful means to modulate intra- and extracellular signals. Drugs can inhibit enzymes either by competing with the chemical substrate on which the enzyme normally acts or by binding to regulatory sites on the enzyme (Figure 21-4). A drug that interferes with AChE (e.g., physostigmine) would prolong the action of the transmitter agent.

Drug Actions not Mediated by Receptors

Examples include chelating agents (drugs that bind to divalent cations and metals to effectively reduce the concentration of those elements free in solution); ions themselves, such as lithium, magnesium, and potassium; and drugs that act through their colligative properties rather than through specific chemical structure. Examples include some diuretics and some general anesthetics.

PHARMACOLOGIC TOOLS AND THEIR ACTIONS IN THE COCHLEA

With that background, one can begin to consider the application of pharmacologic tools in the study of normal cochlear function. Sites, mechanisms, and consequences of drug action in the cochlea display many similarities to processes already discussed, with some adaptations related to the unique nature of the chemical environment and the specialized functions of the cochlear machinery. The effective use of pharmacologic tools in the cochlea has special constraints that are reviewed in the following sections.

Chemical Composition of Cochlear Fluids

The two specialized types of extracellular fluid in the inner ear are perilymph and endolymph. A more detailed description of the sources, chemical composition, volumes, and flow characteristics of those fluids may be found in Salt and Konishi (1986). General characteristics of the electrochemical environment of the cochlea are considered here.

Perilymph, a fluid with a chemical composition grossly similar to that of other extracellular fluids in the body, fills the scala vestibuli and scala tympani and bathes most of the structures of the organ of Corti, including the dendritic endings of the auditory nerve fibers, the basolateral surfaces of the hair cells (but not the apical surfaces or stereocilia), and the spiral ligament (Figure 21-5). The perilymph of scala tympani is in diffusional continuity with the cerebrospinal fluid (CSF) via the cochlear aqueduct and is generally similar in ionic composition to CSF.

Endolymph, a fluid unlike any other extracellular fluid in the body, is similar in cationic composition to intracellular fluid, having a high K+ concentration and a low Na+ concentration. It fills the greater fluid space of scala media, bathing the apical surfaces of the hair cells, but does not have access to their basolateral surfaces. The cells that line the endolymph fluid compartment of scala media are connected with tight junctions that separate the unique electrochemical environments of the perilymph- and endolymph-containing compartments. That separation of the two fluids

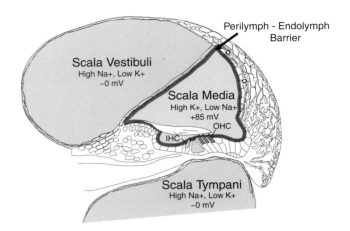

Figure 21-5. Fluid spaces in the cochlea. Epithelial cells lining the endolymph-filled cochlear duct (scala media) are connected by tight junctions (denoted by heavy line surrounding scala media; red in color plates), forming a barrier separating this fluid compartment from those containing perilymph (scala vestibuli and scala tympani). Note that perilymph diffuses through the basilar membrane; thus, basolateral surfaces of hair cells are in contact with perilymph, while apical surfaces and stereocilia see endolymph.
Anatomy and Embryology, 191, Kikuchi et al., Gap junctions in the rat cochlea: immunohistochemical and ultrastructural analysis, 101–118 (1995). With kind permission of Springer Science and Business Media.

bathing hair cells is an important element in their function as transducers in that they maintain electrical and chemical gradients for current flow.

The electrochemical environment of the cochlear scalae allows the hair cells to transduce acoustic stimulation by modulating a steady-state current flowing from scala media through the hair cells. Gating of the mechanotransducer channels located near the tips of the hair cell stereocilia permits the current to flow into the cell from the surrounding endolymph. The channel is a nonselective cation channel, but most of the current is carried by potassium, which exits the basolateral surface of the hair cell down an electrochemical gradient. Thus, energy expenditure in the stria vascularis relieves the hair cells of expending a great deal of energy in ionic balance during transduction.

Getting Drugs to Inner Ear Targets

Systemic Drug Delivery

In the cochlea, most drug targets of interest are located in the perilymph and endolymph fluid compartments. The challenge is getting drugs to intended inner ear targets in the form and concentration desired without unwanted effects. With careful dosing, some systemically applied drugs have met those challenges. However, systemically delivered drugs often do not achieve a necessary level of selectivity and control to be useful as probes of inner ear function. Even if not systemically toxic, a compound with desirable activity within the cochlea may not be absorbed, may be altered by metabolic processes in the liver, or may not gain access to the inner ear because of its chemical properties. That limited access is due to the presence of a physicochemical barrier to drugs entering the inner ear called the blood-cochlea (blood-labyrinth) barrier.

Blood-Cochlea Barrier

For many drugs, local delivery to the fluids of the inner ear is necessary because of the presence of a blood-cochlea drug barrier, which protects the cochlear fluid spaces and the structures within from the systemic circulation. Though the blood-cochlea barrier has not been as extensively characterized as the blood-brain barrier, it appears to operate similarly. Through the presence of tight junctions between adjacent cells in the inner ear end organs, substances outside those organs encounter substantial physical barriers to entry. The ability of drugs to enter the organs is correlated with their ability to enter into and pass out of the individual cells that form the barrier. Such barriers discriminate molecules on the basis of their size and charge, their solubility in the lipid bilayer, and their association with specific transport molecules. These barriers undoubtedly protect the inner ear and brain from exposure to potentially toxic substances; however, their presence also complicates delivery of substances intended as pharmacologic probes or even as therapeutic agents. Prime candidates for exclusion from the cochlea after systemic injection are complex molecules, such as proteins and peptides, as well as any molecule that is not lipid (fat) soluble. Moreover, access of positively charged drugs into the endolymph is further restricted because of the relatively large (+85 mV) electrical potential in the endolymph. Thus, systemic administration is unsuitable for many pharmacologic manipulations to the inner ear.

Those biochemical features of the cochlea, together with the highly specialized nature of and restricted access to cochlear transduction processes and the cells that support them, pose challenges for those who would use drugs to dissect the function of the various cells and systems of the cochlea. Because of these complications, drug delivery, *per se*, and particularly local drug delivery, has received a fair amount of attention in pharmacologic studies of cochlear function.

Local Drug Delivery

Local drug application by transtympanic perfusion of the middle ear (with the goal of diffusion through the round window membrane (RWM) into the fluid spaces of the inner ear) has been used for many years to deliver both investigative and therapeutic drugs (Schuknecht, 1956). Modifications of this technique attempting to optimize or extend drug contact with the RWM have included placement of drug-containing polymer (Pasic & Rubel, 1989) or drug-soaked Gelfoam (Chen et al., 2004; Heydt et al., 2004) against the RWM or placing the outlet port of a drug delivery pump near the round window niche (Lang et al., 2003; Schmiedt et al., 2002). Such local application has advantages over systemic drug delivery in that drugs so applied can reach their desired targets at higher concentrations and without unwanted systemic side effects. Chronic studies that do not require rigorous control of dosage or separate application of control solutions within an experiment can make good use of such techniques to deliver drugs to the cochlea. Precise control of the amount of drug that diffuses through the membrane and into the inner ear, however, is not possible. This becomes even more problematic when considering delivery of complex macromolecules with limited diffusion coefficients (Salt & Ma, 2001) and those that might require sequenced delivery. To avoid such difficulties, drugs can be infused directly into the fluid spaces of the cochlea (Figure 21-6).

The practice of placing drugs of interest within cochlear perilymphatic spaces via a perfusion technique is a method with a long history of successful application (Fex, 1968; Bobbin & Konishi, 1971; Konishi, 1972; Galley, 1973; Nuttall et al., 1982; Puel et al., 1994; Kujawa et al., 1992a, 1992b, 1993, 1994; Sridhar et al., 1995, 1997). When carefully administered, the technique itself has little effect on a variety of gross cochlear and neural potentials as recorded from sites within and near the cochlea (Kujawa et al., 1994; see also Figures 21-8 and 21-9). This mode of delivery bypasses the blood-cochlea barrier, allowing drugs to reach their intended targets more directly in the form

and concentration desired and with fewer nonspecific actions. Drugs are largely unaltered by metabolic changes that inevitably occur with other routes of administration. Drugs perfused into the perilymph compartment of scala tympani have ready access to the hair cells and the synaptic regions of hair cells, a view supported by investigations in which various stains demonstrated ready access to structures within the organ of Corti when introduced via the scala tympani perilymph compartment (Tonndorf et al., 1962). Additionally, comparisons of the concentrations of cholinergic antagonists required to block the cochlear efferents *in vivo* (Kujawa et al., 1994; Sridhar et al., 1995) and those effective at *in vitro* isolated OHCs (Erostegui et al., 1994) show remarkably close agreement.

In such applications, intracochlear perfusions typically are of short duration (minutes) with effects on cochlear and auditory nerve function assayed at short postperfusion times. The desire for chronic or sequential delivery of compounds has resulted in the development of techniques for the chronic intracochlear perfusion of the perilymphatic space (Chen et al., 2005; Kingma et al., 1992; Brown et al., 1993; Carvalho & Lalwani, 1999). Investigators have shown that with very slow delivery of very small quantities of drug into scala tympani, delicate structures and functions of the cochlea can be preserved while delivering sufficient drug to produce intended effects. Investigations also are under way in which chronic drug delivery will be accomplished via a cochlear implant electrode assembly (Shepherd & Xu, 2002; Paasche et al., 2003). The ultimate objective of these investigations is therapeutic delivery of various neurotrophic agents to support nerve survival in profoundly impaired ears; however, it is easy to imagine that newer short electrode configurations (Gantz & Turner, 2003) could provide a valuable tool for drug delivery to a cochlea with hearing remaining through a portion of its range.

In vitro Drug Delivery

Perhaps the most direct approach to getting drugs exactly where they are intended is to place them directly in contact with the cells of interest and only with the cells of interest. *In vitro* methods sequester

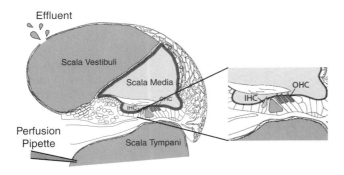

Figure 21-6. Schematic of the cochlear perfusion. Control solutions and drug are commonly introduced into the cochlear perilymph through a hole placed in basal turn scala tympani. A hole in basal turn scala vestibuli allows the effluent to escape. Gap junction barriers are noted by heavy line surrounding scala media (red in color plates). *Anatomy and Embryology*, 191, Kikuchi et al., Gap junctions in the rat cochlea: immunohistochemical and ultrastructural analysis, 101–118 (1995). With kind permission of Springer Science and Business Media.

tissues of interest and place them in a chemically controlled environment in which they can be maintained for acute (or semiacute) pharmacologic, electrophysiologic, or biomechanical study.

In vitro techniques can be as simple as monitoring from and applying drugs to acutely isolated hair cells (Art et al., 1985; Housley & Ashmore, 1992; Erostegui et al., 1994; Dallos et al., 1997; Blanchet et al., 2000; Ricci et al., 2000; Fuchs, 2002) and auditory neurons (Ruel et al., 1999; Trussell, 1999; Parks, 2000), and as complicated as using *in vitro* cochlea preparations that isolate and monitor portions or whole turns of the organ of Corti (Le Calvez & Ulfendahl, 2000; Oliver et al., 2003; He et al., 2004; Chan & Hudspeth, 2005; Goutman et al., 2005).

In vitro systems allow drugs to be added directly to the media, bathing the cells. If more control of timing and concentration is required, drugs can be rapidly injected onto the cell itself; or for drugs with a charged ionic group, an electrical current (iontophoresis) can be used to time delivery. Indeed, very elaborate drug delivery systems have been devised to examine the rapid desensitization that follows application of glutamate agonists to the AMPA receptors that reside on auditory neurons (Trussell, 1999).

In vitro analysis of single cells has its problems, and one must carefully choose the appropriate question for their use. Hair cells removed from the cochlea, for example, no longer have separate fluid media on their apical versus basolateral surfaces. It is possible to pull the apical surface into a microchamber (Evans et al., 1989; Dallos et al., 1997), although doing so removes access to the stereocilia. The ability to displace the stereocilia in isolated hair cells allows one to generate and analyze transduction in the organ (Corey & Hudspeth, 1983).

Some of the problems with isolated hair cells can be overcome by using *in vitro* tissue preparations. The lateral line organ of *Xenopus laevis* has, for decades, served as a model for studying the pharmacology of hair cell organs (Russell & Sellick, 1976; Sewell et al., 1978; Bobbin et al., 1985; Bledsoe et al., 1989; Sewell & Starr, 1991; Dawkins et al., 2005). The lateral line organ is a reasonable model for the auditory system since it codes afferent fiber discharge as a temporal modulation of the mechanical stimulus (although it

responds to much lower frequencies than auditory organs). The primary advantage of this preparation is that the hair cells sit on the surface of the skin and afferent nerve discharge is easily monitored while drugs are perfused over the synapse. Anatomical and physiological conditions for hair cells and nerve fibers are preserved, while improved access allows separate perfusion of apical and basal surfaces of the sensory epithelium if one desires. The preparation will last for hours, discharging spontaneously and responding to movement of the cupula into which the hair cell stereocilia are embedded. That has allowed analysis of the effects of drugs (and generation of dose-response curves) on discharge patterns in single nerve fibers.

Another preparation that has proved valuable for pharmacological analysis is the isolated organ of Corti (Oliver et al., 2003; Goutman et al., 2005). In this preparation, whole sections of the organ of Corti are isolated from the rat cochlea and placed on a microscope for electrophysiological monitoring of hair cell or afferent fiber activity. Drugs can be perfused and efferent fibers or hair cells depolarized with perfusion of solutions containing high concentrations of potassium.

Monitoring Drug Effects on Cochlear Function

Electrophysiological and biomechanical assessments are an integral part of studies involving pharmacologic manipulation of auditory function. Two types of electrical potentials are available for monitoring effects of drugs on the cochlea: resting potentials and stimulus-related potentials. The so-called "resting" (nonstimulus-related) potentials (cell membrane potential, Em; endocochlear potential, EP) are properties of electrochemical events occurring within cells and within the electrochemical environment of the cells that comprise the organ of Corti (see detailed review by Santos-Sacchi, 1988).

The EP provides the energy needed to drive the exquisite sensitivity of the cochlea to sound. This approximately +85 mV potential, measured in the fluid space into which the tips of the sensory cells protrude, is unique in the body. It provides a driving current, the mechanical modulation of which yields the stimulus-related cochlear potentials (cochlear microphonic (CM) and summating potential (SP); see Dallos, 1973). The CM, an AC stimulus-related potential, is an extracellular manifestation of the response to displacement of primarily OHCs. The SP is a stimulus-related DC potential that usually appears as a shift in the baseline of the CM. The polarity of this potential varies depending on the frequency and intensity of stimulation and the recording site and likely reflects IHC and OHC contributions (Durrant et al., 1998). Neural outflow from the cochlear end organ reflects contributions from both hair cell subsystems and can be assayed by recording single afferent unit activity and the ensemble activity of the auditory nerve as reflected in the compound action potential (CAP). Auditory brainstem responses (ABRs) often are used to monitor function when noninvasive testing is required.

Drugs acting at certain mechanically sensitive structures in the cochlea (e.g., the OHCs) can shape the normal, nonlinear cochlear mechanical response to sound. Distortion product otoacoustic emissions are acoustic signals that can be detected noninvasively in the ear canal. The distortion product corresponding to the frequency 2f1-f2 is quite robust and is commonly used as a metric of cochlear and, in particular, OHC function.

Sensitivity of these responses to drug manipulations is highly dependent on numerous variables of stimulation and recording, as well as on the health of the system into which the drugs are introduced. A drug that targets OHCs, for example, will have a limited range of effect in an ear with OHCs previously damaged by some other ototrauma.

Perturbing Hearing Function: Drugs That Affect the Cochlear Battery

The generation of the EP in the stria vascularis requires interactions of a variety of transporters, providing several opportunities for altering the potential with drug. An additional advantage is that the cells using these transporters are isolated from the blood-cochlear barrier and, thus, are accessible to drugs delivered into the systemic circulation. The stria vascularis, which generates the EP, has high concentrations of Na,K-ATPase, an enzyme that regulates the

sodium and potassium concentrations in cells. Na,K-ATPase is susceptible to block by drugs such as ouabain, although the agents don't easily reach the stria vascularis after delivery to the cochlea and can be toxic after systemic delivery. Metabolic inhibitors, which affect all processes that rely on aerobic metabolism, include cyanide and 2,4-dinitrophenol. Those drugs are not necessarily selective for actions on endolymph production. However, because the stria vascularis has such a high metabolic rate and is in diffusional contact with the systemic circulation, effects on EP are often more dramatic than those on other cochlear processes.

The most commonly used pharmacological probes for EP manipulation are the high ceiling, or loop-inhibiting, diuretics, such as furosemide and ethacrynic acid (Sewell, 1984), which specifically block the NKCC1 channel to prevent the transport of potassium and chloride into the marginal cell. This blocks the fundamental drive for generating the EP, leading to a rapid drop. These drugs can be administered systemically and are rapidly acting, and their effects are usually reversible.

Perturbing Hearing Function: Drugs That Affect Hair Cells

Transduction in the hair cells requires movement of ions through channels at the tips of the stereocilia. The channel is a relatively nonselective cation channel: it allows any number of positively charged ions to pass through the channel's pore. The transduction channel can be blocked by perfusing the apical surface of the hair cell with tetramethylammonium or by lowering endolymph calcium concentration to less than 10 μM (Corey & Hudspeth, 1979). The aminoglycoside antibiotics (see below) also are known to block transduction, presumably by virtue of their properties of large cations.

Clinicians are well aware that there are many pharmacologic agents (e.g., ototoxic antibiotics and antineoplastic agents) that can damage or destroy hair cells, as they are quite vulnerable elements in the cochlea (see review by Dallos, 1992). As normally administered, however, such drugs do not often make particularly good pharmacologic tools as their selectivity for specific cells and processes is poor. In some applications, however, the agents have proven to be valuable tools. Aminoglycoside antibiotics have well-described associations with hearing and balance dysfunction. Carefully applied, however, they can be employed as (1) blockers of the hair cell mechanosensitive transduction channel (Konishi, 1979; Ohmori, 1985; Jaramillo & Hudspeth, 1991; Kimitsuki & Ohmori, 1993) and (2) modulators of the cation current flowing through nicotinic cholinergic receptors (nAChRs)of the OHCs (Blanchet et al., 2000; Rothlin et al., 2000). In addition, kanamycin has been successfully employed in attempts to selectively damage OHCs (Ryan & Dallos, 1975; Dallos & Harris, 1978). The antineoplastic agent, carboplatin, when used in a chinchilla model, selectively targets IHCs while sparing OHCs (Takeno et al., 1994; Wake et al., 1994; Liberman et al., 1997).

Such compounds have been employed in creating, as nearly as possible, OHC-less or IHC-less preparations so that the functional contributions of each of the hair cell subsystems to normal hearing sensitivity and frequency selectivity can be characterized. Moreover, such preparations could provide opportunities to sample the activity and potential roles of structures not normally accessible (e.g., to record responses from type II afferents to OHCs in the absence of IHCs and their associated afferents; see Liberman et al., 1997).

Perturbing Hearing Function: Drugs That Affect Afferent Synaptic Transmission

The hair cell releases a neurotransmitter to excite afferent nerve fibers. Some drugs act on the nervous system because they resemble, at the molecular level, the endogenous neurotransmitter. They exert their actions through the same postsynaptic receptor, and the same postsynaptic events result from their action.

In the study of the pharmacology of this neurotransmission or in efforts to characterize the functional consequences of receptor activation, perhaps the most powerful and commonly used tools are those that selectively antagonize (block) the endogenous transmitter's actions. And here, work with antagonists of glutamatergic transmission has provided significant support for the notion that effects of the hair cell transmitter are probably mediated via glutamate receptors on afferent fibers. Three types of glutamate receptors are present on auditory nerve fibers. Moment-by-moment transmission of auditory information is mediated by the AMPA subtype of glutamate receptor. This receptor is blocked by the quinoxalinediones DNQX and CNQX (Littman et al., 1989). NMDA and metabotropic receptor subtypes also are present, although their function is presently unclear.

The release of neurotransmitter from the hair cells requires an influx of calcium via voltage-sensitive calcium channels. Those channels are L-type calcium channels that can be blocked by a class of calcium channel blockers that include nimodipine and nifedipine, as well as by more traditional general calcium channel blockers such as cobalt and magnesium.

Perturbing Hearing Function: Drugs That Affect Efferent Synaptic Transmission

The cochlea is innervated by two groups of efferent nerve fibers. Large myelinated efferent fibers originate near the medial nucleus of the trapezoid body and synapse predominantly on OHCs, and small unmyelinated efferent fibers originate in the hilus of the lateral superior olivary complex and terminate predominantly on the radial afferent fibers that innervate the IHCs. Those two efferent groups are respectively termed the medial and lateral efferents. The major neurotransmitter used by the medial efferent fibers is acetylcholine. Binding of ACh on the OHC nAChR results in calcium influx through the integral ion channel of this ionotropic receptor. This calcium influx stimulates a large outward $K+$ current through $Ca2+$-activated $K+$ channels, hyperpolarizing the hair cell. The nicotinic AChR on the OHC is a little unusual pharmacologically in that it can be blocked by a broad variety of cholinergic drugs, even those that typically block the muscarinic subtype of acetylcholine receptor. In addition, it is blocked by both strychnine and bicuculline, usually thought of as specific glycine and GABA receptor blockers, respectively. Another means of blocking efferent action is to block the KCa channels that are activated after the nAChR is opened. Those channels are thought to be a subtype of KCa channel called the SK, or small conductance K channel. They are sensitive to block by a peptide in bee venom called apamin and by a smaller molecule called dequalinium.

The lateral efferents contain, in addition to acetylcholine, an assortment of neuropeptides, including enkephalins, dynorphins, and CGRP (see reviews by Altschuler & Fex, 1986; Eybalin, 1993). The actions of those peptides in the cochlea are, for the most part, unknown, although opioid receptor activation suppresses adenylate cyclase activity in the cochlea (Eybalin et al., 1987).

Perturbing Hearing Function: Where Is This Drug Acting?

Scientists and clinicians are fortunate to have a number of very well-characterized and sensitive metrics of function for a variety of cochlear cell systems and subsystems. In recent work characterizing drug distribution in the mouse cochlea using a new drug infusion technique (Chen et al., 2006), the authors

monitored the effects of two drugs with well-characterized actions in the cochlea, using two indicants of cochlear sensitivity and function: OHC-based DPOAEs and ABRs. Drugs (salicylate, 5 mM; CNQX, 100 μM) were introduced via an infusion line placed in a single hole carefully drilled in the basal turn.

Because CNQX blocks glutamatergic transmission between the IHCs and the auditory nerve, it should block the ABR, which requires synchronous auditory nerve activity. It should not, on the other hand, alter the DPOAEs, which are produced by the OHCs. Consistent with a site of action at the IHC-afferent fiber synapse, local infusion of CNQX into the mouse cochlea elevated ABR thresholds and reduced suprathreshold amplitudes while leaving DPOAEs unaltered (Figure 21-7). Responses to high-frequency stimuli were altered first and most, followed progressively by involvement of responses to mid- and then lower-frequency stimuli. Those frequency-sensitive drug effects are to be expected from the basal cochlear site of drug entry. Over the period of infusion, changes were seen as far apically as 5.6 kHz, although they were much smaller than those at basal

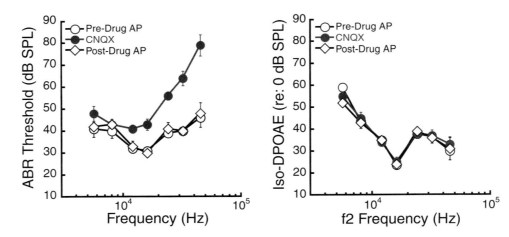

Figure 21-7. Infusion of CNQX. CNQX (100 μM for 175 min infused at 1 μl/hr) elevated ABR thresholds without affecting low-level DPOAEs, consistent with its action to block afferent transmission. Effects were greatest at highest frequencies, consistent with the basal site of drug entry and were completely reversible with washing. Data are plotted as means ± S.E. (n = 5 animals) and are compared to values obtained during control artificial perilymph (AP) infusion periods before and after drug infusion.
J Neuroscience Methods, 150, Chen et al., A method for intracochlear drug delivery in the mouse, 67–73 (2006).

frequencies. Following termination of CNQX infusion and reintroduction of the AP, responses returned to predrug levels.

Salicylates are well known to interfere with OHC electromotility (Brownell, 1990) and would be expected, therefore, to alter *both* ABRs and DPOAEs. Consistent with that expectation, salicylate reversibly altered both ABR thresholds and low-level iso-DPOAEs, as displayed in Figure 21-8. Those effects of intracochlear salicylate infusion in the mouse are similar to the ones observed previously during acute perilymphatic perfusion of salicylate in the guinea pig (Kujawa et al., 1992a).

In those experiments, CNQX and salicylate not only confirmed drug action at intended targets and the lack of nonspecific traumatic effects of the infusion, *per se*, but also documented spread of infused agents from the basal site of drug entry toward the cochlear apex. That is, the very well-characterized, tonotopic organization of the cochlea, in which responses to high-frequency tones arise from the base and low-frequency tones from the apex allowed these responses to be used to assay distribution of delivered drug along the length of the cochlea.

Perturbing Hearing Function: The Pharmacology of Contralateral Suppression of DPOAEs

To illustrate a number of the concepts presented in this chapter, it may be informative here to describe the successful use of a pharmacologic tool in confirming and exploring the efferent nature of a phenomenon that should be familiar to all audiologists: contralateral sound suppression of otoacoustic emissions. At the point when these studies were undertaken, numerous investigations in both animal models and humans had demonstrated that the presentation of an acoustic signal to one ear could suppress sound-evoked activity (e.g., otoacoustic emissions) recorded at the opposite ear (Siegel & Kim, 1982; Mott et al., 1989; Puel & Rebillard, 1990; Moulin et al., 1993; Berlin et al., 1994). This suppression was suggested to be efferent mediated: Medial olivocochlear (MOC) efferent neurons respond to

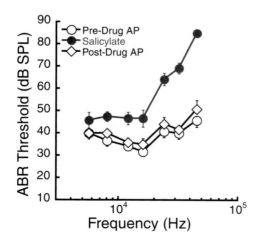

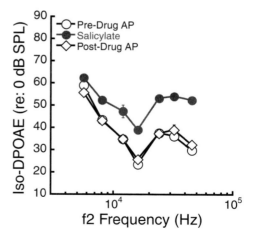

Figure 21-8. Infusion of salicylate. Salicylate (5 mM for 165 min, infused at 1 μl/hr) elevated ABR thresholds and low-level iso-DPOAEs. Highest frequencies were again affected most. The magnitude of the high frequency shifts in DPOAEs are underestimated in this plot because postdrug responses in many animals reached the stimulus level ceiling for frequencies above 24 kHz. Data are plotted as means ± S.E. (n = 6 animals) of responses recorded after predrug AP, salicylate, and postdrug AP infusions.
J Neuroscience Methods, 150, Chen et al., A method for intracochlear drug delivery in the mouse, 67–73 (2006).

sound and release their neurotransmitter directly on their OHC targets, altering the cochlear mechanics and reducing DPOAEs (Figure 21-9). Thus, contralateral sound-evoked release of the endogenous neurotransmitter (ACh) onto OHCs was proposed to underlie the observed changes in the ipsilaterally recorded, OHC-based DPOAEs. Direct tests of this hypothesis were not possible in humans. Moreover, because moderately high levels of contralateral noise were necessary to elicit the suppression, study of the phenomenon in the human was complicated by the potentially contaminating influences of middle ear muscle activation and transcranial crossover of the noise, both of which (through ipsilateral response suppression) could produce effects on emissions that looked very similar to those proposed to be efferent mediated.

In animal models, however, evidence for efferent involvement in the contralateral sound effects was strong. There was ample evidence that ACh was the primary neurotransmitter of the MOC efferents to the OHCs (Barron & Guth, 1987; Bobbin & Konishi, 1974; Galley et al., 1973). Indeed, the sound-evoked effect (DPOAE suppression by contralateral noise) could be mimicked pharmacologically by intracochlear ACh, (Kujawa et al., 1992b). Additionally, it was blocked by known antagonists of olivocochlear activity (Kujawa et al., 1993) and could be prevented as well by sectioning the olivocochlear bundle (Liberman, 1989). Those demonstrations could be made in animals where complicating issues surrounding crossover and middle ear muscle activation could be avoided altogether: crossover could be quantified directly and signals chosen to avoid that possibility. Acoustic reflex activation could be avoided by sectioning the middle ear muscles.

With that knowledge in hand, Kujawa et al. (1994) employed contralateral sound suppression of

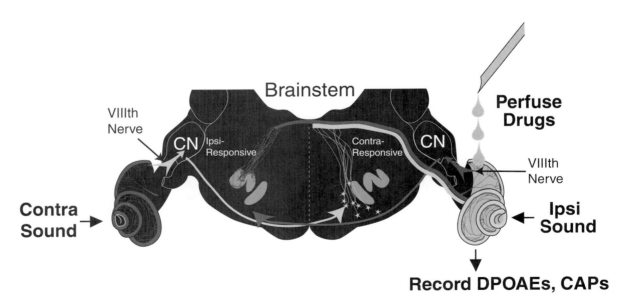

Figure 21-9. Schematic of the medial olivocochlear (MOC) reflex pathway to one ear, showing the afferent inputs to CN, outputs that cross the brainstem midline, and the origins and projections of ipsilaterally and contralaterally responsive MOC units. Pharmacologic antagonists of the OHC receptor were introduced ipsilaterally, and effects were assayed using contralateral sound stimulation of ipsilaterally stimulated DPOAEs. Drug effects on ipsi-recorded DPOAEs and CAPs without contra sound also were monitored to rule out nonspecific or traumatic effects of the perfusion. *J Neurophysiol*, 79, M. C. Brown, S. G. Kujawa, and M. L. Duca, Single Olivocochlear Neurons in the Guinea Pig. I. Binaural Facilitation of Responses to High-Level Noise, 3077–3087 (1998).

DPOAEs as an assay to characterize, *in vivo,* the pharmacology of the inhibitory MOC efferent influence on DPOAEs. Contralateral suppression of DPOAEs was blocked dose-responsively by a constellation of antagonists that suggested the sound-evoked effects were mediated by a novel nicotinic cholinergic receptor (nAChR); see also Fuchs and Murrow (1992). Scientists now know that that pharmacologic profile closely resembles the alpha9 nAChR subtype (Elgoyhen et al., 1994). The results were consistent with *in vitro* studies of the pharmacology of the nAChR mediating the effects of acetylcholine in mammalian OHCs (Erostegui et al., 1994).

In the years since, molecular biological studies have provided ongoing characterization of the nature of this novel nAChR (Elgoyhen et al., 1994, 2001; Weisstaub, 2002) and are now yielding mouse models (e.g., alpha9 and alpha10 receptor knockouts and overexpressors; Vetter et al., 1999; Maison et al., 2002; May et al., 2002) to provide additional information about the nature and consequences of OC efferent neurotransmission. Such powerful techniques are used ever more frequently in conjunction with traditional pharmacology to uncover the basic mechanisms of biological function and dysfunction.

New Tools to Dissect Function

Historically, most drugs were either extractions from or synthetic variations on natural products. More recent developments have arisen from efforts to target specific proteins that play key roles in biological processes. Breakthroughs in molecular biology and genetic engineering have facilitated the creation of new pharmacologic tools. Compounds have been identified that can more selectively target cell constituents, with the goal of uncovering processes that support the cell in health and those that underlie alterations with aging, trauma, and disease. Cell signaling pathways have undergone extensive characterization, and potential targets of drug action have been identified. Such clarification of the molecular mechanisms and consequences of drug action contributes not only to an understanding of basic biological processes, but also to the development of therapeutic (perhaps even individualized) designer drugs to modify the processes in disease.

Benefits from Drug Discovery Efforts

The physiologist/pharmacologist has benefited from drug discovery efforts. The pharmaceutical industry's need to identify or synthesize drugs with therapeutic properties that can act more specifically and at lower concentrations also has uncovered novel ligands that can be employed as informative probes of function. Large-scale screening of existing compounds and generation of novel ligands using structure-based drug design strategies will yield new and increasingly selective ways to manipulate proteins and pathways (Caporale, 1995; Breaker, 2004; Dahl & Sylte, 2005).

Combined Pharmacologic-Genetic Approaches

The availability of mouse models with specific alterations to their genetic makeup (e.g., point mutations and nulls) as well as the ability to create targeted modifications (knockout and knock-in) has provided powerful models for studying function (see review by Parkinson & Brown, 2002; Zuo, 2002). Using such methods, researchers can study the functional consequences of alterations to protein components of hair cells (Verpy et al., 2000; Liberman et al., 2002; Cheatham et al., 2004), ion channels (Parkinson et al., 2001), transporters (Shimizu et al., 2005), receptors (Vetter et al., 1999; Maison et al., 2002), and other components of cells and systems.

New fields of investigation (pharmacogenetics and chemical genetics) are combining the tools of the pharmacologist with those of the chemist and geneticist with goals that range from identifying key proteins in complicated cellular pathways to addressing issues related to individual differences in drug response. Such cross-discipline collaborations will likely result in the creation of new tools that are valuable to both the researcher and the clinician (Heller, 2002; Strausberg & Schreiber, 2003).

The identification of specific protein targets involved in inner ear function, as well as in development, maintenance, and possibly regeneration of sensory cells, provides hope for the development of specific pharmacological tools with which to probe these processes. One can expect that in the near future, a broad array of pharmacological probes will be available for analysis of hearing.

SUMMARY

Drugs perturb cellular function. Their actions can be toxic, they can be therapeutic or, through their interactions with specific cellular constituents, they can help scientists understand the functioning of cells and systems. This chapter considers drugs as tools to dissect physiological and biochemical processes supporting normal function in general and cochlear function in particular.

Most drugs exert their biological actions by interacting with receptors. The term *receptor* in this context refers to those cellular macromolecules that function specifically and directly to mediate chemical signaling between and within cells. Receptors are almost always membrane proteins. The binding of an endogenously-occurring ligand (e.g., neurotransmitter or hormone) with its receptor results in a change in cellular activity. In a similar fashion, exogenously-applied drugs can interact with receptors and effect changes in cellular activity. Those that bind to the receptor and mimic the endogenous compound are called agonists, and those that prevent the endogenous compound from acting are called antagonists. Drugs that act at very low concentrations are more likely to act selectively. It is important to remember that virtually all drugs will act nonselectively at high concentrations and that their value as probes of function will be limited.

Both the specificity of the drug-receptor interaction and the transduction system employed in initiating the cellular response are determined by the structure of the receptor. Ionotropic receptors are those that comprise an ion channel. The receptor spans the membrane, forming a pore. Ligand binding opens the pore, allowing certain ions to flow and resulting in a change in electrical activity of the cell. Metabotropic receptors are those that include a

G protein binding site. In that case, ligand binding leads to activation of GTP-binding proteins that may then directly or indirectly (via intracellular second messengers) effect changes within the cell. Other receptor types exist as well. Some membrane proteins either possess or link to an enzyme; some interact with DNA to produce their effects.

In the cochlea, most drug targets of interest are located in the perilymph and endolymph fluid compartments; for example, at the level of the sensory hair cells, their afferent or efferent innervation, and the stria vascularis. At those sites, mechanisms and consequences of drug action are similar in many respects to those described for other systems. The challenge, however, is in getting drugs into the cochlea in the form and concentration desired and without unwanted (nonspecific and toxic) effects. Drug access to cochlear targets is limited by the presence of a blood-cochlea barrier that discriminates molecules on the basis of their size and charge, their solubility in the lipid bilayer, and their association with specific transport molecules. This barrier undoubtedly protects the inner ear from exposure to potentially toxic substances that may be present in the systemic circulation; however, its presence also complicates delivery of substances intended as pharmacologic probes or even as therapeutic agents. Methods to circumvent this barrier include *in vitro* preparations in which drugs can be applied directly to desired tissues and techniques suitable for *in vivo*, local delivery to the cochlea.

New fields of investigation (pharmacogenetics and chemical genetics) are combining the tools of the pharmacologist with those of the chemist and geneticist. Such cross-discipline collaborations will likely result in the creation of new and powerful tools to study inner ear function and to treat dysfunction.

REFERENCES

Altschuler, R. A. & Fex, J. (1986). Efferent neurotransmitters. In R. A. Altschuler, R. P. Bobbin, & D. W. Hoffman (Eds.), *Neurobiology of Hearing: The Cochlea* (pp. 383–396). New York: Raven Press.

Art, J. J., Crawford, A. C., Fettiplace, R., & Fuchs, P. A. (1985). Efferent modulation of hair cell tuning in the cochlea of the turtle. *J Physiol, 360,* 397–421.

Barron, S. E., & Guth, P. S. (1987). Uses and limitations of strychnine as a probe in neurotransmission. *Trends Pharmacol Sci, 8,* 204–206.

Berlin, C. I., Hood, L. J., Hurley, A., & Wen, H. (1994). The First Jerger Lecture. Contralateral suppression of otoacoustic emissions: An index of the function of the medial olivocochlear system. *Otolaryngol Head Neck Surg, 110,* 3–21.

Blanchet, C., Erostegui, C., Sugasawa, M., & Dulon, D. (2000). Gentamicin blocks ACh-evoked K+ current in guinea-pig outer hair cells by impairing Ca2+ entry at the cholinergic receptor. *J Physiol, 525,* 641–654.

Bledsoe, S. C., Jr., Sinard, R. J., & Allen, S. J. (1989). Analysis of histamine as a hair-cell transmitter in the lateral line of Xenopus laevis. *Hear Res, 38,* 81–93.

Bobbin, R. P., Bledsoe, S. C., Jr., Winbery, S., Ceasar, G., & Jenison, G. L. (1985). Comparative actions of GABA and acetylcholine on the Xenopus laevis lateral line. *Comp Biochem Physiol C, 80,* 313–318.

Bobbin, R. P., & Konishi, T. (1971). Acetylcholine mimics crossed olivocochlear bundle stimulation. *Nature New Biol, 231,* 222–223.

Bobbin, R. P., & Konishi, T. (1974). Action of cholinergic and anticholinergic drugs at the crossed olivo-cochlear bundle-hair cell junction. *Acta Otolaryngol, 77,* 56–65.

Breaker, R. R. (2004). Natural and engineered nucleic acids as tools to explore biology. *Nature, 432,* 838–845.

Brown, J. N., Miller, J. M., Altschuler, R. A., & Nuttall, A. L. (1993). Osmotic pump implant for chronic infusion of drugs into the inner ear. *Hear Res 70,* 167–172.

Brown, M. C., Kujawa, S. G., & Duca, M. L. (1998). Single olivocochlear neurons in the guinea pig. I. Binaural facilitation of responses to high-level noise. *J Neurophysiol, 79,* 3077–3087.

Brownell, W. E. (1990). Outer hair cell electromotility and otoacoustic emissions. *Ear Hear, 11,* 82–92.

Caporale, L. H. (1995). Chemical ecology: A view from the pharmaceutical industry. *Proc Natl Acad Sci USA, 92,* 75–82.

Carvalho, G. J., & Lalwani, A. K. (1999). The effect of cochleostomy and intracochlear infusion on auditory brainstem response threshold in the guinea pig. *Am J Otol, 20,* 87–90.

Chan, D. K., & Hudspeth, A. J. (2005). Ca2+ current-driven nonlinear amplification by the mammalian cochlea in vitro. *Nat Neurosci, 8,* 149–155.

Cheatham, M. A., Huynh, K. H., Gao, J., Zuo, J., & Dallos, P. (2004). Cochlear function in Prestin knock-out mice. *J Physiol, 560,* 821–830.

Chen, Z., Ulfendahl, M., Ruan, R., Tan, L., & Duan, M. (2004). Protection of auditory function against noise trauma with local caroverine administration in guinea pigs. *Hear Res, 197,* Chen, Z., Kujawa, S.G., McKenna, M.J., Fiering, J.O., Mescher, M.J., Borenstein, J.T., Swan, E.E. & Sewell, W.F. (2005). Inner ear drug delivery via a reciprocating perfusion system in the guinea pig. *J Control Release,* 110(1):, 1–19.

Chen, Z., Mikulec, A. A., McKenna, M. J., Sewell, W. F., & Kujawa, S. G. (2006). A method for intracochlear drug delivery in the mouse. *J Neurosci, 150*(1), 67–73.

Corey, D. P., & Hudspeth, A. J. (1979). Ionic basis of the receptor potential in a vertebrate hair cell. *Nature 281,* 675–677.

Corey, D. P., & Hudspeth, A. J. (1983). Kinetics of the receptor current in bullfrog saccular hair cells. *J Neurosci, 3,* 962–976.

Dahl, S. G., & Sylte, I. (2005). Molecular modeling of drug targets: The past, the present and the future. *Basic Clin Pharmacol Toxicol, 96,* 151–155.

Dallos, P. (1973). *The auditory periphery: Biophysics and physiology.* New York: Academic Press.

Dallos, P. (1992). The active cochlea. *J Neurosci, 12,* 4575–4585.

Dallos, P., & Harris, D. (1978). Properties of auditory nerve responses in the absence of outer hair cells. *J Neurophysiol, 41,* 365–383.

Dallos, P., He, D. Z. Z., Lin, X., Sziklai, I., Mehta, S., & Evans, B. N. (1997). Acetylcholine, outer hair cell electromotility, and the cochlear amplifier. *J Neurosci, 17,* 2212–2226.

Dawkins, R., Keller, S. L., & Sewell, W. F. (2005). Pharmacology of acetylcholine-mediated cell signaling in the lateral line organ following efferent stimulation. *J Neurophysiol, 93,* 2541–2551.

Durrant, J. D., Wang, J., Ding, D. L., & Salvi, R. J. (1998). Are inner or outer hair cells the source of summating potentials recorded from the round window? *J Acoust Soc Am, 104,* 370–377.

Elgoyhen, A. B., Johnson, D. S., Boulter, J., Vetter, D. E., & Heinemann, S. (1994). Alpha 9: An acetylcholine receptor with novel pharmacological properties expressed in rat cochlear hair cells. *Cell, 79,* 705–715.

Elgoyhen, A. B., Vetter, D. E., Katz, E., Rothlin, C. V., Heinemann, S. F. & Boulter, J. (2001). Alpha 10: A determinant of nicotinic cholinergic receptor function in mammalian vestibular and cochlear mechanosensory hair cells. *Proc Natl Acad Sci USA, 98,* 3501–3506.

Erostegui, C., Norris, C. H., & Bobbin, R. P. (1994). In vitro pharmacologic characterization of a cholinergic receptor on outer hair cells. *Hear Res, 74,* 135–147.

Evans, B. N., Dallos, P., & Hallworth, R. (1989). Asymmetries in motile responses of outer hair cells in simulated in vivo conditions. In J. P. Wilson & D. T. Wilson (Eds.), *Cochlear Mechanisms* (pp. 205–206). New York: Plenum.

Eybalin, M. (1993). Neurotransmitters and neuromodulators of the mammalian cochlea. *Physiol Rev, 73,* 309–373.

Eybalin, M., Pujol, R., & Bockaert, J. (1987). Opioid receptors inhibit the adenylate cyclase in guinea pig cochleas. *Brain Res, 421,* 336–342.

Fex, J. (1968). Efferent inhibition in the cochlea by the olivocochlear bundle. In A. V. S. DeReuck & J. Knight (Eds.), *Hearing Mechanisms in Vertebrates* (pp. 169–181). Boston: Little, Brown & Co.

Fuchs, P. (2002). The synaptic physiology of cochlear hair cells. *Audiol Neurootol, 7,* 40–44.

Fuchs, P. A., & Murrow, B. W. (1992). A novel cholinergic receptor mediates inhibition of chick cochlear hair cells. *Proc Biol Sc, 248,* 35–40.

Galley, N., Klinke, R., Oertel, W., Pause, M., & Storch, W. H. (1973). The effect of intracochlearly administered acetylcholine-blocking agents on the efferent synapses of the cochlea. *Brain Res, 64,* 55–63.

Gantz, B. J., & Turner, C. W. (2003). Combining acoustic and electrical hearing. *Laryngoscope, 113,* 1726–1731.

Goutman, J. D., Fuchs, P. A., & Glowatzki, E. (2005). Facilitating efferent inhibition of inner hair cells in the cochlea of the neonatal rat. *J Physiol, 566,* 49–59.

He, D. Z., Jia, S., & Dallos, P. (2004). Mechanoelectrical transduction of adult outer hair cells studied in a gerbil hemicochlea. *Nature, 429,* 766–770.

Heller, S. (2002). Application of physiological genomics to the study of hearing disorders. *J Physiol, 543,* 3–12.

Heydt, J. L., Cunningham, L. L., Rubel, E. W., & Coltrera, M. D. (2004). Round window gentamicin application: An inner ear hair cell damage protocol for the mouse. *Hear Res, 192,* 65–74.

Housley, G. D., & Ashmore, J. F. (1992). Ionic currents of outer hair cells isolated from the guinea-pig cochlea. *J Physiol, 448,* 73–98.

Jaramillo, F., & Hudspeth, A. J. (1991). Localization of the hair cell's transduction channels at the hair bundle's top by iontophoretic application of a channel blocker. *Neuron, 7,* 409–420.

Kikuchi, T., Kimura, R. S., Paul, D. L., & Adams, J. C. (1995). Gap junctions in the rat cochlea: Immunohistochemical and ultrastructural analysis. *Anatomy and Embryology, 191,* 101–118.

Kimitsuki, T., & Ohmori, H. (1993). Dihydrostreptomycin modifies adaptation and blocks the mechano-electric transducer in chick cochlear hair cells. *Brain Res, 624,* 143–150.

Kingma, G. G., Miller, J. M., & Myers, M. W. (1992). Chronic drug infusion into the scala tympani of the guinea pig cochlea. *J Neurosci Methods, 45,* 127–134.

Konishi, T. (1972). Action of tubocurarine and atropine on the crossed olivocochlear bundles. *Acta Otolaryngol, 74*(4), 252–264.

Konishi, T. (1979). Effects of local application of ototoxic antibiotics on cochlear potentials in guinea pigs. *Acta Otolaryngol, 88,* 41–46.

Kujawa, S. G., Fallon, M., & Bobbin, R. P. (1992a). Intracochlear salicylate reduces low-intensity acoustic and cochlear microphonic distortion products. *Hear Res, 64,* 73–80.

Kujawa, S. G., Glattke, T. J., Fallon, M., & Bobbin, R. P. (1992b). Intracochlear application of acetylcholine alters sound-induced mechanical events within the cochlear partition. *Hear Res, 1992, 61*(1–2), 106–116.

Kujawa, S. G., Glattke, T. J., Fallon, M., & Bobbin, R. P. (1993). Contralateral sound suppresses distortion product otoacoustic emissions through cholinergic mechanisms. *Hear Res, 68*(1), 97–106.

Kujawa, S. G., Glattke, T. J., Fallon, M., & Bobbin, R. P. (1994). A nicotinic-like receptor mediates suppression of distortion product otoacoustic emissions by contralateral sound. *Hear Res, 74,* 122–134.

Lang, H., Schulte, B. A., & Schmiedt, R. A. (2003). Effects of chronic furosemide treatment and age on cell division in the adult gerbil inner ear. *J Assoc Res Otolaryngol, 4,* 164–175.

Le Calvez, S., & Ulfendahl, M. (2000). An in vitro preparation to access cellular and neuronal components in the mouse inner ear. *J Neurocytol, 29,* 645–652.

Liberman, M. C. (1989). Rapid assessment of sound-evoked olivocochlear feedback: Suppression of compound action potentials by contralateral sound. *Hear Res, 38,* 47–56.

Liberman, M. C., Chesney, C. P., & Kujawa, S. G. (1997). Effects of selective inner hair cell loss on DPOAEs in carboplatin-treated chinchillas. *Auditory Neurosci, 3,* 255–268.

Liberman, M. C., Gao, J., He, D. Z., Wu, X., Jia S., & Zuo, J. (2002). Prestin is required for electromotility of the outer hair cell and for the cochlear amplifier. *Nature, 419,* 300–304.

Littman, T., Bobbin, R. P., Fallon, M., & Puel, J. L. (1989). The quinoxalinediones DNQX, CNQX and two related congeners suppress hair cell-to-auditory nerve transmission. *Hear Res, 40,* 45–53.

Maison, S. F., Luebke, A. E., Liberman, M.C., & Zuo, J. (2002). Efferent protection from acoustic injury is mediated via alpha9 nicotinic acetylcholine receptors on outer hair cells. *J Neurosci, 22,* 10838–10846.

May, B. J., Prosen, C. A., Weiss, D., & Vetter, D. (2002). Behavioral investigation of some possible effects of the central olivocochlear pathways in transgenic mice. *Hear Res, 171,* 142–157.

Mott, J. B., Norton, S. J., Neely, S. T., & Warr, W. B. (1989). Changes in spontaneous otoacoustic emissions produced by acoustic stimulation of the contralateral ear. *Hear Res, 38*(3), 229–242.

Moulin, A., Collet, L., & Duclaux, R. (1993). Contralateral auditory stimulation alters acoustic distortion products in humans. *Hear Res, 65,* 193–210.

Nuttall, A. L., LaRoure, M. J., & Lawrence, M. (1982). Acute perilymphatic perfusion of the guinea pig cochlea. *Hear Res, 6,* 207–221.

Ohmori, H. (1985). Mechano-electrical transduction currents in isolated vestibular hair cells of the chick. *J Physiol, 359,* 189–217.

Oliver, D., Knipper, M., Derst, C., & Fakler, B. (2003). Resting potential and submembrane calcium concentration of inner hair cells in the isolated mouse cochlea are set by KCNQ-type potassium channels. *J Neurosci, 23,* 2141–2149.

Paasche, G., Gibson, P., Averbeck, T., Becker, H., Lenarz, T., & Stover, T. (2003). Technical report: Modification of a cochlear implant electrode for drug delivery to the inner ear. *Otol Neurotol, 24,* 222–227.

Parkinson, N., & Brown, S. D. (2002). Focusing on the genetics of hearing: You ain't heard nothin' yet. *Genome Biol, 3*(6).

Parkinson, N. J., Olsson, C. L., Hallows, J. L., McKee-Johnson, J., Keogh, B. P., Noben-Trauth, K., Kujawa, S. G., & Tempel, B. L. (2001). Mutant beta-spectrin 4 causes auditory and motor neuropathies in quivering mice. *Nat Genet, 29,* 61–65.

Parks, T. N. (2000). The AMPA receptors of auditory neurons. *Hear Res, 147,* 77–91.

Pasic, T. R., & Rubel, E. W. (1989). Rapid changes in cochlear nucleus cell size following blockade of auditory nerve electrical activity in gerbils. *J Comp Neurol, 283,* 474–480.

Puel, J. L., Pujol, R., Tribillac, F., Ladrech, S., & Eybalin, M. (1994). Excitatory amino acid antagonists protect cochlear auditory neurons from excitotoxicity. *J Comp Neurol, 341,* 241–256.

Puel, J. L., & Rebillard, G. (1990). Effect of contralateral sound stimulation on the distortion product 2F1–F2: Evidence that the medial efferent system is involved. *J Acoust Soc Am, 87,* 1630–1635.

Ricci, A. J., Crawford, A. C., & Fettiplace, R. (2000). Active hair bundle motion to fast transducer adaptation in auditory hair cells. *J Neurosci, 20,* 7131–7142.

Rothlin, C. V., Katz, E., Verbitsky, M., Vetter, D. E., Heinemann, S. F., & Elgoyhen, A. B. (2000). Block of the alpha9 nicotinic receptor by ototoxic aminoglycosides. *Neuropharmacology, 39,* 2525–2532.

Ruel, J., Chen, C., Pujol, R., Bobbin, R. P., & Puel, J. L. (1999). AMPA-preferring glutamate receptors in cochlear physiology of adult guinea-pig. *J Physiol, 518*(Pt. 3), 667–680.

Russell, I. J., & Sellick, P. M. (1976). Measurement of potassium and chloride ion concentrations in the cupulae of the lateral lines of Xenopus laevis. *J Physiol, 257*, 245–255.

Ryan, A., & Dallos, P. (1975). Absence of cochlear outer hair cells: Effect on behavioural auditory threshold. *Nature 253*, 44–46.

Salt, A. N., & Konishi, T. (1986). The cochlear fluids: Perilymph and endolymph. In R. A. Altschuler, R. P. Bobbin, & D. W. Hoffman (Eds.), *Neurobiology of Hearing: The Cochlea* (pp. 109–122). New York: Raven Press.

Salt, A. N., & Ma, Y. (2001). Quantification of solute entry into cochlear perilymph through the round window membrane. *Hear Res, 154*, 88–97.

Santos-Sacchi, J. (1988). Cochlear physiology. In A. F. Jahn & J. Santos-Sacchi (Eds.), *Physiology of the Ear* (pp. 271–293). New York: Raven Press.

Schmiedt, R. A., Okamura, H. O., Lang, H., & Schulte, B. A. (2002). Ouabain application to the round window of the gerbil cochlea: A model of auditory neuropathy and apoptosis. *J Assoc Res Otolaryngol, 3*, 223–233.

Schuknecht, H. F. (1956). Ablation therapy for the relief of Meniere's disease. *Laryngoscope, 66*, 859–870.

Sewell, W. F. (1984). The effects of furosemide on the endocochlear potential and auditory nerve fiber tuning curves in cats. *Hearing Research, 14*, 305–314.

Sewell, W. F., Norris, C. H., Tachibana, M., & Guth, P. S. (1978). Detection of an auditory nerve-activating substance. *Science, 202*(4370), 910–912.

Sewell, W. F., & Starr, P.A. (1991). Effects of calcitonin gene-related peptide and efferent nerve stimulation on afferent transmission in the lateral line organ. *J Neurophysiol, 65*, 1158–1169.

Shepherd, R. K., & Xu, J. (2002). A multichannel scala tympani electrode array incorporating a drug delivery system for chronic intracochlear infusion. *Hear Res, 172*, 92–98.

Shimizu, Y., Hakuba, N., Hyodo, J., Taniguchi, M., & Gyo, K. (2005). Kanamycin ototoxicity in glutamate transporter knockout mice. *Neurosci Lett, 380*, 243–246.

Siegel, J. H., & Kim, D. O. (1982). Efferent control of cochlear mechanics? Olivocochlear bundle stimulation affects cochlear biomechanical non-linearity. *Hear Res, 6*, 171–182.

Sridhar, T. S., Brown, M. C., & Sewell, W. F. (1997). Unique postsynaptic signaling at the hair cell efferent synapse permits calcium to evoke changes on two time scales. *J Neurosci, 17*, 428–437.

Sridhar, T. S. Liberman, M. C., Brown, M. C., & Sewell, W. F. (1995). A novel cholinergic "slow effect" of efferent stimulation on cochlear potentials in the guinea pig. *J Neurosci, 15*, 3667–3678.

Strausberg, R. L., & Schreiber, S. L. (2003). From knowing to controlling: A path from genomics to drugs using small molecule probes. *Science, 300*, 294–295.

Takeno, S., Harrison, R. V., Mount, R. J., Wake, M., & Harada, Y. (1994). Induction of selective inner hair cell damage by carboplatin. *Scanning Electron Microscopy, 8*, 97–106.

Tonndorf, J., Duvall, A. J., & Reneau, J. P. (1962). Permeability of intracochlear membranes to various vital stains. *Ann Otol Rhinol Laryngol, 71*, 801–841.

Trussell, L. O. (1999). Synaptic mechanisms for coding timing in auditory neurons. *Annu Rev Physiol, 61*, 477–496.

Verpy, E., Leibovici, M., Zwaenepoel, I., Liu, X. Z., Gal, A., Salem, N., Mansour, A., Blanchard, S., Kobayashi, I., Keats, B. J., et al. (2000). A defect in harmonin, a PDZ domain-containing protein expressed in the inner ear sensory hair cells, underlies Usher syndrome type 1C. *Nat Genet 26*, 51–55.

Vetter, D. E., Liberman, M. C., Mann, J., Barhanin, J., Boulter, J., Brown, M. C., Saffiote-Kolman, J., Heinemann, S. F., & Elgoyhen, A. B. (1999). Role of alpha9 nicotinic ACh receptor subunits in the development and function of cochlear efferent innervation. *Neuron 23*, 93–103.

Wake, M., Takeno, S., Ibrahim, D., & Harrison, R. (1994). Selective inner hair cell ototoxicity induced by carboplatin. *Laryngoscope, 104*, 488–493.

Weisstaub, N., Vetter, D. E., Elgoyhen, A. B., & Katz, E. (2002). The alpha9alpha10 nicotinic acetylcholine receptor is permeable to and is modulated by divalent cations. *Hear Res, 167*(1–2), 122–135.

Zuo, J. (2002). Transgenic and gene targeting studies of hair cell function in mouse inner ear. *J Neurobiol, 53*, 286–305.

CHAPTER
22

Staying Current: Web Sites and Resources for Pharmaceutical Information

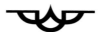

Robert M. DiSogra, AuD
Director, Audiology Associates of Freehold
Freehold, NJ
Instructor, Pharmacology/Ototoxicity
School of Audiology, Pennsylvania College of Optometry
Elkins Park, PA

INTRODUCTION

Every day in clinical practice, audiologists are confronted by patients who, besides voicing communication complaints, present themselves with other medical problems that are currently being managed with prescription medications. Audiologists' knowledge of patients' nonhearing/balance disorder might be considered "general" at best. For example, audiologists may be somewhat knowledgeable about visual disorders, but they are not optometrists (and vice versa).

They are not expected to fully understand the biochemistry, pharmacokinetics, or pharmacodynamics of every drug that patients take. However, the Web provides a wealth of information that, in the past, was not easily accessible to audiologists, let alone to the consumer. Audiologists' ability to access information quickly from their office or home computer has expedited finding answers to almost any question on any topic—and consumers now have access to the same information and databases that were once restricted to a limited group of interested parties. The educational community has developed distance learning courses that a person can take online, leading to a college degree or another advanced degree.

For consumers, the medical and pharmaceutical communities have also made information available for free on their Web sites. Visitors can learn more about their health conditions, possible treatment options, and prescription drugs as well as herbal and nutritional supplements and homeopathic medicines. The sites even contain links to other professional, commercial, and/or consumer Web sites where a person can obtain additional health information, including support group Web sites, for most disorders and medical conditions.

This chapter addresses using the Internet to research trustworthy, legitimate, and preferred Web sites for drug information available to the professional and the consumer.

Note: *The author, editor, and publisher do not endorse or have any vested interest in any of the commercial sites listed. Rather, this chapter lists a sampling of sites for drug information from sources considered to be of interest to audiologists and active at the time this book went to press.*

GETTING TO WHERE YOU WANT TO GO FAST

Basic Internet research is achieved in the following way. Simply type a keyword (or keywords) in a browser (AOL, Yahoo, etc.) search window, and in a few seconds, numerous Web sites are listed using that keyword. Those Web sites give the researcher a myriad of places to visit—and information to learn.

To make the most of one's time on the Internet, specificity is very important in selecting keyword(s). For example, entering the word *drugs* in the browser's search window seems easy. However, using America Online, that word brings up a list of over 1,240,000 Web sites for review. Clearly, more specific terminology is needed. Audiologists just need to add specific words, as shown in the following examples:

- *Ototoxic drugs* identifies 369 sites, thus reducing reading time from several months to several days.

- *Ototoxic drug side effects* identifies 421 sites—still, a few days of reading.

- *Pediatric ototoxic drug side effects* identifies 103 sites.

- *Fatal pediatric ototoxic drug side effects* identifies twenty-nine sites.

- *Fatal European pediatric ototoxic drug side effects* yields eight sites.

- *Fatal over-the-counter European pediatric ototoxic drug effects* identifies just one site.

INTERNET WEB SITE BASICS

Visitors to any Web site should be given information, navigational direction, and tools needed to make effective use of content. The American Medical Association (AMA) (http://www.ama-assn.org) provides medical and health information of high quality via its Web site. The AMA recommends that the visitor ask the following questions when viewing a medical-related Web site:

- *Whose site is it?* Site ownership, including affiliations, strategic alliances, and significant investors, should be clearly indicated on the home page or directly accessible from a link on the home page.

- *Viewer access.* Does this site require a fee to view? If so, how are payments to be made? Is the Web site secure for financial information if payments are made? What is its privacy policy? Can anyone enter this site? Is a password needed, and does the site have password protection (if applicable)?

- *Is this site funded?* Funding, sponsorship funding, or other sponsorship for any specific content should be clearly indicated. Content should be easily distinguished from any advertising.

- *Is the language clear?* Is the language complexity of the content appropriate for the site's audience?

- *Are the dates of revising and updating and timeliness of editorial content posted?* Information from a site whose last posted update was a few years ago may be useless.

- *Reference material* should be cited in a manner appropriate for the site's audience.

- *Are there intrasite and/or intersite links?* These links easily assist the visitor in locating additional information on a specific topic.

- *Can files be downloaded to a computer?* If content can be downloaded in a portable document file (PDF) format, instructions regarding how to download the PDF file and how to obtain the necessary software should be provided and easy to find. A link to such software should also be provided.

- *Is there a site map (or another site organizational guide)?* This helps visitors get to where they want to go faster. Also, is there a frequently-asked-questions (FAQ) page? A useful tool is the "Contact Us" feature. This feedback mechanism puts the visitor in touch with a product specialist to answer questions.

Drug Manufacturers' Web Sites

The following is a sample "tour" of a pharmaceutical company's Web site. The information that appears on the site can be quite informative and educational. Once an individual becomes familiar with touring one site, he or she will generally find the methods for touring other sites similar.

In the browser's search window, type the name of the company. The home page will then appear, which is where the visitor is first introduced to the company. Some companies use the home page to inform visitors of current news, stock information (for publicly traded companies), and product highlights. Recent press releases are also linked here.

Legal notices and disclaimers are usually found on the home page. These notices include copyright and trademark information. Disclaimers essentially hold the company harmless from any liability if the visitor is harmed or injured by the information presented on or linked from the Web page. The Bristol-Myers Squibb (http://www.bms.com) disclaimer reads as follows:

> *This site may contain from time to time information related to various health, medical and fitness conditions and their treatment. Such information is not meant to be a substitute for the advice provided by a physician or other medical professional. You should not use the information contained herein for diagnosing a health or fitness problem or disease. You should always consult a physician and medical advisers. This site may provide links or references to other Web sites not affiliated with Bristol-Myers Squibb. Bristol-Myers Squibb is not responsible for the content of such other sites and shall not be liable for any damages or injury arising from users' access to such sites. Links to other sites are provided only as a convenience to users of our site.*

The About Us tab provides the visitor with information about the company's administration. In general, such information includes the names of the president and members of the board of directors (including medical consultants). Also listed are the company's corporate address and phone numbers, its New York Stock Exchange listing (if applicable), the number of employees, global sales figures, donations, businesses (i.e., pharmaceuticals, infant and children's nutritional products, etc.), and a sample list of the company's key products. Other links on this page may take the visitor to the company's history, any awards it has received, special committees, other Web sites it maintains (i.e., international), and any business links.

Visitors may see a News, Newsroom, or Press Release tab. Those areas provide the most recently issued press releases issued by the company. Some sites even allow visitors to access the Press Release archives. A contact name and phone number might be listed, too. Another link on the home page might be to company publications (brochures, information sheets, etc.), including the company's annual report. Most can be downloaded in PDF format.

The site will probably include a Products tab where visitors can read about the company's over-the-counter (OTC) medications and/or its medications that have been approved by the Food and Drug Administration (FDA). There may even be a dedicated Web site for a particular drug and a link to any of the company's other Web sites. By clicking a product name, visitors are sent to a new home page for that product, where they will find both consumer-friendly information and health care professional information.

The consumer section provides the visitor with information written in plain language, usually accompanied by several photographs and other illustrations. From there, information packets, brochures, and other educational information can be ordered directly. FAQs, a common tab found on Web sites, usually answers more common questions about a drug. The health care professionals section offers technical information such as prescribing recommendations, professional journal references for published research about a drug, adverse drug reactions, drug interactions, and other critical information.

Usually, this section includes a search window for getting more specific information. An Index tab may also be available with a variety of related topics to the drug in question. A very useful tab is Contact Us. A person can e-mail a question or express a concern about a product directly to the company. Usually, within a few days, he or she will receive a reply from the company's public relations/public information department or product specialist.

The following is a sample inquiry from an audiologist:

I am an audiologist in private practice. I have a 75-year-old male patient who has been using _____ for two months now. This is his only medication, and he does not take any herbals.

The patient reports tinnitus bilaterally within 30 minutes of taking his daily pill. The ringing usually lasts for a few hours but is not debilitating, just annoying. I note that tinnitus (or any other aural disturbance) is not listed as an adverse drug reaction in the latest edition of the Physician's Desk Reference (PDR) or on your drug's dedicated Web site.

Do you have any subsequent post-FDA approval data (including incidence figures) on tinnitus as an ADR of this medication?

Thank you.

The audiologist should always include his or her full name; degree; title; and business/hospital name, address, and telephone and fax numbers. The Contact Us tab is the best way to get the most current consumer and professional information or to express a concern about a particular product. Companies are generally very responsive to these e-mails.

Another tab of interest might be Research and Development, or R&D. It is here that the visitor learns about the ongoing FDA clinical trials for drugs under investigation by the company. Information about the locations of the research sites around the world may also be listed.

A variety of information may be available. For publicly traded companies on the New York Stock Exchange (http://www.nyse.com) or the American Stock Exchange (http://www.amex.com), investors can access investment information that includes financial reports, Securities and Exchange Commission (SEC) filings (http://www.sec.gov), stockholder services, and stock trading history. Some companies have an e-mail service to which visitors can subscribe to get the latest stock information via e-mail. The site might even offer a Job Opportunities/Careers/Employment section that takes visitors to the appropriate page listing available jobs and provides information about how to apply online. Finally, most sites usually include a keyword search window. The window is useful if a visitor is unsuccessful in locating the information he or she seeks from the company using its other tabs. From the keyword search, the visitor should be guided to the area of interest.

Important Web Sites and Sources of Information

Any person can set up a Web site and offer information on any topic, including health care and treatment strategies for a specific disease or disorder. The reader should first visit the U.S. Food and Drug Administration's (FDA) Web site. The following federal agencies offer credible information on drugs for consumers and professionals since all prescription drugs must be approved by the FDA. The information on these sites is updated regularly.

Food and Drug Administration (FDA)

The FDA (http://www.fda.gov) is an agency within the Department of Health & Human Services (DHHS) that comprises eight centers/offices, which are listed in Table 22-1. Selecting a center/office will take visitors to its home page. Visitors may also view the agency's organizational charts, read an overview about the FDA, and learn about the agency's work in protecting public health. The FDA Web site has organized its main page to assist visitors in accessing the information provided.

The FDA is responsible for protecting public health by assuring the safety, efficacy, and security of human and veterinary drugs, biological products, medical devices, the nation's food supply, cosmetics, and products that emit radiation. The FDA is also responsible for advancing public health by expediting innovations that make medicines and foods more effective, safer, and more affordable and helping people get the accurate, science-based information they need to use medicines and foods to improve their health.

For audiologists, one of the most useful FDA sites is CDER. This organization promotes and protects the health of Americans by assuring that all prescription and OTC drugs are safe and effective. CDER evaluates all new drugs before they are sold and serves as a consumer watchdog for the more than 10,000 drugs on the market to ensure that they continue to meet the highest standards. The center routinely monitors TV, radio, and print drug ads to ensure that they are truthful and balanced. CDER also plays a critical role in providing health professionals and consumers with information about how to use drugs appropriately and safely.

The center depends on a cadre of experienced physicians, toxicologists, chemists, statisticians, mathematicians, project managers, and other highly qualified and dedicated professionals. In 2002, the center launched important initiatives to remove barriers to innovation in drug development and to facilitate the modernization of U.S. drug manufacturing. CDER continues to enhance its drug safety program to help ensure that drugs are used safely once they are approved. The center is collaborating with a broad spectrum of groups to improve information for both health care providers and consumers. CDER continues to facilitate development of new drugs and new uses for already approved drugs that could be used as medical countermeasures.

Table 22-1. FDA Center/Office Web Sites

Center for Biologics Evaluation and Research (CBER)	http://www.fda.gov
Center for Devices and Radiological Health (CDRH)	http://www.fda.gov
Center for Drug Evaluation and Research (CDER)	http://www.fda.gov
Center for Food Safety and Applied Nutrition (CFSAN)	http://vm.cfsan.fda.gov
Center for Veterinary Medicine (CVM)	http://www.fda.gov
National Center for Toxicological Research (NCTR)	http://www.fda.gov
Office of the Commissioner (OC)	http://www.fda.gov (Conduct a search using the keywords *Office of the Commissioner.*)
Office of Regulatory Affairs (ORA)	http://www.fda.gov

When visiting the FDA's CDER Web site, visitors will find Quick Info Links such as Drugs@FDA. There visitors can access the complete catalog of FDA-approved drug products (both brand names and generic names) and tentatively approved prescription, OTC, and discontinued drugs. They can learn about a particular drug by typing its brand name or generic name in the "Search by Drug Name or Active Ingredient" window. For example, typing *cisplatin*, a known ototoxic drug, will identify its two brand names (Platinol and Platinol-AQ) in addition to the generic name (cisplatin). The active ingredient is also listed. By clicking on the word *cisplatin*, visitors go to an Overview page that lists the form (injectable) and strengths available (10mg/vial; 1mg/ML; 50mg/vial) and the marketing status (prescription). Visitors can then identify the manufacturers of the generic version of cisplatin (AM Pharm Partners, Bedford, Pharmachemie, and Sicor Pharms) or the brand name manufacturer (Bristol-Meyers).

The site also provides a Glossary of Terms throughout; all a user has to do is click on the already highlighted word.

National Library of Medicine (NLM)

The National Library of Medicine (NLM) (http://www.nlm.nih.gov) is the world's largest medical library. The library collects materials in all areas of biomedicine and health care, as well as works on biomedical aspects of technology; the humanities; and the physical, life, and social sciences. The collections stand at more than 7 million items—books, journals, technical reports, manuscripts, microfilms, photographs, and images. NLM is a national resource for all U.S. health science libraries through a National Network of Libraries of Medicine.

For 125 years, the library published the Index Medicus, a monthly subject/author guide to articles in 4,000 journals. Today that information is available in the database MEDLINE, the major component of PubMed, freely accessible via the World Wide Web. PubMed has more than 12 million MEDLINE journal article references and abstracts going back to the mid-1960s, with another 1.5 million references back to the early 1950s. Consumers can access this site through MedlinePlus (http://medlineplus.gov).

MedlinePlus has extensive information from the National Institutes of Health (NIH) (and other sources) on over 650 diseases and conditions. There are also lists of hospitals and physicians, a medical encyclopedia and a medical dictionary, health information in Spanish, extensive information on prescription and nonprescription drugs, health information from the media, and links to thousands of clinical trials. MedlinePlus is updated daily. The site contains no advertising, nor does MedlinePlus endorse any company or product.

Information on thousands of prescription and OTC medications can be obtained from the Drug Information section. The information is provided through two drug resources—MedMaster, a product of the American Society of Health-System Pharmacists (ASHP), and the USP DI and Advice for the Patient, a product of the U.S. Pharmacopeia (USP).

MedWatch—FDA Safety Information and Adverse Event Reporting Program

MedWatch (available through http://www.fda.gov) serves health care professionals and the medical product-using public. It provides important and timely clinical information about safety issues involving medical products, including prescription and OTC drugs, biologics, medical and radiation-emitting devices, and special nutritional products (e.g., medical foods, dietary supplements, and infant formulas).

Medical product safety alerts, recalls, withdrawals, and important labeling changes that may affect the health of all Americans are quickly disseminated to the medical community and the general public via this Web site and MedWatch E-list. By selecting *Safety Information*, visitors can see reports, safety notifications, and labeling changes posted to the Web site since 1996.

MedWatch even allows health care professionals and consumers to report serious problems that they suspect are associated with drugs and medical devices they prescribe, dispense, or use. Reporting can be done online or over the telephone or by submitting the MedWatch 3500 form by mail or fax. Forms can be easily downloaded. Continuing education articles, FDA bulletins, and articles from the FDA's *Consumer* magazine can also be printed out. The site is very easy to navigate.

MedWatch Safety Alerts can be delivered by e-mail. By subscribing (for free), consumers and health care professionals obtain directly from the FDA clinically important medical product safety alerts and concise, timely information about the drugs and devices they use, prescribe, or dispense every day. Each e-mail contains a summary of the safety alert. When a visitor needs to know more, a hyperlink in the e-mail directs him or her to more detailed information. The MedWatch E-list is an automated message delivery system; it does not allow users to post or reply to messages.

National Institute on Deafness and Other Communication Disorders (NIDCD)

This site (http://www.nidcd.nih.gov) contains information about the National Institute on Deafness and Other Communication Disorders (NIDCD), one of the institutes that comprise the NIH. NIDCD supports and conducts research in and distributes information on the disorders of human communication to improve the lives of millions of individuals with communication disorders.

NIDCD Directory of Organizations

The NIDCD directory (http://www.nidcd.nih.gov) lists organizations that are national in scope and that focus on health issues relating to hearing, balance, smell, taste, voice, and speech. The directory is designed to encourage networking among individuals and organizations that have an interest in deafness and communication disorders. Clicking on the Health Info link provides more information on these topics.

Pharmacopeias

Pharmacopeias are nonprofit standards setting organizations. Several worldwide pharmacopeias provide consumers and professionals with a wealth of research information about medications, their ingredients, and dietary supplements. Pharmacopeias are generally good sources of reliable information that do not have a commercial slant.

U.S. Pharmacopeia (USP)

The USP (http://www.usp.org) is a nongovernmental, standards setting organization that advances public health by ensuring the quality and consistency of medicines, promoting the safe and proper use of medications, and verifying ingredients in dietary supplements. USP standards are developed by a unique process of public involvement and are accepted worldwide. In addition to standards development, USP's other public health programs focus on promoting optimal health care delivery (discussed in the following paragraph). USP achieves its goals through the contributions of volunteers representing pharmacy, medicine, and other health care professions, as well as science, academia, the U.S. government, the pharmaceutical industry, and consumer organizations.

Are Your Patients Involved in a Clinical Study?

Clinical trials are voluntary research studies conducted in humans. They are designed to answer specific questions about the safety and/or effectiveness of drugs, vaccines, other therapies, or new ways of using existing treatments. (More information can be found at http://www.fda.gov, using the keywords *clinical trials*.)

In areas of the country where major drug manufacturers conduct their research, audiologists should be aware that a patient's communication complaints might be related to a drug that the patient is evaluating as part of an FDA-approved study. The case history questions should address that possibility. Chapter 4 addresses clinical trials in detail.

The USP's Drug Quality and Information (DQI) Program (http://www.uspdqi.org) provides technical assistance in drug quality assurance, develops and disseminates unbiased drug and therapeutic information, trains health care workers to better use medicines, and provides scientific evidence for health care decision making in developing countries. USP DQI is supported by a cooperative agreement with the United States Agency for International Development (USAID) (http://www.usaid.gov) and USP. Thus far, the USP DQI Program has established a presence in the Mekong region of Vietnam, Mozambique, Nepal, Russia and the New Independent States (NIS), and Senegal. The program is advancing strategies to improve drug quality and the appropriate use of drugs and is expanding to other regions.

British Pharmacopoeia (BP)

The British Pharmacopoeia (BP), according to its Web site (http://www.pharmacopoeia.co.uk), is "the most up-to-date and authoritative resource on standards for medicinal substances and pharmaceutical products in the United Kingdom (UK)." The BP contains many new monographs, both British and those from the European Pharmacopoeia (EP). The BP has essential information for anyone concerned with the quality of medicines, including pharmaceutical and chemical industries, quality control personnel, analysts, government regulators, academics, and students of pharmacy.

American Herbal Pharmacopoeia (AHP)

The mission of the AHP (http://www.herbal-ahp.org) is to promote the responsible use of herbal medicines and ensure that they are used with the highest achievable degree of safety and efficacy. AHP's primary method to accomplish that is through the development of standards of identity, purity, and analysis for botanicals, as well as the critical review of traditional and scientific data regarding their efficacy and safety. Those works are disseminated through a variety of AHP publications including monographs, textbooks, and other educational materials; workshops and conferences; electronic media; and other appropriate avenues of distribution.

While herbal medicines are well integrated into the health care systems of many other nations, that is not the case in the United States. Authoritative information regarding proper use and manufacture of herbal medicines is lacking. The AHP and Therapeutic Compendium was founded to address that deficiency.

In 1994, the AHP began developing qualitative and therapeutic information on botanicals, including many of the Ayurvedic (http://www.niam.com) (Indian), Chinese, and Western herbs most frequently used in the United States. These monographs represent the most comprehensive and critically reviewed body of information on herbal medicines in the English language and serve as a primary reference for academicians, health care providers, manufacturers, and regulators.

FDA's Role with Herbals. For decades, the FDA regulated dietary supplements as foods, in most circumstances, to ensure that they were safe and wholesome and that their labeling was truthful and not misleading. An important facet of ensuring safety was the FDA's evaluation of the safety of all new ingredients, including those used in dietary supplements, under the 1958 Food Additive Amendments to the Federal Food, Drug, and Cosmetic (FD&C) Act. However, with passage of the Dietary Supplement Health and Education Act of 1994 (DSHEA) (information can be found at http://www.fda.gov, using the keyword *DSHEA*), Congress amended the FD&C Act to include several provisions that apply only to dietary supplements and dietary ingredients of dietary supplements. As a result of those provisions, dietary ingredients used in dietary supplements are no longer subject to the premarket safety evaluations required of other new food ingredients or for new uses of old food ingredients. They must, however, meet the requirements of other safety provisions.

The DSHEA acknowledges that millions of consumers believe dietary supplements may help to augment daily diets and provide health benefits. Congress's intent in enacting the DSHEA was to meet the concerns of consumers and manufacturers to help ensure that safe and appropriately labeled products remain available to those who want to use them. In the findings associated with the DSHEA, Congress stated that there may be a positive relationship between sound dietary practice and good health and that although further scientific research is needed, there may be a connection between dietary supplement use, reduced health care expenses, and disease prevention.

The provisions of the DSHEA define dietary supplements and dietary ingredients, establish a new framework for assuring safety, outline guidelines for literature displayed where supplements are sold, provide for use of claims and nutritional support statements, require ingredient and nutrition labeling, and grant the FDA the authority to establish good manufacturing practice (GMP) regulations. The law also requires formation of an executive level Commission on Dietary Supplement Labels and an Office of Dietary Supplements within the NIH. An excellent review of this legislation is at http://www.cfsan.fda.gov. Also, see Section XII.

European Pharmacopeia (EP)

Founded by eight countries (Belgium, France, Germany, Italy, Luxembourg, the Netherlands, Switzerland, and the UK) in 1964 and based in Strasbourg, France, the EP (http://www.pheur.org) is also known as the European Directorate for the Quality of Medicines (EDQM). The EDQM evolved from the EP; this evolution was necessary because new responsibilities and activities had developed. The success of the biological standardization program for medicines for human use, run by the EP Secretariat, led to initiating further collaboration between the Commission of the European Communities and the Council of Europe in the area of the quality control of medicines. The EDQM is part of the administrative structure of the Council of Europe. The EP's Web site is not easy to navigate unless one has a scientific background.

International Organizations and Associations

Around the world, nations have recognized the need to share health care information. The Web provides quick access to information twenty-four hours a day without regard to time zones. Although the following list is not comprehensive, the major Web sites for health and pharmaceutically related information are provided below.

World Health Organization (WHO)

Worldwide, nations have pooled their resources to assist one another in the dissemination of accurate information about medications and in providing consumer education. It is the World Health Organization (WHO) (http://www.who.it) that oversees public health issues. WHO is the United Nations (UN) specialized agency for health issues. Established in 1948, WHO's objective is the attainment by all people of the highest possible level of health. The WHO coordinates programs aimed at solving health problems and helping all people attain the highest possible level of health. It works in areas such as immunizations, health education, and the provision of essential drugs.

Pan American Health Organizations (PAHO)

With headquarters in Washington, D.C., the Pan American Health Organization (PAHO) (http://www.paho.org) is an international public health agency with one hundred years of experience in working to improve health and living standards of the countries of North, Latin, and South America. It serves as the specialized organization for health of the Inter-American System. It also serves as the regional office for the Americas of the World Health Organization and enjoys international recognition as part of the UN system.

Drug Programme of Health Canada

Health Canada (http://www.hc-sc.gc.ca) is the federal department, in partnership with provincial and territorial governments, that provides national leadership to develop health policy, enforce health regulations, promote disease prevention, and enhance healthy living for all Canadians. Health Canada ensures that health services are available and accessible to First Nations and Inuit communities. It also works closely with other federal departments, agencies, and health stakeholders to reduce health and safety risks to Canadians.

Through its administration of the Canada Health Act, Health Canada is committed to maintaining Canada's world-renowned health insurance system, which is universally available to permanent residents, comprehensive in the services it covers, accessible without income barriers, portable within and outside the country, and publicly administered. Health Canada's Web site also includes the Notices of Compliance and the Canadian Drug ID Codebook.

Product Quality Research Institute (PQRI)

The Product Quality Research Institute (PQRI) (http://www.pqri.org) is a collaborative process involving FDA's CDER, industry, and academia. The mission of PQRI is to conduct research to generate scientific information to support regulatory policy. This initiative will help identify the types of product quality information that should be submitted in a regulatory filing to CDER. The outcomes of PQRI are focused on research projects whose results provide a continuing scientific basis for regulatory policy.

The institute comprises the following organizations: American Association of Pharmaceutical Scientists (AAPS), Consumer Healthcare Products Association (CHPA), Generic Pharmaceutical Association (GPhA, formerly GPIA, NPA, ad NAPM), Parenteral Drug Association (PDA), Pharmaceutical Research and Manufacturers of America (PhRMA), FDA/CDER, International Pharmaceutical Aerosol Consortium on Regulation & Science (IPAC-RS), International Pharmaceutical Excipients Council of the Americas (IPEC-Americas), International Society for Pharmaceutical Engineering (ISPE), and USP.

MedicAlert

Founded in 1956, MedicAlert (http://www.medicalert.org) is one of the world's largest nonprofit membership organizations that saves lives in emergencies by providing member identification and medical information to doctors, nurses, and other medical personnel. Over 4 million members worldwide rely on the MedicAlert Service to protect them, regardless of where they live or travel. MedicAlert is known for its bracelet and pendant alerting device. Its popular television advertisement shows an elderly woman lying on her living room floor, saying, "Help! I've fallen and I can't get up!"

MedicAlert's Emergency Response Center handles more than 3,000 emergency calls annually. It provides instant access to identification and vital information. The 24-Hour Emergency Response Center provides translation support in more than 140 languages to meet today's demand for transmission of personal medical information.

Pharmaceutical Industry

The pharmaceutical manufacturers have organized worldwide to have a "common ground" for R&D and education. Worldwide, there are over seventy organizations. The list includes many state associations. The following list shows the variety of organizations associated with the pharmaceutical industry.

- *The Association of the British Pharmaceutical Industry* (http://www.abpi.org.uk) is a trade association of companies in the UK that produces prescription medicines; the Web site offers information about the society and statistics.

- *Belgian Pharmaceutical Industry Association (AGIM)* (http://pharma.be) presents information about the pharmaceutical industry and medicines in Belgium and about AGIM and her member companies, figures, publications, position statements, and ethical code.

- *British Institute of Regulatory Affairs (BIRA)* (http://www.bira.org.uk) is the foremost association for drug registration professionals.

- *Drug Information Association* (http://www.diahome.org) provides information on the discovery, development, evaluation, and utilization of medicines and related health care technologies.

- *European Federation of Pharmaceutical Industries and Associations (EFPIA)* (http://www.efpia.org) represents the research-based pharmaceutical industry operating in Europe. Members comprise twenty-nine national pharmaceutical industry associations (in addition to six associations with liaison status) and forty-three leading pharmaceutical companies involved in the research, development, and manufacturing of medicinal products in Europe for human use.

- *Health Research Association* (http://www.health-research.org) provides names of well-trained, experienced physicians/researchers in any medical specialty; the researchers work with state-of-the-art equipment and have a huge patient pool.

- *Institute For Safe Medication Practices (ISMP)* (http://www.ismp.org) provides information about adverse drug events and their prevention to health care practitioners and institutions, regulatory agencies, professional organizations, and the pharmaceutical industry; the Web site includes research findings, books and publications, an electronic discussion forum, and links to related sites.

- *International Pharmaceutical Federation* (http://www.fip.nl) is a worldwide federation of national pharmaceutical (professional and scientific) associations that represents and serves pharmacy and pharmaceutical sciences around the globe.

- *Pharmaceutical Marketing Club of Quebec* (http://www.pmcq.qc.ca) has more than 400 members connected to the pharmaceutical and biotech industry.

- *PhRMA* (http://www.phrma.org) represents the country's leading research-based pharmaceutical and biotechnology companies. In 2003, the companies invested more that $33.2 billion in discovering and developing new medicines, marking the thirty-third straight year the industry has increased its investment in R&D. PhRMA conducts effective advocacy for public policies that encourage discovery of important new medicines

for patients by pharmaceutical/biotechnology research companies.

- *PQRI* (http://www.pqri.org) conducts research to generate scientific information to support regulatory policy.

Worldwide, there are over 140 pharmaceutical companies. Each company has its own Web site, and most maintain a Web site for the individual drugs they produce. Each Web site contains general and educational information a well as advertising. Pharmaceutical companies take great pride in presenting their public image in a way that is both professional and friendly.

Professional Web Sites

In medicine and allied health fields, professional associations exist to unify each profession to achieve goals and objectives germane to the individual specialty. The following list of professional organizations can also be a source of drug-related information. Most of these sites are user-friendly and have a Contact Us link.

American Medical Association (AMA)

The AMA (http://www.ama-assn.org) is the professional organization for all physicians in the United States. The organization serves as the steward of medicine and leader of the medical profession. The AMA's envisioned future is to be an essential part of the professional life of every physician and an essential force for progress in improving the nation's health. The AMA has the national voice and the reputation and the stature to be a strong advocate for physicians and their patients. Through active advocacy at all levels of the private and public sectors, the AMA is working to protect the patient-physician relationship, which is at the heart of medicine. Advocacy takes many forms, including public health initiatives, legislation, marketplace interventions, and strengthening physician leverage in negotiations. As an activist physician organization, the AMA is dedicated to ensuring that the patient-physician bond is kept vital and that physicians retain the freedom to practice the science and art of medicine in its purest form.

Parental Drug Association (PDA)

Since its founding in 1946, PDA (http://www.pda.org) has been a nonprofit association that does not perform consulting services for individual companies. PDA's membership includes microbiologists, chemists, pharmacists, engineers, and others sharing a common interest in pharmaceutical manufacturing and quality. Members include employees of pharmaceutical companies, suppliers of goods and services to the pharmaceutical industry, academia, government agencies, and independent consultants.

American Academy of Otolaryngology—Head and Neck Surgery (AAO-HNS)

The American Academy of Otolaryngology—Head and Neck Surgery (AAO-HNS) (http://www.entnet.org) is a nonprofit association that represents the interests of ear, nose, and throat specialists and their patients to the public, government, other medical specialists, and related organizations. It is the world's largest organization representing specialists who treat the ear, nose, throat, and related structures of the head and neck. The organization represents more than 10,000 otolaryngologists.

The organization's Web site is not consumer friendly for information about drugs and their side effects. Professionals will find limited information. However, there is a link to the DHSS (http://www.hhs.gov). On that site, visitors can find many pages of articles dealing with drug side effects. Most of the articles are consumer-oriented.

American Academy of Audiology (AAA)

The American Academy of Audiology (AAA) (http://www.audiology.org) is the world's largest professional organization of, for, and by audiologists. The active membership of more than 9,600 audiologists join together to provide the highest quality of hearing health care service to children and adults described by its national slogan "Caring for America's Hearing." There is a drug and herbal side effects reference publication; however, it is available only to AAA members.

American Speech-Language-Hearing Association (ASHA)

Membership in the American Speech-Language-Hearing Association (ASHA) (http://www.asha.org) comprises speech-language pathologists and audiologists. The Web site is more "professional friendly" than "consumer friendly." If a consumer types in *side effects* or *drug* in the search window, over 60 articles that mention drug side effects and over 300 articles for drugs are posted. Specific topics are not separated. Unfortunately, some articles cannot be accessed unless a visitor is a member.

Commercial Web Sites

The Internet has provided companies directly or indirectly associated with the pharmaceutical industry with new avenues of marketing. Several commercial sites are noteworthy. Again, however, the site visitor should consider the source and determine whether any information is biased.

Drugs.com

The site http://www.drugs.com is intended for viewing by the U.S. audience only. If a person is in another country, local laws may not permit access to the medical information contained in the site.

Drugs.com is a drug information resource online. The site provides fast, easy searching of over 24,000 FDA-approved medications (including OTC products).

Drugs.com states that it is not an online pharmacy; nor does it condone the sale of prescription medicines over the Internet without a prescription. Drugs.com provides a free drug-information service to help visitors better understand how medicines work: their uses, side effects, and potential to interact with other medicines. For information on purchasing prescription medicines online Drugs.com suggests the FDA's "Buying Prescription Medicines Online: A Consumer Safety Guide" (http://www.fda.gov). In the right column of the FDA web site, a visitor clicks the Buying Medicines Online link under "Hot Topics." Under "Drugs,", he or she clicks the link that reads "Buying Prescription Medicines Online: A Consumer Safety Guide."

The "Latest News" and "FDA Drug Alerts" sections are written by Drugs.com's in-house staff of health care journalists. The topical health information presented under "Categories" is sourced from Micromedex and summarized by the staff pharmacists at Drugs.com.

Unlike many drug information sites, Drugs.com is not affiliated with any pharmaceutical companies. The only funding it receives from pharmaceutical companies is by way of advertisements that occasionally appear on the Drugs.com Web site. It states that that advertising in no way affects the content of the drug information it supplies.

Visitors can search for a drug by name by typing it in the search window or selecting from the A–Z links. Most alphabetical selections have multiple pages. Brand names and generic names are listed.

Searching for cisplatin, a known ototoxic drug, provides not only a brief description of the drug and its brand name(s), but also detailed consumer information in the form of FAQs. The same is true for all drugs listed. Some FAQs include the following:

- What is the most important information I should know about cisplatin?

- What is cisplatin?

- Who should not use cisplatin?

- How should I use cisplatin?

- What happens if I miss a dose?

- What happens if I overdose?

- What should I avoid while using cisplatin?

- What are the possible side effects of cisplatin?

- What other drugs will affect cisplatin?

- Where can I get more information?

Additional information includes a link to the Internet for the drug, a link for Spanish-speaking visitors, information from the PDR (http://www.pdr.net), and news and related articles.

Cable News Network (CNN)

The Cable News Network (CNN) site (http://www.cnn.com) is among the world's leaders in online news and information delivery. Staffed twenty-four hours, seven days a week by a staff in CNN's world headquarters in Atlanta, Georgia, and in bureaus worldwide, CNN.com relies heavily on CNN's global team of almost 4,000 news professionals. CNN.com features the latest multimedia technologies, from live video streaming to audio packages to searchable archives of news features and background information. The Health tab links visitors to a page that is affiliated with the Mayo Clinic (http://www.mayoclinic.com) in Rochester, Minnesota.

The CNN.com Health Centers section has several headings titled "Family Health," "Women's Health," "Men's Health," "Senior's Health," "Fitness and Nutrition," "Working Life," and "Pain Management." All sections are extremely thorough in coverage and written in plain language. The Condition Centers section identifies five major areas where visitors can address specific issues: AIDS/HIV & Immune System, Arthritis, Cancer, Digestive System, and Mental Health.

Drug InfoNet

Based in East Syracuse, New York, this site (http://www.druginfonet.com) will simplify one's search for health care information. Visitors can review the Drug InfoNet pages containing information and link to other health care sites on the Internet. This site provides a wide range of health care information, coupled with easy access. There are special tabs for FAQs, drug information, disease information, drug manufacturers (both prescription and OTC), health news, general health information, medical references, U.S. government sites, selected hospital Web sites by region, and selected medical schools worldwide.

Deafness/Hard of Hearing

The site http://www.deafness.about.com deals with deafness and hearing loss and has an excellent section on ototoxicity. By clicking on the Hearing Loss Basics link under the Topics menu in the left column, then clicking "Causes of Hearing Loss," and then selecting "Ototoxicity," visitors will find a list of different articles, resources, and links for more information. There is also a link for more information about ototoxicity. This page provides a more detailed explanation of ototoxicity and has a small list of ototoxic drugs; a longer, more detailed list is easily accessible. After the category description, a graph identifies ototoxicity, vestibulotoxicity, the toxic levels, and the percent of toxicity. There are advertisements and links to different sites. The negative aspect of the site is that it is focused mainly on the hard-of-hearing and deaf populations. Consequently, only a limited amount on information is available about ototoxicity.

eMedicine

eMedicine (http://www.emedicine.com) is an excellent source for medical and limited consumer information. This site links visitors to a variety of sources including medical journal abstracts (*Journal of the American Medical Association, New England Journal of Medicine*, and *British Medical Journal*), MEDLINE, and "Drug Information Look-up," as well as maintains a professional and consumer journal index. The opportunity to e-mail questions or comments to the author is a useful feature.

The Web site covers very specific topics related to ototoxicity and the effects on the inner ear. The bibliography section includes a link to MEDLINE so visitors can obtain the latest journal articles relating to ototoxicity and effects of medications known to be ototoxic to the cochlea and vestibular system. MEDLINE charges a fee to obtain the articles referenced. The site also provides a concise overview of cochleovestibular toxicity.

Perhaps the most useful link on this site is the patient education section. That section is very easy to understand for a person with no medical background.

Family Practice Notebook

Family Practice Notebook (http://www.fpnotebook.com) has 4,316 topics within 616 chapters and 31 subspecialty books. The author of the Family Practice Notebook is a board-certified family physician. The site's information has been gathered from resources such as lectures, workshops, peer-reviewed articles, bulletins, and texts. Links and patient education materials can be found. Information is referenced, and supporting studies are provided.

However, advertisers and the site's author fund the site. Advertising is evident. The site claims to have over 750,000 visitors per month. The site includes a disclaimer stating that there is an ongoing effort to limit errors and that the visitor should to use his or her own judgment when implementing strategies. Visitors are encouraged to e-mail the site's author if they find any errors.

Institute for Safe Medical Practices (ISMP)

The ISMP (http://www.ismp.org) is a nonprofit organization that works closely with health care practitioners and institutions, regulatory agencies, professional organizations, and the pharmaceutical industry to provide education about adverse drug events and their prevention. The organization provides an independent review of medication errors that have been voluntarily submitted by practitioners to a national Medication Errors Reporting Program (MERP) operated by the USP in the United States. Information from the reports may be used by the USP to impact drug standards. All information derived from the MERP is shared with the FDA and pharmaceutical companies whose products are mentioned in reports.

ISMP is an FDA MedWatch partner and regularly communicates with the FDA to help prevent medication errors. ISMP encourages the appropriate reporting of medication errors to the MedWatch program. ISMP is dedicated to the safe use of medications through improvements in drug distribution, naming, packaging, labeling, and delivery system design. The organization has established a national advisory board of practitioners to assist in problem solving.

MDLinx

Based in Washington, D.C., MDLinx (http://www.mdlinx.com—click on "PharmacistLinx" under the Healthcare Professionals section) is a network of medical Web sites and e-newsletters that provide pharmaceutical and health care companies with direct access to health care professionals and patients interested in the latest patient-focused news. MDLinx owns and operates a network of 34 Web sites and over 700 different daily e-mail newsletters. For health care professionals, MDLinx has a network of comprehensive sites for each medical specialty and therapeutic category. MDLinx recently launched PatientLinx, a free Web site that provides reliable clinical updates for patients. The site also has a section that contains published articles dealing with adverse drug reactions. Visitors must register to access this free site.

Medscape

For an excellent source of drug information, consumers and professionals can link to the American College of Physicians and access abstracts and/or buy chapters. This site (http://www.medscape.com) has a section on Best Dx/Best Rx—point-of-care recommendations. A fee is required to obtain pertinent, concise medical information in various media forms. Visitors can link to various pages depending on their medical specialty.

The home page tabs include News and CME (continuing medical education, but no section for audiologists, that leads to broader subjects). Resource Centers provides a broad range of information (e.g., basic medical information, nutrition, patient safety, business, and law). There is a section on pharmacological management of pain, which links to various options under continuing education.

MedicineNet, Inc.

MedicineNet, Inc. (http://www.medicinenet.com) is an online health care media publishing company. The site provides easy-to-read, in-depth, authoritative medical information for consumers. MedicineNet is a robust, user-friendly, interactive Web site.

RxList

The content of this site (http://www.rxlist.com) is similar to that of Drugs.com for drug information.

This site also offers additional information such as RxList Search to search the RxList database for brand name, generic name, and pharmacologic category. Many of the most popular entries have links to professional- and/or patient-oriented material. The site provides a keyword search that allows visitors to search the body of the professional monographs and the RxList Alternatives content for topics such as interactions, side effects, and foreign brand names. A unique feature of this site is the RxList-ID (Imprint) search. Many tablets and capsules have alphanumeric characters printed on them for identification. Using this search, visitors can identify drugs by the characters printed (imprint codes) on tablets and capsules. A Drug FAQs/Patient monographs section allows visitors to search drug information written in plain English. Finally, a medical dictionary is available— the complete Taber's Medical Encyclopedia of more than 55,000 medical terms.

SafeMedication.com

The site http://www.safemedication.com features complete, easy-to-read information on more than 700 drugs. It is based on the ASHP's drug information resources, which are developed independently by pharmacists and other medication experts.

Sound-Alike Drugs

Sound-Alike Drugs (http://www.nacds.org) is the official site of the National Association of Chain Drug Stores. This site lists a large number of drugs whose names sound alike. It is interesting to see how many drugs sound alike but are prescribed for different ailments, which can cause confusion for both patients and providers.

WebMD

WebMD (http://www.webmd.com) provides services that help physicians, consumers, and providers navigate the complexity of the health care system. WebMD includes providers of online health information, as well as leaders in the areas of electronic data interchange services and practice management software and services to the health care industry. Several key operations include:

- *WebMD Health:* WebMD Health is the leading consumer-focused health care information Web site with 20 million visitors each month. Consumers can access health and wellness news, support communities, interactive health management tools, and more. The site includes online communities and special events that allow consumers to participate in real-time discussions with experts and with other people who share similar health conditions and concerns.

- *Medscape from WebMD:* This site provides clinical information and educational tools that are objective, credible, and relevant to members, their patients, and their practice. With over 575,000 members registered as physicians and 1.6 million allied health care professionals worldwide, the Medscape from WebMD portal claims to reach more health care providers than any other online professional destination.

Ototoxicity/Vestibulotoxicity Web Sites

Many prescription medications have side effects that can cause hearing loss or vestibular problems. Internet information for both the professional and consumer abound on this topic. Several sites are concise and well organized (including easily understood graphs and charts) and offer numerous useful links. However, Web sites owned by nonphysicians, audiologists, oncology nurses, etc., must be viewed cautiously. Some sites, although generally informative, serve as an advertising platform for the owners, whose goal is to sell their books, pamphlets, and OTC remedies.

Ototoxic Medications

Ototoxic Medications (http://www.tchain.com) is a personal Web site by Timothy C. Hain, MD. For detailed information on ototoxic drugs, visitors can click on "Information for dizzy patients," then open "Educational information (primarily for patients)." From there, they click on "Otoxic drugs." The author

states that this Web site is for information purposes and does not replace an examination by a physician. The Web site clearly states that the other Web sites linked within are neither endorsed nor maintained by the author of this Web site.

The site lists ototoxic medications in table format. Each chart identifies what the class of drug is, whether it is vestibulotoxic or cochleotoxic, and what the ototoxicity level is. The site provides seven tables dedicated to chemotherapy agents, antibiotics with good evidence of ototoxicity, antibiotics for which there is suspicion for ototoxicity, antibiotics considered safe, ototoxic diuretics, quinine derivatives, and miscellaneous ototoxic drugs. The site also has a section for ototoxins that are not medications, such as mercury, lead, and noise. Links at the end of the Web site to related articles are a great resource for research related to cochlear and vestibulotoxic drugs.

Occupational Ototoxins

The site http://chppm-www.apgea.army.mil provides a thorough listing of potential ototoxic chemicals in the occupational environment. This site emanates from the U.S. Army Center for Health Promotion and Preventive Medicine.

Ototoxicity

The Web site http://www.vestibular.org provides a practical review of ototoxicity written by P. J. Haybach, who is a registered nurse. The information is easy to read. The site is user friendly, even for the nonprofessional.

The Web site http://www.personal.umich.edu includes an excellent overview of ototoxic drugs for professionals and consumers. A link to the FDA's Medwatch Web site is also provided. The author reviews information to help visitors understand both the generic form of the drug and the propriety or brand name. Visitors to the site can also access a pharmacology link to look up a particular drug. Another section reviews ototoxic antibiotics. Other medical problems and ototoxic drug correlates are also reviewed.

Vertigo

The site http://www.ivertigo.net is an excellent source for information on vertigo and its causes, treatment, and management. The site is a reprint of a book chapter published by the site's author, a former Professor and Chair of Neurology at Wake Forest University School of Medicine. Despite the simple graphics, the information is useful for consumers as well as professionals.

Meniere's Disease

The Web site http://www.menieresinfo.com is maintained by individuals who are patients and not medical professionals. For examination, diagnosis, and treatment, the site advises that visitors should consult licensed and qualified medical professionals. The information and links at this site are provided "at your own risk." None of the information or links at this site is warranted in any manner, including accuracy, reliability, timeliness, and completeness. The site's stated mission is "to provide the single most accurate, comprehensive, and understandable site for general information about Meniere's disease." The site also provides links to authoritative sources on the World Wide Web.

Meniere's Society

The Meniere's Society (http://www.menieres.org.uk) was founded in 1984 by Mrs. Marie Nobbs MBE of the UK to support people with Meniere's disease and those who care for them. The society acquired charitable status in 1987; and by 1995, membership had grown to 2,200. With increased publicity about Meniere's disease and the improved services the organization offers, membership now stands at over 5,500. Members are found in all parts of the UK, with a small number from other countries including Ireland, Spain, Australia, and the United States.

Meniere's Disease

The Web site http://www.menieres.org is a consumer information site whose disclaimer states that the site maintainers have no medical credentials.

Therefore, no medical advice is included. Medical advice should be obtained only from licensed physicians. None of the information or links at this site is warranted for accuracy or reliability. Consequently, visitors should be circumspect in utilizing the information obtained, as with all sites. The purpose of this site is to support patients with Meniere's disease and their families, not to provide medical information.

Hearing Loss Resources for Consumers

Any person with a medical diagnosis who has access to the Internet will be sure to find numerous sites pertaining to diagnosis, treatment plans, and management strategies. Some sites are medically based; others are nationwide consumer-oriented listing support groups that provide information and other forms of support to patients and their families.

Hearing-impaired Internet users are no different than people with other medical disorders in seeking information. Patients and their families come from a wide variety of backgrounds and have a wide variety of needs. Not all of these Web sites contain pharmaceutical information. However, audiologists should be aware of them, not only to access themselves, but also to be familiar with Web sites that their patients are probably accessing for information.

The following are examples of the variety of sites for information about hearing loss and deafness.

Acoustic Neuroma Association (ANA)

The Acoustic Neuroma Association (ANA) (http://www.anausa.org) provides information and support to patients who have been diagnosed with or have experienced an acoustic neuroma or another benign problem affecting the cranial nerves. Patient-founded in 1981, ANA is an incorporated, nonprofit organization, recognized as such by the IRS, and is supported by contributions from its members. The association furnishes information on patient rehabilitation to physicians and health care personnel; promotes research on acoustic neuroma; and educates the public regarding symptoms suggestive of acoustic neuroma, thus promoting early diagnosis and successful treatment.

Alexander Graham Bell Association for the Deaf and Hard of Hearing (A. G. Bell)

The Alexander Graham Bell Association for the Deaf and Hard of Hearing (A. G. Bell) (http://www.agbell.org) is a membership-based information center on hearing loss, emphasizing the use of technology, speech, speech reading, residual hearing, and written and spoken language. A.G. Bell focuses specifically on children with hearing loss, providing ongoing support and advocacy for parents, professionals, and other interested parties. A.G. Bell publishes a variety of useful materials on hearing loss.

American Society for Deaf Children (ASDC)

The American Society for Deaf Children (ASDC) (http://www.deafchildren.org) is a national organization of families and professionals committed to educating, empowering, and supporting parents and families of children who are deaf or hard of hearing. The ASDC helps families find meaningful communication options, particularly through the competent use of sign language in their homes, schools, and communities.

American Society of Health-System Pharmacists (ASHP)

The Web site http://www.safemedicine.com does not show drug manufacturer sponsorship, which could help provide unbiased information on more than 800 drugs. The resources for the information are pharmacists and other medication experts. The site is user friendly for both consumers and professionals.

American Tinnitus Association (ATA)

The mission of the American Tinnitus Association (ATA) (http://www.ata.org) is to silence tinnitus through education, advocacy, research, and support. This nonprofit organization provides the latest information and resources to tinnitus patients, promotes tinnitus awareness to the general public and the medical community, and funds some tinnitus research.

Association of Late-Deafened Adults Inc. (ALDA)

The Association of Late-Deafened Adults Inc. (ALDA) (http://www.alda.org) serves as a resource center providing information and referrals, self-help, and support groups for people deafened as adults. ALDA works to increase public awareness of the special needs of deafened adults. Over thirty links are listed, but they are not endorsed by ALDA.

AudiologyNet

AudiologyNet (http://www.audiologynet.com) is an audiology and hearing health care informational Web site. It is dedicated to providing links pertaining to audiology for patients, family members, students, and health care providers. The information and Web links listed are intended for informational purposes only and do not substitute for medical consultation with a personal physician or hearing health care provider. The information in each link is provided by an independent Web server and cannot be guaranteed with respect to accuracy and timeliness of the material. This site provides annotated audiology links for consumers and professionals.

Auditory-Verbal International, Inc. (AVI)

Auditory-Verbal International, Inc. (AVI) (http://www.auditory-verbal.org) is a private nonprofit international organization whose mission is to provide the choice of listening and speaking as the way of life for children and adults who are deaf or hard of hearing. According to the Web site, "AVI's goals are to heighten public awareness of the Auditory-Verbal approach, ensure certification standards for Auditory-Verbal clinicians and teachers, provide quality educational opportunities for parents and professionals, and facilitate networking among the professional and lay communities. The goal of the Auditory-Verbal approach is for children who are deaf or hard of hearing to grow up in regular classrooms and living environments and to become independent, participating citizens in mainstream society."

Boys Town National Research Hospital

The mission of Boys Town National Research Hospital is to "help heal America's children and operate the nation's leading clinical research center for childhood hearing loss and related disorders." Its Web sites—http://www.boystownhospital.org and http://www.babyhearing.org—offer information on the causes of hearing loss in children, as well as information on hearing testing.

The Web sites were created by the Boys Town National Research Hospital to answer parents' questions about infant hearing screening and follow-up testing and to provide information about the steps to take after diagnosis of hearing loss, hearing loss and hearing aids, language and speech, and parenting issues. The sites were developed with support from the NIDCD (http://www.nidcd.nih.gov).

Cochlear Implant Association, Inc. (CIAI)

Cochlear Implant Association, Inc. (CIAI) (http://www.cici.org) is a nonprofit organization that provides information and support to cochlear implant users, health professionals, and the general public. CIAI distributes educational materials, organizes national and international meetings and conventions, promotes cochlear implant technology and deafness research, and advocates on all governmental levels for the rights and services of people who have impaired hearing. The CIAI will soon be a division of the Hearing Loss Association of America (HLAA) (http://www.hearingloss.org).

DeafZONE

DeafZONE (http://www.deafzone.com) is a clearinghouse for information on deafness, sign language, closed captioning, and related topics. The site includes a great deal of useful information on hearing loss. However, users are cautioned that some may find the jokes section to be inappropriate.

Deafness and Family Communication Center (DFCC) at the Children's Hospital of Philadelphia

The Deafness and Family Communication Center (DFCC) (http://www.raisingdeafkids.org) is an organization dedicated to helping parents make better decisions for their deaf and hard-of-hearing children. The Web site has a wealth of information and resources on hearing loss. This site is made possible by a grant from the NIDCD.

HearingExchange

HearingExchange (http://www.hearingexchange.com) is a discussion Web site established by a deaf attorney who has a hearing-impaired child. The site addresses a variety of hearing loss-related and communication issues. The Resource Directory link lists over forty organizations and other hearing loss-related Web sites.

Hearing Loss Association of America (HLAA)

In 2006, Self Help for Hard of Hearing People (SHHH) changed its name to the Hearing Loss Association of America (HLAA) (http://www.hearingloss.org). This consumer organization is an international volunteer organization comprised of people who are hard of hearing and their relatives and friends. SHHH is a nonprofit, nonsectarian educational organization devoted to the welfare and interests of those who cannot hear well but are committed to participating in the hearing world.

The HLAA is the nation's largest membership and advocacy organization for people with hearing loss. Founded in 1979, it provides information, education, advocacy, and support to people with hearing loss. It publishes a bimonthly magazine, *Hearing Loss*. The support network includes the national office in Maryland, 13 state organizations, and 250 local chapters. The CIAI, mentioned earlier, will soon be a division of this association.

Hyperacusis Network

The Hyperacusis Network (http://www.hyperacusis.net) consists of individuals who have a reduced tolerance to sound. This site is a support network. As a network, it works at ways to improve the condition of and educate the medical community about hyperacusis, recruitment, and hyperacute hearing. No membership fees are required to receive the newsletter, although donations are accepted to help defray costs of mailings and Web site maintenance.

KidsHealth

Created by The Nemours Foundation Center for Children's Health Media, this site (http://www.kidshealth.com) provides easy-to-read children's health information. KidsHealth has separate areas for parents, children, and teens. Each section has its own design and age-appropriate content. The parents' section has basic information on cochlear implants and an explanation of the different tests used by audiologists to evaluate hearing. The information is simply written, but no supporting images help make the information easier to understand.

League for the Hard of Hearing

The League for the Hard of Hearing (http://www.lhh.org) was founded in New York in 1910. Its Web site states that the organization "is the oldest and foremost hearing rehabilitation and human services agency in the world for infants, children, adults and seniors who are hard of hearing, deaf and deaf-blind, and their families." The organization offers people who are hard of hearing or deaf access to diagnostic, rehabilitation, counseling, and education programs. The mission of this nonprofit agency is to improve the quality of life for people with all degrees of hearing loss and to offer comprehensive services regardless of age or mode of communication.

MedlinePlus

The National Library of Science manages this site. The site (http://www.medlineplus.gov) provides a wealth of health and prescription (and nonprescription) drug information for consumers and professionals. Special access for Spanish-speaking visitors is included. The site is easy to navigate to find information about drugs and their side effects. The site also provides a link to CDER (http://www.fda.gov/cder)

National Association of the Deaf (NAD)

Established in 1880, the National Association of the Deaf (NAD) (http://www.nad.org) is the nation's largest consumer organization safeguarding the accessibility and civil rights of 28 million deaf and hard–of-hearing Americans in education, employment, health care, and telecommunications. The NAD focuses on grassroots advocacy and empowerment, captioned media, deafness-related information and publications, legal assistance, policy development and research, public awareness, certification of interpreters, and youth leadership development.

National Center for Hearing Assistive Technology (NCHAT)

The National Center for Hearing Assistive Technology (NCHAT) (http://www.hearingloss.org) promotes the use of technology to maximize the residual hearing of people who are hard of hearing. The Web site has a reference list of articles dealing with cochlear implants, hearing aids, and other technologies. There are commercial sponsors with links to their Web sites.

National Information Center on Deafness (NICD)

The National Information Center on Deafness (NICD) (http://www.gallaudet.edu) is a part of Gallaudet University in Washington, D.C. The center is a centralized source for accurate, up-to-date objective information on topics dealing with deafness and hearing loss. NICD responds to a wide range of questions from the general public and from deaf and hard-of-hearing people, their families, and professionals who work with them. NICD collects, develops, and disseminates information on deafness, hearing loss, and services and programs related to people with hearing loss.

Pharmacy Times

This site was created for pharmacists. Pharmacy Times (http://www.pharmacytimes.com) is a resource for information relating to the pharmacy profession.

According to the Web site, *"Pharmacy Times* is dedicated to providing pharmacists with practical, authoritative information with the ultimate goal of improving patient care. Primarily focused on providing clinical information that pharmacists can use in their everyday practice when counseling patients and interacting with physicians, *Pharmacy Times* has recently expanded its coverage to include pharmacy technology and health-systems pharmacy. Accredited by the Accreditation Council for Pharmacy Education (ACPE) as a provider of continuing pharmacy education, important topics include drug errors, drug interactions, pharmacy technology, disease state management, patient counseling, and pharmacy law. *Pharmacy Times* strictly follows the educational standards set forth in the ACPE Criteria for Quality and seeks to fulfill these important educational needs in the pharmacy profession."

Rochester Institute of Technology (RIT) Libraries

Rochester Institute of Technology (RIT) Libraries (http://wally.rit.edu) is a comprehensive Web site for information on hearing loss, deafness, cochlear implants, deaf culture, and related information. The site emanates from RIT's Wallace Library. RIT Libraries are comprised of Wallace Library, the Cary Library, and RIT Archives and Special Collections. RIT's Wallace Library is the primary information resource center on campus. It offers traditional collections, electronic resources, and flexible study space.

Telecommunications for the Deaf and Hard of Hearing, Inc. (TDI)

Founded in 1968, Telecommunications for the Deaf and Hard of Hearing, Inc. (TDI) (http://www.tdi-online.org) is an active national advocacy organization focusing its energies and resources on addressing equal access issues in telecommunications and media for four constituencies in deafness and hearing loss—specifically people who are deaf, hard of hearing, late-deafened, or deaf-blind.

Herbal and Alternative Medicine Web Sites and Resources

The following sites are provided to assist audiologists seeking information on herbal and other alternative medicines. Many patients avail themselves of alternative treatments that may interact with other drugs they are taking. Further, some nutritional supplements have auditory effects. While this listing is not comprehensive, it does provide audiologists with a starting point in their search for information.

Dietary Supplement and Health Education Act of 1994 Public Law 103-417

The site http://www.fda.gov contains the complete text of the law that deals with labeling and other herbal/dietary supplement issues (see "Pharmacopeias"). Under "Reference Room," visitors can click on "Laws FDA Enforces" and find the link to Dietary Supplement Health and Education Act of 1994.

Alternative Medicine Foundation

Based in Maryland, the Alternative Medicine Foundation (http://www.amfoundation.org) is a nonprofit 501(c)(3) organization founded in 1998 to provide responsible and reliable information about alternative medicine to the public and health professionals. The Information Resource Guides section provides a wealth of information and additional Web sites on alternative medicine topics. Topics included are as widely varied as acupuncture, Ayurveda, energy work, herbal medicines, homeopathy, manual therapies, mind/body medicine, and Tibetan and Chinese medicine.

National Center for Complementary and Alternative Medicine (NCCAM)

The National Center for Complementary and Alternative Medicine (NCCAM) (http://nccam.nih.gov) is one of the twenty-seven institutes and centers that make up the NIH. The NIH is one of eight agencies under the Public Health Service (PHS) (http://www.usphs.gov) in the DHHS (www.hhs.gov).

NCCAM is dedicated to exploring complementary and alternative healing practices in the context of rigorous science, training complementary and alternative medicine (CAM) researchers, and disseminating authoritative information to the public and professionals.

U.S. Department of Health and Human Services (DHHS)

The DHHS (http://www.hhs.gov) is the U.S. government's principal agency for protecting the health of all Americans and providing essential human services, especially for those who are least able to help themselves. The organization includes more than 300 programs covering a wide spectrum of activities including preventing disease and assuring food and drug safety.

U.S. Public Health Service (PHS)

The mission of the Public Health Service (PHS) (http://www.usphs.gov) Commissioned Corps is to provide highly trained and mobile health professionals who carry out programs to promote the health of the nation, aid in understanding and preventing disease and injury, assure safe and effective drugs and medical devices, deliver health services to federal beneficiaries, and furnish health expertise in time of war or other national or international emergencies.

Veterans Administration

This medical Web site (http://www.myhealth.va.gov) emanates from the Veterans Administration. The information is available for all to use. Visitors can access the site by creating a user ID and password. However, they do not have to enter identifying information afterward unless they choose to do so. This site provides a useful medications interaction option in the package. A visitor can conduct a search for a medication not listed, including some common herbals. The information in the package is from Micromedex material. The site also provides worthwhile links, including MedlinePlus and federal sites.

World Council on Hearing Health

World Council on Hearing Health (http://www.wchh.com) is the public education and advocacy arm of the Deafness Research Foundation (DRF). Its charge is to provide the strategies and tactics and to implement programs to fulfill the mission of the DRF.

The above site automatically directs visitors to the DFR's Web site (http://www.drf.org). The DRF is a source of private funding for basic and clinical research in hearing science. According to its Web site, "DRF is committed to making lifelong hearing health a national priority by funding research and implementing

education projects in both the government and private sectors."

DRF created the National Temporal Bone Banks Program (NTBB) to encourage individuals with ear disorders to pledge their temporal bones at death to scientific research. This program was a crucial step in the establishment of the National Temporal Bone Hearing and Balance Pathology Resource Registry by the NIDCD.

Other Sites of Interest

The following sites contain information that may be useful to audiologists and their patients for a variety of reasons. Some patients may want to purchase their medications on the Web and need more information about the advantages and disadvantages of that approach. Other patients may have special dietary concerns. The sites reviewing quackery and false medical claims may help audiologists assist their most vulnerable patients. Patients and their families may become so distraught or desperate for help that they waste their resources on "useless treatments." Audiologists may not be trained to provide all of the information their patients need in every arena. However, they can help themselves and others access the needed information.

Joint Institute for Food Safety and Applied Nutrition (JIFSAN)

The Joint Institute for Food Safety and Applied Nutrition (JIFSAN) (http://www.jifsan.umd.edu) was established between the FDA and the University of Maryland (UM) in 1996. The organization is a jointly administered, multidisciplinary research and education program. It includes research components from the FDA's CFSAN, from the CVM, and from the UM.

Buying Drugs Online

A comprehensive consumer-oriented article from the FDA that looks at risks of buying medication online can be found at http://www.fda.gov. The article is found by conducting a search for "Use Caution Buying Medical Products Online."

Edumacation

The real value of http://www.edumacation.com is that it lists many Web sites promoting unproven medical products and other sites that "help you to tell what's for real and what isn't." To gain additional information, visitors must register. Ownership information is not provided on the main page, just the privacy policy. There is a link to "Balance Bracelets Benefits," but it takes the visitor to a list of commercial sites where the bracelets can be purchased. The site is not professional-looking; but, again, the quackery Web list is useful.

Fraud and Quackery

Questionable medical products, devices, "potions," etc., have been around for years. Pseudo-medical information, which, of course, is "free," can be marketed in a way that makes the product sound like the "cure-all product" of the twenty-first century.

When words such as *secret formula, proven effective, miracle, breakthrough, works overnight,* and *guaranteed to work* appear on the home page, the visitor needs to understand that he or she is about to enter a site whose credibility should be questioned immediately.

Some sites are watchdog Internet sites that report any quackery or fraud. Those sites are quite helpful and should be referred to as often as one would visit the FDA's Web site (http://www.fda.gov).

Quack Watch

Quackwatch (http://www.quackwatch.org), which was a member of the Consumer Federation of America from 1973 through 2003, is a nonprofit corporation whose purpose is to combat health-related frauds, myths, fads, and fallacies. Its primary focus is on quackery-related information that is difficult or impossible to get elsewhere. Founded in 1969 as the Lehigh Valley Committee Against Health Fraud, it was incorporated in 1970. In 1997, it assumed its current name and began developing a worldwide network of volunteers and expert advisors. Its activities include investigating questionable claims, answering inquiries about products and services, advising quackery victims, distributing reliable publications, reporting illegal marketing, assisting or generating consumer protection lawsuits, improving the quality of health information on the Internet, and attacking misleading advertising on the Internet.

National Council Against Health Fraud

The National Council Against Health Fraud (http://www.ncahf.org) was founded in 1977 as a nonprofit, tax-exempt voluntary health agency that focuses its attention on health fraud, misinformation, and quackery as public health problems. It is private, nonpartisan, and nonsectarian. Its members are health professionals, educators, researchers, attorneys, and other concerned citizens. The site contains hundreds of articles that can help people evaluate health claims.

National Fraud Information Center of the National Consumers League

This Washington, D.C.-based group (http://www.fraud.org) will assist visitors in reaching their state's attorney general office if they believe they have been a victim of medical fraud. The National Consumer's League Web site (http://www.ncl.org) provides useful information on health-related topics with associated links.

SUMMARY

Access to medical information previously was limited to people directly involved in medicine or allied health; now it is accessible to the consumer. The Web provides many excellent sources for reliable and accurate information that should promote a positive dialogue between the patient and the physician and/or other health care provider.

The FDA—and its affiliated agencies—as well as other federal agencies in the United States and around the world have a recognized system of evaluation, clinical trials, analysis, and interpretation of scientific and statistically based data indicating that a chemical compound is safe (for the general population) to cure or slow the disease process.

The pharmacy profession (as well as the pharmaceutical industry) has opened its doors for consumers to learn more about FDA-approved products, clinical trials, and the process to report any adverse event after taking a particular medication. In other words, there has been a sharing of information that, in the past, was thought to be out of the reach of the average person.

Professional associations have expanded their Web sites to include consumer information. The information is provided free of charge in most cases to people directly involved with patients.

Information from support groups exists that focuses on having a better understanding of specific diseases and disorders. However, reading the disclaimer statements is vital to determining the usefulness of the information offered.

Numerous commercial Web sites provide drug information gleaned from federal Web sites. However, that information is usually supported by private companies having direct or no direct association with the drug. Superfluous nonmedical information can be a distraction.

Federal laws exist concerning herbal medicines and the claims made by their manufacturers. Consumers can read this legislation and access other Web sites that provide objective scientific data to support the claims made by the manufacturer of these OTC products. The information should help consumers make an informed decision about the herbal medicine in question.

However, regardless of a Web site's ownership, all sites state that the information provided is intended "for informational purposes only and does not substitute for proper medical care." That statement must be taken seriously by anyone looking for "free" medical information.

See Appendix A for a comprehensive list of Web sites mentioned in this chapter.

Appendix A: Online Resources Summary

Acoustic Neuroma Association:
  http://www.anausa.org
Alexander Graham Bell Association for the Deaf and
  Hard of Hearing: http://www.agbell.org
Alternative Medicine Foundation:
  http://www.amfoundation.org
American Academy of Audiology:
  http://www.audiology.org
American Academy of Otolaryngology—Head and
  Neck Surgery: http://www.entnet.org
American Herbal Pharmacopoeia:
  http://www.herbal-ahp.org
American Medical Association:
  http://www.ama-assn.org
American Society for Deaf Children:
  http://www.deafchildren.org
American Society of Health-System Pharmacists:
  http://www.ashp.org
American Speech-Language-Hearing Association:
  http://www.asha.org
American Stock Exchange: http://www.amex.com

American Tinnitus Association: http://www.ata.org
The Association of the British Pharmaceutical
  Industry: http://www.abpi.org.uk
Association of Late-Deafened Adults Inc.:
  http://www.alda.org
AudiologyNet: http://www.audiologynet.com
Auditory-Verbal International, Inc.:
  http://www.auditory-verbal.org
Belgian Pharmaceutical Industry Association:
  http://pharma.be
Boys Town National Research Hospital:
  http://www.boystownhospital.org
  http://www.babyhearing.org
British Institute of Regulatory Affairs:
  http://www.bira.org.uk
British Pharmacopoeia:
  http://www.pharmacopoeia.co.uk
Cable News Network: http://www.cnn.com
Cochlear Implant Association, Inc.: http://www.cici.org
Deafness and Family Communication Center:
  http://www.raisingdeafkids.org

Deafness/Hard of Hearing:
    http://www.deafness.about.com
DeafZONE: http://www.deafzone.com
Department of Health & Human Services:
    http://www.hhs.gov
Drug InfoNet: http://www.druginfonet.com
Drug Information Association:
    http://www.diahome.org
Drug Programme of Health Canada:
    http://www.hc-sc.gc.ca
Drugs.com: http://www.drugs.com
eMedicine: http://www.emedicine.com
European Directorate for the Quality of Medicines:
    http://www.pheur.org
European Federation of Pharmaceutical Industries
    and Associations: http://www.efpia.org
Family Practice Notebook:
    http://www.fpnotebook.com
Health Research Association:
    http://www.health-research.org
HearingExchange:
    http://www.hearingexchange.com
Hearing Loss Association of America:
    http://www.hearingloss.org
The Hyperacusis Network:
    http://www.hyperacusis.net
Institute for Safe Medication Practices:
    http://www.ismp.org
International Pharmaceutical Federation:
    http://www.fip.nl
Joint Institute for Food Safety and Applied Nutrition:
    http://www.jifsan.umd.edu
KidsHealth: http://www.kidshealth.com
League for the Hard of Hearing:
    http://www.lhh.org
MDLinx: http://www.mdlinx.com
MedicAlert: http://www.medicalert.org
MedicineNet, Inc.: http://www.medicinenet.com
MedlinePlus: http://www.medlineplus.gov
Medscape: http://www.medscape.com
Meniere's Disease: http://www.menieresinfo.com
    http://www.menieres.org
Meniere's Society: http://www.menieres.org.uk
National Association of the Deaf:
    http://www.nad.org

National Center for Complementary and Alternative
    Medicine: http://nccam.nih.gov
National Center for Hearing Assistive Technology:
    http://www.hearingloss.org
National Consumer's League: http://www.ncl.org
National Council Against Health Fraud:
    http://www.ncahf.org
National Fraud Information Center of the National
    Consumers League: http://www.fraud.org
National Information Center on Deafness:
    http://www.gallaudet.edu
National Institute of Ayurvedic Medicine:
    http://niam.com
National Institute on Deafness and Other
    Communication Disorders:
    http://www.nidcd.nih.gov
New York Stock Exchange: http://www.nyse.com
National Library of Medicine:
    http://www.nlm.nih.gov
Ototoxic Medications: http://www.tchain.com
Pan American Health Organizations:
    http://www.paho.org
Parenteral Drug Association: http://www.pda.org
Pharmaceutical Marketing Club of Quebec:
    http://www.pmcq.qc.ca
Pharmaceutical Research and Manufacturers of
    America: http://www.phrma.org
Pharmacy Times: http://www.pharmacytimes.com
Product Quality Research Institute:
    http://www.pqri.org
Public Health Service: http://www.usphs.gov
Quackwatch: http://www.quackwatch.org
Rochester Institute of Technology: http://wally.rit.edu
RxList: http://www.rxlist.com
SafeMedication.com:
    http://www.safemedication.com
Securities and Exchange Commission:
    http://www.sec.gov
Sound-Alike Drugs: http://www.nacds.org
Telecommunications for the Deaf and Hard of
    Hearing, Inc.: http://www.tdi-online.org
U.S. Agency for International Development:
    http://www.usaid.gov
U.S. Food and Drug Administration:
    http://www.fda.gov

U.S. Pharmacopeia: http://www.usp.org

U.S. Pharmacopeia's Drug Quality and Information Program: http://www.uspdqi.org

Vertigo: http://www.ivertigo.net

Vestibular Disorders Association: http://www.vestibular.org

Veterans Administration: http://www.myhealth.va.gov

WebMD: http://www.webmd.com

World Council on Hearing Health: http://www.wchh.com

World Health Organization: http://www.who.it

GLOSSARY

Acetyl-L-carnitine—Amino acid-like substance that occurs naturally in the brain.

Actin—Protein that is abundant in microfilaments and active in muscular contraction, cellular movement, and maintenance of cell shape.

Actin-binding sequence—Specific region of an actin-binding protein, such as myosin or α-actinin, that associates with actin monomers or filaments and modifies their properties.

Actinomycetes—Type of gram-positive soil bacteria that often produces pharmacologically useful compounds.

Actins—Protein complexes that provide structural stiffness, for example, to the stereocilia of cochlear and vestibular hair cells.

Acyl-CoA synthetase—An enzyme that catalyzes the formation of acyl CoA from a fatty acid and coenzyme A (CoA). Acyl-CoA is subsequently carried by carnitine into the mitochondrion for beta-oxidation.

Adenosine triphosphate (ATP)—The primary energy source used by tissue. Chemically, it is called a nucleotide. A nucleotide contains three parts: an organic base, a five-carbon sugar molecule called a pentose, and a phosphate group. ATP has three phosphate groups. Deoxyribonucleic acid (DNA) and ribonucleic acid (RNA) contain nucleotides with one phosphate group. In DNA, the pentose sugar molecule is deoxyribose. In ATP and RNA, the pentose sugar is ribose. The nucleotide containing deoxyribose in place of ribose is represented by placing a *d* before the abbreviation. Thus, deoxyadenosine triphosphate contains deoxyribose and is represented as dATP.

Adenylate cyclase—Membrane-bound enzyme that catalyzes the formation of cyclic AMP, an important signaling molecule, from ATP. Adenylate cyclase is activated by other proteins, such as the G proteins; also called adenylyl cyclase.

Adverse effect—Undesired and usually unintended or negative effects of a drug. Severe adverse effects may also be referred to as toxicities. The term *side effect* usually relates to more predictable and minor negative effects that may be dose-related.

Aerobic—Organism such as bacteria that requires molecular oxygen to live.

Affinity—How well a drug binds to its receptor.

Agonist—Drug capable of binding with a receptor to activate a response or molecules that bind to receptors to activate that receptor. All neurotransmitters are agonists at their respective receptor sites. Some drugs can mimic the actions of a naturally occurring agonist.

Airborne transmission—Manner of spreading disease through exposure to microorganisms suspended in the air as droplet residue or dust particles.

Aliphatic solvents—Solvents that are made from petroleum and that have a straight chain carbon backbone.

Allergic rhinitis—Inflammation of the nasal mucous membranes associated with environmental and seasonal allergies/hay fever.

Alpha lipoic acid—A vitamin-like substance and powerful antioxidant that dissolves in both fat and water, which is why it is sometimes referred to as the "universal antioxidant."

American Conference of Governmental Industrial Hygienists (ACGIH)—Nonprofit organization that recommends exposure guidelines for chemical and physical agents in the workplace.

Amino-Amino groups (-NH2)—Part of amino acids and other organic compounds, imparting a basic character.

Aminoglycoside—Class of antibiotics including gentamicin, tobramycin, amikacin, streptomycin, neomycin, kanamycin, paromomycin, netilmicin, and spectinomycin that are known to have nephrotoxic and ototoxic properties. This group of antibiotics is produced primarily by species of soil-dwelling Actinomycetes. Aminoglycosides work via multiple cellular effects, including blockage of protein synthesis. They are most effective against gram-negative bacteria. They inhibit the bacterial 30s ribosomal subunit and protein synthesis to treat many gram-negative bacterial infections.

Amoxicillin—Penicillin antibiotic. It has a wider spectrum than penicillin, with activity similar to ampicillin, with greater oral bioavailability.

Ampicillin—Penicillin antibiotic. It has a wider spectrum than penicillin G, as well as E. coli, H. influenza, P. mirabilis, and Shigella.

Anaerobic—Microorganism such as bacteria that does not require oxygen to live.

Anaphylaxis—Immediate allergic reaction characterized by the contraction of smooth muscle and dilation of capillaries due to release of pharmacologically active substances (such as histamine and serotonin).

Antagonist—Drug molecule capable of binding to a receptor, but the interaction does not activate the receptor to produce a response and will prevent an agonist from binding to produce an action. An antagonist can block or reduce the action of the natural agonist at the respective receptor site. For example, beta-receptor antagonists (beta-blockers) are a group of drugs that affect blood pressure and heart rate by blocking the effect of norepinephrine (the agonist).

Anticholinergics—Medications such as atropine that are antagonistic to the action of parasympathetic or other cholinergic nerve fibers.

Antihistamine—Drug having an action antagonistic to that of histamine; used in the treatment of allergy symptoms.

Antioxidant—Chemical that slows or prevents oxidation. Oxidation is defined as "the process whereby a molecule loses electrons." Antioxidants are said to scavenge free radicals and prevent them from doing damage to cellular components such as DNA. Glutathione and ascorbic acid (vitamin C) are examples of antioxidants.

Apoptosis—Natural process of programmed cell death through initiation of cell-destroying enzymes; cell suicide. This type of programmed cell death (PCD) is characterized morphologically by cell shrinkage; membrane blebbing; chromatin condensation; intracellular fragmentation associated with membrane-enclosed cellular fragments called apoptotic bodies, causing an increased electron density of the cytoplasm; and intranucleosomal DNA fragmentation. Those effects are largely achieved by activation of a cascade of events involving the activation of a group of enzymes called caspases that cleave proteins (i.e., proteases).

Apoptosome complex—Protein complex formed by the apoptotic protease-activating factor (Apaf-1), dATP, cytochrome c, and procaspase-9 that activates procaspase-9 to form caspase-9.

Aromatic solvents—Diverse group of organic chemicals based on a benzene ring structure. These agents are useful in dissolving a wide range of materials that are not soluble in water, such as grease, paints, and glues. Aromatic solvents can depress the central nervous system and are sometimes abused (sniffed, for example) because they give a high. They also can damage the brain with frequent use.

Ataxic gait—Uncoordinated wide-base gait pattern that is commonly associated with a variety of disorders including cerebellar disease and bilateral peripheral vestibular loss.

ATP—Adenosine 5′-triphosphate, a nucleotide composed of adenosine, ribose, and three phosphate groups. Hydrolysis of each of the two high-energy phosphoanhydride bonds in ATP releases a large amount of free energy that can be used to "power" other biochemical processes.

Auditory brainstem response (ABR)—Measurement of auditory threshold using computer-averaged electric responses produced by the auditory nerve and the brainstem during the first few milliseconds after the onset of each signal. It is an electrophysiologic measure of auditory function up through the level of the brainstem.

Auditory toxicity—Hearing loss, tinnitus, and/or aural fullness that result from exposure to toxins.

Autolysis—Death of a cell because of the breakdown of intracellular structures due to enzymes within the cell that results in the appearance of vacuoles in the cytoplasm with an intact cell membrane.

Autoreceptor—Receptor located on the presynaptic nerve terminal membrane that is activated by the same neurotransmitter that is released by that terminal.

Axon hillock—Specialized region between the soma and the axon of a neuron that has a high density of voltage-gated sodium channels and a low threshold for initiating an action potential; also called the spike initiation zone.

Azelastine (Astelin)—Topically administered antihistamine via a nasal spray.

Bacteria (singular: bacterium)—Life forms consisting of a single DNA molecule suspended in cytoplasm encased within a thin cell wall.

Bacteriocidal—Causing death to bacteria.

Bacteriostatic—Inhibiting or retarding the growth of bacteria.

Bacterium (plural: bacteria)—Life form potentially capable of causing disease, consisting of a single DNA molecule capable of independently executing all functions and processes necessary for survival.

Basal lamina—Thin sheet of extracellular matrix material that separates a layer of cells (epithelial, muscle, or fat) from connective tissues; also called a basement membrane.

Bcl-2 family of proteins—Proteins involved in the mitochondrial apoptosis pathway. There are at least fifteen members of the Bcl-2 family; they have been divided into three subfamilies: Group I are anti-apoptotic (e.g., Bcl-2 and Bcl-XL), Group II are pro-apoptotic (e.g., Bax, Bak, and Bok), and Group III are pro-apoptotic (e.g., Bad, Bid, Bik, and Bim).

Bell's palsy—Unilateral weakness or paralysis of the facial nerve, leading to unilateral weakness or paralysis of facial muscles.

Benzodiazepines—Sedative hypnotic medications. May be utilized in the treatment of anxiety, sleep disorders, and seizure disorder and as anesthetics and muscle relaxants.

Biliary excretion—Secondary and usually minor route of elimination of some medications separate from renal elimination. Drugs and metabolites may be processed by the liver, which also forms bile and bile acids, and released directly through the bile duct, emptying into the intestine for eventual elimination from the body.

Bioavailability—Fraction (percentage of the quantity) of a drug reaching systemic circulation after administration. Equation: $$\text{bioavailability} = \frac{\text{quantity of drug in systemic circulation}}{\text{quantity of drug administered}}.$$

Bipolar neuron—Neuron having only two neural processes projecting from the soma (cell body). In the auditory system, bipolar neurons (type I spiral ganglion neurons) connect hair cells in the organ of Corti to neurons in the cochlear nucleus of the brainstem.

Blood lead levels—Common way of measuring exposure to lead. Adverse health effects have been associated with blood lead levels of $10\mu g/dl$ (10 micrograms per deciliter of blood).

Buccal—Oral mucosa is thin with significant blood flow. To assist in drug absorption, some drugs can be placed between the gum and cheek (e.g., nicotine gum and smokeless tobacco), which is referred to as buccal administration.

C (carboxyl) terminus—End, or tail domain, of a polypetide chain that consists of a free carboxyl group.

Ca^{2+}/calmodulin-dependent kinase—Enzyme that is activated by high levels of calcium and calmodulin (a ubiquitous calcium-binding protein) in a cell. The activated kinase regulates other molecules by phosphorylating them and is therefore an important component of signal transduction processes.

Calcium (Ca^{2+})-ATPase—Transport protein that carries calcium out of a cell, using energy derived from the hydrolysis of ATP; also called a calcium pump.

Calmodulin—Ubiquitous protein that binds calcium and stimulates the activity of calmodulin-dependent kinases.

Calpains—Calcium-dependent cysteine proteases that are involved in cellular function and that have been implicated in various diseases.

cAMP- stimulated kinase—Enzyme that is maximally active in catalyzing the transfer of the phosphate of ATP to serine or threonine hydroxyl groups in proteins in the presence of cyclic nucleotides.

Carbon monoxide—Toxic gas that is generated as a by-product of combustion. Carbon monoxide (CO) is the most common cause of fatal toxic chemical exposure.

Cascade—Series of steps in which the protein catalyzing each step is activated (or inhibited) by the product of the preceding step. The whole system is regulated by the initiator molecule. In this book, the molecule called CD95L is the initiator ligand of the caspase cascade. In addition, the cascade involves amplification so that each step produces more active molecules than the preceding step. Thus, one initiator ligand molecule (e.g., CD95L) can result in thousands of active molecules (e.g., caspase-3) at the final step in the cascade.

Caspases—Groups of cysteine proteases (protein-cleaving enzymes) essential for apoptotic signaling. Caspases include a family of at least 14 cysteine-dependent and aspartate-specific proteases (thus, the term *caspase*) that includes initiator caspases (e.g., caspase-8; caspase-9, and caspase-10) and effector or executioner caspases (e.g., caspase-3, caspase-6, and caspase-7).

Cassava—Plant widely consumed around the world. If not properly prepared, cassava consumption may result in significant cyanide exposure.

Cathepsins—Lysosomal proteolytic enzymes that nonspecifically cleave various intracellular proteins (i.e., proteolytic).

Cefazolin—First-generation cephalosporin prototype. It is a bacteriocidal beta-lactam inhibitor of cell wall synthesis. Active against gram-positive cocci, E. coli, and K. Pneumoniae. It does not cross the blood-brain barrier.

Ceftriaxone—Third-generation cephalosporin antibiotic. It does cross the blood-brain barrier. Active against gram-negative bacteria including gonocci and H. influenza.

Cell cycle—Reproductive cycle of a cell: the orderly sequence of events by which a cell duplicates its contents and divides into two. The cell cycle includes the complete series of events from one cell division to the next whereby cells grow and divide into new cells.

Cetirizine (Zyrtec)—Second-generation antihistamine. These drugs do not cross the blood-brain barrier and thus have decreased CNS side effects; therefore, they are less sedating compared to first-generation antihistamines.

Checkpoint—Point in eukaryotic cell cycle where progress through the cycle can be halted until conditions are suitable for the cell to produce to the next phase.

Chemical asphyxiants—Class of agents that reduce the delivery of oxygen to tissue or the utilization of oxygen by tissues.

Chlorpheniramine (Chlor-Timetron)—A sedating antihistamine. An H1 receptor blocker prototype.

Chromatin—Strands in the nucleus of a cell containing DNA and protein.

Cimetidine (Tagamet)—H2 blocker prototype. Used to treat acid reflux disease.

Cinchonism—Hallmark set of symptoms of acute quinine toxicity that includes tinnitus along with hearing loss, dizziness, headache, nausea, and vision changes.

Ciprofloxacin—Flouroquinolone antibiotic. It is bactericidal. Active against many gram-negative rods including E. coli, H. influenza, Capylobacter, Enterobacter, Pseudomonas, and Shigella.

c-Jun N-terminal kinases (JNKs)—Family of proteins, also known as stress-activated protein kinase (SAPK), within the mitogen-activated protein kinase (MAP kinase, MAPK) family that phosphorylate transcription factors such as c-Jun and c-Fos. The c-Jun and c-Fos form activation protein-1 (AP-1), which can trigger rapid transcriptional activity. AP-1 has been implicated in the regulation of many important biological processes including both survival signaling and apoptosis. In general, the role of JNK in cell death remains unclear since both pro-apoptotic and prosurvival effects have been reported.

Cleaning—Removing gross contamination without necessarily killing germs.

Clearance (CL)—The ability of the body or organs (usually kidneys and liver) to remove a drug from the blood. Expressed as a volume per unit of time.

Clindamycin—Bacteriostatic inhibitor of protein synthesis. It is active against gram-positive cocci.

Clinical Test of Sensory Integration and Balance (CTSIB)—Postural control screening test in which postural sway in four of the six conditions (Conditions 1, 2, 4, and 5) included in CDP is evaluated.

Clostridium difficile—Species of gram-positive anaerobic bacteria that can infect the human intestine, leading to diarrhea and inflammation. Their toxins can also inhibit certain apoptotic pathways.

Cocaine—Indirectly acting sympathomimetic, meaning it blocks amine reuptake into nerve endings. A local anesthetic.

Cochleotoxic—Agent such as a drug that causes damage to the cochlea, resulting in a sensorineural hearing loss and/or tinnitus.

Collagen—Family of fibrous proteins that are the major components of the extracellular matrix and connective tissue.

Contact transmission—Manner of spreading disease through exposure to microorganisms by way of touching or coming in contact with potentially infections objects. Also see *Airborne transmission, Direct contact transmission, Droplet contact transmission, Indirect contact transmission, Vectorborne transmission,* and *Vehicle transmission*.

Corrective saccade—Rapid eye movement that moves the eye to the correct position to maintain clear vision when head movement velocity exceeds the capability of the VOR.

Critical instruments—Reusable instruments that are invasive and directly introduced into the blood stream (i.e., needles); noninvasive and come in contact with mucous membranes and/or bodily substances (i.e., curette used for cerumen removal); or noninvasive and penetrate skin surfaces from use or misuse (i.e., curette used for cerumen removal).

Cubic distortion product (CDP)—One of many otoacoustic emissions (OAEs) generated by a healthy cochlea when it is stimulated simultaneously by two pure tones, f_1 and f_2, having a frequency ratio between 1.1 and 1.3. Because the CDP is the largest amplitude distortion product generated by the cochlea, it is the one that is most commonly measured to assess outer hair cell function in clinical practice. The frequency of the CDP is $2f_1–f_2$.

Cushingnoid—Resembling the signs and symptoms of Cushing's disease or syndrome, including buffalo hump, obesity, striations, adiposity, hypertension, diabetes, and osteoporosis, usually due to exogenous corticosteroids.

Cyanide—Toxic gas that is generated by the burning of plastics and certain fibers. In addition to being toxic, cyanide is also used in the purification of certain metals, in the pharmaceutical industry, and for other chemical processes.

Cyclic nucleotides—Molecules such as cyclic adenosine monophosphate (cAMP) and cyclic guanosine monophosphate (cGMP) that function as second messengers in cell signaling. cAMP is generated from ATP in response to stimulation of many types of cell surface receptors; it activates cyclic-AMP-dependent kinase (protein kinase A, PKA) and is hydrolyzed to AMP by a phosphodiesterase.

Cyclin—Any of a group of proteins active in controlling the cell cycle and initiating DNA synthesis. These proteins periodically rise and fall in concentration in step with the eukaryotic cell cycle. Cyclins activate crucial cyclin-dependent kinases, thereby helping to control progression from one phase of the cell cycle to the next.

Cyclin-dependent kinase—Protein kinases that control cell cycle progression in all eukaryotes and require physical association with cyclins to achieve full enzymatic activity. Cyclin-dependent kinases are regulated by phosphorylation and dephosphorylation events.

Cyclin-dependent kinase inhibitor (CKI)—Protein that binds to and inhibits cyclin-dependent kinase complexes, primarily involved in the control of G1 and S phases.

Cyclitols—Five- or six-membered carbon rings with hydroxyl groups on the ring atoms.

Cytochromes—Proteins in the membrane of mitochondria that are used to transport electrons in the electron transport apparatus.

Cytocochleogram—Graphical representation of the number of intact and missing hair cells along the length of the cochlea.

dATP—Abbreviation for deoxyadenosine triphosphate, a nucleotide that contains the sugar deoxyribose in place of ribose, which is present in the nucleotide adenosine triphosphate (ATP). Nucleotides containing deoxyribose are found in DNA, while nucleotides containing ribose are found in RNA.

Death-inducing signaling complex (DISC)—complex formed by CD95L (ligand), CD95 (receptor), and FADD (adapter protein) that recruits and activates pro-caspase molecules to initiate the caspase cascade.

Death receptor—Protein complex in the outer membrane of a cell that reacts with a ligand such as CD95L to initiate an apoptosis cascade.

Death receptor apoptosis pathway—Extrinsic cell death pathway that is activated through receptors in the cell membrane that are a subset of the tumor necrosis factor receptor (TNF-R) family containing intracellular death domains (DD). Examples of death receptors are CD95 (also known as Fas or APO-1), TNF-R1, DR3, DR4, DR5, and NGFRp75. CD95L (Fas L) is a ligand that activates death receptors such as CD95.

Decussation—Crossing over of nerve fibers from one side of the brain or spinal cord to the other side.

Deoxy-—Prefix referring to the deficiency of an oxygen atom in comparison to a closely related (or parent) compound.

Dexamethasone—Long-acting glucocorticoid without any mineral corticoid activity.

Dietary Supplement Health and Education Act (1994)—Created the "dietary supplements" category of agents that the FDA regulates as to labeling and therapeutic claims, but does not require safety and effectiveness testing. Herbal medicines are covered under provisions of this act.

Dimerization—Union of two chemically identical molecules.

Diphenhydramine (Benadryl)—Sedating antihistamine. An H1 receptor blocker prototype frequently used in the treatment of hay fever, motion sickness, and dystonias.

Direct contact transmission—Form of contact transmission where exposure to microorganisms occurs by coming in contact with potentially infectious microbes without intervening persons, barriers, or conditions.

Disinfecting—Process of killing germs.

Distortion product otoacoustic emission (DPOAE)—Otoacoustic emission that occurs due to the presentation of a series of two simultaneous tones.

DNA (Deoxyribonucleic acid)—Nucleic acid containing a series of molecules called nucleotides that contain the deoxyribose sugar that provides the genetic code for the synthesis of various mRNAs and proteins in a cell.

Dopamine—One of several catecholamine neurotransmitters derived from the amino acid tyrosine. Dopamine is synthesized from dopa in a reaction catalyzed by dopa-decarboxylase, and it is converted to norephinephrine in a reaction catalyzed by dopamine b-hydroxylase.

Dose-response curve—Describes the level of response (positive or negative) and the relationship of a given dose to the desired or adverse effect in a population. For example, aminoglycosides have a steep response curve, meaning the dose to treat the disease is very close to the dose required to cause an adverse effect.

Doxycycline—Tetracycline antibiotic that works via protein synthesis inhibition.

Droplet contact transmission—Form of contact transmission where exposure to microorganisms occurs when droplets expelled briefly in the air come in direct contact with mucous membranes (i.e., lining of the eyelids, nose, or mouth).

Drug—Any chemical agent or molecule that can affect the processes of living. Commonly binds to receptors or enzymes to cause a biochemical and physiological effect. Drugs can be legal prescriptions, nonprescriptions (over-the-counter drugs), illicit substances, social substances (caffeine and nicotine), or natural products such as alternative herbal medicine or dietary supplements and vitamins. Although broadly defined as "a chemical substance that affects living processes in a positive or negative manner," a working definition for health care use is "a chemical used in the diagnosis, prevention, or treatment of disease."

Drug action—Underlying biochemical or physiological mechanism by which chemicals produce their response in living organisms.

Drug effect—Observed consequences of a drug's action.

Durham-Humphrey Amendment (1951)—Act that specified how prescription drugs were to be ordered and dispensed. Required "Caution: Federal law prohibits dispensing without prescription" to be on the label of all prescription medications and created a second group of drugs listed as over-the-counter medications.

Dynorphins—One of three families of endogenous opioid peptides that function as neurotransmitters, neuromodulators, or neurohormones.

Efficacy—Drug's ability to elicit its maximum response/effect at a certain dose or the drug's ability to treat a disease state. Sometimes expressed as a percentage value, such as "most antidepressants are approximately 70% efficacious in treating depression at all doses." Efficacy can compare agents with different mechanisms of action to treat a given disease state. For example, morphine is more efficacious than acetaminophen in treating postsurgical pain.

Electron transport apparatus—A series of molecules in the inner membranes of mitochondria that consumes oxygen in the process of generating ATP.

Endocochlear potential—Measure of stria vascularis function.

Endolymphatic hydrops—Disorder characterized by the loss of normal fluid regulation within the inner ear. The disorder may be primary and idiopathic (e.g., so-called Meniere's disease) or secondary (e.g., occurring in response to an underlying disease process or other causative event).

Endoplasmic reticulum—System of membrane-enclosed cavities within a cell.

Enkephalins—One of three families of endogenous opioid peptides that function as neurotransmitters, neuromodulators, or neurohormones. Enkephalins include met-enkephalin (with methionine at one end) and leu-enkephalin (with leucine at one end).

Enterococcal—Infection by any of the bacterial genus Enterococcus, which generally are sensitive to vancomycin and ampicillin treatment.

Enzyme—Protein molecule that is used by the body to catalyze biochemical reactions. An enzyme may be used to produce or break down different compounds in the body or activate or inhibit various chemicals, neurotransmitters, or physiological processes in the body. Enzymes are common drug targets.

Epidemiology—Scientific discipline that focuses on the association between exposure and medical outcome in populations.

Epiglottitis—Inflammation of the epiglottis that may cause respiratory obstruction.

Epithelial cells—Cells that pack closely together to form tissue that covers internal organs and that lines other surfaces of the body. Epithelial cell types include columnar cells, cuboidal cells, squamous cells, and the hair cells in the organ of Corti.

Exocytosis—Process whereby substances contained in vesicles are discharged from the nerve terminal into the synaptic cleft after fusion of the vesicular membrane with the cell membrane.

Extracellular matrix—Noncellular portion of animal tissues comprised of three major components: fibrous elements (e.g., collagen), link proteins (e.g., fibronectin and laminin), and space-filling molecules (usually glycosaminoglycans). The extracellular matrix can influence cellular behavior in important ways. The basal lamina is a common extracellular matrix.

False positive rate—Failure on a test/response that should have been passed.

Famotidine (Pepcid)—H2 blocker. Used to treat acid reflux disease.

Federal Food, Drug, and Cosmetic Act (1938)—Federal legislation requiring safety testing for new drugs and accurate and complete labeling of drugs.

Federal Pure Food and Drug Act (1906)—Act passed by Congress that required drug manufacturers to list ingredients on labels and to limit false and misleading claims about therapeutic effectiveness. It also required registration of preparations containing dangerous or addicting drugs (e.g., morphine, heroin, alcohol, cocaine, and opium).

Fexofenadine (Allegra)—Second-generation antihistamine. These drugs do not cross the blood-brain barrier and thus have decreased CNS side effects; therefore, they are less sedating compared to first-generation antihistamines.

Fibrocytes—Flattened, irregular, branched, motile cells that form, secrete, and maintain the extracellular collagen and mucopolysaccharide of connective tissue in vertebrates.

First-pass metabolism—Delivery of a drug to the liver via portal circulation from the gastrointestinal tract after absorption but before entry to the systemic circulation. Serves to detoxify potentially toxic substances (including drugs) before they are exposed to the rest of the body. Contributes to the reduced bioavailability of many drugs after oral administration.

Five- or six-membered sugars—Carbohydrates with a skeleton consisting of five (e.g., pentose) or six (e.g., glucose) carbon atoms.

Food and Drug Administration (FDA)—U.S. federal regulatory agency that is responsible for assuring safety of drugs and foods.

Free radical scavengers—Usually antioxidants that scavenge free radicals and protect cells from their deleterious effects. Examples of antioxidants include glutathione, vitamin E, and vitamin C.

Free radicals—Molecules that have an extra or an unpaired electron. These chemical entities are unstable and tend to react rapidly with a range of cellular constituents including the membranes that make up cells and with DNA. An example is the superoxide molecule (O_2^-) generated by the electron transport apparatus.

Fungus (plural fungi)—Diverse group of organisms potentially capable of causing disease; they thrive or grow in wet or damp areas.

Gain constant, VOR—Peak eye velocity divided by peak head velocity as a function of frequency.

Gene therapy—Treatment of a disease caused by malfunction of a gene by stably transfecting the cells of the organism with the normal gene.

Gene—Section of DNA in the nucleus that contains the code for specific RNA, called messenger RNA (mRNA); each mRNA is used to code for a specific protein.

Genomics—Branch of biotechnology concerned with applying the techniques of genetics and molecular biology to the genetic mapping and DNA sequencing of sets of genes or the complete genomes of selected organisms using high-speed methods, with organizing the results in databases, and with applying the data.

Gentamicin—Aminoglycoside prototype. It is a bacteriocidal antibiotic (via protein synthesis inhibition). It is active against many gram-negative bacteria. Side effects include ototoxicity and renal dysfunction.

Glomerular filtration rate—Early step in the renal elimination and urine formation process by which blood is filtered through the kidneys for removal of waste products and foreign substances. Usually expressed as a rate of volume cleared per minute.

Glucose—Monosaccharide $C_6H_{12}O_6$ that is the principal circulating sugar in the blood and the major energy source of the body.

Glutamine synthetase—Enzyme that catalyzes the formation of glutamine from glutamate.

Glycerol phospholipid—Molecule comprised of fatty acids, a negatively charged phosphate group, and an alcohol (glycerol) backbone. Phospholipids, along with glycolipids and cholesterol, are major components of biological membranes. It is also called glycerophospholipid.

Glycoproteins—Group of conjugated proteins that contain a carbohydrate (sugar) as the non-protein component. The sugars may be bound to OH side chains (O-linked) or to the amide nitrogen of asparagine side chains (N-linked).

Glycosidic linkage—Connection between two sugars consisting of a -C-O-C- bridge.

Gram-negative—Referring to bacteria not stained by Gram staining, indicating a lack of peptidoglycan in the cell wall, which is generally thinner than that of gram-positive bacteria.

Gram-positive—Referring to bacteria stained by Gram staining, indicating the presence of peptidoglycan in the cell wall.

Gram stain—Method for differential staining of bacteria. Smears of bacteria are fixed by flaming, stained in a solution of crystal violet, treated with iodine solution, rinsed, decolorized, and then counterstained with safranin. Gram-positive organisms stain purple, and gram-negative organisms stain pink. Staining is useful in bacterial taxonomy and classification and identification.

Growth factor—Complex family of polypeptide hormones or biological factors that are produced by the body to control growth, division, and maturation of blood cells. They regulate the division and proliferation of cells and influence the growth rate of some cancers.

Habenula perforatae—Holes in the bony shelf (osseous spiral lamina) beneath the medial portion of the basilar membrane through which nerve fibers enter the organ of Corti.

Hair cells—Sensory receptors of the membranous labyrinth and cochlea.

Half-life—Time it takes for a drug's concentration in the body to decrease by 50%.

Histamine—Amine that plays a role in allergic reactions, neurotransmission, and stomach acid secretion. In allergic reactions, it is released from mast cells in response to IgE-mediated reactions.

Hydrogen cyanide—Form of cyanide gas that has high toxicity. It is composed of hydrogen and cyanide (HCN).

Hydro-ionic homeostasis—State of chemical and electrical balance achieved through the automatic regulation of fluid and ionic composition despite the tendency for fluctuations to occur.

Hydrolysis—Chemical reaction that breaks a covalent bond through the addition of hydrogen from a water molecule.

Hydrophilicity—Level or degree to which a molecule or drug is attracted to water or is water soluble. The affinity for water due to the polar nature of a compound, making it readily soluble in water but impeding its diffusion across natural membranes.

Hydroxyl—Functional (-OH) group on organic compounds.

Hypoxia—State of reduced oxygen delivery that occurs when chemical asphyxiants are applied.

Hypoxic hypoxia—Reduction of oxygen concentration in inspired air typically achieved by diluting air with nitrogen.

Iatrogenic adverse effect—Induced inadvertently by a physician or surgeon or by medical treatment or diagnostic procedures For example, an adverse effect that is not usually related to a specific dose of a drug and is more unpredictable due to this seemingly lack of a dose-response relationship. May also refer to an allergic reaction.

Idiopathic—Referring to a disease of unknown cause.

Indirect contact transmission—Form of contact transmission where exposure to microorganisms occurs by coming in contact with a contaminated object.

Industrial hygiene—Applied discipline that seeks to limit exposure to agents with adverse health effects by means of reengineering the environment (e.g., shielding equipment to reduce noise levels) or by providing protective clothing and equipment (e.g., sound attenuating ear plugs).

Infection control—Organized management of the clinical environment for purposes of minimizing or eliminating the spread of disease.

Inner hair cells—Receptor cells of the cochlea that transduce mechanical energy associated with acoustic stimulation into chemical energy that modulates the activity of the primary auditory neurons (type I spiral ganglion cells) that synapse with them.

Intersubject—Between or among subjects.

Intrasubject—Within the same subject.

Ion—Atom or molecule with a net electrical charge. Positively charged ions are called cations; negatively charged ions are called anions.

Iontophoresis—Method of applying neurotransmitters or other drugs in very small quantities to cells or the fluid surrounding them to study the effects of their application.

Ischemia—Cessation or blockage of blood flow to a tissue, which can lead to ischemic tissue damage.

Jun-kinase—Member of protein kinases that responds to a number of cellular stresses by activating specific transcription factors as part of apoptotic signaling.

Kainic acid—2S-(2 alpha,3 beta,4 beta)-2-Carboxy-4-(1-methylethenyl)-3-pyrrolidineacetic acid, a potent excitatory amino acid agonist at some types of excitatory amino acid receptors. Kainic acid has been used as a way to discriminate among amino acid receptor subtypes and as a tool for creating neurotoxic lesions in the cochlea and central nervous system.

Kefauver-Harris Drug Amendment (1962)—Act requiring drug manufacturers to prove both safety and effectiveness to the FDA before new drugs are allowed on the market. It also requires effectiveness testing for all drugs marketed after the 1938 Federal Food, Drug, and Cosmetic Act.

Kinase—Enzyme that transfers the terminal phosphate group of ATP to a specific amino acid of a target protein.

Lactate dehydrogenase—Enzyme involved in the conversion of lactate and NAD to pyruvate and NADH in the final step of anaerobic glycolysis.

Lansoprazole—(Prevacis): Irreversible blocker of $H+/K+$ ATPase proton pump in parietal cells of the stomach. Used to treat gastroesophageal reflux disease (GERD).

Lecithin—Fatty substance produced naturally in the body; it is a rich source of the B vitamin choline.

Ligand—Any molecule that binds to another, in normal usage; a naturally occurring soluble molecule such as a hormone or neurotransmitter that binds to a receptor and activates it. May also be an agonist. A ligand is usually a small molecule that chemically interacts with a protein to produce a conformational change in the protein that in turn induces subsequent events. An example is the hormone epinephrine (the ligand) that is released from the adrenal gland into the blood stream to arrive at and interact with epinephrine receptor proteins in the membranes of fat storage cells to release fatty acids into the blood stream.

Light chain—Smaller of the two types of polypeptide chains in immunoglobulins, consisting of an antigen-binding portion with a variable amino acid sequence and a constant region with a relatively unchanging amino acid sequence.

Lipophilic—Having the property of dissolving preferentially in fatty materials such as oils.

Lipophilicity—Level or degree to which a molecule or drug is attracted to and possibly stored in fat or lipid compartments. A lipophilic substance will dissolve more easily in organic oil-based or lipid mediums than in water and may be called fat soluble.

Loratidine (Claritin)—Second-generation antihistamine. These drugs do not cross the blood-brain barrier and thus have decreased central nervous system (CNS) side effects; therefore, they are less sedating compared to first-generation antihistamines.

Lymphocytes—Type of white blood cell (leukocyte) that is responsible for providing the immune response.

Lysosomes—Intracellular structure (i.e., organelle) that contains enzymes that digest molecules in the cell.

Macrolide—Group of drugs including the antibiotics erythromycin and azithromycin whose structure includes a many-membered lactone ring (macrolide).

Macrophage—White blood cell derived from a monocyte that leaves the circulation and enters tissues. These cells are important in nonspecific phagocytosis and in regulating, stimulating, and "cleaning up" after immune responses.

Manganese dioxide (MnO2)—Insoluble form of manganese with many commercial uses, including the production of dry cell batteries.

Megalin—Transmembrane protein of the lipoprotein-receptor family postulated to be involved in aminoglycoside transport in renal cells.

Melatonin—Produced by the pineal gland, it is a hormone that plays an essential role in managing the sleep/wake cycles.

Membrane potential ($\Delta\Psi m$)—Difference in voltage between the inside and outside of a membrane. These voltages or potential differences are measured across a cell membrane and arise as a result of unequal distributions of ions and fluids in intracellular and extracellular fluid compartments.

Meta-analysis—Statistical procedure for pulling together the results of multiple experiments in an attempt to overcome the weakness of any given report to provide an overarching conclusion.

Metabotropic (G-protein-linked) receptors—Relatively slow-acting membrane receptors that initiate intracellular biochemical responses through a second messenger system. Second messenger formation is stimulated by the binding of a first messenger (neurotransmitter or neurohormone) to a G-protein-coupled cell surface receptor. Common second messengers are cAMP; cGMP; and inositol-1, 4, 5-triphosphate.

Methylene chloride—Paint stripping chemical that has been used, for example, in cleaning furniture. Because it is turned into carbon monoxide in the body, it can produce severe toxicity. Thus, warning labels call for its use in well-ventilated areas.

Methylmercury—Organic form of the metal mercury, which has severe neurotoxic effects.

Metronidazole—Antiprotozoal antibiotic.

Microbiology—Study of living organisms that cannot be readily seen with the naked eye.

Micromonospora—Genus of gram-positive bacteria, various species of which are sources of aminoglycosides.

Microvilli—Thin fingerlike protrusions from the surface of epithelial cells.

Micturate—To urinate.

Mitochondria—Intracellular organelle that is responsible for the synthesis of most of the energy utilized by the cell in the form of adenosine triphosphate (ATP). Mitochondria have an inner membrane in addition to an outer membrane. Mitochondria contain the electron transport apparatus, which is a series of molecules, including cytochromes (e.g., cytochrome c) constructed in the inner membrane, that uses molecular oxygen to generate ATP. In the process of generating ATP, the apparatus generates a small number of superoxide molecules (O_2^-). Those are also called free radicals because they have an extra unpaired electron.

Mitochondrial apoptosis pathway—Intrinsic cell death pathway that is activated extensively in cells in response to extracellular and intracellular triggers. It is characterized by an increase in mitochondrial permeability (i.e., pore formation), a change in the mitochondrial membrane potential, and release of cytochrome c from the mitochondria.

Mitosis—Division of the nucleus of a eukaryotic cell, involving condensation of the DNA into visible chromosomes, and separation of the duplicated chromosomes to form two identical sets. This process takes place in the nucleus of a dividing cell and typically involves a series of steps consisting of prophase, metaphase, anaphase, and telophase, resulting in the formation of two new nuclei, each having the same number of chromosomes as the parent nucleus.

Mode of transmission—General method by which microorganisms are transmitted from their temporary resting place to a susceptible host.

Muscarinic—Producing an effect similar to muscarine, mimicking postganglionic parasympathetic stimulation, or stimulating the postganglionic parasympathetic receptor.

Muscatine receptor—One of two major types of acetylcholine receptors; slow-acting metabotropic receptors agonized (stimulated) by muscarine and antagonized (blocked) by atropine.

Mycobacterial—Any of a number of rod-shaped bacteria, including those that cause tuberculosis and leprosy.

Myo7a gene (sh-1)—Mouse gene that codes for myosin VIIA protein. Mutation of the *myo7a* gene is responsible for the shaker-1 (sh-1) phenotype in mice, characterized by circling/waltzing and a form of sensorineural hearing loss.

Myosin 7A—Protein molecule that reacts with actin to form actinomycin for contraction or stabilization of the filaments.

Myosin VIIA protein—Protein made by the MYO7A gene in humans (homologous to the *myo7a* gene in mice), produced mainly in the inner ear and the retina. This protein is part of a large family of actin-binding myosin proteins that are important for cell shape and movement. In the inner ear, myosin VIIA protein is thought to transport proteins that are critical for the development and maintenance of the stereocilia.

Myosins—Superfamily of proteins that function as molecular motors or translocating proteins. Myosins bind to actin and use energy derived from ATP hydrolysis to generate force and movement along actin filaments. They generally consist of heavy chains that are involved in locomotion and light chains that are involved in regulation.

Na⁺,K⁺,2Cl- cotransport—Coupled membrane transport process in which the transport of one molecule depends on the simultaneous or sequential transfer of other molecules.

Nafcillin—Penicillinase-resistant penicillin prototype. Not active against methycillin-resistant staphylococci.

National Institute for Occupational Safety and Health (NIOSH)—U.S. federal agency that is charged with developing basic research knowledge used to protect workers' health. NIOSH commonly makes recommendations limiting exposure to potentially dangerous agents.

Necrosis—Death of a cell due to passive cellular events and characterized by the formation of vacuoles in the cytoplasm, mitochondrial swelling, dilation of the endoplasmic reticulum, cellular debris, and disintegration or a loss of plasma membrane integrity and organelle membrane integrity. Necrosis generally results in localized pathologic death of body tissue.

Nerve conduction time—Speed with which a nerve impulse is transmitted.

Neurotransmitter-gated receptors—Membrane proteins that are activated by the binding of chemicals released by a presynaptic nerve terminal.

Nodes of Ranvier—Periodically spaced regions of a myelinated axon where the myelin sheath thins and the density of voltage-gated sodium ion channels is high. Sodium ion influx at the nodal region supports action potential propagation.

Nonsteroidal anti-inflammatory drugs (NSAIDs)—Class of medications used to reduce inflammation. Actions are likely mediated through inhibition of prostaglandin production. Possible cause of otoxicity. Examples include ibuprofen, naproxen, and celecoxib.

N-terminal head (or motor) domain—End of a protein chain that carries the free alpha-amino group.

Nystagmus—To-and-fro movement of the eyes that in the context of the VOR, has a slow (vestibular) component and a fast (central) component. In vestibular function testing, the speed (velocity) of the slow component is typically measured and the direction of the nystagmus is described according to the fast component.

Objective measures—Test methods for acquiring ear and hearing information that do not require the patient to actively respond, such as tympanometry, acoustic reflexes, ABR, and OAE.

Occupational Safety & Health Administration (OSHA)—U. S. federal regulatory agency charged with establishing safe work practices.

Omeprazole (Prilosec)—Irreversible blocker of H+/K+ ATPase proton pump in parietal cells of the stomach. Used to treat gastroesophageal reflux disease (GERD).

Oncogene—Altered gene whose product can act in a dominant fashion to help make a cell cancerous. Typically, an oncogene is a mutant form of a normal gene involved in the control of cell growth or division.

Opportunistic infection—Infection caused by a commonplace microorganism that does not produce infection in individuals with intact immune systems, but takes the opportunity to infect a body with some form or degree of immunocompromise.

Organelle—Small structure within a cell that carries out a given task.

Organic solvents—Organic molecules based on hydrogen-carbon bonds that are widely used to dissolve materials that are not soluble in water.

Organotoxins—Chemicals such as pesticides, solvents, and certain plastics that are toxic to tissues and organisms.

Oscillopsia—Illusory movement of viewed stationary objects or surroundings that occurs with head movement. The perceived object movement is on the same plane as the head movement and in the opposite direction. This subjective sensation of visual field "bobbing" occurs in response to movement of the head or body. It occurs when moderate to severe VOR loss prevents stabilization of the ocular globes (eyeballs).

Osmotic disequilibrium—Condition wherein the number of water molecules on one side of a membrane does not equal the number on the other side of the membrane. That results in water moving to the side with fewer water molecules, accompanied by the swelling or expansion of the compartment receiving the water.

Otoacoustic emissions (OAEs)—Sounds that originate in the cochlea and propagate through the middle ear and into the ear canal, where they can be measured using a sensitive microphone.

Otocyst—Embryonic vesicle from which the parts of the internal ear of vertebrates are developed.

Ototoxic—Any substance that is destructive to inner ear tissues.

Ototoxicity—Damage to the structure and function of the inner ear (auditory, vestibular, or both) that results from exposure to toxins.

Outer hair cells—Specialized postmitotic cells of the cochlea that are essential for normal sensitivity and frequency resolution through their ability to elongate and contract in response to acoustic stimulation. Outer hair cells are heavily innervated by efferent fibers from the medial superior olivary region of the brainstem and sparsely innervated by afferent fibers of type II spiral ganglion cells.

Over-the-counter (OTC)—Describes medications deemed by the FDA to be safely used without direct medical supervision or prescription.

Oxidative stress—Overproduction of unstable and highly reactive forms of oxygen that can damage cells.

P0 (myelin basic protein)—Most abundant protein in the myelin sheath and produced by Schwann cells in the peripheral nervous system. Myelin basic protein is required for the proper formation and maintenance of myelin. It acts like a molecular glue (adhesion molecule) and plays a role in myelin compaction. It is also called myelin protein zero.

Pantoprazole (Protonix)—Irreversible blocker of $H+/K+$ ATPase proton pump in parietal cells of the stomach. Used to treat gastroesophageal reflux disease (GERD).

Parasite—Organism that may potentially cause disease; it exists and functions at the expense of a host organism without contributing to the survival of the host.

Parenteral—Systemic administration other than through the alimentary canal.

Parts per million—Measure of concentration commonly used for chemical contaminants in air.

Penicillin G—Penicillin prototype. It is active against common streptococci, gram-positive bacilli, gram-negative cocci, and spirochetes and in conjunction with aminoglycosides against enterococci. It is penicillinase-susceptible.

Peptide/polypeptide/protein—A peptide, also known as a polypeptide, is an organic compound containing amino acids linked by peptide bonds. According to some definitions, when the length of the peptide exceeds thirty amino acids, the peptide can be called a protein.

Peripheral myelin protein 22 (PMP22)—Major component of myelin produced primarily by Schwann cells. PMP22 plays a crucial role in the development and maintenance of myelin.

Permissible exposure levels (PELs)—Legal limit established by OSHA for exposure to chemicals and physical factors in the workplace.

Pharmacodynamics—Action of a drug upon the body. Pharmacodynamics is commonly related to a drug's mechanism of action, including the study of site and mechanism of interaction with physiological systems. Essentially what the drug does to the body.

Pharmacogenetics—Branch of pharmacology that analyzes the body's genetic response to specific drugs.

Pharmacogenomics—Study of individual genetic variability in the variable response of individuals to drugs.

Pharmacokinetics—Study of how drugs are acted upon by physiological systems, including absorption, distribution in the body, biotransformation/metabolism, and excretion. Essentially what the body does to the drug.

Pharmacology—Study of the interactions of drugs or chemicals with living systems.

Phase I hepatic enzymes—Major route of drug metabolism by the liver, utilizing enzymatic processes to change the structure or nature of a drug to make it easier for the body to eliminate. Some examples of these enzymatic reactions include oxidation and demethylation. A common group of Phase I enzymes is known as the cytochrome P450 enzymes.

Phosphoinositide—One of a family of lipids containing phosphorylated inositol derivatives, which are important in signal transduction in eucaryotic cells; also called inositol phospholipid.

Phosphoprotein phosphatases—Group of enzymes that remove serine- or threonine-bound phosphate groups from a wide range of phosphoproteins, including a number of enzymes that have been phosphorylated by kinases.

Phosphorylation—Reaction in which a phosphate group becomes covalently coupled to another molecule.

Phosporylate—Transfer of an inorganic phosphate group to an organic molecule. An example is the process used by enzyme proteins called kinases (e.g., JNKs) to transfer an inorganic phosphate group to a protein (the transcription factors c-Jun and c-Fos).

Polyamine-like—Compound similar to polyamines, which are composed only of carbon, nitrogen, hydrogen, and several amino groups.

Polymorphism—Variation, or mutation, in the expression of a gene that could be responsible for certain enzymes, receptors, or other endogenously created material.

Polyneuropathies—Nerve damage that can result from chemical exposure or from disease.

Potency—Amount (dose/concentration) of drug required to produce 50% of the maximal potential response. For example, morphine is more potent than codeine. Both may be equally effective.

Precursor—Substance, cell, or cellular component from which another substance, cell, or cellular component is formed especially by natural processes.

Prednisone—Glucocorticoid prototype.

Prion—Newer class of infectious agents consisting of an abnormal protein particle that is thought to be acquired through ingesting contaminated or diseased meat, handling contaminated objects following medical procedures, or injecting growth hormone. Much information remains unknown.

Programmed cell death (PCD)—Death of a cell due to naturally occurring, active events in the cell that involves the triggering of a set of molecular events preprogrammed into the molecular machinery of the cell. PCD is also known as genetic cell death because gene products (i.e., proteins) are necessary for the process to occur. PCD notably occurs during human development.

Prostaglandins—any member of a group of lipid compounds that are derived from fatty acids and have important functions in the animal body. Every prostaglandin contains 20 carbon atoms, including a 5-carbon ring. They are mediators and have a variety of strong physiological effects; although they are technically hormones, they are rarely classified as such.

Protease—Class of enzymes that cleave protein molecules (i.e., proteolysis) by breaking certain peptide bonds that hold together the amino acids in the protein. In this book, caspases are generally proteases that break peptide bonds occurring after the amino acid aspartate in the protein. Essentially proteases are enzymes that digest other proteins.

Proton pump inhibitors—Drugs that specifically bind and block ATP-dependent proton pumps (acid-secreting enzymes) of the stomach's parietal cells.

Pruritis—Itching.

Pseudomonas—Genus of ubiquitous plant- and animal-pathogenic bacteria mostly benign to humans but able to cause problems for the immune-compromised patient; the most prevalent bacteria in the lungs of cystic fibrosis patients.

Rabeprazol (Aciphex)—Irreversible blocker of H+/K+ ATPase proton pump in parietal cells of the stomach. Used to treat gastroesophageal reflux disease (GERD).

Ranitidine (Zantac)—H2 blocker. Used to treat acid reflux disease.

Reactive oxygen species (ROS)—Highly chemically reactive state of oxygen, such as the superoxide anion radical (O_2^-) formed from molecular oxygen by mitochondria. The mitochondrial O_2^- can lead to the production of additional ROS, such as hydrogen peroxide (H_2O_2), and the highly reactive hydroxyl radical (OH^-).

Receiver-operator characteristic (ROC) curves—Sensitivity or hit rates for a range of criterion threshold shifts that are plotted as a function of the corresponding false positive rate.

Receptor—Proteins in membranes that interact with ligands, generating changes in the protein that initiate subsequent events in the cell. Drugs bind to these macromolecules, which are tissue constituents, to produce their physiologic actions.

Relative risk—Term commonly used in epidemiology to represent an increase or decrease in risk of some health outcome due to a specific exposure.

Reperfusion—Restoration of blood flow to an organ or tissue after a period of blockage that creates ischemia.

Rhinitis—Inflammation of the nasal mucous membranes.

Rhinorrhea—Discharge from the nasal mucous membranes.

Rosenthal's canal—Canal following the course of the bony spiral lamina of the cochlea and containing the spiral ganglion that houses the spiral ganglion cells that innervate the cochlear hair cells.

Route of transmission—Port of entry through which microorganisms enter or gain passage into the body.

Second Messenger—Generally, a type of direct or indirect signaling and conveyance of a ligand-receptor (first messenger) or drug-receptor agonistic binding and response. Common in G-protein-coupled receptors. The target site is often a cytosolic effector. An example is cyclic adenosine-3', 5'-monophosphate (cAMP).

Sensitive range for ototoxicity (SRO)—Shortened test protocol that targets the uppermost frequency (R) with a threshold of $\leq$ 100 dB SPL followed by the adjacent six lower frequencies in 1/6-octave steps, R-1 through R-6 (all $\leq$ 100 dB SPL).

Sensitivity—How accurate a test is at correctly identifying the presence of a condition or result.

Serum half-life—Time required for a compound in serum to fall to half of its peak level.

Sherley Amendment (1912)—Federal legislation that prevented fraudulent claims about therapeutic medications.

Side effect—Secondary effect of a drug not related to the primary beneficial effect.

Signal transduction—Biochemical reaction(s) initiated by a signal such as a hormone or another chemical messenger.

Sodium, potassium (Na^+,K^+)-ATPase—Transmembrane carrier protein that removes sodium from a cell and carries potassium into a cell, using the energy derived from hydrolysis of ATP; also called a sodium pump.

Specificity—How accurate a test is at correctly identifying the absence of a condition or result.

Splash surface—Area that may be hit with blood, bodily fluids, or other secretions from a potentially contaminated source.

Staphylococcus aureus—Species of bacteria leading to abscesses, boils, endocarditis, osteomyelitis, and pneumonia.

Steady state—Point in time when the amount of a drug going into the body is equal to the amount of the drug being eliminated. Usually occurs after five half-lives of the specific drug if the dosing interval is equal to the drug's half-life. For example, if a drug has a $t_{1/2}$ = 6 hours, then steady state is usually achieved after 5 doses in approximately 30 hours.

Stem cells—Relatively undifferentiated cells of the same lineage (family type) that retain the ability to divide and cycle throughout postnatal life to provide cells that can become specialized and take the place of those that die or are lost.

Sterilization—Process of killing 100% of germs, including endospores resistant to the process of disinfecting.

Stimulus frequency otoacoustic emission (SFOAE)—Otoacoustic emission elicited by a single-tone stimuli.

Stria vascularis—Structure within the cochlea containing a rich supply of blood vessels. The stria vascularis plays a critical role in maintaining the ionic difference between the endolymph and perilymph fluids of the cochlea.

Styrene—Aromatic organic solvent that is commonly used in making certain rigid plastics (polystyrene).

Succinate dehydrogenase—Enzyme located on the mitochondrial membrane that catalyzes the conversion of succinate to fumarate with the simultaneous conversion of an FAD cofactor into FADH2.

Telomerase—Enzyme that elongates telomere sequences in DNA.

Telomere—End of a chromosome associated with a characteristic DNA sequence that is replicated in a special way. Counteracts the usual tendency of the chromosome to shorten with each round of replication.

Tetracycline—Tetracycline prototype antibiotic. It is a bacteriostatic inhibitor of protein synthesis.

Therapeutic effect—Drug's desired primary beneficial effect.

Therapeutic index—Ratio of toxic dose to treatment dose of a given drug. The narrower the index and smaller the ratio, the smaller the difference between a drug's treatment dose to the dose that will cause toxicity. The larger the number or ratio, the safer a medication is considered to be. Often depicted as LD_{50}/ED_{50}. Examples of agents with narrow therapeutic indices include aminoglycosides and warfarin. Examples of agents with wide therapeutic indices include penicillin and acetaminophen.

Therapeutic window—Describes the dosage range and effect of a drug when efficacy is achieved without causing adverse effects or toxicity.

Threshold limit values (TLVs)—Suggested maximal exposure limit values that are established by the ACGIH.

Time constant, VOR—Time taken for slow-phase eye velocity to decline to 37% of its initial value.

Tinnitus—Perception of sound in the absence of an external stimulus.

Toluene—One of the most common aromatic organic solvents used as a degreaser and as a carrier for paints and glues. It is also one of the most commonly abused solvents.

Tonic influence—Sustained low-level activity of the efferent fibers that occurs in the absence of acoustic stimulation and influences the gain of the cochlear amplifier.

Touch surface—Area that may come in direct or indirect contact with hands.

Toxic oxidative stress—State of a cell where the concentrations of ROS in the mitochondria increase to levels that are too great to be overcome by the antioxidants and antioxidant enzymes in the cell.

Toxicity—Describes the often irreversible and dangerous effect of a drug, including death. It is usually dose-related. Ototoxicity describes both reversible and irreversible hearing impairment.

Toxicology—Study of toxic or unwanted effects of drugs on physiological systems.

Transcription factor NF-κB—Family of dimeric proteins that activate the transcription of (primarily) survival protein pathways. The compounds that combine with specific segments of the DNA to initiate or enhance the transcription of DNA into RNA.

Transcription factor—Any of various proteins that bind to DNA and play a role in the regulation of gene expression by promoting transcription. These molecules bind to regions of genetic DNA called promoter regions and activate a gene to produce new mRNA and protein molecules. For example, activation protein-1 (AP-1) formed by c-Fos and c-Jun triggers rapid transcriptional activity and, thus, protein synthesis. In genetic terms, it is the production of RNA molecules (mRNA) that are complementary to an area of genetic DNA that codes for a specific protein. The mRNA carries the message for the construction of the protein by the cell at structures called ribosomes. Essentially transcription is the process of constructing a messenger RNA molecule by using a DNA molecule as a template with resulting transfer of genetic information to the messenger RNA.

Transdifferentiation—Change of a cell or tissue from one differentiated state to another without cell division.

Transfection—Introduction of DNA into a recipient eukaryote cell and its subsequent integration into the recipient cells chromosomal DNA.

Transgenic—Refers to an organism whose genome has been artificially altered by inserting new genes or replacing existing genes.

Transgenic mouse—Mouse whose genetic code has been altered by the insertion of a foreign gene.

Transient evoked otoacoustic emission (TEOAE)—Otoacoustic emission that occurs due to the presentation of a broad spectrum stimulus to the ear, usually a click or tone burst, producing a robust response.

Translation—In genetic terms, it is the production of a protein in the ribosome based on the code given by the mRNA molecule.

Tumor suppressor gene—Gene that appears to prevent cancer formation. Loss-of-function mutations in such genes enhance susceptibility to cancer.

Type 1 hair cells—One of two types of vestibular hair cells. Type 1 cells are flask-shaped with a neck area that is constricted by an afferent nerve that cups the cell.

Type I spiral ganglion neurons (SGNs)—Large spiral ganglion neurons that have only two processes extending from the cell body. The distal, or peripheral, process enters the organ of Corti to innervate inner hair cells; the proximal, or central, process travels within the eighth cranial nerve to the cochlear nucleus in the brainstem.

Type II spiral ganglion neurons (SGNs)—Small pseudounipolar neurons located in the spiral ganglion that make contact with outer hair cells in the cochlea and presumably project to neurons of the central nervous system. The function of the type II SGNs has not yet been established.

Ultra-high frequency—Frequency extending beyond conventional test frequencies of 8000 Hz and includes the highest frequencies heard by humans (9000–20000 Hz).

Urticaria—Eruption of itching wheals, usually of systemic origin; it may be due to a state of hypersensitivity to foods or drugs, infection, or physical agents (heat, cold, or friction). Hives.

Vancomycin—Bacteriocidal antibiotic that inhibits the synthesis of cell wall precursor building blocks. Used for methicillin-resistant staphylococci infections.

Vectorborne transmission—Manner of spreading disease whereby insects or animals carrying a pathogenic agent transfer disease by interacting with a susceptible host.

Vehicle transmission—Transfer of a microorganism to a susceptible host via contaminated food or water.

Vertigo—Abnormal sensation of movement (of self or surroundings) in a situation where no movement is actually occurring.

Vesiculated—Containing membrane-bound structures (vesicles) filled with neurochemicals.

Vestibular ototoxicity—Vestibular symptoms (e.g., dizziness and oscillopsia) that result from exposure to toxins.

Vestibulo-ocular reflex (VOR)—Rotational VOR: Compensatory nystagmus (slow phase in opposite direction of head movement) produced by stimulation of the semicircular canals in response to head rotations (active or passive). Translational VOR: Compensatory eye movements driven by the otolith organs in response to head linear accelerations.

Vestibulotoxic—Agent that causes damage to the vestibular system, located in the inner ear, that is important for balance. Symptoms may include disequilibrium, inability to maintain a steady visual field, or vertigo.

V-gated channel—Membrane protein that forms a pore that is permeable to particular ions when the membrane voltage induces an appropriate change in protein conformation.

Virus—Smallest known organism consisting of either DNA or RNA, but not both. The organism is potentially capable of causing disease. It cannot reproduce or metabolize independently and, therefore, is designed to take over the genetic machinery of other cells for purposes of reproduction.

Visual sensitivity—Condition in which activity in the environment, especially in the peripheral visual field, causes symptom onset or exacerbation of symptoms.

Volatile organic solvents—In industrialized societies, often as mixtures or blends, they are used extensively in home-cleaning products; in paints, thinners, and glues; and in industry.

Volume of distribution—Apparent amount of water or size of a compartment that would account for the total amount of drug in the body if it were present throughout the body at the same concentration found in the serum.

Washout period—Usual time it takes for most of a drug to leave the body. Considered to be at least 5 times the half-life of the drug. For example, if a drug has $t_{1/2} = 24$ hours, then the washout period is approximately 5 days.

Xylene—Common high-production organic solvent having many different uses.

Zymogen—Inactive form of an enzyme that must have a portion of its protein structure removed for it to be active. In this book, pro-caspases are zymogens.

INDEX

W

X

Z